Handbook of Antimicrobial Agents

Handbook of Antimicrobial Agents

Edited by **Leslie Hunt**

Callisto Reference

New York

Published by Callisto Reference,
106 Park Avenue, Suite 200,
New York, NY 10016, USA
www.callistoreference.com

Handbook of Antimicrobial Agents
Edited by Leslie Hunt

International Standard Book Number: 978-1-63239-368-5 (Hardback)

Printed in China.

Contents

	Preface	IX
Chapter 1	**Natural Antimicrobial Peptides from Eukaryotic Organisms** Renaud Condé, Martha Argüello, Javier Izquierdo, Raúl Noguez, Miguel Moreno and Humberto Lanz	1
Chapter 2	**Antibacterial Activity of Naturally Occurring Compounds from Selected Plants** Olgica Stefanović, Ivana Radojević, Sava Vasić and Ljiljana Čomić	23
Chapter 3	**Future Antibiotic Agents: Turning to Nature for Inspiration** Nataša Radić and Tomaž Bratkovič	47
Chapter 4	**Antibacterial Activity of Novel Sulfonylureas, Ureas and Thioureas of 15-Membered Azalides** Mirjana Bukvić Krajačić and Miljenko Dumić	73
Chapter 5	**Antimicrobial Activity of Condiments** André Silvério and Maria Lopes	97
Chapter 6	**The Susceptibility of *Staphylococcus aureus* and *Klebsiella pneumoniae* to Naturally Derived Selected Classes of Flavonoids** Johannes Bodenstein and Karen Du Toit	117
Chapter 7	**An Alternative Approaches for the Control of Sorghum Pathogens Using Selected Medicinal Plants Extracts** Varaprasad Bobbarala and Chandrasekhar K. Naidu	129

Chapter 8 **Antimicrobial Activity of Lectins from Plants** 145
Aphichart Karnchanatat

Chapter 9 **Mechanisms Determining Bacterial Biofilm Resistance to Antimicrobial Factors** 179
Kamila Myszka and Katarzyna Czaczyk

Chapter 10 **Antimicrobial Activity of Endophytes from Brazilian Medicinal Plants** 205
Chirlei Glienke, Fabiana Tonial, Josiane Gomes-Figueiredo, Daiani Savi, Vania Aparecida Vicente, Beatriz H. L. N. Sales Maia and Yvelise Maria Possiede

Chapter 11 **The Natural Antimicrobial Chromogranins/Secretogranins-Derived Peptides - Production, Lytic Activity and Processing by Bacterial Proteases** 221
Ménonvè Atindehou, Rizwan Aslam, Jean-François Chich, Youssef Haïkel, Francis Schneider and Marie-Hélène Metz-Boutigue

Chapter 12 **Quinolones: Synthesis and Antibacterial Activity** 255
Pintilie Lucia

Chapter 13 **Superbugs: Current Trends and Emerging Therapies** 273
Amy L. Stockert and Tarek M. Mahfouz

Chapter 14 **Antibacterial Agents in Dental Treatments** 295
Saeed Rahimi, Amin Salem Milani, Negin Ghasemi and Shahriar Shahi

Chapter 15 **From Synthesis to Antibacterial Activity of Some New Palladium(II) and Platinum(IV) Complexes** 307
Ivana D. Radojević, Verica V. Glođović, Gordana P. Radić, Jelena M. Vujić, Olgica D. Stefanović, Ljiljana R. Čomić and Srećko R. Trifunović

Chapter 16 **The Prophylactic Use of Acidifiers as Antibacterial Agents in Swine** 329
V. G. Papatsiros and C. Billinis

Chapter 17 ***Andrographis paniculata* (Burm.f) Wall. ex Ness: A Potent Antibacterial Plant** 345
Qamar Uddin Ahmed, Othman Abd. Samah and Abubakar Sule

Chapter 18 **Antibacterial Agents in Textile Industry** **361**
Sheila Shahidi and Jakub Wiener

Chapter 19 **Antibacterial Agents from Lignicolous Macrofungi** **381**
Maja Karaman, Milan Matavulj and Ljiljana Janjic

Chapter 20 **Silver Nanoparticles: Real Antibacterial Bullets** **407**
G. Thirumurugan and M. D. Dhanaraju

Permissions

List of Contributors

Preface

An antimicrobial agent is an agent that kills microorganisms or restricts their growth. This book talks about a wide range of topics, stressing on various antibacterial agents with clinical outlook and options to artificial antibacterial agents through thorough reviews of illnesses and their management using substitute approaches. It attempts to explain bacterial ailments and their management through synthetic drugs replaced by chemicals procured from various natural sources which provide a new path in the pharmaceutical industry. This book aims to bring to notice, the upcoming cost effective and eco-friendly medicines that are free of side effects, having been observed in the intersecting disciplines of medicinal chemistry, biochemistry, microbiology and pharmacology.

The researches compiled throughout the book are authentic and of high quality, combining several disciplines and from very diverse regions from around the world. Drawing on the contributions of many researchers from diverse countries, the book's objective is to provide the readers with the latest achievements in the area of research. This book will surely be a source of knowledge to all interested and researching the field.

In the end, I would like to express my deep sense of gratitude to all the authors for meeting the set deadlines in completing and submitting their research chapters. I would also like to thank the publisher for the support offered to us throughout the course of the book. Finally, I extend my sincere thanks to my family for being a constant source of inspiration and encouragement.

Editor

1

Natural Antimicrobial Peptides from Eukaryotic Organisms

Renaud Condé, Martha Argüello,
Javier Izquierdo, Raúl Noguez, Miguel Moreno and Humberto Lanz
Centro de Investigación Sobre Enfermedades Infecciosas,
Instituto Nacional de Salud Pública
Mexico

1. Introduction

Antimicrobial peptides (AMP) are usually described as being short (less than 100 a.a.), gene encoded, ribosome synthesized, polypeptide substances that have antimicrobial activity. For simplicity reasons, we will exclude peptaibol and other non-ribosomaly synthetized antibiotic from our classification.

The first peptidic antibiotic was described in 1968 coming from the *Manduca sexta* and was of linear nature; since then the number of antimicrobial peptide discovered have grown asymptotically. Though loose homology has been found between certain set of antimicrobial peptides; it has proven difficult to classify the AMP through their primary structure. Antimicrobial peptides show a great diversity of primary structures, and their short size do not permit robust evolutionary classification, but for the most close related peptides. The primary structures signature of the different AMP families may have arisen independently, and in some case these structures homology are the result of convergent evolution rather than a common ancestry. Nevertheless in order to classify the new components, general classification methods have been established. So far this has been done regardless of evolutionary relationship, source or activity. The criteria that have been commonly used are the number of disulfide bridges and particular amino-acid composition. In 2005 P. Bullet and co-workers suggested a 3 categories classification namely: α-Helical host defense peptides (HDPs), β-Sheet HDPs, Flexible HDPs rich in certain amino acids (Bulet et al., 1999). Though most AMP would fit in this classification, little insight about function can be inferred from the class relation; nor does it give any comparative information between peptides belonging to the same class.

More recently Tomas Ganz proposed a structural classification of the AMP based on their secondary structure (Ganz, 2003b). The classes proposed included antimicrobial peptides with 4 disulfide bridges with alpha helix and beta sheet mixed structures, 3 disulfide bridges with alpha helix and beta sheet mixed structures, 3 disulfide bridges with beta sheet motif, 3 disulfide bridges with two alpha helix and beta sheet mixed structures, 2 disulfide bridges with beta-sheet structures, one disulfide bridge cyclic peptide and alpha helical peptides.

The classification proposed here contains 9 different peptide structure families. The last group consider hybrid structure peptide possessing structural features of more than one AMP class.

1.1 The lineal amphipathic alpha-helix antimicrobial peptide

1.1.1 General properties

The first peptide of this family discovered is the cecropin A from the pupae of the moth *Hyalophora cecropiae* (Steiner et al., 1981; Hultmark et al., 1982). This structure of AMP has been encountered in virtually all the multi-cellular organisms. Even if their sequences show some similarity, they are not all evolutionary linked. As such, they cannot be aligned as a whole, and are commonly separated in structural subclasses: Cecropin, magainin and dermaseptin AMP. This AMP class do share general common features: the lack of cysteine bridges, the tendency to form alpha helical secondary structure in relatively hydrophobic solvent, the net positive charge at neutral pH and hydrophobic residues interspersed every 3 amino acid, giving them an amphipatic nature. Indeed, basic amino acid side chains face predominantly one side of the alpha helix and hydrophobic residues are generally on the other side of the molecule. A global alignment of the linear peptides separates three different classes that could be broadly characterised as Dermaseptin, magainin and cecropin class of lineal amphipathic AMP. Most of these peptides share the present a glycine near the middle of their peptidic sequence.

1.1.2 Dermaseptins peptides

These peptides were extracted from Phyllomedusa genus frog skin secretions. Some of them present a proline-induced kink in the middle of the alpha helix (Shin et al., 2001). Others have a glycine in the same relative position that has been suggested to give the flexibility needed for the membrane lysis activity (Xiao et al., 2006). This structural plasticity has been defined as a molecular determinant for the antimicrobial vs eucaryont membrane specificity (Shin et al., 1999; Shin et al., 2000; Shin et al., 2001), together with overall net positive charge and hydrophibic moment. They present hydrophobic and positively charged amino acid in an alternate pattern. Though mature dermaseptin amino acid sequences are highly variable, their acidic pro-peptides are strikingly conserved (Azevedo Calderon et al., 2010).

1.1.3 Cecropin peptides

Cecropin peptides were first purified from insect hemolymph, and their expression is usually inducible. Cecropins structural conformations were determined by NMR. Circular dichroism and NMR (Nuclear Magnetic Resonance) data have shown that in aqueous solvent the cecropin structure is largely disordered; but they adopt a stable alpha-helical secondary structure in more hydrophobic environment. This makes the insertion of these peptides in the lipidic membranes entropically favorable. Cecropin usually present a glycine in the middle of their amino acid sequence. This glycine has been proposed to induce a kink between the alpha helical structures that these peptides form in hydrophobic solvent. In turn the deletion of this glycine or its replacement by another amino acid do not eliminate the antimicrobial activity; instead it endows these mutant peptides with hemolytic and cytolytic activity (Moore et al., 1996). The cecropin usually present a tryptophan in one of the first two amino acid position as well as a glycine in the first position.

1.1.4 Magainin/scorpions AMP/cathelicidin peptides

Magainin peptides come from the frog genus Xenopus (Duclohier et al., 1989). In this AMP class arthtropod AMP like Opistoporin-2 from Scorpion *Opistophthalmus carinatus* are also included (Moerman et al., 2002) as well as cathelicidin peptides (Travis et al., 2000) and the fly cecropin from *Stomoxys calcitrans* (Boulanger et al., 2002). This phylogenetically heterogeneous group present lysine/argine doublet repeats that could be considered as a structural signature. These peptides do not present the conserved glycine present in the other 2 lineal amphipatic AMP subclasses. Their positive general formal charge at neutral pH is higher than the one of the cecropin and dermaseptin AMP. They also present a conserved aspartic acid residue at the amino side of these peptides.

1.2 Proline rich peptides

This AMP class has been first described in mammals, in the intestine of *Sus scrofa*, (Agerberth et al., 1991). They are also present in Hymenoptera, Lepidoptera and diptera. Some of these peptides from this AMP class have been studied extensively, like drosocin from *D. melanogaster* (Bulet et al., 1993), pyrrhocoricin from the European sap- sucking bug *Pyrrhocoris apterus* (Cociancich et al., 1994) apidaecins from the *Apis mellifera* (Casteels-Josson et al., 1993), and formaecin from the ant *Myrmecia gulosa* (Mackintosh et al., 1998). Mature proline-rich antimicrobial peptides vary in length from 12 to 54 amino acid, and have few common structural feature. Some authors distinguish between glycine/proline rich and alanine/proline rich peptides. The variety of sequence does not allow for straightforward sequence signature recognition for these peptides. Therefore, their antibacterial activity/specificity is not deducible from the sequence analysis.

On the other hand, some of these peptides are able to penetrate the microbial cytoplasm without inducing bacterial lysis, and do not present hemolytic or cytolitic activities (Knappe et al., 2010). Model PR peptides have been designed, using the Ac-(Arg-Pro-Pro-Phe)n-NHCH3 framework, and some essential structural feature, necessary for antimicrobial activity have been determined. The ability to form poly(proline)-II structure in aqueous solution, as well as a critical peptide length are essential for antimicrobial activity (Niidome et al., 1998).

1.3 Glycine/arginine rich peptides

The first purification of glycine rich peptide was done in 1991 (Bulet et al., 1991). As for the proline rich antimicrobial peptide class, the glycine rich peptides have variable sizes and do not show clear sequence signature, apart from the high proportion of glycine in their primary sequence. These peptides are in general longer than AMP from other classes. Between 25 to 50% of their amino acid are glycines. They have disordered structure in water, and tend to self-order when in contact with artificial membranes (Bruston et al., 2007). The structure of bombinin H resembles the influenza hemagglutinin fusion peptide (Zangger et al., 2008). When binding to DPC micelles, a helix is formed that have a glycine ridge on one side. There is an helix-helix interaction that leads to a multimerization process in the bacterial membrane (Zangger et al., 2008).

1.4 Brevinin (hook structure) peptides

This class of peptides is characterized by having a short amino acid sequence, and a carboxyloterminus disulfide bridge. Some brevinin peptides show post-translational modification. The amino acids included in the carboxyloterminus loop are determinant for the specificity of the antimicrobial activity as well as the length of the loop (Lee et al., 2002) .

The brevinin show alpha helical structure in sodium dodecyl sulfate solution (Lee et al., 2002). Antibacterial activity is favored by structure that group the cationic amino acids of the molecule with on one side an hydrophobic stretch of amino acids and on the other side streches of apolar amino acids (Kumari and Nagaraj, 2001). Liposome disruption activity of the brevinins correlates with the anti-Gram positive bacterial activity, suggesting a lytic activity. None of the peptides showed hemolytic activity making brevinins attractive prospects for broad-spectrum antimicrobial peptide design (Lee et al., 2002).

1.5 Defensins (cysteine knot structure)

1.5.1 General properties

This class of peptide is characterized by its rigid structure, given by the presence of 3 to 4 disulfid bridges. They are sub-classified through their cysteines connectivity and their secondary structure.

By virtue of the cysteine knot motif that stabilize them, all these peptides show a rigid secondary structure. Defensin are amphipatic molecules with a common defined beta sheet motif secondary structure. Indeed there is a gamma-core motif (GXCX(3-9)C), considered the structural signature of the disulfide-stabilized antimicrobial peptides that present two beta strands with an interposed loop (Sagaram et al., 2011). This motif has one hydrophobic and one hydrophilic side. The hydrophilic side of these peptides is usually constituted by several lysine or arginine aminoacids. This gives them a general positive charge at physiological pH. They are resistant to degradation and peptidase digestion because of their compact structure. As for the other antimicrobial peptide classes, there are few phylogenetic relationships even within each defensin subclass. The first three defensins class described were found exclusively in mammals.

1.5.2 Alpha defensins

This type of defensins is found in mammals. Their cysteine are connected between the cysteines 1-6 2-4 3-5. They show a structure of triple-stranded beta-sheet stabilized by a conserved triple disulfide bridges array (Hadjicharalambous et al., 2008). Alpha defensin sequence present more arginine than lysine residues, and it has been suggested that this high arginine content endows the alpha-defensin with a higher antibacterial activity in high salt conditions (Llenado et al., 2009).

P. hamadryas alpha-defensin ACYCRIPACFAGERRYGTCFYLGRVWAFCC

1.5.3 Beta defensins

The beta defensin have a cysteine connectivity of 1-5 2-4 3-6. They present the consensus sequence of Xn-C-X2-4-G-X1-2-CX3-5CX9-10CX5-6CCXn (Ganz, 2003a) (C=cysteine and G=Glycine). They present a tri dimensional structure of a triple stranded beta sheet. The glycine invariant is also present in alpha defensin. This glycine is necessary for the beta bulge structure to be formed, and the protein is unable to fold if it is replaced by any other natural amino acid (Xie et al., 2005).

Sus scrofa beta-defensin 1 SVSCLRNKGVCMPGKCAPKMKQIGTCGMPQVKCCKRK

1.5.4 θ defensins

θ defensin are macrocyclic octadeca peptides connected head to tail. These peptides are present in monkeys but absent in human. There are θ-defensin ortholog pseudo genes in the human genome but the Theta-defensin genes contain a premature stop codon that aborts translation. (Cole et al., 2002) (Cole et al., 2004). Their synthesis implies a head to tail circularization of an octa-peptide (Selsted, 2004). They were found to be active against *S. aureus, E. coli, and C. albicans* as well as HIV virus (Cole et al., 2002). This type of defensins also present a disulfide bridges stabilized amphipathic beta sheet structure.

P. hamadryas theta-defensin-1 RCVCRRGVCRCVCTRGFC

1.5.5 Insect defensins

The insect defensin class have an alpha-helix secondary structure bound to the beta sheet. Their structures are similar to another arthropod peptide class: the scorpion potassium channel blocker toxins (Bontems et al., 1991). Study of the structural features involved in the antimicrobial activity of longicin, a defensin from the hard tick *Haemaphysalis longicornis*, showed that the beta sheet alone was sufficient for antimicrobial activity. This part of the insect peptide is positively charged at neutral pH, as does the alpha helix of the same, nevertheless the role of the alpha-helix, at the antimicrobial level, seems to be restricted to maintain the globular shape of the peptide (Rahman et al., 2009).

R. prolixus insect defensin B
ATCDLLSFRSKWVTPNHAGCAAHCLLRGNRGGHCKGTICHCRK

1.5.6 Plant defensins

Plant defensin antimicrobial peptide class present 4 disulfide bridges with a cysteine connectivity of 1-8, 2-5, 3-6, and 4-7. Their three-dimensional structures are similar to the insect defensin structure in that they have a disulfide bonds stabilized alpha-helix. Their structure also show a triple anti-parallel beta-strands. (Sagaram et al., 2011). The strong antifungal activity of the plant defensin has been associated with their alpha helix motif, in a similar fashion as for insect defensin (Lamberty et al., 2001). Conversely, heliomycin, a defensin from *Heliothis virescens*, has more structural communality with plant defensin than with insect defensin (Lamberty et al., 2001).

P. sylvestris defensin 1

RMCKTPSGKFKGYCVNNTNCKNVCRTEGFPTGSCDFHVAGRKCYCYKPCP

1.6 Tachyplesin

This class of AMP was first found in horseshoe crab (*Polyphemus litoralis*). Gomesin is a tachyplesin type of antimicrobial peptide found in tarantula hemocyte (Silva et al., 2000); and androctonin has been extracted from scorpion hemolymph (Mandard et al., 1999). This type of antimicrobial structure is broadly distributed amongst the genus. The AMP related to this class of peptide present a beta sheet secondary structure stabilized by two disulfide bridges (Nakamura et al., 1988). Tachyplesin have a rigid conformation of antiparallel beta-sheet connected by a beta-turn (Iwanaga et al., 1994). The tachyplesin family of AMP adopts beta-hairpin-like structures when in contact with hydrophobic solvent. NMR studies revealed a largely unordered structure in water, but a transition to a regular beta-hairpin backbone conformation in the presence of dodecylphosphocholine micelles. The cysteine null mutant of protegrin, a mammal tachyplesin type peptide, revealed that the cystein bridges were not necessary for antimicrobial activity. Aside from their antimicrobial activity, tachyplesin have also a scavenger capability. They bind lipo-polysacharide with high affinity (Niwa et al., 1990). The structure of tachyplesin I also interacts with Vesicular stomatitis virus envelope, inactivating the virus (Murakami et al., 1991).

Tachyplesin III *Tachypleus gigas*: KWCFRVCYRGICYRKCR

1.7 Tryptophan rich antimicrobial peptides

The archetypical W rich peptide is the indolicin, this peptide comes from *Bos Taurus* neutrophils and is the result of proteolysis. Unlike the amphipathic alpha helical structure of the cecropin class of peptides, their linear structure (no disulfid bridges) has no particular secondary structure in water. Indolicin is globular and amphipathic in aqueous solution, while it adopts a wedge shape when in contact with micelles. Indolicin shows a high affinity for neutral POPC and anionic POPG vesicles(Hsu et al., 2005). The author suggests that the structure changes and the strong membrane affinity are key to the antimicrobial activity of indolicin (Ladokhin and White, 2001). Tryptophan rich AMP contains more than 25% of the aminoacid. Indolicin, the archetypical tryptophan rich antimicrobial peptide, has a globular secondary structure in water, but show a wedge shape when in contact with in lipid micelles (Rozek et al., 2000). This peptide has the ability to permeate bacterial membranes and, depending of its tridimensional shape, inhibits DNA synthesis by binding to it (Hsu et al., 2005).

Indolicin: H-ILPWKWPWWPWRR-NH2

1.8 Histidine rich glycoprotein peptides

Histidine-rich amphipathic cationic peptides are peptides with ¼ of their amino acids represented by histidine. They show a global cationic amphipathic helical structure. They trigger microorganism membrane disruption when the peptide adopts an alignment parallel to the membrane surface. Even though, pore formation is not essential for their high antimicrobial activity (Mason et al., 2009). Clavinin and daptomycin are other studied members of this antimicrobial peptide class. Some Histine rich peptide, like LH4, also have the capability to enhance transfection, a feature that is related to membrane perturbation capability (Georgescu et al., 2010).

1.9 Mixed structure peptides

Some peptides share structural communality with more than one class of AMP; the sum of the different AMP part activity are not additive; and these peptides classes do show unique activity not present in the separated structural part of the molecule. Scorpine type AMP represent a class on its own, as several homologous proteins have been found. The structural defensin part of the molecule resembles the insect peptides. It has been determined in later studies that once separated from the linear cecropin-like amino terminus, this peptide could effectively block these channels. Even though, the antimicrobial activity of the complete molecule was dependent of the presence of this toxin/defensin motif (Diego-Garcia et al., 2008).

The penaeidin class of peptide consist in proline-rich N-terminus and of a C-terminus containing six cysteine residues engaged in three disulfide bridges (Destoumieux et al., 2000). The proline-rich domain of penaeidin class AMP suffices to confer target specificity and antimicrobial activity of penaeidin (Cuthbertson et al., 2004). The carboxyl end cysteine-rich domain consists of an amphipathic helix linked to the upstream and the downstream coils by two disulfide bonds. The peptide shows a highly hydrophobic core of globular and compact structure, that has 2 arginines exposed on each side (Yang et al., 2003).

Another example of hybrid antimicrobial peptide is Hyastatin, isolated from the spider crab (*Hyas araneus*) hemocytes (Cuthbertson et al., 2008). This AMP combines a Glycine rich motif N-terminal region, a short Pro/Arg-rich region, and a panaeidin like C-terminal region containing 3 disulfid bridges (Sperstad et al., 2009).

The chicken beta defensin 11 is formed by the repeat of two defensin motif, therefore having 6 disulfid bridges. This defensin show a nanomolar range of anti *E.coli* activity, being one of the most effective antimicrobial peptide for this microorganism (Herve-Grepinet et al., 2010).

Microplusin, is a *Rhipicephalus* (*Boophilus*) microplus anti-microbial peptide (AMP). Microplusin has a cysteine-rich AMPs structure with histidine-rich regions at the N- and C-termini. Microplusin consists of five alpha-helix and has been shown to bind copper and iron (Silva et al., 2009).

2. Antimicrobial mechanisms of AMP

The activity of AMPs must start at the cytoplasmic membrane since most AMPs permeabilize microbial membranes. Several models have been proposed on how AMPs insert into the membrane leading to the formation of ion channels, transmembrane pores or extensive membrane rupture. These models are: 1) transmembrane pore models and 2) nonpore models activity. Here we will also review other antimicrobial mechanisms that have been found. For example, the antimicrobial mechanisms of apidaecin do not rely on pore forming activity, this peptide does have antimicrobial activity at a concentration at least four order of magnitude below the concentration that disturbs the bacterial membrane. Peptides from each structural family have been reported to rely on antimicrobial mechanism that would not imply membrane depolarization of the target microorganism, suggesting internal molecular determinant. Certain peptides are unable to cause membrane depolarization at the minimal inhibitory concentration, while other cause maximal depolarization well below the MIC (Minimal Inhibitory Concentration) value. Evidences are mounting that involve particular macromolecules as well as intracellular functions as the final target for antimicrobial activity of the AMP. Even though, bacterial membranes are a necessary entry path for the AMP, therefore determining part of the AMP selectivity as well as efficiency.

2.1 Transmembrane pore models of AMPs

There are more than 1,000 known AMPs (Brahmachary et al., 2004; Wang and Wang, 2004; Fjell et al., 2007), and for the majority of them, there is little or no evidence for transmembrane pores (Wimley, 2010). Instead, there is compelling evidence that many AMPs function by binding to membrane surfaces and disrupting the packing and organization of the lipids in a nonspecific way. The simplest models of membrane permeation by peptides involve the formation of membrane-spanning pores. These pores have been studied in lipid bilayers and have been proposed to be the major cause of bacterial membrane depolarization. As bacteria ATP synthesis is linked to the trans-membranal potential of the cell, any perturbation of the ion partition may potentially lead to the cell death. The structure of these peptides induced pores have been analyzed and several pore structure were proposed.

The barrel stave pore model (Rapaport and Shai, 1991) involves a mechanism where the peptides interact laterally with one another to form a specific structure enclosing a water-filled channel, much like a protein ion channel. Bioinformatic analysis of protegrin 1 insertion in membranes concluded that this model was most consistant with the observed energy of insertion of the peptide in artificial membranes (Langham et al., 2008). Furthermore the electrophysiology record analysis of Ceratotoxin and pleuricidin peptides inserted in lipid bilayers show that they form a peptide filled pore isolated from the lipids from the membranes. The pore formation dynamics correlates with their antimicrobial activity (Bessin, 2004).

In the toroidal pore model (Ludtke et al., 1996), specific peptide–peptide interactions are not present Instead, the peptides affect cooperatively the local curvature of the membrane, forming a peptide lipid toroid pore in the membrane. The cathelicidin peptide LL 37 (an amphipathic, alpha-helical, antimicrobial peptide) appears to form such kind of pore in the microbial membranes. NMR spectra studies of LL 37 shows that its pore channel is filled with the membrane lipids phosphate heads. The resulting ionic leakage ultimately leads to bacterial membrane depolarization (Henzler Wildman et al., 2003). The pore formation of cateslytin, a beta sheet conformation peptide, has been studied through patch clamp and NMR experiments, and has been found to fit a pore formation model involving transient dissymmetry between the phospholipid leafs of the membrane as a key ingredient to explain the formation of the pore (Jean-Francois et al., 2008)

The carpet model for AMP antimicrobial activity , originally described by Shai (Gazit et al., 1996), is the most commonly cited model of membrane destabilization by AMPs. The carpet/detergent model proposes that the accumulation of the peptides imbedded in the microbial membrane provoques perturbation in the membrane integrity. Antimicrobial peptides accumulate on the membrane surface with an orientation that is parallel to the membrane untill peptide concentration has reached a critical level (i.e., a peptide-rich "carpet" has formed on the membrane surface). Then permeabilization occurs, via global bilayer destabilization. PMAP-23, a cationic peptide member of the cathelicidin family, is considered to induce membrane permeability according to the Shai-Matsuzaki-Huang "carpet" model (Bocchinfuso et al., 2009). Cecropin P1, another alpha helical AMP, imbedded in reconstituted phospholipid bilayer is preferentially oriented nearly parallel to the surface of the lipid membranes, a position that is incompatible with the proteinaceous pore model, as demonstrated by polarized ATR-FTIR spectroscopy analysis(Gazit et al., 1996) The detergent model is also often cited to explain the catastrophic collapse of membrane integrity, observed with some AMPs at high peptide concentration (Ostolaza et al., 1993; Hristova et al., 1997; Bechinger and Lohner, 2006). Some authors combine the carpet and detergent models into a single idea in which the catastrophic collapse of membrane integrity includes membrane fragmentation. Others distinguish between the two models based on whether or not the peptide-induced leakage efficiency depends on the size of the entrapped solutes (Ostolaza et al., 1993). Bechinger and Lohner (Bechinger and Lohner, 2006; Salnikov et al., 2009) recently discussed molecular shape models in which AMP lipid interactions could be depicted with phase diagrams to describe the propensity of an AMP to permeabilize a membrane by disrupting the lipid packing. Epand and colleagues have proposed a lipid clustering model in which AMPs induce clustering or phase separation of lipids, with leakage occurring due to boundary defects (Epand et al., 2009; Epand et al., 2010). Almeida and colleagues have described AMP activity in terms of binding, insertion and perturbation using the sinking raft model, which they recently augmented by adding a formal thermodynamic analysis to predict activity (Pokorny and Almeida, 2004; Gregory et al., 2008; Almeida and Pokorny, 2009; Gregory et al., 2009; Almeida and Pokorny, 2010). Interfacial activity is defined as the propensity of an imperfectly amphipathic peptide to partition into the bilayer interface and drive the vertical rearrangement of the lipid polar and non polar groups. The disruption of the normally strict segregation of polar and nonpolar groups causes membrane permeabilization.

While these models, and others, have been useful in discussing AMPs, the molecular organization of the lipid bilayer undergoing solutes leakage in the presence of AMPs is still very much unknown. Without this knowledge, it remains challenging to predict structure-sequence activity relationships; thus, it also remains challenging to engineer or *de novo* design AMPs.

2.2 Non membrane mediated models of AMP activity

In addition to the pore models described above, AMP activity has been described using antimicrobial mechanism that do not involve bacterial membrane permeability impairement. For instance PR-39, a porcine proline-arginine-rich antibacterial peptide was found to lyse the microbes through a non pore forming mechanism, altering the microbe division and septum formation (Shi et al., 1996). Small Anionic antimicrobial peptides have been found in ovine lungs, that appear to function without the need for the initial electrostatic interaction with the bacterial membranes, and kill the bacteria through intracellular content flocculation (Brogden et al., 1998). Mersacindin, a lantibiotic, has been shown to inhibits bacterial cell wall formation (Brotz et al., 1997). Some antimicrobial peptides like the pleurocidin and dermaseptin inhibit bacterial DNA synthesis while buforin II and tachyplesin bind to nucleic acid in general (Yonezawa et al., 1992). The proline rich AMP family target proteicious or nucleic acid intracellular molecules (Park et al., 2008), indeed members of the proline-rich AMP family like Drosocin, pyrrhocoricin, and apidaecin have been shown to act on bacterial GRO EL and Dna K proteins(Otvos et al., 2000).

3. AMP classical functions

The classical function of AMP has been their role as major effectors of the innate immune system; AMPs complement the highly specific but relatively slow adaptive immune system. Unlike the acquired immune mechanisms, endogenous AMPs, which are constitutively expressed or induced, provide fast and effective means of defense. Most of these gene-encoded peptides are mobilized shortly after microbial infection and act rapidly to neutralize a broad range of microbes (bacteria, virus and protozoa). The ubiquitous nature of antimicrobial peptides suggests that their role in nature has been long standing and must have contributed to an organism's fitness. Many of these molecules exert mechanisms of action that appear to be unique and highly complex. However, AMPs exhibit varying, and in some cases, significant degrees of host cytotoxicity, reflecting non-selective cell targeting (Shin et al., 1999). It is likely that distinct antimicrobial peptides have evolved to function within specific physiologic and anatomic contexts to minimize their potential to concomitantly injuring the host cells. An intensive area of focus regarding antimicrobial peptide biochemistry relates to the precise mechanisms by which these molecules cause cell death. A long-held paradigm for microbicidal action has been that AMPs kill microorganisms by initiating multiple injuries in target microbial cell membranes. The principal theory suggest that peptides may create membrane pores in the organism, making a leakage of some metabolites, ensuing depolarization, loss of membrane-coupled respiration and biopolymer synthesis, and ultimately cell death. However, other authors suggest additional mechanisms, , where membrane permeabilization alone appears to be insufficient to cause cell death. These evidences come from studies documenting a clear dissociation between membrane perturbation and cell death. In these cases, cell killing may proceed in the absence of significant disruption in membrane architecture, due rather to disruptions in cellular function (Zhang et al., 2000). The functional integrity of the cytoplasmic membrane is crucial to essential functions of microbial pathogens, including gradient formation and selective permeability, cellular energetics, and synthesis of bio-molecules (Yeaman et al., 1998).

The general membrane effects of AMP are the membrane perturbation however alone may be insufficient for microbicidal effects of certain peptides. Permeabilization alone does not invariably result in staphylococcal death due antimicrobial peptides. Different peptides with varying staphylocidal potencies exhibited disparate capacities of membrane permeabilization and cell killing (Koo et al., 2001). Similar studies showed that gramicidin S rapidly depolarizes *Pseudomonas aeruginosa,* but did not kill it, suggesting that the concept of membrane perturbation and eventual cell killing may be independent (Zhang et al., 2000). Bacterial membrane energetic also appears to be involved in AMP mechanisms of action (Yeaman et al., 1998). It is now widely recognized that the AMP concept could play a promising role in fighting the presently raging microbial resistance to conventional antibiotics.

4. Unconventional function of AMP

4.1 Regulatory activities of AMPs.

Besides the role of endogenous antibiotics, the antimicrobial peptides have other functions in the inflammation; wound healing and regulation of the response immune response, of which are described below.

Microbial infection of the mucosa and skin induces production of large quantities of small antimicrobial peptides, including defensins and cathelicidins, (Zasloff, 2002; Ganz, 2003a; Yang et al., 2004). They can act as chemokines, such as some β-defensins chemoattract immature iDC and other effector cells through the CCR6 receptor (Biragyn et al., 2002); (Niyonsaba et al., 2004) or human cathelicidin LL-37 recruits neutrophils, monocytes and mast cells via human formyl peptide receptor-like 1, FPRL1 (De et al., 2000) (Agerberth et al., 2000; Niyonsaba et al., 2002). Defensins can also activate effector cells that can work together with the complement system to destroy microbial invaders. The α-defensins HNP1~3 have been reported to increase the production of TNFa and IL-1 while decreasing the production of IL-10 by monocytes (De et al., 2000). Some α-defensins enhance expression of adhesion molecules including ICAM-1, CD11b, and CD11c by neutrophils and facilitate the recruitment and enhance the microbicidal activity (Van Wetering et al., 1997; Chaly et al., 2000; Di Nardo et al., 2003) (FÈger et al., 2002). β-defensins induce mast cell degranulation and release of histamine and prostaglandin D2 (Yamashita and Saito, 1989; Befus et al., 1999; Niyonsaba et al., 2001) increase the expression of CXCL8 and CXCL5 (Van Wetering et al., 1997; van Wetering et al., 2002). Furthermore, murine β-defensin 2 has been shown to act directly on immature DCs as an endogeneous ligand for Toll like receptor 4 (TLR-4), inducing up regulation of co-stimulatory molecules and DC maturation, triggering robust, Th1 polarized adaptive immune responses in vivo (Biragyn et al., 2002). However, the mechanisms that regulate these functions are not well studied. Defensins attract inflammatory cells as neutrophils, B lymphocytes and macrophages. All these cells release inflammatory mediators such as IL-8, IFNγ, IL-6, IL-10 and LTB4. It is interesting that defensins may also have anti-inflammatory activity by the induction of IL-10 or SLPI.(Durr and Peschel, 2002; Zasloff, 2002).The synthesis of β-defensins by epithelial cells and the recruitment of peripheral blood granulocytes α-defensin-rich site of inflammation generates a high concentration of them. Also have direct antimicrobial effects, defensins facilitate and amplify the subsequent immune response. Indeed, spleen cells stimulated with α-defensins increase the production of human cytokines and lymphocyte proliferation. This same type of defensins, when administered to mice, produces increased serum IgG1, IgG2 and IgG2b. In addition, small amounts of HNP extend the antibody response against a singenic tumor (Tani et al., 2000).

These results indicate, without doubt, the AMPs have a role in the regulation of the immune response. On the other hand, recent studies have identified several structurally diverse endogenous mediators of innate immunity with certain features: firstly, they are rapidly released in response to infection or tissue injury; secondly, they have both chemotactic and activating effects on APCs; and thirdly, they exhibit particularly potent *in vivo* immunoenhancing activity and enhance DC differentiation from DC precursors. This subset of mediators alerts host defenses by augmenting innate and adaptive immune responses to tissue injury and/or infection. On the basis of their unique activities, they are called 'alarmins' (Oppenheim and Yang, 2005). Innate-immune mediators possessing alarmin activity include defensins, cathelicidin, eosinophil-derived neurotoxin (EDN), and high mobility group box protein 1 (HMGB1) (Oppenheim and Yang, 2005). The concept of alarmins is very interesting. This has only been observed in mammals, but is likely to exist in other groups of animals including insects. It has been observed over-expression of antimicrobial peptides during infection with various pathogens and even damage to the cuticle. Many groups of insects have been used to understand the basic characteristics of the innate immunity. However, surprisingly, the study of AMPs in insects has been limited study of their bactericidal or antiparasitic activity and virtually no information on the alternative role that could have the AMPs on the immune response in these organisms.

Differential analyses after bacterial or fungal challenge showed the regulation of more than a 100 molecules in adult *Drosophila* hemolymph (Levy et al., 2004). Using differential

MALDI-TOF MS, 28 peptides with a molecular mass below 15 kDa and belonging to different structural families were identified and could be classified into two groups. The first group contains the AMPs and their different isoforms. DIMs belonging to this group are likely to be effectors molecules of the immune response through their antimicrobial activity. The second group contains molecules for which the lack of similarity to any peptide prevents the proposition of any precise function. These peptides are suspected to serve as chemokines during the *Drosophila* immune response but the different approaches for investigating their role have so far been unsuccessful (Levy et al., 2004). On the other hand, our group has analyzed the peptides in the hemolymph of mosquitoes *An. albimanus* infected with malaria parasites. We found a complex pattern of peptides, including cecropin, which are released into the hemolymph. Similarly, gambicin, cecropin, and defensin are over-expressed in the intestinal epithelium and fat body of mosquitoes infected with *Plasmodium*. However, it is unknown whether these peptides participate in the elimination of the parasite. Cecropin has been consider an important AMP against Plasmodium, but in vitro assays with synthetic cecropin did not affect *Plasmodium* viability (unpublished results), but this peptide is over-expressed in mosquitoes infected with the parasite (Herrera-Ortiz, A. et al., 2010.). It would be interesting to analyze the peptides released into the hemolymph of these insects and their role in regulating the immune response.

4.2 Anti-inflammatory (Anti-endotoxin) roles of host defense peptides

Bacterial lipopolysaccharides (LPS), also known as endotoxins, are major structural components of the outer membrane of Gram-negative bacteria that serve as a barrier and protective shield between them and their surrounding environment. LPS is considered to be a major virulence factor as it strongly stimulates the secretion of pro-inflammatory cytokines which mediate the host immune response and culminating in septic shock.

Early experiments determined that a number of host defense peptides from various sources bound to LPS from diverse Gram-negative bacteria and reduced LPS-induced release of pro-inflammatory cytokines (e.g. TNF-α, IL-1, IL-6) and nitric oxide from monocyte or macrophages and protected mice from LPS lethality (Larrick et al., 1994; Larrick et al., 1995; VanderMeer et al., 1995; Kirikae et al., 1998). Initial studies focused on the unprocessed form of cathelicidin, hCAP- 18 (Kirikae et al., 1998); however, it was later found that the LPS-binding properties of the peptide were contained within the processed 37-amino acid C-terminal domain, LL-37 (Turner et al., 1998). It has been proposed that the anti-endotoxic properties of these peptides are the result of the inhibition of binding of LPS to CD14 (Nagaoka et al., 2001) and lipopolysaccharide binding protein (LBP) (Scott et al., 2000), and/or indirect effects on cells (Scott et al., 2002). LL-37 has been shown to block a number of LPS-induced inflammatory responses, including contractility and (nitric oxide) NO release in aortic rings (Ciornei et al., 2003), pro-inflammatory cytokine production in a macrophage cell line and in animal models (Scott et al., 2000; Ohgami et al., 2003), suppression of leukocyte infiltration in a model of endotoxin-induced uveitis (Ohgami et al., 2003) and lethality in animal models of sepsis (Scott et al., 2002). These effects occur at concentrations in the physiological range for LL-37 (1–5 μg/ml) and may reflect a natural role for LL-37 in the body (e.g. balancing of the potential stimulus by endotoxin from commensals). This anti-endotoxin activity appears to correlate with an ability to dampen the pro-inflammatory effects of the Gram-positive surface molecule lipoteichoic acid (Scott et al., 2002; Gutsmann et al., 2010) designed a new class of peptides synthetic anti-LPS peptides (SALPs). SALPs were originally based on the LPS-binding domain of the *Limulus* anti-LPS factor (LALF) but were substantially changed in length and primary sequence for optimal binding to the lipid A portion of LPS. They observed that these peptides are highly efficient in neutralization of LPS and blockage of its immunopathological consequences *in vitro* and *in vivo*. SALPs combine excellent selectivity for LPS, with high neutralizing activity *in vitro* and potent protection to septic shock using the murine model *in vivo*. They also demonstrate the biological efficacy of rationally designed new synthetic antilipopolysaccharide peptides (SALPs) based on the *Limulus* anti-LPS factor for systemic application. Efficient inhibition of LPS-induced cytokine release and protection from lethal septic shock *in vivo* was analyzed, whereas cytotoxicity was not observed under physiologically relevant conditions and concentrations. It seems that the lipid A part of LPS is converted from its "endotoxic conformation," the cubic aggregate structure, into an inactive multilamellar structure. These observations suggest a novel therapeutic role of AMPs.

4.3 Anti-viral activity

Apart from the antibacterial activity, AMPs also possess antiviral activity. For example, the α-defensins target the human immunodeficiency virus (HIV) activity by directly inactivating viral particles and affecting the ability of the virus to replicate within CD4 cells. Human α-defensins HNP-1 to -3 and HD-5 have been shown to block papillomavirus infection. Retrocyclin 2, a synthetic θ-defensin peptide that humans do not synthesize due to a mutation in the corresponding human gene, has the capacity to block influenza virus infection. Human β-defensins can also block HIV-1 replication, and interestingly, a single nucleotide polymorphism in a β-defensin gene has been associated with clinical manifestation of HIV-1 infection, suggesting that the human β-defensins play an important role in host defense against HIV. Cathelicidins, in contrast, have an inhibitory effect on lentiviral replication in vitro, and LL-37 appears capable of interfering with vaccinia virus replication in vitro and in mice. Dermaseptin S4, a 28-residue AMP isolated from frog skin, attenuates HIV infection in vitro. Other AMPs from frog skin including caerin 1.1, caerin 1.9, and maculatin 1.1 have also demonstrated inhibition of HIV in vitro(Albiol Matanic and Castilla, 2004).(Daher et al., 1986; Sinha et al., 2003; Yasin et al., 2004). Our group has worked with the peptide named scorpine from the venom of *Pandinus imperator* scorpion, where we observed a very interesting anti-virus dengue and anti-plasmodium activity (Carballar-Lejarazu et al., 2008). Scorpine is an antimicrobial peptide whose structure resembles a hybrid between a defensin and a cecropin. It exhibits antibacterial activity and inhibits the sporogonic development of parasites responsible for murine malaria. The recombinant expressed scorpine (RScp) in *Anopheles gambie* cells showed antibacterial activity against *Bacillus subtilis* and *Klebsiella pneumoniae*, at 5 and 10 μM, respectively. It also produced 98%mortality in sexual stages of *Plasmodium berghei* at 15 μM and 100% reduction in *Plasmodium falciparum* parasitemia at 5 μM. RScp also inhibited virus dengue-2 replication in C6/36 mosquito cells. In addition, we generated viable and fertile transgenic *Drosophila* that over-expresses and correctly secretes RScp into the insect hemolymph, suggesting that the generation of transgenic mosquitoes resistant to different pathogens may be viable. However, there is no knowledge of their mechanics, action. It is necessary to extend these studies with other peptides during infection induced with virus dengue and other pathogens.

5. Evolutionary perspective on antimicrobial peptides

In this chapter, we proposed a structural classification of antimicrobial peptide families considering the diversity of their structures and then we reviewed the traditional function and biological activities. Finally, we propose new insights into the functions of antimicrobial peptides that could provide a large body of research to create new classes of antimicrobial therapeutics. AMPs are widespread molecules throughout the animal and plant taxa, this fact suggest its relevance in the evolution of immune response. Traditionally, their basic molecular and biochemical nature is related to the disruption of membrane potential and/or structure with the ensuing cell death. However, the diversity in the structure and biological properties (above mentioned) of AMPs within and between species suggest that these molecules have different functions in immune response.

The immune system of living organisms is formed by a set of cells, molecules and reactions. All of these features are continuously evolving to resist (attack and eliminate) pathogen invasion and to limit the negative (in terms of host survival and reproduction, i.e. fitness) consequences of the infection (Hoffmann and Reichhart, 2002). On the other hand, pathogens success depends upon overcoming the selective immune pressures brought about by the host. As a consequence, both, host and pathogens, evolve traits and strategies to increase the fitness of each one. Van Valen (Van Valen, 1973) proposed this co-evolutionary arm races as an evolutionary theory called "The Red Queen Hypothesis". The theory was proposed citing Lewis Carrol's Red Queen, where it takes all the running somebody can do to keep in the same place. Given this situation, immunologically, there is never a "best" solution to pathogens infection. To understand this scenario, we must consider (1) pathogen's short generational cycles, that may provide enough time to adapt to the host's immune response. As an outcome there will be grounds for high variability in immune response. (2) Differences in the kind and burden of pathogens, where divergent host-pathogen interactions for each species are possible and can be reflected in the course of action of taxa immune response (Read and Taylor, 2001). (3) Virulence differences, where there can or cannot be a harm imposed on a host (for example *Bacillus anthracis* vs. commensal microbiota). As long Hypothesis, an immune effecter that has the ability to be produced under different infection circumstances could have a selective advantage, antimicrobial peptides could have this property, as the host has to deal with the problem of maximizing fitness under the Red Queen pressure.

6. References

Agerberth, B., Charo, J., Werr, J., Olsson, B., Idali, F., Lindbom, L., Kiessling, R., J√∂rnvall, H., Wigzell, H. and Gudmundsson, G.H., 2000. The human antimicrobial and chemotactic peptides LL-37 and Œ±-defensins are expressed by specific lymphocyte and monocyte populations. Blood, 96:3086-3093.

Agerberth, B., Lee, J.Y., Bergman, T., Carlquist, M., Boman, H.G., Mutt, V. and Jornvall, H., 1991. Amino acid sequence of PR-39. Isolation from pig intestine of a new member of the family of proline-arginine-rich antibacterial peptides. Eur J Biochem, 202:849-854.

Albiol Matanic, V.C. and Castilla, V., 2004. Antiviral activity of antimicrobial cationic peptides against Junin virus and herpes simplex virus. International Journal of Antimicrobial Agents, 23:382-389.

Almeida, P.F. and Pokorny, A., 2009. Mechanisms of antimicrobial, cytolytic, and cell-penetrating peptides: from kinetics to thermodynamics. Biochemistry, 48:8083-8093.

Almeida, P.F. and Pokorny, A., 2010. Binding and permeabilization of model membranes by amphipathic peptides. Methods Mol Biol, 618:155-169.

Azevedo Calderon, L., Silva Ade, A., Ciancaglini, P. and Stabeli, R.G., 2010. Antimicrobial peptides from Phyllomedusa frogs: from biomolecular diversity to potential nanotechnologic medical applications. Amino Acids, 40:29-49.

Bechinger, B. and Lohner, K., 2006. Detergent-like actions of linear amphipathic cationic antimicrobial peptides. Biochim Biophys Acta, 1758:1529-1539.

Befus, A.D., Mowat, C., Gilchrist, M., Hu, J., Solomon, S. and Bateman, A., 1999. Neutrophil Defensins Induce Histamine Secretion from Mast Cells: Mechanisms of Action. The Journal of Immunology, 163:947-953.

Bessin, Y., Saint, N., Marri, L., Marchini, D. and Molle, G., 2004. Antibacterial activity and pore-forming properties of ceratotoxins: a mechanism of action based on the barrel stave model. Biochim Biophys Acta, 1667:148-156.

Biragyn, A., Ruffini, P.A., Leifer, C.A., Klyushnenkova, E., Shakhov, A., Chertov, O., Shirakawa, A.K., Farber, J.M., Segal, D.M., Oppenheim, J.J. and Kwak, L.W., 2002. Toll-Like Receptor 4-Dependent Activation of Dendritic Cells by ŒF<-Defensin 2. Science, 298:1025-1029.

Bocchinfuso, G., Palleschi, A., Orioni, B., Grande, G., Formaggio, F., Toniolo, C., Park, Y., Hahm, K.S. and Stella, L., 2009. Different mechanisms of action of antimicrobial peptides: insights from fluorescence spectroscopy experiments and molecular dynamics simulations. J Pept Sci, 15:550-558.

Bontems, F., Roumestand, C., Gilquin, B., Menez, A. and Toma, F., 1991. Refined structure of charybdotoxin: common motifs in scorpion toxins and insect defensins. Science, 254:1521-1523.

Boulanger, N., Munks, R.J., Hamilton, J.V., Vovelle, F., Brun, R., Lehane, M.J. and Bulet, P., 2002. Epithelial innate immunity. A novel antimicrobial peptide with antiparasitic activity in the blood-sucking insect Stomoxys calcitrans. J Biol Chem, 277:49921-49926.

Brahmachary, M., Krishnan, S.P., Koh, J.L., Khan, A.M., Seah, S.H., Tan, T.W., Brusic, V. and Bajic, V.B., 2004. ANTIMIC: a database of antimicrobial sequences. Nucleic Acids Res, 32:D586-589.

Brogden, K.A., Ackermann, M. and Huttner, K.M., 1998. Detection of anionic antimicrobial peptides in ovine bronchoalveolar lavage fluid and respiratory epithelium. Infect Immun, 66:5948-5954.

Brotz, H., Bierbaum, G., Reynolds, P.E. and Sahl, H.G., 1997. The lantibiotic mersacidin inhibits peptidoglycan biosynthesis at the level of transglycosylation. Eur J Biochem, 246:193-199.

Bruston, F., Lacombe, C., Zimmermann, K., Piesse, C., Nicolas, P. and El Amri, C., 2007. Structural malleability of plasticins: preorganized conformations in solution and relevance for antimicrobial activity. Biopolymers, 86:42-56.

Bulet, P., Cociancich, S., Dimarcq, J.L., Lambert, J., Reichhart, J.M., Hoffmann, D., Hetru, C. and Hoffmann, J.A., 1991. Insect immunity. Isolation from a coleopteran insect of a novel inducible antibacterial peptide and of new members of the insect defensin family. J Biol Chem, 266:24520-24525.

Bulet, P., Dimarcq, J.L., Hetru, C., Lagueux, M., Charlet, M., Hegy, G., Van Dorsselaer, A. and Hoffmann, J.A., 1993. A novel inducible antibacterial peptide of Drosophila carries an O-glycosylated substitution. J Biol Chem, 268:14893-14897.

Bulet, P., Hetru, C., Dimarcq, J.L. and Hoffmann, D., 1999. Antimicrobial peptides in insects; structure and function. Dev Comp Immunol, 23:329-344.

Carballar-Lejarazu, R., Rodriguez, M.H., de la Cruz Hernandez-Hernandez, F., Ramos-Castaneda, J., Possani, L.D., Zurita-Ortega, M., Reynaud-Garza, E., Hernandez-Rivas, R., Loukeris, T., Lycett, G. and Lanz-Mendoza, H., 2008. Recombinant scorpine: a multifunctional antimicrobial peptide with activity against different pathogens. Cell Mol Life Sci, 65:3081-3092.

Casteels-Josson, K., Capaci, T., Casteels, P. and Tempst, P., 1993. Apidaecin multipeptide precursor structure: a putative mechanism for amplification of the insect antibacterial response. EMBO J, 12:1569-1578.

Chaly, Y.V., Paleolog, E.M., Kolesnikova, T.S., Tikhonov, II, Petratchenko, E.V. and Voitenok, N.N., 2000. Neutrophil alpha-defensin human neutrophil peptide modulates cytokine production in human monocytes and adhesion molecule expression in endothelial cells. Eur Cytokine Netw, 11:257-266.

Ciornei, C.D., Egesten, A. and Bodelsson, M., 2003. Effects of human cathelicidin antimicrobial peptide LL-37 on lipopolysaccharide-induced nitric oxide release from rat aorta in vitro. Acta Anaesthesiologica Scandinavica, 47:213-220.

Cociancich, S., Dupont, A., Hegy, G., Lanot, R., Holder, F., Hetru, C., Hoffmann, J.A. and Bulet, P., 1994. Novel inducible antibacterial peptides from a hemipteran insect, the sap-sucking bug Pyrrhocoris apterus. Biochem J, 300 (Pt 2):567-575.

Cole, A.M., Hong, T., Boo, L.M., Nguyen, T., Zhao, C., Bristol, G., Zack, J.A., Waring, A.J., Yang, O.O. and Lehrer, R.I., 2002. Retrocyclin: a primate peptide that protects cells from infection by T- and M-tropic strains of HIV-1. Proc Natl Acad Sci U S A, 99:1813-1818.

Cole, A.M., Wang, W., Waring, A.J. and Lehrer, R.I., 2004. Retrocyclins: using past as prologue. Curr Protein Pept Sci, 5:373-381.

Cuthbertson, B.J., Bullesbach, E.E., Fievet, J., Bachere, E. and Gross, P.S., 2004. A new class (penaeidin class 4) of antimicrobial peptides from the Atlantic white shrimp (Litopenaeus setiferus) exhibits target specificity and an independent proline-rich-domain function. Biochem J, 381:79-86.

Cuthbertson, B.J., Deterding, L.J., Williams, J.G., Tomer, K.B., Etienne, K., Blackshear, P.J., Bullesbach, E.E. and Gross, P.S., 2008. Diversity in penaeidin antimicrobial peptide form and function. Dev Comp Immunol, 32:167-181.

Daher, K.A., Selsted, M.E. and Lehrer, R.I., 1986. Direct inactivation of viruses by human granulocyte defensins. J. Virol., 60:1068-1074.

De, A.K., Kodys, K.M., Yeh, B.S. and Miller-Graziano, C., 2000. Exaggerated human monocyte IL-10 concomitant to minimal TNF-alpha induction by heat-shock protein 27 (Hsp27) suggests Hsp27 is primarily an antiinflammatory stimulus. J Immunol, 165:3951-3958.

Destoumieux, D., Munoz, M., Bulet, P. and Bachere, E., 2000. Penaeidins, a family of antimicrobial peptides from penaeid shrimp (Crustacea, Decapoda). Cell Mol Life Sci, 57:1260-1271.

Di Nardo, A., Vitiello, A. and Gallo, R.L., 2003. Cutting Edge: Mast Cell Antimicrobial Activity Is Mediated by Expression of Cathelicidin Antimicrobial Peptide. The Journal of Immunology, 170:2274-2278.

Diego-Garcia, E., Abdel-Mottaleb, Y., Schwartz, E.F., de la Vega, R.C., Tytgat, J. and Possani, L.D., 2008. Cytolytic and K+ channel blocking activities of beta-KTx and scorpine-like peptides purified from scorpion venoms. Cell Mol Life Sci, 65:187-200.

Duclohier, H., Molle, G. and Spach, G., 1989. Antimicrobial peptide magainin I from Xenopus skin forms anion-permeable channels in planar lipid bilayers. Biophys J, 56:1017-1021.

Durr, M. and Peschel, A., 2002. Chemokines meet defensins: the merging concepts of chemoattractants and antimicrobial peptides in host defense. Infect Immun, 70:6515-6517.

Epand, R.F., Maloy, W.L., Ramamoorthy, A. and Epand, R.M., 2010. Probing the "charge cluster mechanism" in amphipathic helical cationic antimicrobial peptides. Biochemistry, 49:4076-4084.

Epand, R.F., Sarig, H., Mor, A. and Epand, R.M., 2009. Cell-wall interactions and the selective bacteriostatic activity of a miniature oligo-acyl-lysyl. Biophys J, 97:2250-2257.

Fèger, F., Varadaradjalou, S., Gao, Z., Abraham, S.N. and Arock, M., 2002. The role of mast cells in host defense and their subversion by bacterial pathogens. Trends in immunology, 23:151-158.

Fjell, C.D., Hancock, R.E. and Cherkasov, A., 2007. AMPer: a database and an automated discovery tool for antimicrobial peptides. Bioinformatics, 23:1148-1155.

Ganz, T., 2003a. Defensins: antimicrobial peptides of innate immunity. Nat Rev Immunol, 3:710-720.

Ganz, T., 2003b. The role of antimicrobial peptides in innate immunity. Integr Comp Biol, 43:300-304.

Gazit, E., Miller, I.R., Biggin, P.C., Sansom, M.S. and Shai, Y., 1996. Structure and orientation of the mammalian antibacterial peptide cecropin P1 within phospholipid membranes. J Mol Biol, 258:860-870.

Georgescu, J., Munhoz, V.H. and Bechinger, B., 2010. NMR structures of the histidine-rich peptide LAH4 in micellar environments: membrane insertion, pH-dependent mode of antimicrobial action, and DNA transfection. Biophys J, 99:2507-2515.

Gregory, S.M., Cavenaugh, A., Journigan, V., Pokorny, A. and Almeida, P.F., 2008. A quantitative model for the all-or-none permeabilization of phospholipid vesicles by the antimicrobial peptide cecropin A. Biophys J, 94:1667-1680.

Gregory, S.M., Pokorny, A. and Almeida, P.F., 2009. Magainin 2 revisited: a test of the quantitative model for the all-or-none permeabilization of phospholipid vesicles. Biophys J, 96:116-131.

Gutsmann, T., Razquin-Olazaran, I., Kowalski, I., Kaconis, Y., Howe, J., Bartels, R., Hornef, M., Schurholz, T., Rossle, M., Sanchez-Gomez, S., Moriyon, I., Martinez de Tejada, G. and Brandenburg, K., 2010. New Antiseptic Peptides To Protect against Endotoxin-Mediated Shock. Antimicrob. Agents Chemother., 54:3817-3824.

Hadjicharalambous, C., Sheynis, T., Jelinek, R., Shanahan, M.T., Ouellette, A.J. and Gizeli, E., 2008. Mechanisms of alpha-defensin bactericidal action: comparative membrane disruption by Cryptdin 4 and its disulfide-null analogue. Biochemistry, 47:12626-12634.

Henzler Wildman, K.A., Lee, D.K. and Ramamoorthy, A., 2003. Mechanism of lipid bilayer disruption by the human antimicrobial peptide, LL-37. Biochemistry, 42:6545-6558.

Herrera-Ortiz, A., Martìnez-Barnetche, J.s., Smit, N., Rodriguez, M.H. and Lanz-Mendoza, H., 2010. The effect of nitric oxide and hydrogen peroxide in the activation of the systemic immune response of Anopheles albimanus infected with Plasmodium berghei. Developmental & Comparative Immunology, 35:44-50.

Hoffmann, J.A. and Reichhart, J.-M., 2002. Drosophila innate immunity: an evolutionary perspective. Nat Immunol, 3:121-126.

Hristova, K., Selsted, M.E. and White, S.H., 1997. Critical role of lipid composition in membrane permeabilization by rabbit neutrophil defensins. J Biol Chem, 272:24224-24233.

Hsu, C.H., Chen, C., Jou, M.L., Lee, A.Y., Lin, Y.C., Yu, Y.P., Huang, W.T. and Wu, S.H., 2005. Structural and DNA-binding studies on the bovine antimicrobial peptide, indolicidin: evidence for multiple conformations involved in binding to membranes and DNA. Nucleic Acids Res, 33:4053-4064.

Hultmark, D., Engstrom, A., Bennich, H., Kapur, R. and Boman, H.G., 1982. Insect immunity: isolation and structure of cecropin D and four minor antibacterial components from Cecropia pupae. Eur J Biochem, 127:207-217.

Iwanaga, S., Muta, T., Shigenaga, T., Seki, N., Kawano, K., Katsu, T. and Kawabata, S., 1994. Structure-function relationships of tachyplesins and their analogues. Ciba Found Symp, 186:160-174; discussion 174-165.

Jean-Francois, F., Elezgaray, J., Berson, P., Vacher, P. and Dufourc, E.J., 2008. Pore formation induced by an antimicrobial peptide: electrostatic effects. Biophys J, 95:5748-5756.

Kirikae, T., Hirata, M., Yamasu, H., Kirikae, F., Tamura, H., Kayama, F., Nakatsuka, K., Yokochi, T. and Nakano, M., 1998. Protective Effects of a Human 18-Kilodalton Cationic Antimicrobial Protein (CAP18)-Derived Peptide against Murine Endotoxemia. Infect. Immun., 66:1861-1868.

Knappe, D., Piantavigna, S., Hansen, A., Mechler, A., Binas, A., Nolte, O., Martin, L.L. and Hoffmann, R., 2010. Oncocin (VDKPPYLPRPRPPRRIYNR-NH2): a novel antibacterial peptide optimized against gram-negative human pathogens. J Med Chem, 53:5240-5247.

Koo, S.P., Bayer, A.S. and Yeaman, M.R., 2001. Diversity in antistaphylococcal mechanisms among membrane-targeting antimicrobial peptides. Infect Immun, 69:4916-4922.

Kumari, V.K. and Nagaraj, R., 2001. Structure-function studies on the amphibian peptide brevinin 1E: translocating the cationic segment from the C-terminal end to a central position favors selective antibacterial activity. J Pept Res, 58:433-441.

Ladokhin, A.S. and White, S.H., 2001. Protein chemistry at membrane interfaces: non-additivity of electrostatic and hydrophobic interactions. J Mol Biol, 309:543-552.

Lamberty, M., Caille, A., Landon, C., Tassin-Moindrot, S., Hetru, C., Bulet, P. and Vovelle, F., 2001. Solution structures of the antifungal heliomicin and a selected variant with both antibacterial and antifungal activities. Biochemistry, 40:11995-12003.

Langham, A.A., Ahmad, A.S. and Kaznessis, Y.N., 2008. On the nature of antimicrobial activity: a model for protegrin-1 pores. J Am Chem Soc, 130:4338-4346.

Larrick, J., Hirata, M., Balint, R., Lee, J., Zhong, J. and Wright, S., 1995. Human CAP18: a novel antimicrobial lipopolysaccharide-binding protein. Infect. Immun., 63:1291-1297.

Larrick, J., Hirata, M., Zheng, H., Zhong, J., Bolin, D., Cavaillon, J., Warren, H. and Wright, S., 1994. A novel granulocyte-derived peptide with lipopolysaccharide-neutralizing activity. The Journal of Immunology, 152:231-240.

Lee, M.K., Cha, L., Lee, S.H. and Hahm, K.S., 2002. Role of amino acid residues within the disulfide loop of thanatin, a potent antibiotic peptide. J Biochem Mol Biol, 35:291-296.

Levy, F., Rabel, D., Charlet, M., Bulet, P., Hoffmann, J.A. and Ehret-Sabatier, L., 2004. Peptidomic and proteomic analyses of the systemic immune response of Drosophila. Biochimie, 86:607-616.

Llenado, R.A., Weeks, C.S., Cocco, M.J. and Ouellette, A.J., 2009. Electropositive charge in alpha-defensin bactericidal activity: functional effects of Lys-for-Arg substitutions vary with the peptide primary structure. Infect Immun, 77:5035-5043.

Ludtke, S.J., He, K., Heller, W.T., Harroun, T.A., Yang, L. and Huang, H.W., 1996. Membrane pores induced by magainin. Biochemistry, 35:13723-13728.

Mackintosh, J.A., Veal, D.A., Beattie, A.J. and Gooley, A.A., 1998. Isolation from an ant Myrmecia gulosa of two inducible O-glycosylated proline-rich antibacterial peptides. J Biol Chem, 273:6139-6143.

Mandard, N., Sy, D., Maufrais, C., Bonmatin, J.M., Bulet, P., Hetru, C. and Vovelle, F., 1999. Androctonin, a novel antimicrobial peptide from scorpion Androctonus australis: solution structure and molecular dynamics simulations in the presence of a lipid monolayer. J Biomol Struct Dyn, 17:367-380.

Mason, A.J., Moussaoui, W., Abdelrahman, T., Boukhari, A., Bertani, P., Marquette, A., Shooshtarizaheh, P., Moulay, G., Boehm, N., Guerold, B., Sawers, R.J., Kichler, A., Metz-Boutigue, M.H., Candolfi, E., Prevost, G. and Bechinger, B., 2009. Structural determinants of antimicrobial and antiplasmodial activity and selectivity in histidine-rich amphipathic cationic peptides. J Biol Chem, 284:119-133.

Moerman, L., Bosteels, S., Noppe, W., Willems, J., Clynen, E., Schoofs, L., Thevissen, K., Tytgat, J., Van Eldere, J., Van Der Walt, J. and Verdonck, F., 2002. Antibacterial and antifungal properties of alpha-helical, cationic peptides in the venom of scorpions from southern Africa. Eur J Biochem, 269:4799-4810.

Moore, A.J., Beazley, W.D., Bibby, M.C. and Devine, D.A., 1996. Antimicrobial activity of cecropins. J Antimicrob Chemother, 37:1077-1089.

Murakami, T., Niwa, M., Tokunaga, F., Miyata, T. and Iwanaga, S., 1991. Direct virus inactivation of tachyplesin I and its isopeptides from horseshoe crab hemocytes. Chemotherapy, 37:327-334.

Nagaoka, I., Hirota, S., Niyonsaba, F.o., Hirata, M., Adachi, Y., Tamura, H. and Heumann, D., 2001. Cathelicidin Family of Antibacterial Peptides CAP18 and CAP11 Inhibit the Expression of TNF-Œ± by Blocking the Binding of LPS to CD14+ Cells. The Journal of Immunology, 167:3329-3338.

Nakamura, T., Furunaka, H., Miyata, T., Tokunaga, F., Muta, T., Iwanaga, S., Niwa, M., Takao, T. and Shimonishi, Y., 1988. Tachyplesin, a class of antimicrobial peptide from the hemocytes of the horseshoe crab (Tachypleus tridentatus). Isolation and chemical structure. J Biol Chem, 263:16709-16713.

Niidome, T., Mihara, H., Oka, M., Hayashi, T., Saiki, T., Yoshida, K. and Aoyagi, H., 1998. Structure and property of model peptides of proline/arginine-rich region in bactenecin 5. J Pept Res, 51:337-345.

Niwa, M., Hua, H., Iwanaga, S., Morita, T., Miyata, T., Nakamura, T., Aketagawa, J., Muta, T., Tokunaga, F. and Ohashi, K., 1990. Biological activities of anti-LPS factor and LPS binding peptide from horseshoe crab amoebocytes. Adv Exp Med Biol, 256:257-271.

Niyonsaba, F., Iwabuchi, K., Someya, A., Hirata, M., Matsuda, H., Ogawa, H. and Nagaoka, I., 2002. A cathelicidin family of human antibacterial peptide LL-37 induces mast cell chemotaxis. Immunology, 106:20-26.

Niyonsaba, F., Ogawa, H. and Nagaoka, I., 2004. Human β-defensin-2 functions as a chemotactic agent for tumour necrosis factor-α-treated human neutrophils. Immunology, 111:273-281.

Niyonsaba, F., Someya, A., Hirata, M., Ogawa, H. and Nagaoka, I., 2001. Evaluation of the effects of peptide antibiotics human β-defensins-1/-2 and LL-37 on histamine release and prostaglandin D2 production from mast cells. European Journal of Immunology, 31:1066-1075.

Ohgami, K., Ilieva, I.B., Shiratori, K., Isogai, E., Yoshida, K., Kotake, S., Nishida, T., Mizuki, N. and Ohno, S., 2003. Effect of Human Cationic Antimicrobial Protein 18 Peptide on Endotoxin-Induced Uveitis in Rats. Investigative Ophthalmology & Visual Science, 44:4412-4418.

Oppenheim, J.J. and Yang, D., 2005. Alarmins: chemotactic activators of immune responses. Current Opinion in Immunology, 17:359-365.

Ostolaza, H., Bartolome, B., Ortiz de Zarate, I., de la Cruz, F. and Goni, F.M., 1993. Release of lipid vesicle contents by the bacterial protein toxin alpha-haemolysin. Biochim Biophys Acta, 1147:81-88.

Otvos, L., Jr., O, I., Rogers, M.E., Consolvo, P.J., Condie, B.A., Lovas, S., Bulet, P. and Blaszczyk-Thurin, M., 2000. Interaction between heat shock proteins and antimicrobial peptides. Biochemistry, 39:14150-14159.

Park, K.H., Park, Y., Park, I.S., Hahm, K.S. and Shin, S.Y., 2008. Bacterial selectivity and plausible mode of antibacterial action of designed Pro-rich short model antimicrobial peptides. J Pept Sci, 14:876-882.

Pokorny, A. and Almeida, P.F., 2004. Kinetics of dye efflux and lipid flip-flop induced by delta-lysin in phosphatidylcholine vesicles and the mechanism of graded release by amphipathic, alpha-helical peptides. Biochemistry, 43:8846-8857.

Rahman, M., Tsuji, N., Boldbaatar, D., Battur, B., Liao, M., Umemiya-Shirafuji, R., You, M., Tanaka, T. and Fujisaki, K., 2009. Structural characterization and cytolytic activity of a potent antimicrobial motif in longicin, a defensin-like peptide in the tick Haemaphysalis longicornis. J Vet Med Sci, 72:149-156.

Rapaport, D. and Shai, Y., 1991. Interaction of fluorescently labeled pardaxin and its analogues with lipid bilayers. J Biol Chem, 266:23769-23775.

Read, A.F. and Taylor, L.H., 2001. The Ecology of Genetically Diverse Infections. Science, 292:1099-1102.

Rozek, A., Friedrich, C.L. and Hancock, R.E., 2000. Structure of the bovine antimicrobial peptide indolicidin bound to dodecylphosphocholine and sodium dodecyl sulfate micelles. Biochemistry, 39:15765-15774.

Sagaram, U.S., Pandurangi, R., Kaur, J., Smith, T.J. and Shah, D.M., 2011. Structure-activity determinants in antifungal plant defensins MsDef1 and MtDef4 with different modes of action against Fusarium graminearum. PLoS One, 6:e18550.

Salnikov, E.S., Mason, A.J. and Bechinger, B., 2009. Membrane order perturbation in the presence of antimicrobial peptides by (2)H solid-state NMR spectroscopy. Biochimie, 91:734-743.

Scott, M.G., Davidson, D.J., Gold, M.R., Bowdish, D. and Hancock, R.E.W., 2002. The Human Antimicrobial Peptide LL-37 Is a Multifunctional Modulator of Innate Immune Responses. The Journal of Immunology, 169:3883-3891.

Scott, M.G., Vreugdenhil, A.C.E., Buurman, W.A., Hancock, R.E.W. and Gold, M.R., 2000. Cutting Edge: Cationic Antimicrobial Peptides Block the Binding of Lipopolysaccharide (LPS) to LPS Binding Protein. The Journal of Immunology, 164:549-553.

Selsted, M.E., 2004. Theta-defensins: cyclic antimicrobial peptides produced by binary ligation of truncated alpha-defensins. Curr Protein Pept Sci, 5:365-371.

Shi, J., Ross, C.R., Chengappa, M.M., Sylte, M.J., McVey, D.S. and Blecha, F., 1996. Antibacterial activity of a synthetic peptide (PR-26) derived from PR-39, a proline-arginine-rich neutrophil antimicrobial peptide. Antimicrob Agents Chemother, 40:115-121.

Shin, S.Y., Kang, J.H. and Hahm, K.S., 1999. Structure-antibacterial, antitumor and hemolytic activity relationships of cecropin A-magainin 2 and cecropin A-melittin hybrid peptides. J Pept Res, 53:82-90.

Shin, S.Y., Kang, J.H., Jang, S.Y., Kim, Y., Kim, K.L. and Hahm, K.S., 2000. Effects of the hinge region of cecropin A(1-8)-magainin 2(1-12), a synthetic antimicrobial peptide, on liposomes, bacterial and tumor cells. Biochim Biophys Acta, 1463:209-218.

Shin, S.Y., Lee, S.H., Yang, S.T., Park, E.J., Lee, D.G., Lee, M.K., Eom, S.H., Song, W.K., Kim, Y., Hahm, K.S. and Kim, J.I., 2001. Antibacterial, antitumor and hemolytic activities of alpha-helical antibiotic peptide, P18 and its analogs. J Pept Res, 58:504-514.

Silva, F.D., Rezende, C.A., Rossi, D.C., Esteves, E., Dyszy, F.H., Schreier, S., Gueiros-Filho, F., Campos, C.B., Pires, J.R. and Daffre, S., 2009. Structure and mode of action of microplusin, a copper II-chelating antimicrobial peptide from the cattle tick Rhipicephalus (Boophilus) microplus. J Biol Chem, 284:34735-34746.

Silva, P.I., Jr., Daffre, S. and Bulet, P., 2000. Isolation and characterization of gomesin, an 18-residue cysteine-rich defense peptide from the spider Acanthoscurria gomesiana hemocytes with sequence similarities to horseshoe crab antimicrobial peptides of the tachyplesin family. J Biol Chem, 275:33464-33470.

Sinha, S., Cheshenko, N., Lehrer, R.I. and Herold, B.C., 2003. NP-1, a Rabbit {alpha}-Defensin, Prevents the Entry and Intercellular Spread of Herpes Simplex Virus Type 2. Antimicrob. Agents Chemother., 47:494-500.

Sperstad, S.V., Haug, T., Vasskog, T. and Stensvag, K., 2009. Hyastatin, a glycine-rich multi-domain antimicrobial peptide isolated from the spider crab (Hyas araneus) hemocytes. Mol Immunol, 46:2604-2612.

Steiner, H., Hultmark, D., Engstrom, A., Bennich, H. and Boman, H.G., 1981. Sequence and specificity of two antibacterial proteins involved in insect immunity. Nature, 292:246-248.

Tani, K., Murphy, W.J., Chertov, O., Salcedo, R., Koh, C.Y., Utsunomiya, I., Funakoshi, S., Asai, O., Herrmann, S.H., Wang, J.M., Kwak, L.W. and Oppenheim, J.J., 2000. Defensins act as potent adjuvants that promote cellular and humoral immune responses in mice to a lymphoma idiotype and carrier antigens. International Immunology, 12:691-700.

Travis, S.M., Anderson, N.N., Forsyth, W.R., Espiritu, C., Conway, B.D., Greenberg, E.P., McCray, P.B., Jr., Lehrer, R.I., Welsh, M.J. and Tack, B.F., 2000. Bactericidal activity of mammalian cathelicidin-derived peptides. Infect Immun, 68:2748-2755.

Turner, J., Cho, Y., Dinh, N.N., Waring, A.J. and Lehrer, R.I., 1998. Activities of LL-37, a cathelin-associated antimicrobial peptide of human neutrophils. Antimicrob Agents Chemother, 42:2206-2214.

Van Valen, L., 1973. A new evolutionary law. Evolutionary Theory, 1:1-30.

Van Wetering, S., Mannesse-Lazeroms, S.P., Van Sterkenburg, M.A., Daha, M.R., Dijkman, J.H. and Hiemstra, P.S., 1997. Effect of defensins on interleukin-8 synthesis in airway epithelial cells. American Journal of Physiology - Lung Cellular and Molecular Physiology, 272:L888-L896.

van Wetering, S., Mannesse-Lazeroms, S.P.G., van Sterkenburg, M.A.J.A. and Hiemstra, P.S., 2002. Neutrophil defensins stimulate the release of cytokines by airway epithelial cells: modulation by dexamethasone. Inflammation Research, 51:8-15.

VanderMeer, T.J., Menconi, M.J., Zhuang, J., Wang, H., Murtaugh, R., Bouza, C., Stevens, P. and Fink, M.P., 1995. Protective effects of a novel 32-amino acid C-terminal fragment of CAP18 in endotoxemic pigs. Surgery, 117:656-662.

Wang, Z. and Wang, G., 2004. APD: the Antimicrobial Peptide Database. Nucleic Acids Res, 32:D590-592.

Wimley, W.C., 2010. Describing the mechanism of antimicrobial peptide action with the interfacial activity model. ACS Chem Biol, 5:905-917.

Xiao, Y., Dai, H., Bommineni, Y.R., Soulages, J.L., Gong, Y.X., Prakash, O. and Zhang, G., 2006. Structure-activity relationships of fowlicidin-1, a cathelicidin antimicrobial peptide in chicken. FEBS J, 273:2581-2593.

Xie, C., Prahl, A., Ericksen, B., Wu, Z., Zeng, P., Li, X., Lu, W.Y., Lubkowski, J. and Lu, W., 2005. Reconstruction of the conserved beta-bulge in mammalian defensins using D-amino acids. J Biol Chem, 280:32921-32929.

Yamashita, T. and Saito, K., 1989. Purification, primary structure, and biological activity of guinea pig neutrophil cationic peptides. Infect. Immun., 57:2405-2409.

Yang, Y., Poncet, J., Garnier, J., Zatylny, C., Bachere, E. and Aumelas, A., 2003. Solution structure of the recombinant penaeidin-3, a shrimp antimicrobial peptide. J Biol Chem, 278:36859-36867.

Yang, Y.H., Zheng, G.G., Li, G., Zhang, X.J., Cao, Z.Y., Rao, Q. and Wu, K.F., 2004. Expression of bioactive recombinant GSLL-39, a variant of human antimicrobial peptide LL-37, in Escherichia coli. Protein Expr Purif, 37:229-235.

Yasin, B., Wang, W., Pang, M., Cheshenko, N., Hong, T., Waring, A.J., Herold, B.C., Wagar, E.A. and Lehrer, R.I., 2004. {theta} Defensins Protect Cells from Infection by Herpes Simplex Virus by Inhibiting Viral Adhesion and Entry. J. Virol., 78:5147-5156.

Yeaman, M.R., Bayer, A.S., Koo, S.P., Foss, W. and Sullam, P.M., 1998. Platelet microbicidal proteins and neutrophil defensin disrupt the Staphylococcus aureus cytoplasmic membrane by distinct mechanisms of action. J Clin Invest, 101:178-187.

Yonezawa, A., Kuwahara, J., Fujii, N. and Sugiura, Y., 1992. Binding of tachyplesin I to DNA revealed by footprinting analysis: significant contribution of secondary structure to DNA binding and implication for biological action. Biochemistry, 31:2998-3004.

Zangger, K., Gossler, R., Khatai, L., Lohner, K. and Jilek, A., 2008. Structures of the glycine-rich diastereomeric peptides bombinin H2 and H4. Toxicon, 52:246-254.

Zasloff, M., 2002. Innate immunity, antimicrobial peptides, and protection of the oral cavity. Lancet, 360:1116-1117.

Zhang, L., Dhillon, P., Yan, H., Farmer, S. and Hancock, R.E., 2000. Interactions of bacterial cationic peptide antibiotics with outer and cytoplasmic membranes of Pseudomonas aeruginosa. Antimicrob Agents Chemother, 44:3317-3321.

2

Antibacterial Activity of Naturally Occurring Compounds from Selected Plants

Olgica Stefanović, Ivana Radojević, Sava Vasić and Ljiljana Čomić
Labaratory of Microbiology, Department of Biology and Ecology,
Faculty of Science, University of Kragujevac, Kragujevac
Serbia

1. Introduction

Man is in constant contact with a large number of different bacteria which temporarily or permanently inhibit his body creating temporary or permanent community. Relations which are thus established are various and very complex, from those positive to those whose consequences for man are extremely negative. Very often, both on and in man's body, bacteria which have the ability to cause an infection are present. This ability of pathogenic bacteria is reflected in possession of certain pathogenicity factors. A set of factors which enable successful invasion and damage of the host are: toxins, surface structures and enzymes. Between the host and the pathogen very complex relations are established whose income depends on host's characteristics as well as on pathogen's characteristics.

Infections caused by bacteria can be prevented, managed and treated through anti-bacterial group of compounds known as antibiotics. Antibiotics are natural, semi-synthetic or synthetic compounds that kill or inhibit the growth of bacteria. When bacteria are exposed to an antibiotic, they doubly respond: i) they are sensitive what cause the inhibition of their growth, division and death or ii) they can remain unaffected or resistant.

The resistance of bacteria to antibiotics can be natural (intrinsic) or acquired. Natural resistance is achieved by spontaneous gene mutation. The acquired resistence occurs after the contact of bacteria with an antibiotic as a result of adaptation of a species to adverse environmental conditions. In such population, an antibiotic as a selective agent, acts on sensitive individuals, while resistant survive and become dominant. Bacteria gain antibiotic resistance due to three reasons namely: (i) modification of active site of the target resulting in reduction in the efficiency of binding of the drug, (ii) direct destruction or modification of the antibiotic by enzymes produced by the organism or, (iii) efflux of antibiotic from the cell (Sheldon, 2005). The evolution of antibacterial resistance in human pathogenic and commensal microorganisms is the result of the interaction between antibiotic exposure and the transmission of resistance within and between individuals. It is especially interesting the phenomenon of horizontally gene transfer. Extrachromosomal DNA material, so-called plasmids, often carry genes of resistance and can transfer information within and between the individuals of the same or related bacterial species, thus also spreading the resistance. Transformation, transduction and conjugation represent the horizontal gene transfer mechanisms of resistance between the bacteria.

Having in mind the current progress of resistance spreading and resilience of larger and larger number of bacteria to traditional antibiotics as well as a way of transmitting the gene of resistance, above all via plasmids, one can conclude that the ability of obtaining bacterium resistance to antibiotics represents a very dynamic and unpredictable phenomenon. For that reason, bacterial resistance to antibiotics represents a major health problem. Solving this problem and search for new sources of antimicrobial agents is a worldwide challenge and the aim of many researches of scientific and research teams in science, academy institutions, pharmaceutical companies. One of the approaches in solving this issue is testing the biologically active compounds of plant origin.

1.1 Plants as potential antibacterial agents

Healing potential of plants has been known for thousands of years. Medicinal use of plants and their products was passed down from generation to generation in various parts of the world throughout its history and has significantly contributed to the development of different traditional systems of medicine. Even today, the World Health Organization (WHO) has estimated that approximately 80% of the global population relies on traditional herbal medicines as part of standard healthcare (Foster et al., 2005). Many drugs presently prescribed by physicians are either directly isolated from plants or are artificially modified versions of natural products. In Western countries, approximately 25% of the drugs used are of natural plant origin (Payne et al., 1991).

Plants produce a whole series of different compounds which are not of particular significance for primary metabolism, but represent an adaptive ability of a plant to adverse abiotic and biotic environmental conditions. They can have a remarkable effect to other plants, microorganisms and animals from their immediate or wider environment. All these organic compounds are defined as biologically active substances, and generally represent secondary metabolites, given the fact that they occur as an intermediate or end products of secondary plant metabolism. These secondary metabolites, apart from determining unique plant traits, such as: colour and scent of flowers and fruit, characteristic flavour of spices, vegetables, they also complete the functioning of plant organism, showing both biological and pharmacological activity of a plant. Therefore, medicinal properties of plants can be attributed to secondary metabolites (Hartmann, 2008).

1.1.1 Antibacterial secondary metabolites

It is known and proved by *in vitro* experiments that plants produce a great number of secondary metabolites that have antimicrobial activity (Iwu et al., 1999; Cowan, 1999; Rios & Recio, 2005; Cos et al., 2006). These plant-formed antibiotics have been classified as phytoanticipins, which are preformed inhibitory compounds, or phytoalexins, which are derived from precursors via *de novo* synthesis in response to microbial attack (VanEtten et al., 1994). Antibacterial secondary metabolites are usually classified in three large molecule families: phenolics, terpenes and alkaloids.

The phenolics and polyphenols are one of the largest groups of secondary metabolites that have exhibited antimicrobial activity. Important subclasses in this group of compounds include phenols, phenolic acids, quinones, flavones, flavonoids, flavonols, tannins and coumarins. Phenols are a class of chemical compounds consisting of a hydroxyl functional group (-OH) attached to an aromatic phenolic group. The site(s) and number of hydroxyl groups on the phenol group are thought to be related to their relative toxicity to microorganisms, with evidence that increased hydroxylation results in increased toxicity (Geissman, 1963, as cited in Cowan, 1999). Quinones have aromatic rings with two ketone substitutions. Quinones have a potential to form irreversible complex with nucleophilic amino acids in proteins (Stern et al., 1996, as cited in Cowan, 1999). This could explain their antibacterial properties. Probable targets in the microbial cell are surface-exposed adhesins, cell wall polypeptides and membrane-bound enzymes. Flavones are phenolic structures containing one carbonyl group. The addition of a 3-hydroxyl group yields a flavonol. Flavonoids are also hydroxylated phenolic substances but occur as a C6-C3 unit linked to an aromatic ring. Flavones, flavonoids and flavonols have been known to be synthesized by plants in response to microbial infection so it is not surprising that they have been found, *in vitro*, to be effective antimicrobial substances against a wide array of microorganisms (Dixon et al., 1983, as cited in Cowan, 1999). Their activity is probably due to their ability to complex with extracellular and soluble proteins and to complex with bacterial cell walls. Lipophilic flavonoids may also disrupt microbial membranes (Tsuchiya et al., 1996, as cited in Cowan, 1999). Tanins, a group of polymeric phenolic substances, are found in almost every plant part: bark, wood, leaves, fruits and roots. They are divided into two groups, hydrolyzable and condensed tannins. In plant tissue, tannins have been synthesized and accumulated after microbial attack. Their mode of antimicrobial action may be related to their ability to inactivate microbial adhesins, enzymes, cell envelope transport proteins, because of a property known as astringency. Coumarins are benzo-α-pyrones and could be categorised as: simple coumarins and cyclic coumarins (furanocoumarins and pyranocoumarins) (Ojala, 2001). Coumarins have been found to stimulate macrophages, which could have an indirect negative effect on infections (J. R. Casley-Smith & J. R.Casley-Smith, 1997, as cited in Cowan, 1999).

Terpenes are a large and varied class of organic compounds built up from isoprene subunits, while the terpenoids are oxygen-containing analogues of the terpenes. According to number of isoprene subunits, there are monoterpenes (C10), sesquiterpenes (C15), diterpenes (C20), triterpenes (C30), tetraterpenes (C40) and polyterpenes (Kovacevic, 2004). Monoterpenes, diterpenes and sesquiterpenes are the primary constituents of the essential oils. The mechanism of antibacterial action of terpenes is not fully understood but is speculated to involve membrane disruption by the lipophilic compounds. Accordingly, Mendoza et al., 1997 found that increasing the hydrophilicity of kaurene diterpenoids by addition of a methyl group drastically reduced their antimicrobial activity. (Mendoza et al., 1997, as cited in Cowan, 1999).

Alkaloids, one of the earliest isolated bioactive compounds from plants, are heterocyclic nitrogen compounds. They are derived from amino acids, and the nitrogen gives them alkaline properties. The mechanism of antibacterial action is attributed to their ability to intercalate with DNA, inhibition of enzymes (esterase, DNA-, RNA-polymerase), inhibition of cell respiration (Kovacevic, 2004).

1.1.2 Plant extracts as potential antibacterial agents

The screening of plant extracts has been of great interest to scientists for the discovery of new compound effective in the treatment of bacterial infection. Plant extracts exhibit:

- direct antibacterial activity showing effects on growth and metabolism of bacteria
- indirect activity as antibiotic resistance modifying compounds which, combined with antibiotics, increase their effectiveness.

A great number of reports concerning the antibacterial screening of plant extracts have appeared in the literature. Examples of such articles include studies of medicinal plants from different geographical regions: Brazil (Alves et al., 2000), Argentina (Salvat et al., 2000), Columbia (López et al., 2001); India (Perumal et al., 1998; Ahmad & Beg, 2001), China (Zuo et al., 2008), Turkey (Sokman et al., 1999; Uzun et al., 2004); Greece (Skaltsa et al., 2003), Spain (Ríos et al., 1987; Recio et al., 1989), Serbia (Stefanovic et al., 2009a; Stefanovic et al., 2009b, Stanojevic et al., 2010a; Stanojevic et al., 2010b; Stojanovic-Radic et al., 2010; Stefanovic et al., 2011; Stefanovic et al., 2012); Africa (Atindehou et al., 2002; Konning et al., 2004; Chah et al., 2006); Australia (Palombo & Semple, 2001). According to published data, the plant extracts exhibited the activity against a great number of bacterial species (Gram positive and Gram negative strains; sensitive and resistant, pathogens and opportunistic pathogens). The experiments involved the standard strains as well as the clinical isolates of pathogenic bacteria, as more realistic test organisms for estimation of antibacterial activity. Plant extracts were prepared from fresh or dried plant material using conventional extraction methods (Soxhlet extraction, maceration, percolation). Extraction is process of separation of active compounds from plant material using different solvents. During extraction, solvents diffuse into the plant material and solubilise compounds with similar polarity. At the end of the extraction, solvents have been evaporated, so that an extract is a concentrated mixture of plant active compounds. Successful extraction is largely dependent on the type of solvent used in the extraction procedure. The most often tested extracts are: water extract as a sample of extract that primarily used in traditional medicine and extracts from organic solvents such as methanol, ethanol as well as ethyl acetate, acetone, chloroform, dichlormethane (Ncube et al., 2008).

Diffusion and dilution method are two types of susceptibility test used to determine the antibacterial efficacy of plant extracts. Diffusion method is a qualitative test which allows classification of bacteria as susceptible or resistant to the tested plant extract according to size of diameter of the zone of inhibition. In dilution method, the activity of plant extracts is determined as Minimum Inhibitory Concentration (MIC). MIC is defined as the lowest concentration able to inhibit bacterial growth. In broth-dilution methods, turbidity and redox-indicators are most frequently used for results reading. Turbidity can be estimated visually or spectofotometrically while change of indicator colour indicate inhibition of bacterial growth (Cos et al., 2006).

2. Evaluation of antibacterial activity of selected plant species

Considering a large number of still insufficiently or incompletely examined species in the plant world; in inexhaustible possibilities of modifying natural substances, there is a need for systematic research and even greater affirmation of plant antimicrobial compounds. In this study the *in vitro* antibacterial activity of selected plant species was tested and evaluated the potential use of their extracts as a source of antibacterial compounds. The experiment involved water, ethanol, ethyl acetate and acetone extracts from 10 plant species belonging to 4 the most important plant families. The following plants were used: *Cychorium intybus* L. (Asteraceae); *Salvia officinalis* L., *Melissa officinalis* L., *Clinopodium vulgare* L. (Lamiaceae); *Torilis anthriscus* L. (Gmel), *Aegopodium podagraria* L. (Apiaceae); *Cytisus nigricans* L., *Cytisus capitatus* Scop.,

Melilotus albus Medic., *Dorycnium pentaphyllum* Vill. (Fabaceae). In general, the plants are annual or perennial, herbaceous or shrubby, widespread in Europe. They are rich in secondary metabolites from a group of phenols, flavonoids, coumarins, tannins, terpenes. It is known that different solvents extracted different groups of secondary metabolites, hence different types of extracts were prepared. The plants, as potential candidates for antibacterial agents, were selected on the base of three criteria: i) use in traditional medicine as antiseptic agents, ii) random selection followed by chemical screening (ii) insufficient antibacterial scientific data. Detailed description of known traditional uses, *in vitro* found biological activities and the chemical constituent is shown in Table 1.

Plant species	Traditional use	Biological activity	Chemical constituents
Fam. Asteraceae *Cichorium intybus*	improving digestion, for a diarrhea, as diuretic, for cleansing the liver and benefiting the gallbladder (Saric, 1989)	antibacterial, antifungal activity (Petrovic et al., 2004; Rani & Khullar, 2004; Mares et al., 2005)	sesquiterpene lactones (Zidorn, 2008), inulin , flavonoids, coumarins (Dem'yanenko & Dranik, 1971), tannins, phenolic acids (Sareedenchai & Zidorn, 2010)
Fam. Lamiaceae *Salvia officinalis*	for disorders of the digestive system, as antiseptic for sore throats, ulcers, to treat insect bites, mouth and gum infections and vaginal discharge for night sweats (Saric, 1989)	antibacterial, antifungal, antiviral activity (Velickovic et al., 2003; Nolkemper et al., 2006; Horiuchi et al., 2007; Weckesser et al., 2007)	simple phenols, phenolic acids, flavonoids, coumarins, tannins, terpenoids (Lu & Foo, 1999; 2002; Durling et al., 2007)
Melissa officinalis	to reduce indigestion and flatulence, as a mild sedative, to treat headache, migraine, nervous tension and insomnia, to treat cold, fever and cough (Saric, 1989)	antibacterial, antifungal, antiviral activity (Iauk et al., 2003; Ertürk, 2006; Nolkemper et al., 2006)	flavonoids (Herodež et al., 2003; Patora & Klimek , 2002), phenolic acids (Herodež et al., 2003; Canadanović -Brunet et al., 2008), simple phenols, tannins (Hohmann et al., 1999)
Clinopodium vulgare	as a heart tonic, an expectorant, as a diuretic (Saric, 1989) as an antiseptic for wounds and injuries (Opalchenova and Obreshkova, 1999).	antibacterial activity (Opalchenova & Obreshkova, 1999)	polyphenols (Kratchanova et al., 2010), *cis*-cinnamic, *trans*-cinnamic, *p*-coumaric and ferulic acid (Obreshkova et al., 2001), saponins (Miyase & Matsushima, 1997)

Plant species	Traditional use	Biological activity	Chemical constituents
Fam. Apiaceae *Aegopodium podagraria*	for gout and sciatics (Saric, 1989)	antibacterial, antifungal activity (Ojala et al., 2000; Garrod et al., 1979)	furano-coumarins (Ojala et al., 2000), polyacetilenes, falcarindiol (Christensen & Brandt, 2006), flavonoids (Cisowski, 1985)
Torilis anthriscus syn. *Torilis japonica*	an expectorant and tonic (Duke et al., 2002), for flatulence (Manandhar, 2002)	antibacterial activity (Cho et al., 2008), anti-protozoal activity (Youn et al., 2004)	coumarins (3), sesquiterpenoids (guaiane, humulene, germacrane, eudesmane) (Kitajima et al., 2002)
Fam. Fabaceae *Melilotus albus*	as ointments for external ulcers, as an anticoagulant agent (Saric, 1989)	antibacterial activity (Acamovic-Djokovic et al., 2002)	coumarins (Stoker, 1964), saponins (Khodakov et al., 1996)
Dorycnium pentaphyllum	No data	antibacterial activity (Stamatis, 2003)	phenylbutanone glucosides (dorycnioside), flavonoids, (Kazantzoglou et al., 2004)
Cytisus capitatus	No data	No data	alkaloids (l-sparteine, sarothamnine, genisteine, lupanine, oxysparteine) (Wink et al., 1983)
Cytisus nigricans	No data	No data	alkaloids (Wink et al., 1983)

Table 1. Traditional uses, biological activities and chemical constituents of selected plant species

2.1 Materials and methods

2.1.1 Plant material

The aerial parts of *Clinopodium vulgare, Aegopodium podagraria, Torilis anthriscus, Dorycnium pentaphyllum, Melilotus albus, Cytisus nigricans* and *Cytisus capitatus* were collected from the different regions of Serbia, during summer 2006 and 2009 while *Cichorium intybus* (root), *Salvia officinalis* (leaves) and *Melissa officinalis* (leaves) were supplied from the commercial source. Identification and classification of the plant material was performed at the Faculty of Science, University of Kragujevac. The voucher specimens of the plants are deposited in the Herbarium of the Faculty of Science, University of Kragujevac. The collected plant materials were air-dried under shade at room temperature and then ground into small pieces which were stored into paper bags at room temperature.

2.1.2 Extraction

Dried, ground plant material was extracted by direct maceration with water, ethanol, ethyl acetate and acetone. Briefly, 30g of plant material was soaked with 150ml of solvent for 24h at room temperature. During 24 hours, targeted compounds from plant material were extracted by the solvent. After that the resulting extract was filtered through filter paper (Whatman no.1). The residue from the filtration was extracted again, twice, using the same procedure. The filtrates obtained were combined and then evaporated to dryness using a rotary evaporator at 40°C, for water extracts heating on a water bath. The crude plant extracts are stored at -20°C. Before the testing, stock solutions of the crude extracts were obtained by dissolving in dimethyl sulfoxide (DMSO) and then diluted into nutrient liquid medium to achieve a concentration of 10% DMSO. The groups of secondary metabolites which are expected in prepared plant extracts are given in Table 2.

Water extract	Ethanol extract	Ethyl acetate extract	Acetone extract
Simle phenols	Simle phenols	Simle phenols	Simle phenols
Phenolic acids	Phenolic acids	Phenolic acids	Phenolic acids
Flavonoids	Flavonoids	Flavonoids	Flavonoids
Quinones	Quinones	Quinones	Quinones
Tannins	Tannins	Tannins	Tannins
Coumarins	Coumarins		
Saponins	Saponins		

Table 2. The expected groups of plant secondary metabolites (according to Kovacevic, 2004)

2.1.3 Microorganisms

The following bacteria were used: *Staphylococcus aureus* ATCC 25923, *Escherichia coli* ATCC 25922, *Pseudomonas aeruginosa* ATCC 27853 and clinical isolate of *Staphylococcus aureus* (PMFKg-B30), *Bacillus subtilis* (PMFKg-B2), *Enterococcus faecalis* (PMFKg-B22), *Enterobacter cloaceae* (PMFKg-B23), *Klebsiella pneumoniae* (PMFKg-B26), *Escherichia coli* (PMFKg-B32), *Pseudomonas aeruginosa* (PMFKg-B28) and *Proteus mirabilis* (PMFKg-B29). All clinical isolates were a generous gift from the Institute of Public Health, Kragujevac. Bacteria are stored in microbiological collection at the Laboratory of Microbiology (Faculty of Science, University of Kragujevac).

Bacterial suspension were prepared from overnight cultures by the direct colony method. Colonies were taken directly from the plate and suspent into 5ml of sterile 0,85% saline. The turbidity of initial suspension was adjusted comparing with 0,5 Mc Farland standard (0,5 ml 1,17% w/v $BaCl_2 \times 2H_2O$ + 99,5 ml 1% w/v H_2SO_4) (Andrews, 2001). When adjusted to the turbidity of a 0,5 Mc Farland standard, a suspension of bacteria contains about 10^8 colony forming units (CFU)/ml. Ten-fold dilutions of initial suspension were additionally prepared into sterile 0,85% saline to achieve 10^6 CFU/ml.

2.1.4 Microdilution method

Antibacterial activity was tested by determining the minimum inhibitory concentration (MIC) using microdilution plate method with resazurin (Sarker et al., 2007). Briefly, the 96-well microplate was prepared by dispensing 100 μL of Mueller-Hinton broth (Torlak, Belgrade) into each well. A 100 μL from the stock solution of tested extract (concentration of 40mg/ml) was added into the first row of the plate. Then, two-fold, serial dilutions were performed by transferring 100 μl of solution from one row to another, using a multichannel pipette. The obtained concentration range was from 20 mg/ml to 0.156 mg/ml. Ten microlitres of each 10^6 CFU/ml bacterial suspension was added to wells. Finally, 10 μL of resazurin solution was added. Resazurin is an oxidation-reduction indicator used for the evaluation of microbial growth. It is a blue non-fluorescent dye that becomes pink and fluorescent when reduced to resorufin by oxidoreductases within viable cells (Figure 1.). The inoculated plates were incubated at 37°C for 24h. MIC was defined as the lowest concentration of the tested plant extracts that prevented resazurin color change from blue to pink.

Antibiotic cephalexin, dissolved in Mueller-Hinton broth, was used as positive control. Solvent control test was performed to study an effect of 10% DMSO on the growth of bacteria. It was observed that 10% DMSO did not inhibit the growth of bacteria. Each test included growth control and sterility control. All tests were performed in duplicate and MICs were constant.

2.1.5 Statistical analysis

All statistical analyses were performed using SPSS package. Mean differences were established by Student's *t*-test. In all cases p values <0.05 were considered statistically significant.

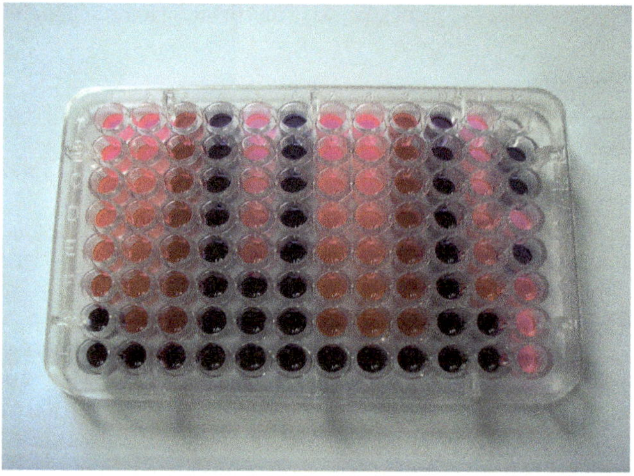

Fig. 1. Plate after 24 h in resazurin assay (pink colour indicates growth and blue means inhibition of growth)

3. Results and discussion

In vitro antibacterial activity of different plant extracts from 10 selected plants was tested in relation to 11 bacterial strains. Intensity of antibacterial activity depended on the species of bacteria, plant species and the type of extract. The MIC values were in range from 0.019 mg/ml to >20mg/ml. In relation to positive control (cephalexin MIC 0. 00156 - >1mg/ml), the extracts showed lower activity. In general, according to obtained results, the following remarks could be made:

- Detectable MICs were noticed in 100% of tested bacteria for *Cichorium intybus*, 70% for *Salvia officinalis*, 90% for *Melissa officinalis*, 83, 33% for *Clinopodium vulgare*, 100% for *Torilis anthriscus*, 33, 33% for *Aegopodium podagraria*, 96, 67% for *Cytisus nigricans*, 76, 67% for *Cytisus capitatus*, 60% for *Melilotus albus* and 96, 67% for *Dorycnium pentaphyllum*.
- Among tested plants, the best inhibitory effects showed acetone extract from *Salvia officinalis*, ethyl acetate and acetone extract from *Cichorium intybus* and ethanol extract from *Aegopodium podagraria*. Moderate antibacterial activity exhibited *Melissa officinalis*, *Clinopodium vulgare* (ethyl acetate and acetone extract), *Torilis anthriscus*, *Cytisus nigricans*, *Cytisus capitatus* and *Dorycnium pentaphyllum* while low activity showed *Clinopodium vulgare* (ethanol extract), *Melilotus albus* and *Aegopodium podagraria* (water and ethyl acetate extract).
- Water extracts were less active than ethanol, ethyl acetate and acetone extracts.
- The antibacterial activity of the tested extracts was closely associated with present secondary metabolites.
- The Gram-positive bacteria were more sensitive than the Gram-negative bacteria. The reason for higher sensitivity of the Gram-positive bacteria than Gram-negative bacteria could be ascribed to their differences in cell wall constituents and their arrangement. The Gram-positive bacteria contain a peptidoglycan layer, which is an ineffective permeability barrier while Gram-negative bacteria are surrounded by an additional outer membrane carrying the structural lipopolysaccharide components, which makes it impermeable to lipophilic solutes and porins constitute a selective barrier to the hydrophilic solutes (Nikaido, 2003).
- Among tested bacteria, the most sensitive bacteria were Gram positive bacteria: *B. subtilis* and *S. aureus* ATCC 25923. Susceptibility of *E. cloaceae*, *Ent. faecalis*, *K. pneumoniae*, *S. aureus*, *Ps. aeruginosa* ATCC 27853 was moderate. Clinical isolate of Gram negative bacteria, *Ps. aeruginosa*, *P. mirabilis*, *E. coli*, exhibited low susceptibility or resistance.

3.1 Antibacterial activity of *Cichorium intybus*

The results of antibacterial activity of ethanol, ethyl acetate and acetone extract from *Cichorium intybus* are presented on the Figure 2. Extracts showed different activity. Ethanol extract acted at concentrations of 2.5 mg/ml to 20mg/ml; ethyl acetate from 1.09 mg/ml to 8.75 mg/ml; acetone extract from 2.5 mg/ml to 5 mg/ml. Antibacterial activity of ethyl acetate and acetone extract is more pronounced than ethanol extract. Similar results were obtained by Nandagopal & Ranjitha Kumari, 2007, among tested extracts, ethyl acetate was one of the more active. Statistic analysis confirms the presented results. Activity of ethyl acetate (p_{EtAc}=0.001) and acetone (p_{AcOH}=0.002) extract was statistically significantly higher that the activity of ethanol extract. Acetone extract was the most active (p=0.018).

The tested bacteria manifested different sensitivity level to the tested extracts. MIC values were ranged from 1.09 mg/ml to 20 mg/ml. The most sensitive bacterium to the tested

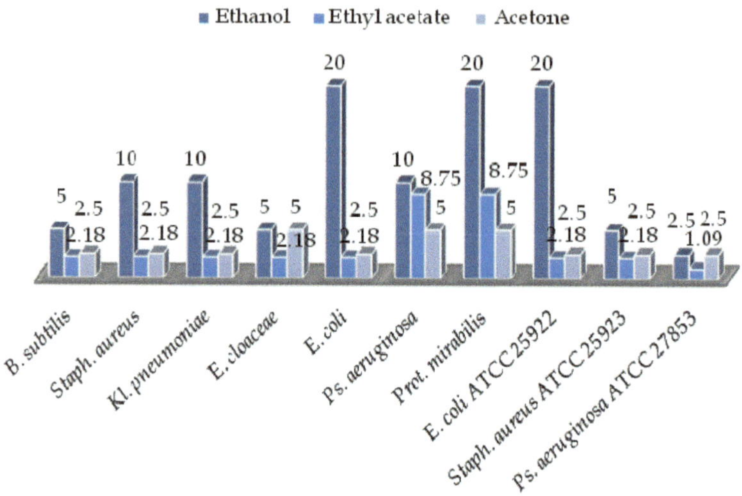

Fig. 2. Antibacterial activity of *Cichorium intybus* extracts expressed as MIC values (mg/ml)

extracts was *Pseudomonas aeruginosa* ATCC 27853. MIC values for this bacterium were 2.5 mg/ml for ethanol and acetone extract, and 1.09 mg/ml for ethyl acetate extract. Bacteria *Bacillus subtilis, Enterobacter cloacae, Staphylococcus aureus* ATCC 25923 with 2.18 mg/ml, 2.5 mg/ml and 5 mg/ml values also manifested significant sensitivity. *Proteus mirabilis, Escherichia coli* ATCC 25922, according to ethanol extract, have showed the least sensitivity (MIC = 20 mg/ml), while they were more sensitive to the other two extracts. Similar results were obtained by other scientists. Petrović et al., 2004 noted the inhibitory effect of chicory extract also on phypopathogenic and human pathigenic bacteria. Acroum et al., 2009 showed the effect of methanol extract on Gram-positive bacteria (*Bacillus subtilis, Bacillus cereus, Staphylococcus aureus*) with the MIC values of 0.010 mg/ml and 0.075 mg/ml while the extract did not act on Gram-negative bacteria *Escherichia coli, Pseudomonas aeruginosa, Klebsiella pneuminiae.*

3.2 Antibacterial activity of *Salvia officinalis*

The acetone extract was the most reactive extract at this testing (p_{EtOH}=0,004; p_{EtAc}=0,001), while there was no statistically significant difference between ethanol and ethyl acetate extracts in acting. Ethanol and ethyl acetate extract showed the activity at concentrations from 2.5 mg/ml to >20 mg/ml, and acetone extract from 0.02 mg/ml to 20 mg/ml (Figure 3.). The reason for good results which acetone extract showed can also be saught in the fact that acetone is a good extractant, of low toxicity and high extractional capacity (Eloff, 1998). Similar results for acetone extract were also obtained by (Horiuchi et al., 2007), MIC values were from 256 µg/ml to 512 µg/ml.

The tested bacteria, except for *Pseudomonas aeruginosa* and *Escherichia coli*, showed a significant sensitivity in relation to acetone extract. MIC values were below 1 mg/ml.

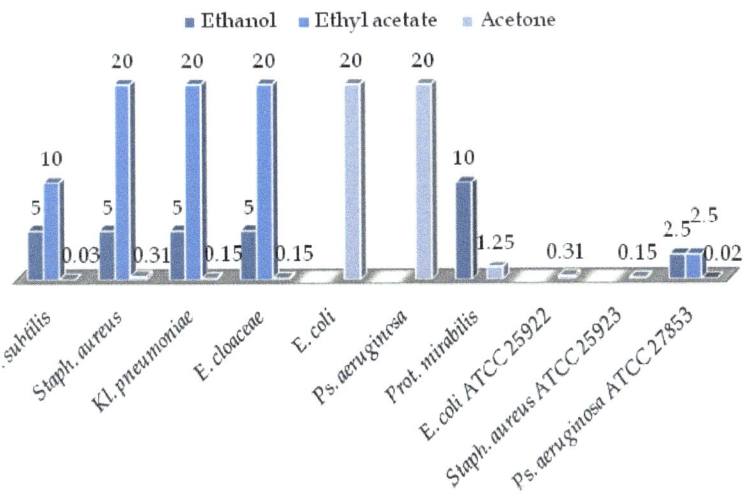

Fig. 3. Antibacterial activity of *Salvia officinalis* extracts expressed as MIC values (mg/ml)

Gram-positive bacteria were more sensitive than Gram-negative bacteria. MICs for *Bacillus subtilis* were showed at 5 mg/ml for ethanol extract, 10 mg/ml for ethyl acetate extract and 0.03 mg/ml for acetone extract. For *Staphylococcus aureus*, MIC of ethanol extract was 5 mg/ml, ethyl acetate 20 mg/ml and acetone 0.31 mg/ml, while *Staphylococcus aureus* ATCC 25923, as G^+ bacterium, only showed sensitivity in relation to acetone extract (MIC = 0.15 mg/ml). Growth of the most of G^- bacteria was not inhibited by action of ethanol and ethyl acetate extract on tested concentrations. Similar results were obtained by Veličković et al., 2003 where ethanol extract reacted poorly on G^- in relation to G^+ bacteria. The exception is *Pseudomonas aeruginosa* ATCC 27853, which is next to *Bacillus subtilis*, the most sensitive bacterium to tested extracts.

3.3 Antibacterial activity of *Melissa officinalis*

The results of antibacterial activity of water, ethanol and ethyl acetate extract from *Melissa officinalis* are presented on the Figure 4. The tested extracts showed equable antibacterial activity, based on the results of statistic analysis, no difference was noted ($p>0.05$). Water extract acted in the interval from 0.31 mg/ml to 20 mg/ml; ethanol extract from 0.62 mg/ml to >20 mg/ml, and ethyl acetate extract from 1.25 mg/ml to 20 mg/ml. Ethanol extract did not act on three species of Gram-negative bacteria. Antimicrobial activity of different *Melissa officinalis* extracts was also tested by other scientists who showed different level of antimicrobial activity with their research (Uzun et al., 2004; Ertürk, 2006; Iauk et al., 2003).

The tested bacteria showed sensitivity at different concentrations. The concentrations were ranged from 0.31 to 20 mg/ml. The greatest sensitivity was noted for standard strains: *Staphylococcus aureus; Escherichia coli* and *Pseudomonas aeruginosa* only to water extract.

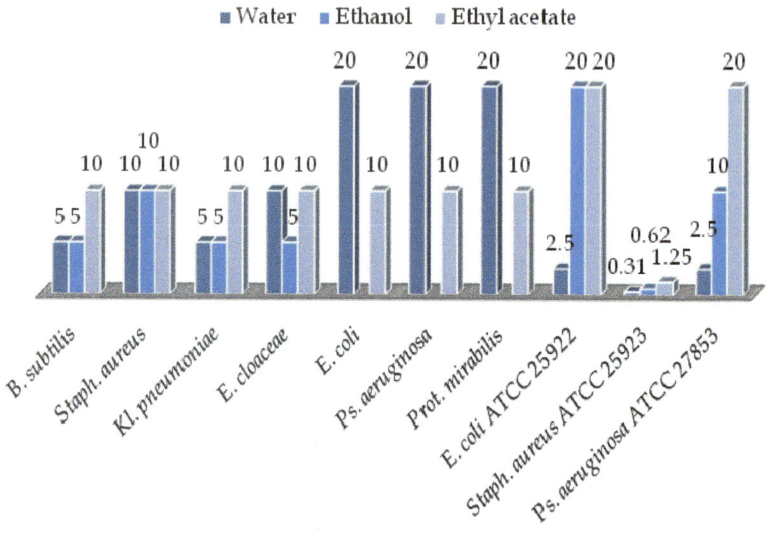

Fig. 4. Antibacterial activity of *Melissa officinalis* extracts expressed as MIC values (mg/ml)

The most tested bacteria showed sensitivity at 10 mg/ml for ethyl acetate extract. *Escherichia coli, Pseudomonas aeruginosa* and *Proteus mirabilis* showed resistance to ethanol extract. Weaker activity of lemon balm to mentioned Gram-negative bacterium was also noted in the work of Canadanović-Brunet et al., 2008.

3.4 Antibacterial activity of *Clinopodium vulgare*

The extracts manifested different level of antibacterial activity, the results are shown on the Figure 5. The ethanol extract acted in concentrations from 1.25 mg/ml to >20 mg/ml, ethyl acetate and acetone extract from 0.62 mg/ml to 20 mg/ml. Ethyl acetate and acetone extract acted better than ethanol extract. Statistically significant difference was noted (p_{EtAc}=0.015 и p_{AcOH}=0.018). Between ethyl acetate and acetone extract no statistically significant difference was noted in the activity (p=0.756).

The tested bacteria in most of the cases showed sensitivity at 10 mg/ml and 20 mg/ml. Gram-positive bacteria *Bacillus subtilis* and *Staphylococcus aureus* ATCC 25923 were the most sensitive to the action of *Clinopodium vulgare* extracts. MIC values were in the interval from 0.62 mg/ml to 2.5 mg/ml. *Klebsiella pneumoniae, Staphylococcus aureus, Enterococcus faecalis, Escherichia coli* and *Pseudomonas aeruginosa* manifested the resistance to the tested concentrations of ethanol extract. Opalchenova & Obreshkova, 1999 showed the action of ethanol extract to G^+ and G^- bacteria but only at 5% of extract's concentration, while Sarac & Ugur, 2007 did not notice the action of ethanol extract to the tested bacteria. These results are in accordance with the shown activity of ethanol extract in this work.

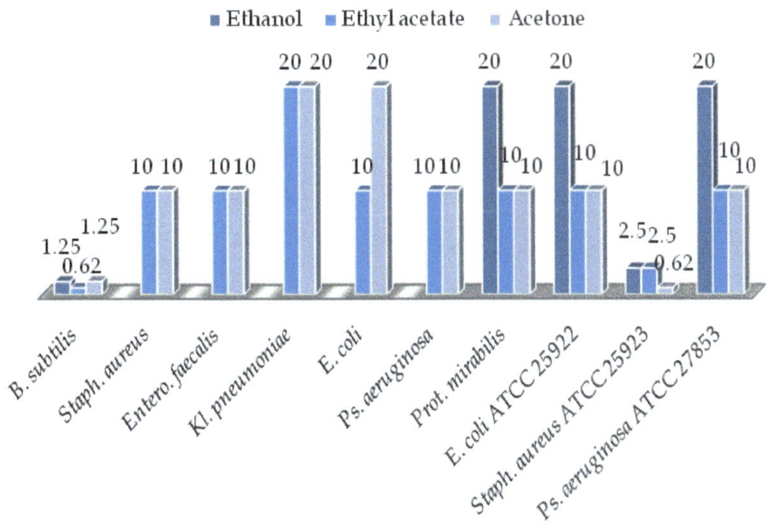

Fig. 5. Antibacterial activity of *Clinopodium vulgare* extracts expressed as MIC values (mg/ml)

3.5 Antibacterial activity of Torilis anthriscus

Among the tested extracts, the most active was ethanol extract, then ethyl acetate, and the weakest water extract. Statistically significant difference was noted between the activity of ethanol extract, on one hand, and ethyl acetate and water extract on the other hand (p_{H20} = 0.008; p_{EtAc} = 0.032). MIC values were ranged in the interval from 1.25 mg/ml to 20 mg/ml. The bacteria showed different level of sensitivity to the tested extracts (Figure 6.). They were the most sensitive to ethanol extract (MIC for most of the bacterium was 5 mg/ml), and then to ethyl acetate extract (MIC for most of the bacterium was 10 mg/ml). Most of the bacteria showed weak sensitivity to water extract with MIC values of 20 mg/ml. For *Staphylococcus aureus* ATCC 25923, *Pseudomonas aeruginosa* ATCC 27853 and *Staphylococcus aureus,* water extract acted at lower concentrations (MIC = 2.5 and 10 mg/ml). The most sensitive bacterium was *Staphylococcus aureus* ATCC 25923, growth inhibition of this bacterium was noted at 1.25 mg/ml and 2.5 mg/ml.

Antibacterial activity of *T. anthriscus* extracts is not explored enough. Inhibitory effect was tested on phytopathogenic bacteria and especially the action of water, ethanol and ethyl acetate extract was shown on *Pseudomonas glycinea* (Brkovic et al., 2006). Methanol extract of fruits slowed germination of spores down and inhibited the growth of vegetative cells of *Bacillus subtilis* (Cho et al., 2008).

3.6 Antibacterial activity of *Aegopodium podagraria*

The results of antibacterial activity of water, ethanol and ethyl acetate extract from *Aegopodium podagraria* are presented on the Figure 7. The extracts showed low antibacterial

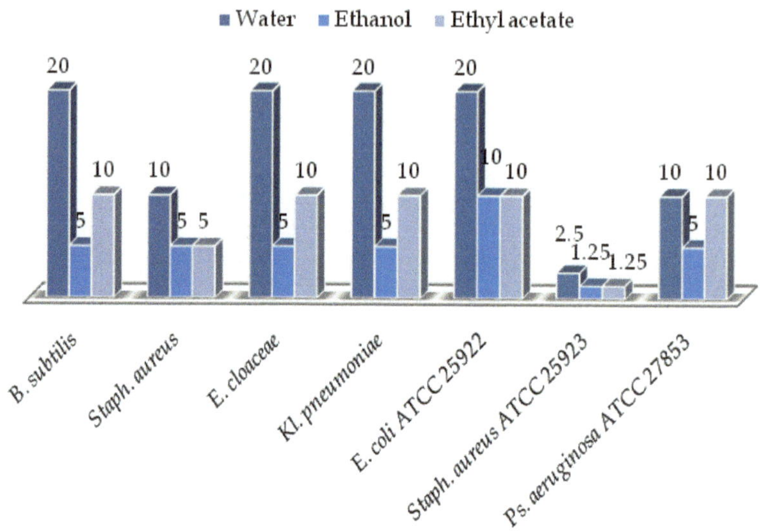

Fig. 6. Antibacterial activity of *Torilis anthriscus* extracts expressed as MIC values (mg/ml)

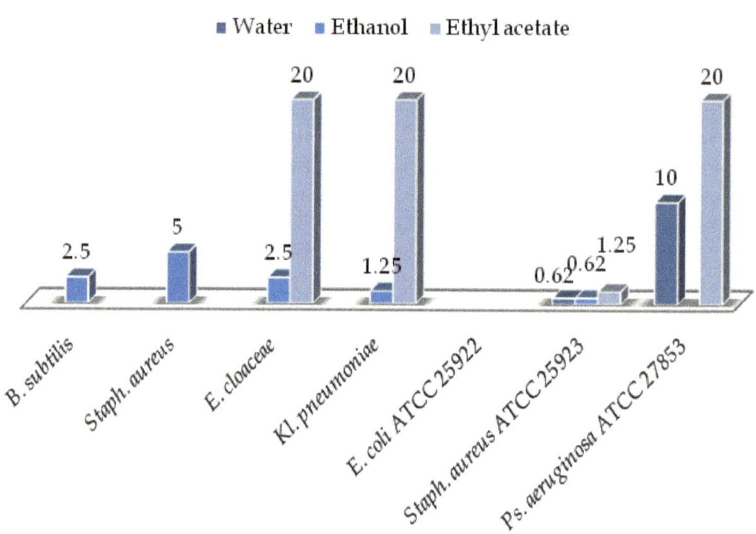

Fig. 7. Antibacterial activity of *Aegopodium podagraria* extracts expressed as MIC values (mg/ml)

activity. Only the ethanol extract activity stands out in relation to water extract, which was confirmed by statistis analysis (p=0.035). Ethanol extract inhibited the growth of most of the bacteria. Water extract only acted on two bacteria, and ethyl acetate extract on four bacteria. Ethanol turned the best extractant of active compounds from this plant.

The tested bacteria showed significant sensitivity to ethanol extract, exceptions were *Escherichia coli* ATCC 25922 and *Pseudomonas aeruginosa* ATCC 27853. Growth inhibition occurred at concentrations from 0.62 mg/ml to 5 mg/ml. All bacteria, except *Pseudomonas aeruginosa* ATCC 27853 and *Staphylococcus aureus* ATCC 25923, were resistant to water extract, while *Escherichia coli* ATCC 25922 was resistant to all three extracts. Bacteria did not show any significant sensitivity to ethyl acetate extract. Ethyl acetate extract acted on *Enterobacter cloacae, Klebsiella pneumoniae, Pseudomanas aeruginosa* ATCC 27853 and *Staphylococcus aureus* ATCC 25923. *Staphylococcus aureus* ATCC 25923 was the most sensitive bacterium to *A. podagraria* extracts.

Ojala et al., 2000 tested methanol extract of *A. podagraria* on G^+, G^- bacteria, yeasts and molds and only partial effect on *Bacillus subtilis, Staphylococcus aureus, Staphylococcus epidermidis* and *Pseudomonas aeruginosa* was noted as well as on *Fusarium culmorum* and *Heterobasidion annosum*, phytopathogenic fungi. Brkovic et al., 2006 also noted the effect on phytopathogenic bacteria. Similar results were obtained for methanol extract (Ojala et al., 2000) and for ethanol extract in this study were expected since the methanol and ethanol are solvents of similar polarity and that there are similar groups of secondary metabolites isolated in extracts.

3.7 Antibacterial activity of *Cytisus nigricans*

Cytisus nigricans extracts showed weaker antibacterial activity than other tested plants. They mostly acted at the highest tested concentration (20 mg/ml). Acetone extract did not act on *Escherichia coli*. There is no statistically significant action difference between extracts (p<0.05).

Bacteria sensitivity to tested extracts is shown on the Figure 8. The most significant results showed the following bacteria: *Bacillus subtilis* (2.5 mg/ml, 5 mg/ml), *Staphylococcus aureus* ATCC 25923 (2.5 mg/ml, 5 mg/ml) and *Pseudomonas aeruginosa* ATCC 27853 (1.25 mg/ml, 5 mg/ml, 10 mg/ml). Growth of other bacteria was inhibited at approximately same concentration (20 mg/ml), and *Escherichia coli* also showed the resistance to *Cytisus nigricans* extracts. Antibacterial activity of this plant was tested for the first time in this study.

3.8 Antibacterial activity of *Cytisus capitatus*

Cytisus capitatus extracts showed equable antibacterial activity. MICs were in the interval from 5 mg/ml to >20 mg/ml for ethanol extract, from 1.25 mg/ml to >20 mg/ml for ethyl acetate extract and from 1.25 mg/ml to >20 mg/ml for acetone extract. Based on statistic analysis no difference was noted in acting between extracts (p<0.05). The obtained results are presented on the Figure 9.

The most sensitive bacteria to tested extracts were *Bacillus subtilis* and *Staphylococcus aureus* ATCC 25923. MIC for *Bacillus subtilis* showed at 5 mg/ml for ethanol extract, 2.5 mg/ml for ethyl acetate extract and 1.25 mg/ml for acetone extract. For *Staphylococcus aureus* ATCC 25923, MIC of ethanol extract was 10 mg/ml, ethyl acetate 1.25 mg/ml and acetone extract 2.5 mg/ml. *Escherichia coli* showed resistance to all three extracts. The results for

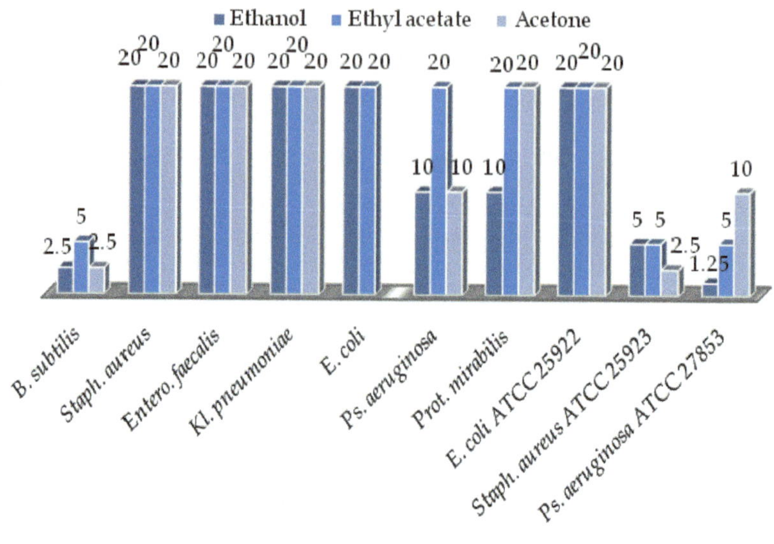

Fig. 8. Antibacterial activity of *Cytisus nigricans* extracts expressed as MIC values (mg/ml)

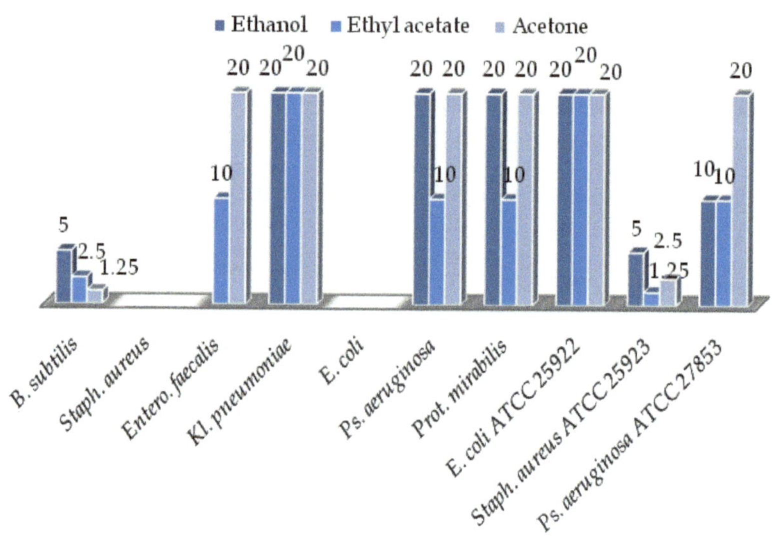

Fig. 9. Antibacterial activity of *Cytisus capitatus* extracts expressed as MIC values (mg/ml)

Staphylococcus aureus and *Enterococcus faecalis* are unexpected since Gram-positive bacteria were more sensitive than Gram-negative bacteria, and in this case they showed resistance or lowered sensitivity. Growth of other bacteria was inhibited at approximately the same concentration. Antibacterial activity of *Cytisus capitatus* was tested for the first time in this study. Based on literary data and other species from *Cytisus* genus are less explored as potential antimicrobial agents. Benaiche, 2007 tested antibacterial activity of *Cytisus purgans* methanol extract in relation to *Staphylococcus aureus, Escherichia coli* and *Pseudomonas aeruginosa*. The biggest zones of inhibition showed at 80 mg/ml.

3.9 Antibacterial activity of *Melilotus albus*

Melilotus albus extracts showed weaker antibacterial activity than other tested plants. Between extracts, the most active one was acetone extract, then ethyl acetate and ethanol extract which was confirmed by statistic analysis (p_{EtOH} = 0,018; p_{EtAc}=0,029). Action interval of extracts was from 1.25 mg/ml to 20 mg/ml (Figure 10). In most of the cases ethanol extracts did not act at tested concentrations.

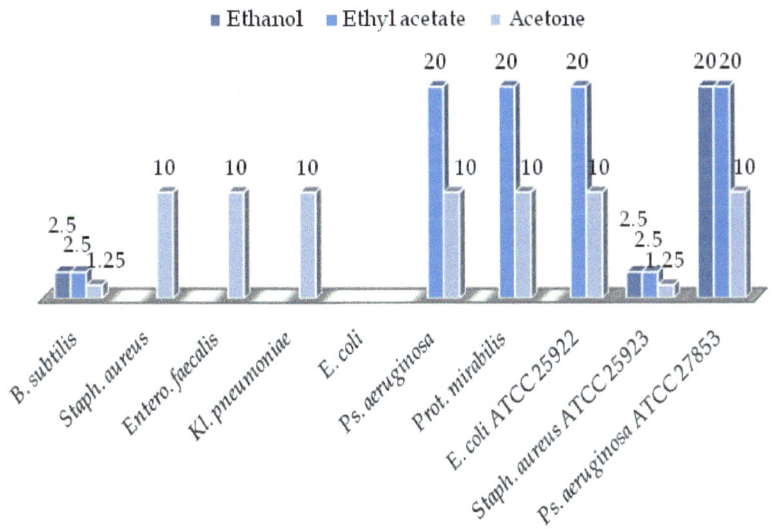

Fig. 10. Antibacterial activity of *Melilotus albus* extracts expressed as MIC values (mg/ml)

Bacillus subtilis, Staphylococcus aureus ATCC 25923 and *Pseudomonas aeruginosa* ATCC 27853 showed sensitivity according to tested extracts where *Bacillus subtilis* and *Staphylococcus aureus* ATCC 25923 were the most sensitive (MIC=1.25; 2.5 mg/ml). *Escherichia coli* showed resistance to all three extracts, while *Klebsiella pneumoniae, Staphylococcus aureus* and *Enterococcus faecalis* showed resistance to ethanol and ethyl acetate extract. *Pseudomonas aeruginosa, Proteus mirabilis* and *Escherichia coli* ATCC 25922 were resistant only to ethanol extract. Aćamović-Đoković et al., 2002 tested antibacterial activity of petrol ether and ethyl acetate extract of *Melilotus officinale, Melilotus albus* and *Melitis melissophyllum* in relation to

Escherichia coli, Proteus mirabilis, Salmonella enteritidis, Pseudomonas aeruginosa, Streptococcus-haemoliticus A, *Staphylococcus aureus* and *Candida albicans. Melilotus albus* extracts were less efficient than other tested plants.

3.10 Antibacterial activity of *Dorycnium penthaphyllum*

Dorycnium penthaphyllum extracts showed different level of antibacterial activity. Ethanol extract acted in the interval from 2.5 mg/ml to 20 mg/ml, ethyl acetate from 1.25 mg/ml to >20 mg/ml, and acetone extract from 1.25 mg/ml to 20 mg/ml (Figure 11.). Between the extracts there was no statistically significant difference in action (p<0.05).

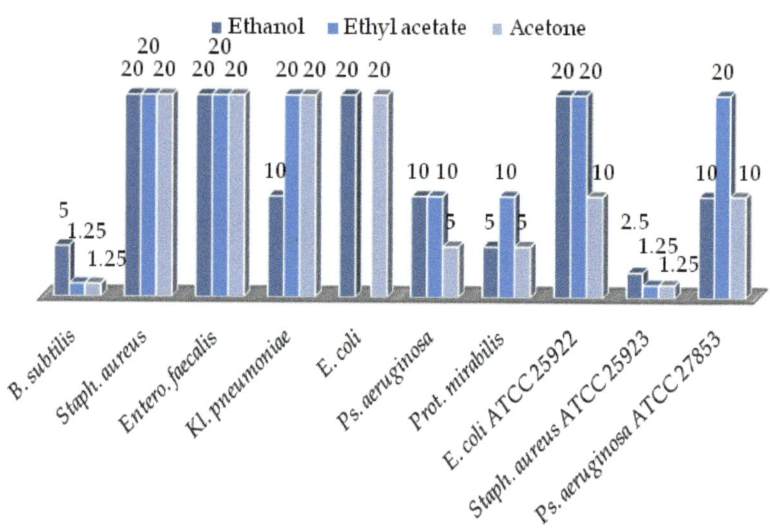

Fig. 11. Antibacterial activity of *Dorycnium penthaphylum* extracts expressed as MIC values (mg/ml)

The most significant results were obtained for *Bacillus subtilis, Staphylococcus aureus* ATCC 25923, *Pseudomonas aeruginosa* and *Proteus mirabilis.* MIC values were between 1.25 mg/ml - 10 mg/ml. Other bacteria showed sensitivity at approximately the same concentrations (20 mg/ml). The exception was *Escherichia coli* which was resistant to ethylaacetate extract. Sensitivity of tested bacteria to the extracts of *D. penthaphylum* was presented for the first time in this study. A group of scientists tested anti - *Helicobacter pilory* effect of medicinal plants of Greek traditional medicine, among which is also *D. penthaphylum,* although they did not note this plant's effect (Stamatis et al., 2003).

4. Conclusion

Plant extracts represent very interesting source of bioactive compounds which provide unlimited opportunities for new antibacterial agents. The results obtained in this study confirm this statement. Significant activities of ethanol extract from *Aegopodium podagraria* and ethyl acetate and acetone extract from *Cichorium intybus*, one of insufficiently explored plants, indicate their use as potential, new antibacterial agents. These results, also, offer a scientific basis for the traditional use of extracts of *Salvia officinalis* and *Melissa officinalis*. The extracts from *Clinopodium vulgare, Torilis anthriscus, Cytisus nigricans, Cytisus capitatus* and *Dorycnium pentaphyllum* showed interesting activity against certain pathogenic bacteria. Mostly, the most sensitive bacteria were *B. subtilis* and *S. aureus* ATCC 25923. Susceptibility of *E. cloaceae, Ent. faecalis, K. pneumoniae, S. aureus, Ps. aeruginosa* ATCC 27853 was moderate while *Ps. aeruginosa, P. mirabilis, E. coli* were resistant. This study represents the first preliminary report on antibacterial activity of the extracts from *Cytisus nigricans, Cytisus capitatus* and *Dorycnium pentaphyllum* and contributes to overall examine antibacterial activity of plant species. Since, the compounds and mechanisms of action responsible for the antibacterial activities of these extracts are currently unclear; the further work will be performed on the isolation and identification of the active compounds and understanding of mechanisms of action.

5. Acknowledgment

This work was supported by the Ministry of Science and Education of the Republic of Serbia (grant number OI173032).

6. References

Alves, T.M., Silva, A.F., Brandão, M., Grandi, T.S., Smânia, E., Smânia Júnior, A. & Zani, C. (2000). Biological Screening of Brazilian Medicinal Plants. Memórias do Instituto Oswaldo Cruz, Vol. 95, No. 3, (May-Jun 2000), pp. 367-373, ISSN 0074-0276

Ahmad, I. & Beg, A.Z. (2001). Antimicrobial and phytochemical studies on 45 Indian medicinal plants against multi-drug resistant human pathogens. Journal of Ethnopharmacology, Vol. 74, No. 2, (February 2001), pp. 113–123, ISSN 0378-8741

Atindehou, K.K., Koné, M., Terreaux, C., Traore, D., Hostettmann, K. & Dosso, M. (2002). Evaluation of the antimicrobial potential of medicinal plants from the Ivory Coast. Phytotherapy Research, Vol. 16, No. 5, (August 2002), pp. 497–502, ISSN 0951-418X

Andrews, J.M. (2001). Determination of minimum inhibitory concentrations. *Journal of Antimicrobial Chemotherapy*, Vol. 48, Suppl. 1, pp. 5-16, ISSN 0305-7453.

Akroum, S., Satta, D. & Lalaoui, K. (2009). Antimicrobial, Antioxidant, Cytotoxic Activities and Phytochemical Screening of Some Algerian Plants. *European Journal of Scientific Research*, Vol. 31, No. 2, pp. 289-295, ISSN 1450-216X

Acamovic-Djokovic, G., Djukic, D., Mandic, L., Kalinic, S. & Boskovic, T. (2002). Antimicrobial activity of the petrol-ether and ethyl-acetate extracts of Melilotus officinalis (L.) Pall, Melilotus albus Medic. and Melitis melissophyllum L. *Lekovite sirovine*, Vol. 22, pp. 59-63, ISSN 0455-6224

Brkovic, D.L., Comic, Lj. & Solujic-Sukdolak, S. (2006). Antibacterial activity of some plants from family Apiaceae in relation to selected phytopathogenic bacteria. *Kragujevac Journal of Science*, Vol. 28, pp. 65-72, ISSN 1450-9636

Benaiche G. (2007). Extraction and GC/MS Analysis of major Alkaloids found in the Family of Fabaceae. Academic Dissertation, Department of Chemistry, Faculty of Sciences and Engineer Sciences, University of M'sila, Algeria, Africa

Cowan, M.M. (1999). Plant Products as Antimicrobial Agents. *Clinical Microbiology Reviews*, Vol. 12, No. 4, (October 1999), pp. 564-582, ISSN 0893-8512

Cos, P., Vlietinck, A.J., Berghe, D.V. & Maes, L. (2006). Anti-infective potential of natural products: How to develop a stronger *in vitro* „proof-of-concept". *Journal of Ethnopharmacology*, Vol. 106, No. 3, (July 2006), pp. 290-302, ISSN 0378-8741

Chah, K.F., Eze, C.A., Emuelosi, C.E. & Esimone, C.O. (2006). Antibacterial and wound healing properties of methanolic extracts of some Nigerian medicinal plants. *Journal of Ethnopharmacology*, Vol. 104, No. 1-2, (March 2006), pp. 164–167, ISSN 0378-8741

Christensen, L.P. & Brandt, K. (2006). Bioactive polyacetylenes in food plants of the Apiaceae family: Occurrence, bioactivity and analysis. *Journal of Pharmaceutical and Biomedical Analysis*, Vol. 41, No. 3, (Jun 2006), pp. 683-693, ISSN 0731-7085

Cisowski, W. (1985). Flavonoid Compounds in the Herb *Aegopodium podagraria. Herba Polonica*, Vol. 31, pp. 135-40, ISSN 0018-0599

Canadanović-Brunet, J., Cetković, G., Djilas, S., Tumbas, V., Bogdanović, G., Mandić, A., Markov, S., Cvetković, D., Canadanović, V. (2008). Radical scavenging, antibacterial and antiproliferative activities of *Melissa officinalis* L. extracts. *Journal of Medicinal Food*, Vol. 11, No. 1, (March 2008), pp. 133-143, ISSN 1096-620X

Cho, W.I., Choi, J.B., Lee, K., Chung, M.S. & Pyun, Y.R. (2008). Antimicrobial activity of torilin isolated from *Torilis japonica* fruit against *Bacillus subtilis*. *Journal of Food Science*, Vol. 73, No. 2, (March 2008), pp. 37-46, ISSN 0022-1147

Dem'yanenko, V.G. & Dranik, LI. (1971). Coumarins from *Cichorium intybus* raceme. *Khimiya Prirodnykh Soedinenii*, Vol. 7, No. 1, pp. 115-118, ISSN 0023-1150

Durling, N.E., Catchpole, O.J., Grey, J.B., Webby, R.F., Mitchell, K.A., Foo, L.Y. & Perry, N.B. (2007). Extraction of phenolics and essential oil from dried sage (*Salvia officinalis*) using ethanol-water mixtures. *Food Chemistry*, Vol. 101, No. 4, pp. 1417-1424, ISSN 0308-8146

Duke, J.A. (2002). *Handbook of Medicinal Herbs*, 2nd ed. CRC Press, ISBN 0849312841, Florida

Eloff, J.N. (1998). Which extractant should be used for the screening and isolation of antimicrobial components from plants? *Journal of Ethnopharmacology*, Vol. 60, No. 1, (February 1998), pp. 1-8, ISSN 0378-8741

Ertürk O. (2006). Antibacterial and antifungal activity of ethanolic extracts from eleven spice plants. *Biologia*, Vol. 61, No. 3, pp. 275-278, ISSN: 0006-3088

Foster, B.C., Arnason, J.T. & Briggs, C.J. (2005). Natural health products and drug disposition. *Annual review of pharmacology and toxicology*, Vol. 45, pp. 203-226, ISSN 0362-1642

Garrod, B., Lea, E. & Lewis, G.B. (1979). Studies on the mechanism of action of the antifungal compound falcarindiol. *New Phytologist*, Vol. 83, No. 2, (September 1979), pp. 463-471, ISSN 0028-646X

Hartmann, T. (2008). The lost origin of chemical ecology in the late 19th century. *Proceedings of the National Academy of Sciences of the United States of America*, Vol. 105, No. 12, (March 2008), pp. 4541-4546, ISSN 0027-8424

Herodež, Š.S., Hadolin, M., Škerget, M. & Knez, Ž. (2003). Solvent extraction study of antioxidants from Balm (*Melissa officinalis* L.) leaves. *Food Chemistry*, Vol. 80, No. 2, (February 2003), pp. 275–282, ISSN 0308-8146

Hohmann, J., Zupkó, I., Rédei, D., Csányi, M.C., Falkay, G., Máthé, I. & Janicsák, G. (1999). Protective effects of the aerial parts of *Salvia officinalis*, *Melissa officinalis* and

Lavandula angustifolia and their constituents against enzyme-dependent and enzyme-independent lipid peroxidation. *Planta Medica,* Vol. 65, No. 6, (August 1999), pp. 576-578, ISSN 0032-0943

Horiuchi, K., Shiota, S., Hatano, T., Yoshida, T., Kuroda, T. & Tsuchiya, T. (2007). Antimicrobial activity of oleanolic acid from *Salvia officinalis* and related compounds on vancomycin-resistant Enterococci (VRE). *Biological & pharmaceutical bulletin*, Vol. 30, No. 6, (Jun 2007), pp. 1147-1149, ISSN 0918-6158

Iwu, M.W., Duncan, A.R. & Okunji, C.O. (1999). New antimicrobials of plant origin, In: *Perspectives on new crops and new uses,* J. Janick, (Ed.), pp. 457–462, ASHS Press, ISBN 0-9615027-0-3, Alexandria, VA

Iauk, L., Lo Bue, A.M., Milazzo, I., Rapisarda, A. & Blandino, G. (2003). Antibacterial Activity of Medicinal Plant Extracts Against Periodontopathic Bacteria. *Phytotherapy Research,* Vol. 17, No. 6, (Jun 2003), pp. 599–604, ISSN 0951-418X

Kovacevic, N. (2004). *Osnovi farmakognozije,* Srpska školska knjiga, ISBN 86-83565-19-X, Beograd

Konning, G.H., Agyare, C. & Ennison, B. (2004). Antimicrobial activity of some medicinal plants from Ghana. *Fitoterapia,* Vol. 75, No. 1, (January 2004), pp. 65-67, ISSN 0367-326X

Kratchanova, M., Denev, P., Ciz, M., Lojek, A. & Mihailov, A. (2010). Evaluation of antioxidant activity of medicinal plants containing polyphenol compounds. Comparison of two extraction systems. *Acta Biochimica Polonica,* Vol. 57, No. 2, pp. 229-234, ISSN 0001-527X

Kitajima, J., Suzuki, N., Satoh, M. & Watanabe, M. (2002). Sesquiterpenoids of *Torilis japonica* fruit. *Phytochemisrty,* Vol. 59, No. 8, (April 2002), pp. 811-815, ISSN 0031-9422

Khodakov, G.V., Akimov, Y.A., Shashkov, A.S., Kintia, P.K. & Grishkovets, V.I. (1996). Triterpene and steroid saponins isolated from two *Melilotus* species. *Advance in Experimental Medicine and Biology,* Vol. 405, pp. 211-222, ISSN 0065-2598

Kazantzoglou, D., Magiatis, P., Panoutsopoulos, G. & Skaltsounis, A.L. (2004). Dorycnioside, a New Phenylbutanone Glucoside from *Dorycnium pentaphyllum* subsp. *herbaceum. Zeitschrift für Naturforschung B,* Vol. 59c, pp. 23-26, ISSN 0932-0776

López, A., Hudson, J.B. & Towers, G.H. (2001). Antiviral and antimicrobial activities of Colombian medicinal plants. *Journal of Ethnopharmacology,* Vol. 77, No. 2-3, (October 2001), pp. 189–196, ISSN 0378-8741

Lu, Y. & Foo L.Y. (1999). Rosmarinic acid derivatives from Salvia officinalis. Phytochemistry, Vol. 51, No. 1, (May 1999), pp. 91-94, ISSN 0031-9422

Lu, Y. & Foo, L.Y. (2002). Polyphenolics of Salvia - a review. *Phytochemistry,* Vol. 59, No. 2, (January 2002), pp. 117-40, ISSN 0031-9422

Miyase T. & Matsushima Y. (1997). Saikosaponin homologues from *Clinopodium* spp. The structures of clinoposaponins XII-XX. *Chemical and Pharmaceutical Bullten,* Vol. 45, No. 9, (September 1997), pp. 1493-1497, ISSN 0009-2363

Manandhar, N. P. & Manandhar, S. (2002). *Plants and People of Nepal,* Timber Press, ISBN 0881925276, Portland, OR

Mares, D., Romagnoli, C.B., Tosi, B., Andreotti, E., Chillemi, G. & Poli, F. (2005). Chicory extracts from *Cichorium intybus* L. as potential antifungals. *Mycopathologia,* Vol. 160, No 1, (August 2005), pp. 85-92, ISSN 0301-486X

Ncube, N.S., Afolayan, A.J. & Okoh, A.I. (2008). Assessment techniques of antimicrobial properties of natural compounds of plant origin: current methods and future trends. *African Journal of Biotechnology,* Vol. 7, No. 12, (June 2008), pp. 1797-1806, ISSN 1684-5315

Nikaido, H. (2003). Molecular Basis of Bacterial Outer Membrane Permeability Revisited. *Microbiology and Molecular Biology Reviews,* Vol. 67, No. 4, (December 2003), pp. 593-656, ISSN 1092-2172

Nandagopal S. & Ranjitha Kumari, B.D. (2007). Phytochemical and Antibacterial Studies of Chicory (*Cichorium intybus* L.) - A Multipurpose Medicinal Plant. *Advances in Biological Research,* Vol. 1, No. 1-2, (January-April 2007), pp. 17-21, ISSN 1992-0067

Nolkemper, S., Reichling, J., Stintzing, F.C., Carle, R. & Schnitzler, P. (2006). Antiviral effect of aqueous extracts from species of the Lamiaceae family against Herpes simplex virus type 1 and type 2 *in vitro. Planta Medica,* Vol. 72, No. 15, (December 2006), pp. 1378-1382, ISSN 0032-0943

Ojala, T., Remes, S., Haansuu, P., Vuorela, H., Hiltunen, R., Haahtela, K. & Vuorela, P. (2000). Antimicrobial activity of some coumarin containing herbal plants growing in Finland. *Journal of Ethnopharmacology,* Vol. 73, No. 1-2, (November 2000), pp. 299-305, ISSN 0378-8741

Ojala, T. (2001). *Biological Screening of Plant Coumarins.* Academic Dissertation, Department Of Pharmacy, Faculty of Science, University of Helsinki, Finland

Opalchenova, G. & Obreshkova, D. (1999). Antibacterial action of extracts of *Clinopodium vulgare* L. curative plant. *Drug development and industrial pharmacy,* Vol. 25, No. 3, (March 1999), pp. 323-328, ISSN 0363-9045

Obreshkova, D.,Tashkov, W. & Ilieva, I. (2001). Phenolcarboxylic acids in *Clinopodium vulgare* L. *Comptes Rendus de l'Academie Bulgare des Sciences,* Vol. 54, No. 1, pp. 57-58, ISSN 0366-8681

Payne, G.F., Bringi, V., Prince, C. & Shuler, M.L. (1991). *Plant Cell and Tissue Culture in Liquid Systems,* Hanser Publishers, ISBN 9783446158306

Perumal Samy, R., Ignacimuthu, S. & Sen, A. (1998). Screening of 34 Indian medicinal plants for antibacterial properties. *Journal of Ethnopharmacology,* Vol. 62, No. 2, (September 1998), pp. 173–182, ISSN 0378-8741

Palombo, E.A. & Semple, S.J. (2001). Antibacterial activity of traditional Australian medicinal plants. *Journal of Ethnopharmacology,* Vol. 77, No. 2-3, (October 2001), pp. 151–157, ISSN 0378-8741

Patora, J. & Klimek, B. (2002). Flavonoids from lemon balm (*Melissa officinalis* L., Lamiaceae). *Acta Poloniae Pharmaceutica,* Vol. 59, No. 2, (March-April 2002), pp. 139-143, ISSN 0001-6837

Petrovic, J., Stanojkovic, A., Comic, Lj. & Curcic, S. (2004). Antibacterial activity of *Cichorium intybus. Fitoterapia,* Vol. 75, No 7-8, (December 2004), pp. 737-739, ISSN 0367-326X

Rios, J.L. & Recio, M.C. (2005). Medicinal plants and antimicrobial activity. *Journal of Ethnopharmacology,* Vol. 100, No. 1-2, (August 2005), pp. 80-84, ISSN 0378-8741

Ríos, J.L., Recio, M.C. & Villar, A. (1987). Antimicrobial activity of selected plants employed in the Spanish Mediterranean area. *Journal of Ethnopharmacology,* Vol. 21, No. 2, (November 1987), pp. 139–152, ISSN 0378-8741

Recio, M.C., Ríos, J.L. & Villar, A. (1989). Antimicrobial activity of selected plants employed in the Spanish Mediterranean area. Part II. *Phytotherapy Research,* Vol. 3, No. 3, pp. 77–80, ISSN 0951-418X

Rani, P. & Khullar, N. (2004). Antimicrobial evaluation of some medicinal plants for their anti-enteric potential against multi-drug resistant *Salmonella typhi*. *Phytotherapy Research*, Vol. 18, No. 8, (August 2004), pp. 670-673, ISSN 0951-418X

Sheldon, A.T. (2005). Antibiotic resistance: a survival strategy. *Clinical laboratory science: Journal of the American Society for Medical Technology*, Vol. 18, No. 3, (summer 2005), pp. 170-180, ISSN 0894-959X

Salvat, A., Antonacci, L., Fortunato, R.H., Suárez, E.Y. & Godoy, H.M. (2004). Antimicrobial activity in methanolic extracts of several plant species from northern Argentina. *Phytomedicine : international journal of phytotherapy and phytopharmacology*, Vol. 11, No. 2-3, (Feb 2004), pp. 230–234, ISSN 0944-7113

Sokmen, A., Jones, B.M. & Erturk, M. (1999). The *in vitro* antibacterial activity of Turkish medicinal plants. *Journal of Ethnopharmacology*, Vol. 67, No. 1, (October 1999), pp. 79-86, ISSN 0378-8741

Skaltsa, H.D., Demetzos, C., Lazari, D. & Sokovic, M. (2003). Essential oil analysis and antimicrobial activity of eight Stachys species from Greece. *Phytochemistry*, Vol. 64, No. 3, (October 2003), pp. 743–752, ISSN 0031-9422

Stefanović, O., Čomić, Lj. & Stanojević, D. (2009). Inhibitory effect of *Torilis anthriscus* on growth of microorganisms. *Central European Journal of Biology*, Vol. 4, No. 4, (September 2009), pp. 493-498, ISSN 189-104X

Stefanović, O., Čomić, Lj., Stanojević, D. & Solujić-Sukdolak, S. (2009). Antibacterial activity of *Aegopodium podagraria* L. extracts and interaction between extracts and antibiotics. *Turkish Journal of Biology*, Vol. 33, No. 2, pp 145-150, ISSN 1300-0152

Stanojević, D., Čomić, Lj. & Stefanović, O. (2010). *In vitro* synergy between *Salvia officinalis* L. and some preservatives. *Central European Journal of Biology*, Vol. 5, No. 4, (August 2010), pp. 491-495, ISSN 1895-104X

Stanojević, D., Čomić, Lj., Stefanović, O. & Solujić-Sukdolak, S. (2010). *In vitro* synergistic antibacterial activity of *Melissa officinalis* L. and some preservatives. *Spanish Journal of Agricultural Research*, Vol. 8, No. 1, pp. 109-115, ISSN 1695-971X

Stojanović-Radić, Z., Čomić, Lj., Radulović, N., Dekić, M., Ranđelović, V. & Stefanović O. (2010). Chemical composition and antimicrobial activity of Erodium species: *E. ciconium* L., *E. cicutarium* L., and *E. absinthoides* Willd. (Geraniaceae). *Chemical papers*, Vol. 64, No. 3, (November 2009), pp. 368-377, ISSN 0366-6352

Stefanovic, O., Stanojevic, D. & Comic, Lj. (2012). Synergistic antibacterial activity of *Salvia officinalis* and *Cichorium intybus* extracts and antibiotics. *Acta Poloniae Pharmaceutica - Drug Research*, Vol. 3, ISSN 0001-6837 (in press)

Stefanovic, O., Stankovic, M.S. & Comic, Lj. (2011). *In vitro* antibacterial efficacy of *Clinopodium vulgare* L. extracts and their synergistic interaction with antibiotics. *Journal of Medicinal Plants Research*, Vol. 5, (September 2011), pp. xxx-xxx, ISSN 1996-0875 (in press)

Sareedenchai, V. & Zidorn, C. (2010). Flavonoids as chemosystematic markers in the tribe Cichorieae of the Asteraceae. *Biochemical Systematics and Ecology*, Vol. 38, No. 5, (October 2010), pp. 935-957, ISSN 0305-1978

Stoker, J.R. (1964). The biosynthesis of coumarin in *Melilotus alba*. Biochemical and Biophysical Research Communications, Vol. 14, No. 1, (December 1964), pp. 17-20, ISSN 0006-291X

Sarker, S.D., Nahar, L. & Kumarasamy, Y. (2007). Microtitre plate-based antibacterial assay incorporating resazurin as an indicator of cell growth, and its application in the *in vitro* antibacterial screening of phytochemicals. *Methods,* Vol. 42, No. 4, (August 2007), pp. 321-324, ISSN 1046-2023

Sarac, N. & Ugur, A. (2007). Antimicrobial activities and usage in folkloric medicine of some Lamiaceae species growing in Mugla, Turkey. *EurAsian Journal of BioSciences,* Vol. 1, No.4, pp. 28-34, ISSN 1307-9867

Stamatis, G., Kyriazopoulos, P., Golegou, S., Basayiannis, A., Skaltsas S. & Skaltsa H. (2003). *In vitro* anti-*Helicobacter pylori* activity of Greek herbal medicines. *Journal of Ethnopharmacology,* Vol. 88, No. 2-3, (October 2003), pp. 175–179, ISSN 0378-8741

Saric, M. (1989). Medicinal Plants of SR Serbia, Serbia Academy of Science and Arts, Belgrade

VanEtten, H.D., Mansfield, J.W., Bailey, J.A. & Farmer, E.E. (1994). Two Classes of Plant Antibiotics: Phytoalexins versus "Phytoanticipins". *Plant Cell,* Vol. 6, No. 9, (September 1994), pp. 1191–1192, ISSN 1191-1192

Uzun, E., Sariyar, G., Adsersen, A., Karakoc, B., Otük, G., Oktayoglu, E. & Pirildar, S. (2004). Traditional medicine in Sakarya province (Turkey) and antimicrobial activities of selected species. *Journal of Ethnopharmacology,* Vol. 95, No. 2-3 (December 2004), pp. 96-287, ISSN 0378-8741

Velickovic, D., Randjelovic, N., Ristic, M., Velickovic, A. & Smelcerovic, A. (2003). Chemical constituents and antimicrobial activity of the ethanol extracts obtained from the flower, leaf and stem of *Salvia officinalis* L. *Journal of Serbian Chemical Society,* Vol. 68, No. 1, pp. 17-24, ISSN 0352-5139

Wink, M., Witte, L., Hartmann, T., Theuring, C. & Volz, V. (1983). Accumulation of Quinolizidine Alkaloids in Plants and Cell Suspension Cultures: General Lupinus, Cytisus, Baptisia, Genista, Laburnum, and Sophora. *Planta Medica,* Vol. 48, No. 8, (August 1983), pp. 253-257, ISSN 0032-0943

Weckesser, S., Engel, K., Simon-Haarhaus, B., Wittmer, A., Pelz, K. & Schempp, C.M. (2007). Screening of plant extracts for antimicrobial activity against bacteria and yeasts with dermatological relevance. *Phytomedicine,* Vol. 14, No. 7-8, (August 2007), pp. 508-516, ISSN 0944-7113

Youn, H.J., Lakritz, J., Rottinghaus, G.E., Seo, H.S., Kim, D.Y., Cho, M.H. & March, A.E. (2004). Anti-protozoal efficacy of high performance liquid chromatography fractions of *Torilis japonica* and *Sophora flavescens* extracts on *Neospora caninum* and *Toxoplasma gondii. Veterinary Parasitology,* Vol. 125, No. 3-4, (November 2004), pp. 409-414, ISSN 0304-4017

Zidorn, C. (2008). Sesquiterpene lactones and their precursors as chemosystematic markers in the tribe Cichorieae of the Asteraceae. *Phytochemistry,* Vol. 69, No. 12, (September 2008), pp. 2270-2296, ISSN 0031-9422

Zuo, G.Y., Wang, G.C., Zhao, Y.B., Xu, G.L., Hao, X.Y., Han, J. & Zhao, Q. (2008). Screening of Chinese medicinal plants for inhibition against clinical isolates of methicillin-resistant *Staphylococcus aureus* (MRSA). *Journal of Ethnopharmacology,* Vol. 120, No. 2, (November 2008), pp. 287–290, ISSN 0378-8741

3

Future Antibiotic Agents: Turning to Nature for Inspiration

Nataša Radić[1,2] and Tomaž Bratkovič[1]
[1]*Department of Pharmaceutical Biology, Faculty of Pharmacy, University of Ljubljana, Ljubljana*
[2]*AB Inovacije d.o.o., Mirna*
Slovenia

1. Introduction

Few drugs have made such a profound impact on modern medicine as antibiotics. With the discovery of sulfonamides, β-lactams, and subsequent antibiotic classes after World War II, bacterial infections with often fatal outcomes literally became curable overnight. These "magic bullets," however, suffer from a serious drawback; the use (and misuse) of antibiotics induces selection pressure resulting in the development of resistance traits in bacterial populations. The process is augmented by short generation times of bacteria enabling rapid mutation and selection of resistant strains, and a horizontal transfer of resistance genes. Bacterial pathogens resistant to more than one, or even most clinically used antibiotics, have become common (Fischbach & Walsh, 2009). Faced with the fact that a renewed pre-antibiotic era might be just around the corner, the World Health Day 2011 campaign "Antimicrobial resistance and its global spread" launched by the WHO offers a strategy to safeguard existing antibiotics for future generations, and contain the spread of antimicrobial resistance (World Health Organization, 2011). However, taking a more sensible approach in prescribing and using available antibiotic drugs will only help to put off the inevitable. In the battle against the ever-increasing multidrug resistance of pathogenic bacteria, we urgently need new alternatives to the currently available broad-spectrum antibiotics. Here we review some current trends in antibiotic discovery focusing on the screening of natural products.

This chapter is composed of four parts. We start by briefly reviewing the history of antibiotic discovery, gradually moving from its most fruitful era in the 1940's and 50's to the unexpected outcome decline in the genomic era. Next, we address two fundamental questions of antibiotic research in the post-genomic age; namely, *where* to look for novel antibiotics and *how*. Finally, we conclude with a concise discussion on the modification of natural scaffolds to be translated into functional drugs.

2. History of antibiotic discovery

2.1 The golden age of antibiotic discovery

Before the discovery of prontosil, the forerunner of sulfonamide chemotherapeutics, the only available measures in combating bacterial infections, apart from practicing proper hygiene, were vaccination and passive immunization. Although these approaches are still invaluable today, the advent of broad-acting antibacterial agents enabled rapid treatment of patients with infections even when the exact causative bacterial pathogen was unknown. Prontosil, later found to be a prodrug releasing folate antimetabolite sulfanilamide upon reduction *in vivo*, was a result of a screening campaign at Bayer, Germany in the early 1930's, aimed at finding synthetic dyes for the potential effect on hemolytic streptococcal infection (Greenwood, 2003). Although the premise that dyes in general should exert antibacterial activity turned out to be incorrect, prontosil paved the way for antimicrobial drugs, becoming the first commercially available antibacterial agent and remained in clinical use for 30 years. Moreover, it inspired new generations of sulfonamide chemotherapeutics, some of which remain on the market today. All major antibiotic classes that form pillars of antibacterial therapy were derived from natural sources – mostly microbial secondary metabolites (Molinari, 2009) – with the exception of sulfonamides and quinolones, inhibitors of bacterial DNA gyrase that were discovered in the 1960's.

The groundbreaking work of Rene Dubois, who studied antibiosis in pairs of soil microorganisms, eventually leading to the discovery of a mixture of peptidic antibiotics collectively termed tyrothricin (its component gramicidin is still in limited use), inspired Selman Waksman and Boyd Woodruff to adopt the principle in systematic search for novel antibiotics (Kresge et al., 2004). It is now well recognized that many microbes produce structurally extremely diverse, small molecules that are involved in complex intra- and interspecies signaling (Shank & Kolter, 2009). Antibiosis is only one of the many possible outcomes of such interaction, but is most readily detected: Waksman and Woodruff looked for growth inhibition zones surrounding single colonies of soil microorganisms cultured under different conditions and then isolated the active substance from pure cultures by activity-guided fractionation (Waksman & Woodruff, 1940). The same route led to the earlier serendipitous discovery of penicillin by Alexander Fleming in 1929 (Fleming, 1929).

It took almost 15 years to scale up penicillin production and demonstrate its efficacy and safety. By that time numerous other antibiotic types were emerging (Fig. 1). The major source of antimicrobials turned out to be soil actinomycetes, such as the *Streptomyces* species, and various fungi. Considering the abundance of soil microbes (there are estimates of 10^9-10^{10} bacteria in a single gram of soil belonging to some 10^4 operational taxonomic units (Curtis et al., 2006; Gans et al., 2005)) the explosion in antibiotic discovery that began in the early 1940's is not surprising from current perspective. However, not all species are equally represented. Moreover, many related bacteria or fungi produce the same or similar secondary metabolites. For example, streptothricin was found in ~10%, streptomycin in ~1%, and tetracycline and actinomycin in ~0.1% of randomly collected soil actinomycetes (Baltz, 2007). So when the most abundant antibiotics were identified the pace of natural antibiotic discovery gradually slowed down (Baltz, 2007, 2008), finally culminating in a 30-year-gap in launching an antibiotic with a novel scaffold to the market (Fig. 1). The situation was exacerbated by ever stricter regulatory demands on safety and efficacy of drugs, the wrongful perception that bacterial infections no longer posed a severe threat to human health, as well as the unfavorable economics of antibacterial development (revenue from antibiotics is significantly lower compared to drugs indicated for chronic diseases), leading to a withdrawal of Big Pharma from the antibiotic business (Brötz-Oesterhelt & Sass, 2010; Fischbach & Walsh, 2009; Projan, 2003). Meanwhile, the development and spread of bacterial resistance was steadily incising into our antibacterial arsenal (Fig. 1).

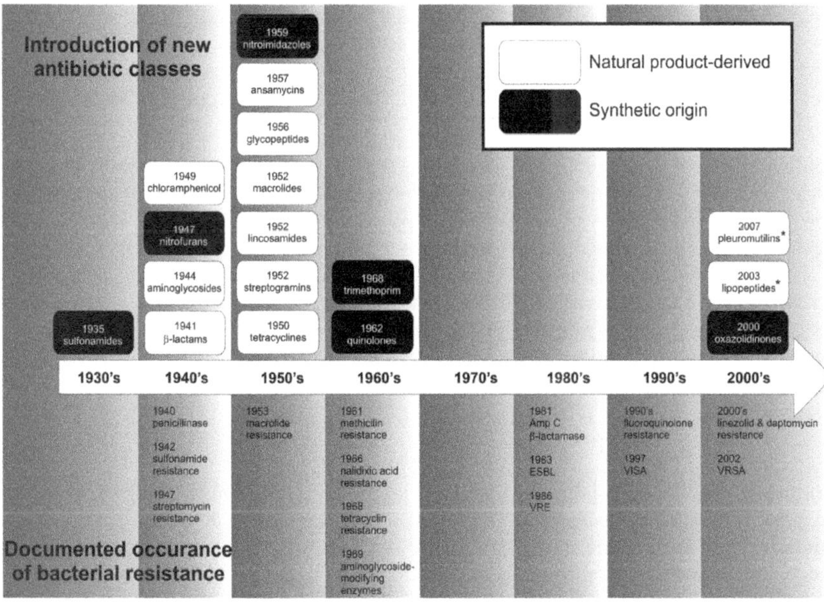

Fig. 1. Timeline for the introduction of major, broad-spectrum antibiotic classes for systemic application in the clinic, and documented occurrence of bacterial resistance (adapted from (Brötz-Oesterhelt & Sass, 2010)). The asterisk denotes two new antibiotic classes with single representatives (i.e., lipopeptide daptomycin, and pleuromutulin retapamulin), both of which are intended for topical application. However, analogues for systemic application (oral or *i.v.*) are being developed (also see section 3.1.4). ESBL - extended spectrum β-lactamase, VISA - vancomycin intermediately resistant *Staphylococcus aureus*, VRE - vancomycin-resistant *Enterococcus*, VRSA - vancomycin highly resistant *S. aureus*.

2.2 The disappointing investment in combinatorial chemistry and high-throughput screening in antibiotic discovery

Rediscovery of known antibiotics from screening microbial extracts and the development of highly effective synthetic (fluoro)quinolones caused a shift in antimicrobial drug R&D strategy in the industry. The search for antibiotics occurring in the environment was mostly abandoned (although semisynthetic modification of natural scaffolds resulted in numerous improved antibiotics (Fischbach & Walsh, 2009)) and the screening efforts were once again invested in synthetic compounds. Since the early 1990's combinatorial chemistry was employed to produce large libraries of compounds that demanded high-throughput assaying for activity. The advent of genomics and bioinformatics raised the hopes for identification of entirely new antibacterial targets by mining bacterial genomes. Genes conserved among bacteria but sharing no homology to eukaryotic counterparts were considered as potential targets, and their activity or expression were manipulated by mutation studies or knockout technology to examine whether their products were indispensable for bacterial survival *in vitro*. Following a functional analysis, selected targets were expressed using recombinant technology and purified. This allowed for setting up miniaturized inhibitory activity assays for screening vast chemical libraries against isolated targets, as well as elucidation of targets' structures to guide the subsequent optimization of leads. Despite enormous efforts in the last 20 years, however, the target-oriented drug discovery approach has not resulted in a single new antimicrobial chemotherapeutic. The reasons for that are multitude (reviewed in detail in (Baltz, 2006; Brötz-Oesterhelt & Sass, 2010; Projan, 2003)).

Firstly, the abandonment of whole-cell assays meant that cell penetrating capabilities were not a selection criterion for hits early in the discovery process. Therefore, most compounds that were highly active against an isolated target possessed no antimicrobial activity. Secondly, it appears that the properties of antibiotics in general do not conform to Lipinski's rule (Lipinski et al., 2001); they are more polar and have a higher molecular weight than drugs for other indications (O'Shea & Moser, 2008). Chemical libraries, on the other hand, had mostly been designed to meet Lipinski's criteria, and were thus likely biased against antibiotic compounds (Payne et al., 2007). Thirdly, inhibiting targets that were validated to be indispensible for bacterial survival *in vitro* does not necessarily lead to antibacterial effect *in vivo*. A prominent example is that of the type II fatty acid synthesis (FASII) pathway, intrinsic to bacteria: bacterial pathogens susceptible to FASII inhibitors *in vitro* were shown to be resistant to them when cultured in the presence of unsaturated fatty acids, or *in vivo* upon infection of rodents (Brinster et al., 2009). This indicates that bacteria can thrive in the nutrient-rich environment of the host by acquiring exogenous fatty acids, fully bypassing FASII pathway inhibition. Similarly, there is no guaranty that a target essential for viability of one bacterial strain will also be indispensible in others – as alternative biochemical pathways may be present that allow the targeted pathway to be circumvented (Gentry et al., 2003).

2.3 Reappraising the natural products

Historically, most drugs were derived from natural products. This trend continues today with ~50% of new small molecule drugs approved between the years 1981 and 2006 being either (semi)synthetic derivatives of compounds isolated from natural sources or synthetic mimetics of pharmacophores found in natural products (Newman & Cragg, 2007). In the field of antibacterial drugs, the trend is even more pronounced. Of 98 new molecular entities that were approved for human therapy in the same time period, only 23 are of totally synthetic origin, most of them (20) belonging to the quinolone group (Newman & Cragg, 2007). A notable exception is linezolid, the first and, to date, the only representative of oxazolidinone chemotherapeutics developed from initial hits of *cell-based* screening efforts for antibacterial activity from a chemical library (Barbachyn & Ford, 2003; Slee et al., 1987). Among the 40 antibacterial compounds currently undergoing clinical trials, 20 are natural product-derived, 18 are synthetic, and 2 are of unknown origin (Butler & Cooper, 2011). Interestingly, while the ratio of natural product-derived vs. synthetic entities is roughly 1:1 in phases I and II, the former predominate in phase III (i.e., 4:1). Moreover, there are more novel antibacterial classes among natural-product derived antibiotics compared to synthetic ones (a total of 7 new chemical scaffolds vs. 4) in the pipeline.

Disappointment from antibacterial drug discovery in the genomic era brought a renewed interest in screening natural products (Baltz, 2008; Davies, 2011; Li & Vederas, 2009; Molinari, 2009). Chemists have been isolating and analyzing secondary metabolites from plants, fungi, and bacteria for over 200 years, yet only a small percentage of species has been addressed (Li & Vederas, 2009). Undoubtedly, the natural supply of small molecules (sometimes referred to as parvome (Davies, 2011), from the Latin *parvus* meaning small) remains vast; however, there is a problem accessing it. A majority (maybe up to 99%) of microbes, renowned for their rich and diverse metabolism, cannot be cultured in a laboratory, at least not under standard conditions (Amann et al., 1995; Li & Vederas, 2009). There are species of microbes that thrive in geographical or ecological niches, such as deep sea and thermal springs, or as symbionts of plants and animals, respectively, that still await to be explored. Besides rediscovery, a major obstacle that can impede natural product research is that some compounds are found in the environment in rather low concentrations, complicating their detection and isolation in quantities allowing structural and functional studies.

Nevertheless, the thesis that the laborious screening for natural products with antibiotic activity is still worth the effort is supported by several facts. The parvome displays structural diversity unmatched by synthetic compounds; secondary metabolites often possess numerous chiral centers and display astonishing steric complexity. Furthermore, many natural antibiotics display complex and multilayer mechanisms of action that might not have been devised by rational design. Last but not least, millions of years of evolution have optimized antibiotics with respect to affinity and specificity for their targets, as well as physicochemical properties to penetrate bacterial envelopes (Butler & Buss, 2006; Pelaez, 2006; Swinney & Anthony, 2011). Encouragingly, owing to the revival of screening for natural antimicrobials or reinspection of collections of old antibiotics in the last decade, we have witnessed attempts to develop antibiotics based on novel chemicals templates, such as lipopeptides, pleuromutilins, ramoplanins, and actinonins (Butler & Buss, 2006; Butler & Cooper, 2011). Drugs based on new scaffolds exerting novel mechanisms of action should be superior to existing antibiotic classes in the fight against multi-drug resistant pathogens (Butler & Buss, 2006). Of note, two such antibiotics have recently been approved for use in humans. Daptomycin, the first member of lipopeptide antibiotics, acts through a complex mechanism involving the disruption of the bacterial membrane leading to inhibition of DNA, RNA, and protein synthesis, and is indicated for the treatment of skin and skin structure infections caused by Gram-positive pathogens (Baltz et al., 2005). Retapamulin, a pleuromutilin type antibiotic with indications similar to those of daptomycin, selectively inhibits the P site of peptidyl transferase centre on the bacterial 50S ribosomal subunit, exhibiting a mechanism that differs from other protein synthesis-inhibiting antibiotics (Dubois & Cohen, 2010; Schlunzen et al., 2004).

It is important to realize that all small molecular weight microbial products are active even though they might not induce antibiosis at concentrations found in the environment, suggesting their role as signaling molecules (Dufour & Rao, 2011; Miao & Davies, 2010; Shank & Kolter, 2009; Wyatt et al., 2010). Remarkably, this holds true even for well established antibiotics; a number of recent studies reported specific modulation of gene expression in different bacteria when exposed to subinhibitory concentrations of various antibiotics (Davies et al., 2006; Fajardo & Martinez, 2008; Linares et al., 2006). Reevaluation of known natural products for traits other than antibiosis might thus present another route leading to antibacterial drug discovery, inhibiting the production of metabolites that provide the producing microbe with an advantage in colonizing a certain niche could prove to be a fruitful approach in designing antimicrobials (Wyatt et al., 2010).

3. Where do we search for natural antibiotics?

The search for new antibiotics compounds goes hand in hand with the discovery of new (micro)organisms producing them. For this purpose the search has continued on land and at sea with great expectations. Soil microorganism exploitation has not subsided and continuous effort is put into the expanding the diversity of actinomycetes and fungi, taking advantage of little explored ecological niches and developing new ways of growing previously uncultivable strains (Harvey, 2000).

Almost all kinds of living things have the ability to produce secondary metabolites with antibiotic properties (Berdy, 2005), although this ability is not equally distributed among different species. Overall, it is clear that unicellular bacteria, eukaryotic fungi, and first of all filamentous actinomyces are the most frequent and most versatile producers. The filamentous actinomycetales species produce over 10,000 bioactive compounds, of which 7600 derived from *Streptomyces* represent the largest group (45%) of bioactive microbial metabolites. Streptomycetes are demonstrably a rich source of compounds, but no more so than other members of the actinobacteria. In 2001 Watve et al. set about to produce a mathematical model that would estimate the number of undiscovered antimicrobials from the genus *Streptomyces* (Watve et al., 2001). They found that there are still around 150,000 antimicrobials to be discovered. Theoretically speaking, this number does sound encouraging and one might expect the antibiotic pipeline to be pouring with new drugs. The reality is quite different. According to Butler and Cooper, in 2011, there were five compounds undergoing phase-III clinical trials, one compound was under NDA/MAA evaluation, 22 compounds were in phase-II, and 12 compounds in phase-I clinical trials (Butler & Cooper, 2011). Twenty of those compounds are derived from natural products. Clinical development of a drug requires certain *in vitro* activity, stability, and pharmacokinetic criteria to be met. It seems that not many of the lead secondary metabolites make it all the way to clinical trials and development and, eventually, drug approval. Nevertheless, finding an effective lead substance remains the most important starting point in antibiotic development. In the following text we give some examples on where some of these lead compounds can and have been found.

3.1 The producing organisms

Natural product resources, including the microbial world, are mainly unexplored both in its dimension and in the respect of geographic, ecological, and environmental points of view. There surely exist, besides the presumed numbers of microorganisms, millions of microbes living in remote and exotic parts of the world, or even the ones living in other organisms as endophytes or symbionts that await discovery and thorough study.

3.1.1 Endophytes

Endophytes reside in tissues between living plant cells. The relationship that they establish with the plant varies from symbiotic to bordering on pathogenic. Of all of the world's plants, it seems that only a few grass species have had their complete complement of endophytes studied, although endophytic fungi have been found in each plant species examined. The estimated number of endophytic fungal species existing in nature is over one million (Petrini, 1991). As a result, the opportunity to find new and interesting endophytes among the myriad of plants is great.

Plant endophytic fungi have a special ability to produce a great number of diverse bioactive compounds, which have been implicated in protection of its host against pathogens and herbivores (Wicklow et al., 2005). These structurally diverse molecules have potential therapeutic value, which is why interest in screening endophytic fungi for discovery of novel metabolites, and more specifically novel antibiotics, has increased. The initial step in discovering secondary metabolites of endophytes is their successful isolation from plant materials. Then, the isolation and characterization of bioactive substances from culture filtrates is done using bioassay guided fractionation and spectroscopic methods (Strobel, 2002). For a detailed explanation on how these endophytic microorganisms are isolated the reader is referred to other publications (Hallmann et al., 2006; Strobel, 2002).

A short selection of substances with antibiotic properties that have been found in endophytic fungi and reported so far is included in Table 1 to provide the reader with an idea of how many potential lead compounds there are presently at our disposal.

Endophytic fungal strain	**Host plant (family)**	**Habitat of the host plant**	**Isolated metabolite(s)**
Colletotrichum gloeosporioides (Penz.) Penz. & Sacc.	*Artemisia mongolica* (Fisch. ex Bess.) Nakai (Asteraceae)	Zijin Mountain, the suburb of Nanjing, China	colletotric acid
Colletotrichum sp.	*Artemisia annua* L. (Asteraceae)	ns	6-isoprenylindole-3-carboxylic acid 3b,5a-dihydroxy-6b-acetoxy-ergosta-7,22-diene 3b,5a-dihydroxy-6b-phenylacetyloxy-ergosta-7,22-diene 3b-hydroxy-ergosta-5-ene; 3-oxo-ergosta-4,6,8(14),22-tetraene 3b-hydroxy-5a,8a-epidioxy-ergosta-6,22-diene
Phomopsis isolate MF6031	*Salix gracilistyla* var. *Melanostachys* (Salicaceae)	acquisition number 237- 71-5282, Wakehurst Place, UK	phomopsichalasin
Phomopsis sp. strain E02018	*Erythrina crista-galli* L. (Fabaceae)	Boraso Stream-Delta del Parana, Argentina.	phomol
unidentified endophytic fungus CR115	*Daphnopsis americana* (Thymelaeaceae)	Guanacaste Conservation Area in Costa Rica	guanacastepenes A-O
Periconia sp. OBW-15	*Taxus cuspidate* Siebold & Zucc (Taxaceae)	Kangwon region, Korea	periconicin A periconicin B
Guignardia sp. IFB-E028	*Hopea hainanensis* Merrill & Chun (Dipterocarpaceae)	Hainan Island, China	monomethylsulochrin rhizoctonic acid guignasulfide
Rhizoctonia sp. strain Cy064	*Cynodon dactylon* (L.) Pers. (Poaceae)	Jiangsu Province, China	rhizoctonic acid monomethylsulochrin ergosterol 3β,5α,6β-trihydroxyergosta-7,22-diene
Aspergillus sp. strain CY725	*Cynodon dactylon* (L.) Pers. (Poaceae)	Sheyang Port on the Yellow Sea	helvolic acid monomethylsulochrin ergosterol 3β-hydroxy-5α,8α-epidioxy- ergosta-6,22-diene

Endophytic fungal strain	Host plant (family)	Habitat of the host plant	Isolated metabolite(s)
Pichia guilliermondii Ppf9	*Paris polyphylla* var. *yunnanensis* (Franch) Hand.-Mazz (Trilliaceae)	Kunming, China	helvolic acid
Xylaria sp. YX-28	*Ginko biloba* L. (Ginkgoaceae)	Jiangsu and Shandong provinces, China	7-amino-4-methylcoumarin
Thielavia subthermophila INFU/Hp/KF/34B	*Hypericum perforatum* L. (Hypericaceae)	Harwan, Jammu and Kashmir, India	hypericin emodin
Twenty-nine unidentified endophytic fungal strains	*Eucommia ulmoides* Oliver (Eucommiaceae)	Sichuan University, Chengdu, Sichuan Province, China	crude ethanol extract of fermentation broth chlorogenic acid
Ampelomyces sp.	*Urospermum picroides* (L.) F.W. Schmidt (Asteraceae)	Alexandria, Egipt	3-O-methylalaternin altersolanol A
Phoma sp. NG-25	*Saurauia scaberrinae* (Actinidiaceae)	central highlands of Papua New Guinea	phomodione usnic acid cercosporamide
Fusarium sp. IFB-121	*Quercus variabilis* Blume (Fagaceae)	southern hillside of the Zijin Mountain in the eastern suburb of Nanjing, China	cerebroside 1 cerebroside 2
Trichoderma ovalisporum PRE-5	*Panax notoginseng* (Burkill) F.H.Chen ex C.Y.Wu & K.M.Feng (Araliaceae)	Yunnan Province, China	koninginin A (E)-2,3-dihydroxypropyl octadec-9-enoate shikimic acid cytosine ribonucleoside a compound considered to be adenine ribonucleoside
Unidentified Ascomycete endophytic fungus strain 6650	*Melilotus dentatus* (Waldst. & Kit.) Pers. (Fabaceae)	coastal area of the Baltic Sea, Ahrenshoop, Germany	4-hydroxyphthalide; 5-methoxy-7-hydroxyphthalide (3R,4R)-cis-4-hydroxymellein
Microsphaeropsis sp. strain 8875	*Lycium intricatum* Boiss. (Solanaceae)	Playa del Ingles, Gomera, Spain	microsphaeropsone A microsphaeropsone C citreorosein enone (oxidized microsphaeropsone A)
Microsphaeropsis sp. strain 7177	*Zygophyllum fortanesii* (Zygophyllaceae)	Gomera, Spain	fusidienol A 8-hydroxy-6-methyl-9-oxo-9H-xanthene-1-carboxylic acid methyl ester
Microdiplodia sp. strain 7092	*Erica arborea* L. (Ericaceae)	Gomera, Spain	3,4-dihydroglobosuxanthone A
Alternaria sp. strain JCM9.2	*Sonneratia alba* J.E. Smith (Sonneratiaceae)	Dong Zhai Gang Mangrove Garden on Hainan Island, China	xanalteric acid I xanalteric acid II altenusin
Chloridium sp. (J.F.H. Beyma) W. Gams & Holubova-Jchova	*Azadirachta indica* A. Juss. (Meliaceae)	Varanasi district, India	javanicin

Table 1. Plant endophytic fungi producing metabolites with antibacterial activity.
ns – not specified.

Another great source of antibiotic producers among endophytes is bacteria. Munumbicins are an example of antibacterial compounds found in these microorganisms. Gary Strobel's research group has isolated and studied the *Streptomyces* NRRL 30562 strain, which is endophytic in the medicinal plant snakevine (*Kennedia nigriscans*), native to the Northern Territory of Australia (Castillo et al., 2002). Bioassay-guided HPLC purification of the culture broth of this endophytic bacterium led to the discovery of four major components. They were characterized as four functionalized peptides named munumbicins A, B, C, and D. The munumbicins possessed widely differing biological activities depending upon the target organism. For instance, munumbicin B had a mimimum inhibitory concentration (MIC) of 2.5 μg/ml against a methicillin-resistant strain of *Staphylococcus aureus* (MRSA), whereas munumbicin A was not active against this organism. In general, the munumbicins demonstrated activity against Gram-positive bacteria such as *Bacillus anthracis* and multidrug-resistant *Mycobacterium tuberculosis*. The most impressive biological activity of any of the munumbicins was that of munumbicin D against the parasite *Plasmodium falciparum*. However, in 2006, they reported that some of the munumbicins are identical to the better known antibiotics, the actinomycins (Castillo et al. 2006). Further effort resulted in the isolation of several novel antibiotics from *Streptomyces* NRRL 30562 with wide-spectrum biological activity that were termed munumbicin E-4 and E-5 (Castillo et al. 2006). Both compounds were tested alongside vancomycin against *Escherichia coli* and MRSA. The MIC of munumbicin E-5 against *E. coli* was 16 μg/ml, while the MIC for vancomycin was 128 μg/ml. The MICs were 16 and 2 μg/ml against MRSA, respectively.

Other antibiotic compounds of different chemical structures such as the bafilomycins (Yu et al., 2011), kakadumycins (Castillo et al., 2003) and many others are also produced by endophytic *Streptomyces* strains, making these bacteria worth investigating. The ability to make bioactive small molecules is not exclusive to microbes. Plants are rich sources of a great variety of compounds, but the original producer of those might be questionable. Opinions on this subject are divided and nobody can say for certain how many microbial metabolites/antibiotics considered today as marine animal or plant products, are produced, in fact, by symbiotic microbes in marine invertebrates and by endophytic fungi or bacteria living in the vascular plants. It has become generally accepted that at least for some compounds isolated from marine invertebrates, and in several cases from higher plants, the actual producers are the symbiotic microbes; bacteria, cyanobacteria, algae, or endophytic fungi. Indeed, several bioactive metabolites (e.g. taxol, bryostatin, theopalauamide, caphalomannin, etc.) have been proven to originate from symbiotic or endophytic microbes and not the "higher" (host) organisms (Berdy, 2005; Newman & Cragg, 2004).

3.1.2 Insects

Insects represent 80% of all fauna and are the most widespread group within the animal kingdom. Furthermore, some of these organisms such as cockroaches live in the filthiest places known to man and thrive in such conditions (Lee et al., 2011).

An investigation of the potential antibacterial activity in various tissues of the desert locust (*Schistocerca gregaria*) and American cockroach (*Periplaneta americana*) was undertaken at the School of Veterinary Medicine and Science, University of Nottingham. Brain lysates of locust and cockroach exhibited powerful broad-spectrum antibiotic properties (>90% bactericidal effects) against MRSA and neuropathogenic *E. coli* K1, strain E44 (a cerebrospinal fluid isolate from a meningitis patient, O18:K1:H7), a spontaneous rifampicin-resistant mutant (Lee et al., 2011). A preliminary test suggested that the active substance is proteinaceous in nature. Brain lysates had no cytotoxic effects on human brain microvascular endothelial cells, suggesting that the putative target(s) is not present in eukaryotic cells. By combining size-exclusion spin columns and fast-performance liquid chromatography, eight different molecules (3–10 kDa in molecular mass) in brain lysates were identified that were toxic both to MRSA and neuropathogenic *E. coli* K1.

Higher insects protect themselves against bacterial infection by rapid synthesis of a battery of potent antibacterial peptides. Antimicrobial peptides (AMPs) have become recognized as important components of the nonspecific host defense or innate immune system in a variety of organisms including bacteria, fungi, plants, insects, birds, crustaceans, amphibians, and mammals (Zasloff, 2002). In order to overcome the problem of multi-resistant pathogenic bacteria, it is imperative to discover and clinically develop agents selectively toxic to bacteria that act on new targets which have not yet experienced selective pressure in the clinical setting. The research group of Laszlo Otvos has prepared derivatives of native proline-rich antibacterial peptides which exhibit these required features. As a lead they used pyrrhocoricin (Fig. 2), a peptide their group originally isolated from the European sap-sucking bug *Pyrrhocoris apterus* (Cociancich et al., 1994). In a couple of publications they report that pyrrhocloricin is non-toxic to eukaryotic cells and healthy mice, has good activity against model bacterial strains *in vitro* and when administered intravenously *in vivo*, and can protect mice from systemic *E. coli* challenge (Cudic et al., 2002; Cudic et al., 2003; Otvos et al., 2000a). Although pyrrhocoricin is toxic to infected animals at a high dose (50 mg/kg), its derivative in which the peptide is protected from exopeptidase cleavage by replacement of the N-terminal Val1 with 1-amino-cyclohexane-carboxylic acid and the C-terminal Asn20 with acetylated 2,3-diamino-propionic acid lacks this high dose toxicity and shows improved protease resistance, while maintaining the *in vitro* and *in vivo* efficacy over a broad concentration and dose range. Even more importantly, pyrrhocoricin and the derivative seem to have a completely new mechanism of action which makes the likelihood of fast accumulation of resistant strains insignificant. Native pyrrhocoricin kills the sensitive species by binding to DnaK, the 70-kDa bacterial heat shock protein (Otvos et al., 2000b). Remarkably, pyrrhocoricin does not bind to the human equivalent protein Hsp70, indicating the potential of this peptide as a drug lead to treat human or animal infections.

A list of antimicrobial peptides in clinical trials was published in 2004 (Andres & Dimarcq, 2004), and to date none of the peptides described has obtained FDA approval for any of the various clinical indications.

3.1.3 Marine (micro)organisms

The annual Marine natural products report has been published continuously since 1984 (until 2002 by John Faulkner (Faulkner, 2002) and later by Blunt et al. (Blunt et al., 2011)). The 2011 report states that 1011 new compounds of marine origin were described in literature in 2009 alone, proving that the oceans are a vast resource of diverse natural products, primarily from invertebrates such as sponges, tunicates, bryozoans, and molluscs, and from marine bacteria and cyanobacteria (Donia & Hamann, 2003).

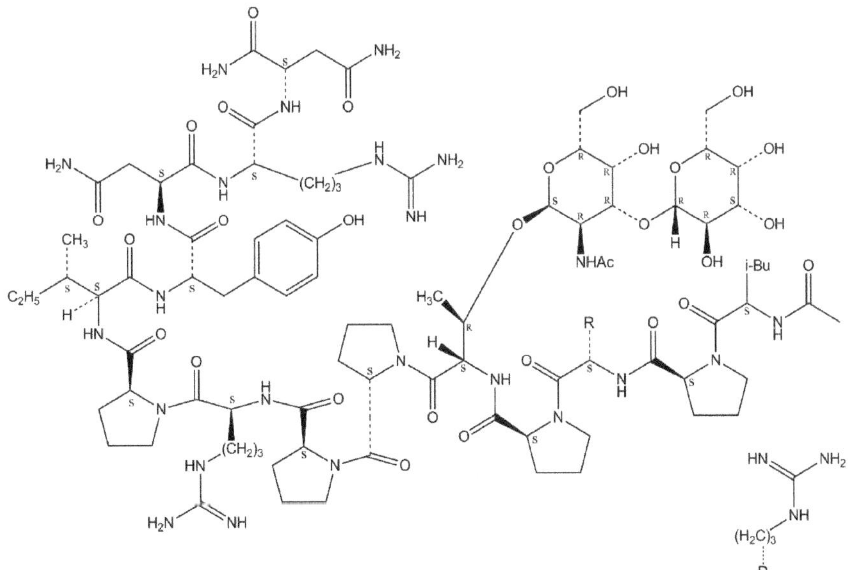

Pyrrhocoricin

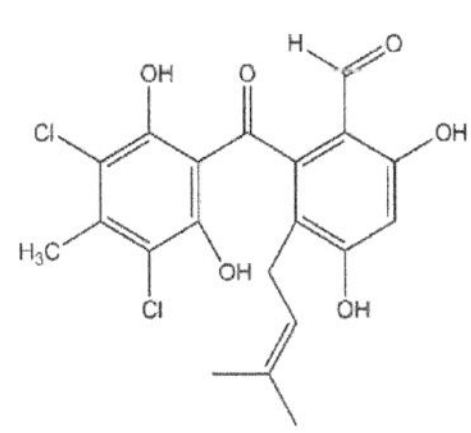

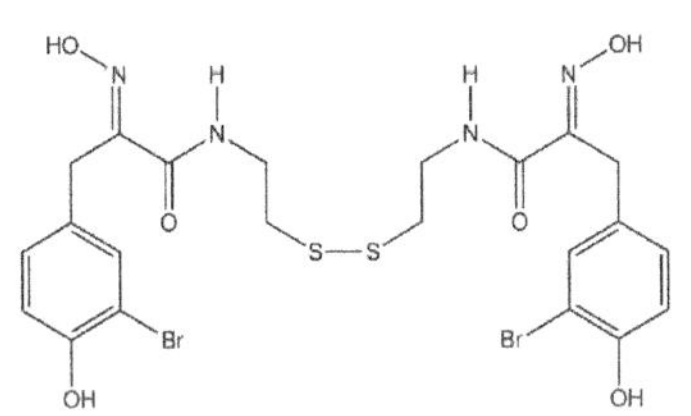

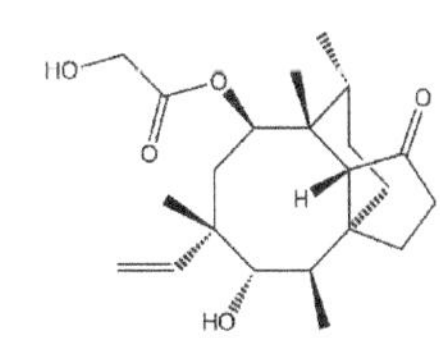

Pestalone Psammaplin A Pleuromutilin

Fig. 2. Structures of pyrrhocoricin, pestalone, psammaplin A, and pleuromutilin.

Research conducted with a marine fungus of the genus *Pestalotia* isolated from the surface of the brown alga *Rosenvingea* sp. collected in the Bahamas, lead to the discovery of pestalone (Fig. 2), a new chlorinated benzophenone antibiotic, which has potent antibiotic activity against MRSA, with a MIC of 37 ng/mL, and vancomycin-resistant *Enterococcus faecium*, with a MIC of 78 ng/mL (Cueto et al., 2001). The potency of this agent toward drug-resistant pathogens suggests that pestalone should be assessed in more advanced infectious diseases animal models. Interestingly, pestalone is produced in the mixed fermentation of a marine fungus, *Pestalotia* sp. (strain CNL-365) and an unidentified, antibiotic-resistant marine bacterium (CNJ-328), highlighting the complex dependence of metabolite biosynthesis on culture conditions and the potential for enhanced antibiotic production through cross-species induction. This observation clearly demonstrates that pestalone is a product of fungal biosynthesis in response to an external trigger, suggesting that this method may have use for drug discovery in the future (Cueto et al., 2001).

Sponges alone produce more than 3300 antibiotics and other bioactive compounds. It is noteworthy to mention that these isolated "animal" compounds very frequently show surprising analogy to microbial or algal products. As with the secondary metabolites produced by plants and their endophytes, it is not surprising that in numerous occasions the active compounds isolated from sponges proved to be derived from the microorganisms living in symbiosis with their host (Berdy, 2005). Marine microbes are particularly attractive because of the high potency required for bioactive compounds to be effective in the marine environment, due to the diluting effect of seawater (Zhang et al., 2005).

Psammaplin A (Fig. 2) is a symmetrical bromotyrosine-derived disulfide natural product isolated from the *Psammaplysilla* sponge (Arabshahi & Schmitz, 1987), with *in vitro* antibacterial activity against MRSA. Based on the structure of psammaplins, Nicolaou et al. produced a library of 3,828 compounds. Six of these optimized antibacterial agents possessed more than 50-fold higher activities than the natural product, demonstrating MIC levels in methicillin-resistant/intermediate vancomycin-resistant strains of *S. aureus* at less than 1μg/ml. In order to construct these heterodimeric disulfide analogues they used a novel combinatorial disulfide exchange strategy, thus demonstrating the power of modern combinatorial techniques when applied to a base active structure from nature (Newman & Cragg, 2004; Nicolaou et al., 2001a; Nicolaou et al., 2001b). Most significantly, a number of these agents exhibited increased selectivity against bacterial cells over fibroblasts and lymphocytes as compared to the natural product.

In similar efforts of the marine natural products community, many antibacterial agents have been identified from sponges (Laport et al., 2009). Despite their high number, none of them has yet been involved in clinical trial as an antibacterial agent.

3.1.4 Higher fungi

Among the eukaryotes, fungal genomes are rich in biosynthetic gene clusters for encoding small molecule production (Miao & Davies, 2010). Fungi are the second largest group of eukaryotes next to insects and exceed not only the bacteria and actinomycetes, but also the higher plants in terms of the number of potential existing species. It looks like the world of fungi is one of the largest reservoirs for isolating further bioactive metabolites (Berdy, 2005).

Besides the discovery of new compounds, the re-evaluation of "old" substances, including microbial metabolites formerly believed to be inactive, have proven to be just as important. On numerous occasions such compounds have been shown to be active in later investigations, or were rediscovered by screening a different stock of microbes, or with specific screening methods. It is unpredictable how many "new" bioactive metabolites will be discovered in this way (Berdy, 2005).

An excellent example of this is pleuromutilin (Fig. 2). It was initially discovered in 1951 in a study of the culture broth of the edible basidiomycete mushroom *Pleurotus multilus* (Kavanagh et al., 1951). After more than 50 years, a derivative of pleuromutilin, named retapamulin, was approved in 2007 by the FDA for the treatment of bacterial skin infections. The low oral bioavailability of retapamulin seems to have been improved in the new derivative named BC-3205, which is being investigated in phase-I clinical trials by Nabriva (Butler & Cooper, 2011). Another pleuromutilin derivative, BC-7013 ([14-O-[(3-hydroxymethyl-phenylsulfanyl)-acetyl]-mutilin]), is in phase-I clinical trials as a topical antibiotic, while BC-3781 successfully completed a phase-II clinical trial for the treatment of acute bacterial skin and skin structure infections (ABSSSI) (US National Institutes of Health, 2011). Nabriva's lead product BC-3781 is the first of a new class of systemically available pleuromutilin antibiotics for the treatment of serious skin infections and pneumonia. BC-3781 is being developed for both oral and intravenous formulations.

4. How do we search for natural antibiotics?

Although the number of antibiotics present in nature may truly be huge, many of them are already known or will not be usable (i.e., will not display selective toxicity to bacteria, will be too weak, or will lack the desired pharmacokinetic properties) (Pelaez, 2006). Yet historically, the development of antibiotics from natural templates has seen an unprecedented gain compared to the *de novo* synthesis. The conventional discovery process of antibiotics from the pool of microbial natural products requires having a given microorganism grown in conditions appropriate to induce the production of (the desired) metabolite, which is then extracted and tested in a screen able to detect it as a hit. Finally, the compound has to be isolated from the original mixture and identified.

Identification of novel antibiotic types that occur in relatively low frequency in nature clearly requires innovative detection and characterization techniques. Numerous promising microbiological approaches supplemented with bioinformatic, genetic, and structural methods have been developed over the last decade to address the issue (Fig. 3).

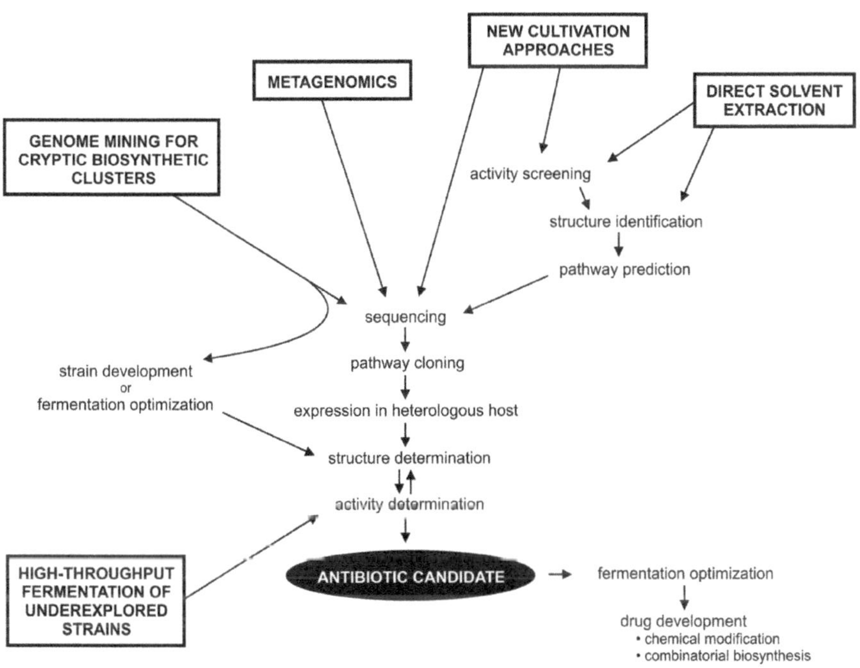

Fig. 3. Postgenomic approaches in antibiotic discovery (adapted from (Davies, 2011)).

These allow for laboratory culturing of previously inaccessible microorganisms as potential antibiotic producers, extracting genomes of uncultivable species from environmental samples or mining for and inducing expression of cryptic biosynthetic clusters to yield yet untapped secondary metabolites, direct solvent extraction and subsequent characterization of low molecular weight compounds from natural samples, and high-throughput fermentation of underexplored bacterial strains. In addition, intelligent strategies to avoid antibiotic rediscovery have been devised. In the following sections, we critically review the recent methodology of antibiotic discovery.

4.1 Improvements in screening platforms

Parallel fermentation coupled with whole-cell assays for antibiotic activity remains the cornerstone of antibiotic discovery. Yet, introduction of certain implementations are vital to detect antibiotic compounds that occur at low concentrations or to prevent rediscovery of old antibiotic types. For example, researchers at Merck developed a highly sensitive assay for detection of inhibitors of β-ketoacyl-[acyl-carrier-protein] synthase II (FabF), a component of FASII pathway, by introducing a plasmid that encodes antisense RNA against the *fabF* transcript in *S. aureus* (S.B. Singh et al., 2007). Thereby, FabF expression is knocked down to growth-limiting levels, resulting in a strain that is hypersensitive to FASII pathway inhibitors. The mutant is assayed in parallel with the control wild-type strain to monitor for differential sensitivity. This combination of target-based and whole-cell screening had a high hit rate of 0.3% and led to discovery of platensimycin, a broad spectrum Gram-positive antibiotic, from a screen of ~250.000 natural product extracts (Wang et al., 2006). Another interesting approach was reported by a team at Cubist Pharmaceuticals. They constructed a model target organism (CM400) by using *E. coli* engineered to harbor multiple resistance markers (conferring resistance to 16 most frequent antibiotics) (Baltz, 2006; Gullo et al., 2006). In this way, the hits are preselected to belong to new antibiotic classes. Additionally, a derivative of CM400 (termed CM435) with increased permeability was created to achieve enhanced sensitivity to antibacterial compounds. However, this strategy requires enormous input of natural products to be tested due to extremely low hit rates.

4.2 High-throughput fermentation focusing on relevant microorganisms

It is absolutely essential to screen extracts of only those organisms that have the capacity to produce complex secondary metabolites. The size of the genome provides a good indication of metabolism complexity; actinomycetes, the most important group of antibiotic producers, have large genomes relative to other bacteria with up to 10% of all genes devoted to production of secondary metabolites, such as nonribosomal peptides and polyketides (Baltz, 2008; Donadio et al., 2007). Using relatively selective antibiotics, bacterial populations can empirically be enriched for rare species (Baltz, 2006 and references cited therein) after which microbial diversity in the remaining population is conveniently assessed by 16S rRNA gene sequencing (Amann et al., 1995; Rajendhran & Gunasekaran, 2011). If the population is considered interesting in terms of secondary metabolite-producing potential, thousands of strains are typically screened for antibiotic activity. This, however, is no trivial task and represents a bottleneck of screening for antibiotics.

An obvious solution to increasing the throughput of fermentation is to miniaturize initial batches (i.e., perform microfermentations), allowing accommodation of larger numbers of strains and/or growth conditions simultaneously. At Cubist Pharmaceuticals they faced the challenge by encapsulating individual environmental microbes in ~2 mm alginate macrodroplets and growing them in media favouring actinomycete growth supplemented with antibiotics against single-cell eubacteria and fungi. This technology supports the fermentation and screening of up to 10 million actinomycetes per year (Baltz, 2006; Gullo et al., 2006). Similarly, a method that couples bacterial encapsulation in gel microdroplets with flow cytometry to detect those beads that contain microcolonies was reported (Zengler et al., 2002). This enables rapid isolation of bacterial strains from environmental samples in order to prepare pure cultures for subsequent studies.

4.3 New cultivation techniques

Since the vast majority of prokaryotes are not amenable to simple cultivation (indeed, only ~0.1% of existing prokaryotes have been cultured so far (Alain & Querellou, 2009)), numerous efforts to develop strategies for efficient bacterial growth *in vitro* have been made. Undoubtedly, expanding the accessible pool of antibiotic producers will raise the odds of discovering novel antimicrobials.

Attempts to recover diverse microorganisms from environmental samples by manipulating growth conditions (e.g. media formulation, light, temperature, agitation) have shown some success (Köpke et al., 2005; Uphoff et al., 2001; Zengler et al., 2002). However, the approach is strictly empirical and the yield is rather unpredictable. Moreover, the projects are often endangered by overgrowth of (common) opportunistic fast-growing microorganisms, especially when using nutrient-rich artificial media (Alain & Querellou, 2009). Furthermore, *in vitro* culturing attempts typically disregard the importance of chemical components or physical conditions of natural growth environments. Culturing *in situ* or under simulated natural conditions was demonstrated to be successful in some instances. For example, new bacteria were isolated from intertidal marine sediments using diffusion chambers and growth in seawater aquarium (Kaeberlein et al., 2002). The membranes of diffusion chambers allow for exchange of chemicals between the chamber and the environment, while restricting cell movement. Interestingly, two isolates easily grown in diffusion chambers could only be maintained in petri dishes in coculture, indicating the requirement for specific signaling between the two species as a marking of a favorable environment. Other studies found specific physical requirements for culturing different strains, such as high hydrostatic pressure (Alain et al., 2002) or carriers for adhesion (Yasumoto-Hirose et al., 2006). Previously uncultured bacteria were successfully recovered from soil, marine sediments or activated sludge by these innovative methods. Unfortunately, they are rather specialized and as a result were not adopted by a wider scientific community.

4.4 Direct isolation of metabolites from environmental samples

Direct sampling of natural products from the environment represents an alternative to microbial strain isolation and fermentation for production of secondary metabolites. In theory, this grants access to the complete metabolome, which cannot be retrieved by classical means because most microbes defy cultivation (see section 4.3). On the other hand, environmental concentrations of numerous antibiotics are too low to be readily detected by conventional analytical methods or activity screening. Modern liquid chromatography-mass spectrometry (LC-MS) instruments combine high resolution and high sensitivity with the power of structure determination, and as such hold great potential for analysis of secondary metabolites in organic extracts of various, complex environmental samples (Davies, 2011).

An exciting new field in natural product research is imaging mass spectroscopy (IMS) (Esquenazi et al., 2009). Application of IMS enables analysis of spatial distribution of compounds in a substrate, such as a plant organ or a marine sponge. This method led to identification of various (endo)symbiotic microorganisms as true producers of secondary metabolites which were initially erroneously attributed to the host organism (Esquenazi et al., 2009; Simmons et al., 2008). Another promising application of IMS is the so-called thin layer agar natural product MALDI-TOF imaging. Here, microorganisms are grown on a thin agar film deposited on a MALDI plate, after which the sample is covered with a matrix and analyzed by MALDI. Thus, a complete set of metabolites produced under different culturing conditions (even in cocultures to trigger interspecies interactions) can be examined (Yang et al., 2009).

Finally, the soaking of potential ligands from environmental extracts into crystals of recombinant proteins was proposed as another method to enrich for and analyze the structures of compounds with desired affinity to bacterial targets (Davies, 2011). Ideally, structural information gathered on the isolated secondary metabolite should assist in identification of the biosynthetic pathway from (meta)genomic library sequences (see sections 4.5 and 4.6).

4.5 Genome mining for cryptic metabolic pathways

In prokaryotes and fungi, gene encoding enzymes involved in secondary metabolite production are often clustered together. Polyketides and nonribosomal peptides (some of which are well established antibiotics) are typically assembled by massive synthetases of modular nature, wherein the modules consist of multiple domains, each being accountable for recognizing and fastening a specific substrate or catalyzing a sequential reaction step (e.g. building block activation, condensation, or tailoring) (Walsh & Fischbach, 2010). Therefore, the products of such assembly lines are said to be templated. Genome sequencing has revealed that certain microbes, especially many actinomycetes, harbor many (20 or more) biosynthetic gene clusters, most of which are cryptic (i.e., direct the production of unknown natural products) (Davies, 2011). This indicates that there are numerous complex secondary metabolites remaining to be discovered. The fact that polyketides and nonribosomal peptides are templated can aid in bioinformatic identification of genomic loci encoding biosynthetic pathways as well as provide clues to the structure and properties of metabolic products that are essential in developing methods for their detection and isolation (Fig. 4). If the product possesses the desired antibiotic activity and has favorable physicochemical properties, it is chosen as drug lead and platforms for sufficient production must be set up in order to support preclinical development. Strategies to elicit cryptic biosynthetic gene expression have been devised but will not be covered here. Readers interested in this topic are referred to two excellent recent reviews (Baltz, 2011; Chiang et al., 2011).

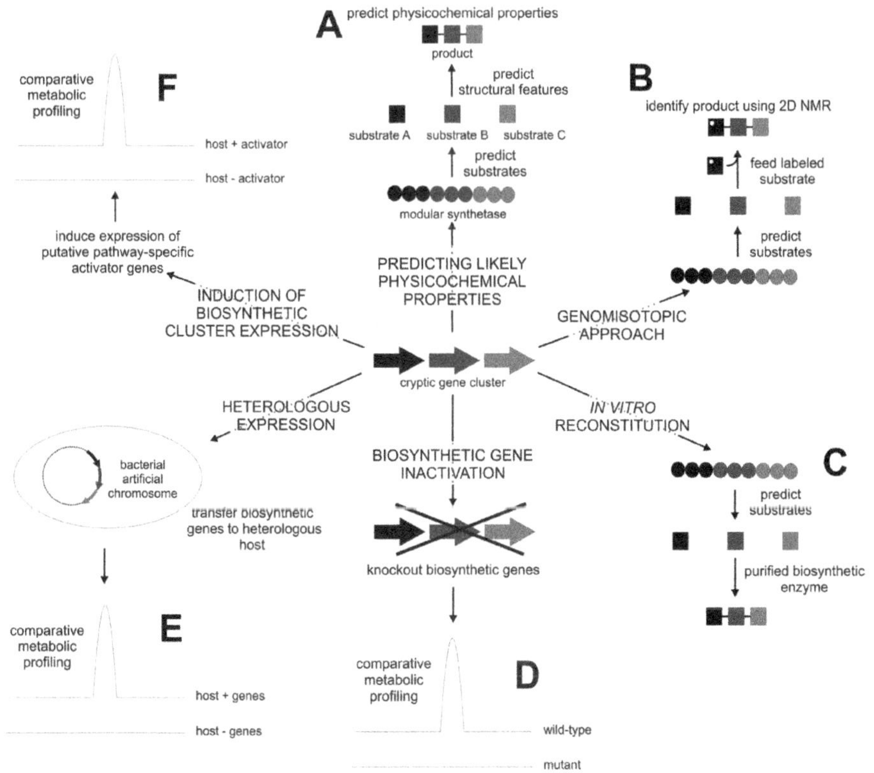

Fig. 4. Strategies for identifying metabolic products of cryptic gene clusters (compiled and adapted from (Challis, 2008)). Based on homology searches, novel biosynthetic gene clusters are predicted from genome sequences. **A**) The modular structure of synthetases allows assumptions on putative substrates, which together define structural and physicochemical features of secondary metabolites that guide the design of isolation procedures. **B**) Alternatively, the organism can be grown on a medium containing putative precursors labeled with stable isotopes to facilitate subsequent identification of final products by 2D NMR. **C**) The predicted synthetase can be expressed using recombinant DNA techniques and used in isolated form to reconstitute the product *in vitro*. **D**) The putative biosynthetic gene cluster can be knocked out and metabolites in culture supernatants analyzed by LC-MS in comparison to the metabolome of the wild-type strain. **E**) Similarly, the entire biosynthetic gene cluster-containing locus can be transferred to a heterologous host. The metabolome of the transgenic strain is compared to the untransformed host. **F**) Attempts to force expression of cryptic biosynthetic genes using induction of various endogenous activators have also been made.

4.6 Metagenomics

The term metagenomics refers to "the application of modern genomic techniques to the study of microbial organisms directly in their natural environments, by-passing the need for isolation and laboratory cultivation of individual species" (Miao & Davies, 2009). At the heart of metagenomics lies the recovery and sequencing of genomes of entire microbial communities occupying diverse ecological niches. Thereby, even the uncultivable microorganisms are addressed. The gathered genetic information is then scanned for potential biosynthetic genes in the hope for identification of novel natural products in a similar way as previously discussed (see section 4.5) (Banik & Brady, 2010; Miao & Davies, 2009). Alternatively, metagenomic expression libraries can also be directly assayed for functional products (Brady, 2007). However, due to methodological obstacles no complex biosynthetic gene clusters have been recovered from environmental DNA (eDNA) to date (Miao & Davies, 2009).

One of the biggest problems in metagenomics is the inefficient cloning of extremely large DNA segments needed to harbor intact gene clusters for preparation of metagenomic libraries. The transformation of vectors such as cosmids or bacterial artificial chromosomes to surrogate hosts is the main factor that limits construction of libraries with acceptable complexity. Moreover, the host might not efficiently express biosynthetic transgenes because of differences in codon usage or incompatibility of promoters (Miao & Davies, 2009; B.K. Singh & Macdonald, 2010). Finally, it is imperative to enrich microbial populations for strains with potential to produce complex secondary metabolites (see section 4.2) (Miao & Davies, 2009) or enrich isolated eDNA samples for genes of interest (Banik & Brady, 2010) before the metagenomic library is constructed to minimize background.

5. Modification of natural scaffolds

Natural resources are and will continue to provide structurally and mechanistically new molecules that serve as useful drugs or lead compounds. One should realize, however, that natural antibiotics rarely possess the appropriate characteristics to be directly considered as drugs. Instead, they typically need to undergo chemical modifications in order to be translated into functional drugs. The goal of such projects may be to improve the pharmacokinetic properties of drug leads (e.g. increase stability and bioavailability) or produce derivatives with higher activity and wider antibiotic spectrum (e.g. by incorporating moieties to evade bacterial efflux pumps or to engage into additional interactions with the bacterial target protein). Both focused rational design and combinatorial chemistry approaches backed up by structural studies of targets complexed with natural or synthetic antibacterials and their derivatives have resulted in numerous optimized antibiotic drugs (Brötz-Oesterhelt & Sass, 2010; Butler & Cooper, 2011; Newman & Cragg, 2007).

Combinatorial biosynthesis is a rapidly expanding field in natural antibiotic optimization (Baltz, 2008; Kopp & Marahiel, 2007). The modular nature of polyketide synthases and nonribosomal peptide synthetases enables generation of natural product variants by exchange or alteration of individual modules within the bioassembly line. Many polyketides and nonribosomal peptides are not amenable to chemical synthesis and semisynthetic modification due to extreme structural complexity. Here, chemoenzymatic approaches represent a viable alternative. One prominent example is the generation of a library of lipopeptides based on the daptomycin structure (Nguyen et al., 2006). The daptomycin biosynthetic pathway was engineered by module and subunit exchange, and inactivation of a tailoring enzyme. Some of the lipopeptide variants produced in fermentations were highly active antibiotics. Another group used error-prone PCR to generate gene mutants of glycosyltransferase that catalyses glucosylation of macrolide antibiotic oleandromycin (Williams et al., 2007). Thereby, they managed to broaden the specificities of the glycosyltransferase for acceptor substrates as well as donor nucleoside diphospho-sugars. Such innovative chemoenzymatic strategies combined with semisynthetic modification of natural products (novel and old) seem to provide a powerful tool for the development of new and improved antibiotics.

6. References

Alain, K., Marteinsson, V.T., Miroshnichenko, M.L., Bonch-Osmolovskaya, E.A., Prieur, D. & Birrien, J.L. (2002). *Marinitoga piezophila* sp. nov., a rod-shaped, thermo-piezophilic bacterium isolated under high hydrostatic pressure from a deep-sea hydrothermal vent. *International Journal of Systematic and Evolutionary Microbiology*, Vol. 52, No. Pt 4, (July 2002), pp. 1331-1339, ISSN 1466-5026

Alain, K. & Querellou, J. (2009). Cultivating the uncultured: limits, advances and future challenges. *Extremophiles*, Vol. 13, No. 4, (July 2009), pp. 583-594, ISSN 1433-4909

Amann, R.I., Ludwig, W. & Schleifer, K.H. (1995). Phylogenetic identification and in situ detection of individual microbial cells without cultivation. *Microbiological Reviews*, Vol. 59, No. 1, (March 1995), pp. 143-169, ISSN 0146-0749

Andres, E. & Dimarcq, J.L. (2004). Cationic antimicrobial peptides: update of clinical development. *Journal of Internal Medicine*, Vol. 255, No. 4, (April 2004), pp. 519-520, ISSN 0954-6820

Arabshahi, L. & Schmitz, F.J. (1987). Brominated tyrosine metabolites from an unidentified sponge. *Journal of Organic Chemistry*, Vol. 52, No. 16, (August 1987), pp. 3584-3586, ISSN 0022-3263

Baltz, R.H., Miao, V. & Wrigley, S.K. (2005). Natural products to drugs: daptomycin and related lipopeptide antibiotics. *Natural Product Reports*, Vol. 22, No. 6, (December 2005), pp. 717-741, ISSN 0265-0568

Baltz, R.H. (2006). Marcel Faber Roundtable: is our antibiotic pipeline unproductive because of starvation, constipation or lack of inspiration? *Journal of Industrial Microbiology and Biotechnology*, Vol. 33, No. 7, (July 2006), pp. 507-513, ISSN 1367-5435

Baltz, R.H. (2007). Antimicrobials from Actinomycetes: back to the future. *Microbe*, Vol. 2, No. 3, (March 2007), pp. 125-131, ISSN 1558-7452

Baltz, R.H. (2008). Renaissance in antibacterial discovery from actinomycetes. *Current Opinion in Pharmacology*, Vol. 8, No. 5, (October 2008), pp. 557-563, ISSN 1471-4892

Baltz, R.H. (2011). Strain improvement in actinomycetes in the postgenomic era. *Journal of Industrial Microbiology and Biotechnology*, Vol. 38, No. 6, (June 2011), pp. 657-666, ISSN 1476-5535

Banik, J.J. & Brady, S.F. (2010). Recent application of metagenomic approaches toward the discovery of antimicrobials and other bioactive small molecules. *Current Opinion in Microbiology*, Vol. 13, No. 5, (October 2010), pp. 603-609, ISSN 1879-0364

Barbachyn, M.R. & Ford, C.W. (2003). Oxazolidinone structure-activity relationships leading to linezolid. *Angewandte Chemie International Edition in English*, Vol. 42, No. 18, (May 2003), pp. 2010-2023, ISSN 1433-7851

Berdy, J. (2005). Bioactive microbial metabolites. *Journal of Antibiotics (Tokyo)*, Vol. 58, No. 1, (January 2005), pp. 1-26, ISSN 0021-8820

Blunt, J.W., Copp, B.R., Munro, M.H., Northcote, P.T. & Prinsep, M.R. (2011). Marine natural products. *Natural Product Reports*, Vol. 28, No. 2, (February 2011), pp. 196-268, ISSN 1460-4752

Brady, S.F. (2007). Construction of soil environmental DNA cosmid libraries and screening for clones that produce biologically active small molecules. *Nature Protocols*, Vol. 2, No. 5, (May 2007), pp. 1297-1305, ISSN 1750-2799

Brinster, S., Lamberet, G., Staels, B., Trieu-Cuot, P., Gruss, A. & Poyart, C. (2009). Type II fatty acid synthesis is not a suitable antibiotic target for Gram-positive pathogens. *Nature*, Vol. 458, No. 7234, (March 2009), pp. 83-86, ISSN 1476-4687

Brötz-Oesterhelt, H. & Sass, P. (2010). Postgenomic strategies in antibacterial drug discovery. *Future Microbiology*, Vol. 5, No. 10, (October 2010), pp. 1553-1579, ISSN 1746-0921

Butler, M.S. & Buss, A.D. (2006). Natural products - the future scaffolds for novel antibiotics? *Biochemical Pharmacology*, Vol. 71, No. 7, (March 2006), pp. 919-929, ISSN 0006-2952

Butler, M.S. & Cooper, M.A. (2011). Antibiotics in the clinical pipeline in 2011. *Journal of Antibiotics (Tokyo)*, Vol. 64, No. 6, (June 2011), pp. 413-425, ISSN 0021-8820

Castillo, U.F., Strobel, G.A., Ford, E.J., Hess, W.M., Porter, H., Jensen, J.B., Albert, H., Robison, R., Condron, M.A., Teplow, D.B., Stevens, D. & Yaver, D. (2002). Munumbicins, wide-spectrum antibiotics produced by *Streptomyces* NRRL 30562, endophytic on *Kennedia nigriscans*. *Microbiology*, Vol. 148, No. Pt 9, (September 2002), pp. 2675-2685, ISSN 1350-0872

Castillo, U., Harper, J.K., Strobel, G.A., Sears, J., Alesi, K., Ford, E., Lin, J., Hunter, M., Maranta, M., Ge, H., Yaver, D., Jensen, J.B., Porter, H., Robison, R., Millar, D., Hess, W.M., Condron, M. & Teplow, D. (2003). Kakadumycins, novel antibiotics from *Streptomyces* sp NRRL 30566, an endophyte of *Grevillea pteridifolia*. *FEMS Microbiology Letters*, Vol. 224, No. 2, (July 2003), pp. 183-190, ISSN 0378-1097

Castillo, U.F., Strobel, G.A., Mullenberg, K., Condron, M.M., Teplow, D.B., Folgiano, V., Gallo, M., Ferracane, R., Mannina, L., Viel, S., Codde, M., Robison, R., Porter, H. & Jensen, J. (2006). Munumbicins E-4 and E-5: novel broad-spectrum antibiotics from Streptomyces NRRL 3052. *FEMS Microbiology Letters*, Vol. 255, No. 2, (February 2006), pp. 296-300, ISSN 0378-1097

Challis, G.L. (2008). Mining microbial genomes for new natural products and biosynthetic pathways. *Microbiology*, Vol. 154, No. Pt 6, (June 2008), pp. 1555-1569, ISSN 1350-0872

Chiang, Y.M., Chang, S.L., Oakley, B.R. & Wang, C.C. (2011). Recent advances in awakening silent biosynthetic gene clusters and linking orphan clusters to natural products in microorganisms. *Current Opinion in Chemical Biology*, Vol. 15, No. 1, (February 2011), pp. 137-143, ISSN 1879-0402

Cociancich, S., Bulet, P., Hetru, C. & Hoffmann, J.A. (1994). The inducible antibacterial peptides of insects. *Parasitology Today*, Vol. 10, No. 4, (April 1994), pp. 132-139, ISSN 0169-4758

Cudic, M., Condie, B.A., Weiner, D.J., Lysenko, E.S., Xiang, Z.Q., Insug, O., Bulet, P. & Otvos, L., Jr. (2002). Development of novel antibacterial peptides that kill resistant isolates. *Peptides*, Vol. 23, No. 12, (December 2002), pp. 2071-2083, ISSN 0196-9781

Cudic, M., Lockatell, C.V., Johnson, D.E. & Otvos, L., Jr. (2003). In vitro and in vivo activity of an antibacterial peptide analog against uropathogens. *Peptides*, Vol. 24, No. 6, (June 2003), pp. 807-820, ISSN 0196-9781

Cueto, M., Jensen, P.R., Kauffman, C., Fenical, W., Lobkovsky, E. & Clardy, J. (2001). Pestalone, a new antibiotic produced by a marine fungus in response to bacterial challenge. *Journal of Natural Products*, Vol. 64, No. 11, (November 2001), pp. 1444-1446, ISSN 0163-3864

Curtis, T.P., Head, I.M., Lunn, M., Woodcock, S., Schloss, P.D. & Sloan, W.T. (2006). What is the extent of prokaryotic diversity? *Philosophical Transactions of the Royal Society of London Series B: Biological Sciences*, Vol. 361, No. 1475, (November 2006), pp. 2023-2037, ISSN 0962-8436

Davies, J., Spiegelman, G.B. & Yim, G. (2006). The world of subinhibitory antibiotic concentrations. *Current Opinion in Microbiology*, Vol. 9, No. 5, (October 2006), pp. 445-453, ISSN 1369-5274

Davies, J. (2011). How to discover new antibiotics: harvesting the parvome. *Current Opinion in Chemical Biology*, Vol. 15, No. 1, (February 2011), pp. 5-10, ISSN 1879-0402

Donadio, S., Monciardini, P. & Sosio, M. (2007). Polyketide synthases and nonribosomal peptide synthetases: the emerging view from bacterial genomics. *Natural Product Reports*, Vol. 24, No. 5, (October 2007), pp. 1073-1109, ISSN 0265-0568

Donia, M. & Hamann, M.T. (2003). Marine natural products and their potential applications as anti-infective agents. *Lancet Infectious Diseases*, Vol. 3, No. 6, (Junuary 2003), pp. 338-348, ISSN 1473-3099

Dubois, E.A. & Cohen, A.F. (2010). Retapamulin. *British Journal of Clinical Pharmacology*, Vol. 69, No. 1, (January 2010), pp. 2-3, ISSN 1365-2125

Dufour, N. & Rao, R.P. (2011). Secondary metabolites and other small molecules as intercellular pathogenic signals. *FEMS Microbiology Letters*, Vol. 314, No. 1, (January 2011), pp. 10-17, ISSN 1574-6968

Esquenazi, E., Yang, Y.L., Watrous, J., Gerwick, W.H. & Dorrestein, P.C. (2009). Imaging mass spectrometry of natural products. *Natural Product Reports*, Vol. 26, No. 12, (December 2009), pp. 1521-1534, ISSN 1460-4752

Fajardo, A. & Martinez, J.L. (2008). Antibiotics as signals that trigger specific bacterial responses. *Current Opinion in Microbiology*, Vol. 11, No. 2, (April 2008), pp. 161-167, ISSN 1369-5274

Faulkner, D.J. (2002). Marine natural products. *Natural Product Reports*, Vol. 19, No. 1, (February 2002), pp. 1-48, ISSN 0265-0568

Fischbach, M.A. & Walsh, C.T. (2009). Antibiotics for emerging pathogens. *Science*, Vol. 325, No. 5944, (August 2009), pp. 1089-1093, ISSN 1095-9203

Fleming, A. (1929). On the antibacterial action of cultures of a Penicillium, with special reference to their use in the isolation of B. influenzae. *British Journal of Experimental Pathology*, Vol. 10, No. pp. 226-236, ISSN 0007-1021

Gans, J., Wolinsky, M. & Dunbar, J. (2005). Computational improvements reveal great bacterial diversity and high metal toxicity in soil. *Science*, Vol. 309, No. 5739, (August 2005), pp. 1387-1390, ISSN 1095-9203

Gentry, D.R., Ingraham, K.A., Stanhope, M.J., Rittenhouse, S., Jarvest, R.L., O'Hanlon, P.J., Brown, J.R. & Holmes, D.J. (2003). Variable sensitivity to bacterial methionyl-tRNA synthetase inhibitors reveals subpopulations of *Streptococcus pneumoniae* with two distinct methionyl-tRNA synthetase genes. *Antimicrobial Agents and Chemotherapy*, Vol. 47, No. 6, (June 2003), pp. 1784-1789, ISSN 0066-4804

Greenwood, D. (2003). Historical introduction, In: *Antibiotic and Chemotherapy* (8th Edition), Finch, R.G., Greenwood, D., Norrby, S.R. & Whitley, R.J., (Ed.), pp. 3-10, Elselvier Science, ISBN 0443071292, Bodmin, Cornwall, UK

Gullo, V.P., McAlpine, J., Lam, K.S., Baker, D. & Petersen, F. (2006). Drug discovery from natural products. *Journal of Industrial Microbiology and Biotechnology*, Vol. 33, No. 7, (July 2006), pp. 523-531, ISSN 1367-5435

Hallmann, J., Berg, G. & Schulz, B. (2006). Isolation procedures for endophytic microorganisms, In: *Microbial Root Endophytes*, Schulz, B.J.E., Boyle, C.J.C. & Sieber, T.N., (Ed.), pp. 299-319, Springer Verlag, ISBN 978-3-540-33525-2, Berlin, Germany

Harvey, A. (2000). Strategies for discovering drugs from previously unexplored natural products. *Drug Discovery Today*, Vol. 5, No. 7, (July 2000), pp. 294-300, ISSN 1878-5832

Kaeberlein, T., Lewis, K. & Epstein, S.S. (2002). Isolating "uncultivable" microorganisms in pure culture in a simulated natural environment. *Science*, Vol. 296, No. 5570, (May 2002), pp. 1127-1129, ISSN 1095-9203

Kavanagh, F., Hervey, A. & Robbins, W.J. (1951). Antibiotic Substances From Basidiomycetes: VIII. Pleurotus Multilus (Fr.) Sacc. and Pleurotus Passeckerianus Pilat. *Proceedings of the National Academy of Sciences of the United States of America*, Vol. 37, No. 9, (September 1951), pp. 570-574, ISSN 0027-8424

Köpke, B., Wilms, R., Engelen, B., Cypionka, H. & Sass, H. (2005). Microbial diversity in coastal subsurface sediments: a cultivation approach using various electron acceptors and substrate gradients. *Applied and Environmental Microbiology*, Vol. 71, No. 12, (December 2005), pp. 7819-7830, ISSN 1098-5336

Kopp, F. & Marahiel, M.A. (2007). Where chemistry meets biology: the chemoenzymatic synthesis of nonribosomal peptides and polyketides. *Current Opinion in Biotechnology*, Vol. 18, No. 6, (December 2007), pp. 513-520, ISSN 0958-1669

Kresge, N., Simoni, R.D. & Hill, R.L. (2004). Selman Waksman: the father of antibiotics. *Journal of Biological Chemistry*, Vol. 279, No. 48, (November 2004), pp. 101-102, ISSN 0021-9258

Laport, M.S., Santos, O.C. & Muricy, G. (2009). Marine sponges: potential sources of new antimicrobial drugs. *Current Pharmaceutical Biotechnology*, Vol. 10, No. 1, (January 2009), pp. 86-105, ISSN 1873-4316

Lee, S., Duce, I., Atkins, H. & Khan, N.A. (2011). Cockroaches and locusts: physicians' answer to infectious diseases. *International Journal of Antimicrobial Agents*, Vol. 37, No. 3, (March 2011), pp. 279-280, ISSN 1872-7913

Li, J.W. & Vederas, J.C. (2009). Drug discovery and natural products: end of an era or an endless frontier? *Science*, Vol. 325, No. 5937, (July 2009), pp. 161-165, ISSN 1095-9203

Linares, J.F., Gustafsson, I., Baquero, F. & Martinez, J.L. (2006). Antibiotics as intermicrobial signaling agents instead of weapons. *Proceedings of the National Academy of Sciences of the United States of America*, Vol. 103, No. 51, (December 2006), pp. 19484-19489, ISSN 0027-8424

Lipinski, C.A., Lombardo, F., Dominy, B.W. & Feeney, P.J. (2001). Experimental and computational approaches to estimate solubility and permeability in drug discovery and development settings. *Advanced Drug Delivery Reviews*, Vol. 46, No. 1-3, (March 2001), pp. 3-26, ISSN 0169-409X

Miao, V. & Davies, J. (2009). Metagenomics and antibiotic discovery from uncultivated bacteria, In: *Uncultivated Microorganisms*, Epstein, S.S., (Ed.), pp. 161-180, Springer Verlag, ISBN 978-3-540-85464-7, New York, USA

Miao, V. & Davies, J. (2010). *Actinobacteria*: the good, the bad, and the ugly. *Antonie Van Leeuwenhoek*, Vol. 98, No. 2, (August 2010), pp. 143-150, ISSN 1572-9699

Molinari, G. (2009). Natural products in drug discovery: present status and perspectives, In: *Pharmaceutical Biotechnology*, Guzman, C.A. & Feuerstein, G., (Ed.), pp. 13-27, Landes Bioscience and Springer Science+Business Media, ISBN 978-1-4419-1131-5, Austin, TX, USA

Newman, D.J. & Cragg, G.M. (2004). Marine natural products and related compounds in clinical and advanced preclinical trials. *Journal of Natural Products*, Vol. 67, No. 8, (August 2004), pp. 1216-1238, ISSN 0163-3864

Newman, D.J. & Cragg, G.M. (2007). Natural products as sources of new drugs over the last 25 years. *Journal of Natural Products*, Vol. 70, No. 3, (March 2007), pp. 461-477, ISSN 0163-3864

Nguyen, K.T., Ritz, D., Gu, J.Q., Alexander, D., Chu, M., Miao, V., Brian, P. & Baltz, R.H. (2006). Combinatorial biosynthesis of novel antibiotics related to daptomycin. *Proceedings of the National Academy of Sciences of the United States of America*, Vol. 103, No. 46, (November 2006), pp. 17462-17467, ISSN 0027-8424

Nicolaou, K.C., Hughes, R., Pfefferkorn, J.A. & Barluenga, S. (2001a). Optimization and mechanistic studies of psammaplin A type antibacterial agents active against methicillin-resistant Staphylococcus aureus (MRSA). *Chemistry*, Vol. 7, No. 19, (October 2001), pp. 4296-4310, ISSN 0947-6539

Nicolaou, K.C., Hughes, R., Pfefferkorn, J.A., Barluenga, S. & Roecker, A.J. (2001b). Combinatorial synthesis through disulfide exchange: discovery of potent psammaplin A type antibacterial agents active against methicillin-resistant *Staphylococcus aureus* (MRSA). *Chemistry*, Vol. 7, No. 19, (October 2001), pp. 4280-4295, ISSN 0947-6539

O'Shea, R. & Moser, H.E. (2008). Physicochemical properties of antibacterial compounds: implications for drug discovery. *Journal of Medicinal Chemistry*, Vol. 51, No. 10, (May 2008), pp. 2871-2878, ISSN 0022-2623

Otvos, L.J., Bokonyi, K., Varga, I., Otvos, B.I., Hoffmann, R., Ertl, H.C., Wade, J.D., McManus, A.M., Craik, D.J. & Bulet, P. (2000a). Insect peptides with improved protease-resistance protect mice against bacterial infection. *Protein Science*, Vol. 9, No. 4, (April 2000), pp. 742-749, ISSN 0961-8368

Otvos, L.J., Insug, O., Rogers, M.E., Consolvo, P.J., Condie, B.A., Lovas, S., Bulet, P. & Blaszczyk-Thurin, M. (2000b). Interaction between heat shock proteins and antimicrobial peptides. *Biochemistry*, Vol. 39, No. 46, (November 2000), pp. 14150-14159, ISSN 0006-2960

Payne, D.J., Gwynn, M.N., Holmes, D.J. & Pompliano, D.L. (2007). Drugs for bad bugs: confronting the challenges of antibacterial discovery. *Nature Reviews Drug Discovery*, Vol. 6, No. 1, (January 2007), pp. 29-40, ISSN 1474-1776

Pelaez, F. (2006). The historical delivery of antibiotics from microbial natural products - can history repeat? *Biochemical Pharmacology*, Vol. 71, No. 7, (March 2006), pp. 981-990, ISSN 0006-2952

Petrini, O. (1991). Fungal endophytes of tree leaves, In: *Microbial Ecology of Leaves*, Andrews, J.H. & Hirano, S.S., (Ed.), pp. 179-197, Springer Verlag, ISBN 3540975799, New York, USA

Projan, S.J. (2003). Why is big Pharma getting out of antibacterial drug discovery? *Current Opinion in Microbiology*, Vol. 6, No. 5, (October 2003), pp. 427-430, ISSN 1369-5274

Rajendhran, J. & Gunasekaran, P. (2011). Microbial phylogeny and diversity: small subunit ribosomal RNA sequence analysis and beyond. *Microbiological Research*, Vol. 166, No. 2, (February 2010), pp. 99-110, ISSN 1618-0623

Schlunzen, F., Pyetan, E., Fucini, P., Yonath, A. & Harms, J.M. (2004). Inhibition of peptide bond formation by pleuromutilins: the structure of the 50S ribosomal subunit from *Deinococcus radiodurans* in complex with tiamulin. *Molecular Microbiology*, Vol. 54, No. 5, (December 2004), pp. 1287-1294, ISSN 0950-382X

Shank, E.A. & Kolter, R. (2009). New developments in microbial interspecies signaling. *Current Opinion in Microbiology*, Vol. 12, No. 2, (April 2009), pp. 205-214, ISSN 1879-0364

Simmons, T.L., Coates, R.C., Clark, B.R., Engene, N., Gonzalez, D., Esquenazi, E., Dorrestein, P.C. & Gerwick, W.H. (2008). Biosynthetic origin of natural products isolated from marine microorganism-invertebrate assemblages. *Proceedings of the National Academy of Sciences of the United States of America*, Vol. 105, No. 12, (March 2008), pp. 4587-4594, ISSN 1091-6490

Singh, B.K. & Macdonald, C.A. (2010). Drug discovery from uncultivable microorganisms. *Drug Discovery Today*, Vol. 15, No. 17-18, (September 2010), pp. 792-799, ISSN 1878-5832

Singh, S.B., Phillips, J.W. & Wang, J. (2007). Highly sensitive target-based whole-cell antibacterial discovery strategy by antisense RNA silencing. *Current Opinion in Drug Discovery & Development*, Vol. 10, No. 2, (March 2007), pp. 160-166, ISSN 1367-6733

Slee, A.M., Wuonola, M.A., McRipley, R.J., Zajac, I., Zawada, M.J., Bartholomew, P.T., Gregory, W.A. & Forbes, M. (1987). Oxazolidinones, a new class of synthetic antibacterial agents: in vitro and in vivo activities of DuP 105 and DuP 721. *Antimicrobial Agents and Chemotherapy*, Vol. 31, No. 11, (November 1987), pp. 1791-1797, ISSN 0066-4804

Strobel, G.A. (2002). Rainforest endophytes and bioactive products. *Critical Reviews in Biotechnology*, Vol. 22, No. 4, (January 2002), pp. 315-333, ISSN 0738-8551

Swinney, D.C. & Anthony, J. (2011). How were new medicines discovered? *Nature Reviews Drug Discovery*, Vol. 10, No. 7, (July 2011), pp. 507-519, ISSN 1474-1784

Uphoff, H.U., Felske, A., Fehr, W. & Wagner-Dobler, I. (2001). The microbial diversity in picoplankton enrichment cultures: a molecular screening of marine isolates. *FEMS Microbiology Ecology*, Vol. 35, No. 3, (May 2001), pp. 249-258, ISSN 1574-6941

US National Institutes of Health (2011). Study comparing the safety and efficacy of two doses of Bc-3781 vs vancomycin in patients with acute bacterial skin and skin structure infection (ABSSSI), August 8th 2011, Available from: http://clinicaltrialsfeeds.org/clinical-trials/show/NCT01119105

Waksman, S.A. & Woodruff, H.B. (1940). The soil as a source of microorganisms antagonistic to disease-producing bacteria. *Journal of Bacteriology*, Vol. 40, No. 4, (October 1940), pp. 581-600, ISSN 0021-9193

Walsh, C.T. & Fischbach, M.A. (2010). Natural products version 2.0: connecting genes to molecules. *Journal of the American Chemical Society*, Vol. 132, No. 8, (March 2010), pp. 2469-2493, ISSN 1520-5126

Wang, J., Soisson, S.M., Young, K., Shoop, W., Kodali, S., Galgoci, A., Painter, R., Parthasarathy, G., Tang, Y.S., Cummings, R., Ha, S., Dorso, K., Motyl, M., Jayasuriya, H., Ondeyka, J., Herath, K., Zhang, C., Hernandez, L., Allocco, J., Basilio, A., Tormo, J.R., Genilloud, O., Vicente, F., Pelaez, F., Colwell, L., Lee, S.H., Michael, B., Felcetto, T., Gill, C., Silver, L.L., Hermes, J.D., Bartizal, K., Barrett, J., Schmatz, D., Becker, J.W., Cully, D. & Singh, S.B. (2006). Platensimycin is a selective FabF inhibitor with potent antibiotic properties. *Nature*, Vol. 441, No. 7091, (May 2006), pp. 358-361, ISSN 1476-4687

Watve, M.G., Tickoo, R., Jog, M.M. & Bhole, B.D. (2001). How many antibiotics are produced by the genus *Streptomyces*? *Archives of Microbiology*, Vol. 176, No. 5, (November 2001), pp. 386-390, ISSN 0302-8933

Wicklow, D.T., Roth, S., Deyrup, S.T. & Gloer, J.B. (2005). A protective endophyte of maize: *Acremonium zeae* antibiotics inhibitory to *Aspergillus flavus* and *Fusarium verticillioides*. *Mycological Research*, Vol. 109, No. Pt 5, (May 2005), pp. 610-618, ISSN 0953-7562

Williams, G.J., Zhang, C. & Thorson, J.S. (2007). Expanding the promiscuity of a natural-product glycosyltransferase by directed evolution. *Nature Chemical Biology*, Vol. 3, No. 10, (October 2007), pp. 657-662, ISSN 1552-4450

World Health Organization (2011). World Health Day - 7th April 2011, Antimicrobial resistance: no action today, no cure tomorrow, July 8th 2011, Available from: http://www.who.int/world-health-day/2011/en/index.html

Wyatt, M.A., Wang, W., Roux, C.M., Beasley, F.C., Heinrichs, D.E., Dunman, P.M. & Magarvey, N.A. (2010). *Staphylococcus aureus* nonribosomal peptide secondary metabolites regulate virulence. *Science*, Vol. 329, No. 5989, (July 2010), pp. 294-296, ISSN 1095-9203

Yang, Y.L., Xu, Y., Straight, P. & Dorrestein, P.C. (2009). Translating metabolic exchange with imaging mass spectrometry. *Nature Chemical Biology*, Vol. 5, No. 12, (December 2009), pp. 885-887, ISSN 1552-4469

Yasumoto-Hirose, M., Nishijima, M., Ngirchechol, M.K., Kanoh, K., Shizuri, Y. & Miki, W. (2006). Isolation of marine bacteria by in situ culture on media-supplemented polyurethane foam. *Marine Biotechnology (NY)*, Vol. 8, No. 3, (May-June 2006), pp. 227-237, ISSN 1436-2228

Yu, Z., Zhao, L.X., Jiang, C.L., Duan, Y., Wong, L., Carver, K.C., Schuler, L.A. & Shen, B. (2011). Bafilomycins produced by an endophytic actinomycete *Streptomyces* sp. YIM56209. *Journal of Antibiotics (Tokyo)*, Vol. 64, No. 1, (January 2011), pp. 159-162, ISSN 0021-8820

Zasloff, M. (2002). Antimicrobial peptides of multicellular organisms. *Nature*, Vol. 415, No. 6870, (January 2002), pp. 389-395, ISSN 0028-0836

Zengler, K., Toledo, G., Rappe, M., Elkins, J., Mathur, E.J., Short, J.M. & Keller, M. (2002). Cultivating the uncultured. *Proceedings of the National Academy of Sciences of the*

United States of America, Vol. 99, No. 24, (November 2002), pp. 15681-15686, ISSN 0027-8424

Zhang, L., An, R., Wang, J., Sun, N., Zhang, S., Hu, J. & Kuai, J. (2005). Exploring novel bioactive compounds from marine microbes. *Current Opinion in Microbiology,* Vol. 8, No. 3, (June 2005), pp. 276-281, ISSN 1369-5274

4

Antibacterial Activity of Novel Sulfonylureas, Ureas and Thioureas of 15-Membered Azalides

Mirjana Bukvić Krajačić[1,2] and Miljenko Dumić[3]
[1]*GlaxoSmithKline Research Centre Zagreb, Zagreb,*
[2]*Galapagos Research Center Ltd., Zagreb,*
[3]*Department of Biotechnology, University of Rijeka, Rijeka,*
Croatia

Dedicated to all our colleagues engaged worldwide in discovery and development of azithromycin, on the occasion of the 30th anniversary of its invention (1981-2011)

1. Introduction

One of the 20th century's significant achievements is a discovery of azithromycin **(1)** and its development to commercial product for effective treatment of various infective diseases. Owing to its exceptional therapeutic and biopharmaceutical properties, it has come to be one of the most successful antibiotics worldwide. For the discovery of azithromycin, in addition to receiving numerous awards, in the year 2000, PLIVA's scientists Slobodan Djokic and Gabrijela Kobrehel together with the representatives from the US-based Pfizer, Gene Michael Bright and Arthur E. Girard, (Anonymous, 2000) were granted the honourable titles of "Heroes of Chemistry" by the American Chemical Society (ACS), a non-profit association of American chemists and chemical engineers, and the largest association of scientists in the world. This prestigious award is taken to be also recognition of the achievement of PLIVA's entire team working on azithromycin. The success of azithromycin has positioned PLIVA among the few pharmaceutical companies in the world that have developed their own blockbuster drug, and has entitled Croatia to join a small group of nations that have developed a new antibiotic.

Nowadays, on the occasion of the 30th anniversary of azithromycin's invention (1981-2011) an increasing prevalence of antibiotic-resistant pathogens suggests that we deeply entered into a "Post-Antimicrobial Era" (Cohen 1992; Travis 1994; Kirst 1996b). Investment in newer anti-infective platforms is essential and urgent in order to achieve a significant progress in our understanding of bacterial resistance and new approaches how to control it.

Macrolides as polyketide class of natural products have a long history as effective therapeutic agents for treating infectious diseases (Schönfeld & Kirst, 2002; G.T. Hansen et al., 2002; T. Kaneko et al., 2006). The popularity of this class of antibiotics, inhibiting bacterial protein synthesis by interfering with ribosome function, is largely due to their spectrum of activity and their relative safety. They are still in the centre of interest of many research groups from academic institutions and pharmaceutical companies and much effort is directed toward the discovery of new macrolide antibiotics by chemical modification of the existing classes of natural derivatives (Sunazuka et al. 2002; Pal 2006). Antibacterial macrolides have attracted considerable attention for two main reasons: (a) the emergence of atypical and/or new pathogens and extensive clinical application of these antibiotics had resulted in an increasing emergence of bacterial resistance, especially among macrolide-resistant *Streptococcus pneumoniae, Streptococcus pyogenes*, and *Staphylococcus aureus* strains, and, therefore, the development of alternative antibacterial agents became essential; (b) macrolide derivatives, especially 14- and 15-membered classes, have also become interesting for treating important chronic diseases, that is, asthma, chronic sinusitis, diffuse panbronchiolitis, cystic fibrosis (Čulić, 2001; Labro, 2000; Labro, 2004), bronchiolitis obliterans syndrome (BOS) (Vanaudenaerde et al., 2008; Culic et al., 2006), etc. Some macrolides proved active in treatment of malaria (Andersen et al., 1994; Kuschner et al., 1994; Andersen et al., 1995; Ohrt et al., 2002; Sidhu et al., 2007) and cancer (Romano et al., 2004; Oyelere et al. 2009; Mwakwari et al. 2010; Bao et al., 2010), showed antiparasitic activity (Lee et al. 2011) or act as motilides, *ie.* macrolides with gastrointestinal motor stimulating activity (Takanashi et al. 2009).

Following this trend, the chemists from PLIVA Pharmaceuticals (Zagreb, Croatia) discovered in 1980 the famous azithromycin molecule, 1 (Fig. 1), characterized by unique 15-membered macrolide ring system, having a basic methylamino group inserted into the erythromycin aglycone (Kobrehel & Djokić 1982;. Kobrehel et al., 1982; Kobrehel & Djokić, 1985; Djokić et al. 1986; Djokić et al. 1987; Djokić et al. 1988). Soon after the publication of PLIVA's Belgian azithromycin patent, researchers at Pfizer (Groton, USA) prepared azithromycin independently, as the results of their own research program (Bright 1984).

Azithromycin was, beside clarithromycin, the leader of the second-generation of macrolides, the first representative of new series of macrolides termed "azalides"(Schönfeld & Mutak 2002; Mutak 2007), and today the golden standard for macrolide antibiotics (Spaventi 2002).

Azithromycin has broad spectrum of activity against all relevant bacteria causing respiratory tract infections, including *Haemophilus influenzae* and *Moraxella catarrhalis* (Mutak, 2007). It also possesses excellent safety and tolerability profiles and is widely prescribed for the treatment of upper and lower respiratory tract infections (Kirst, 1996a; Girard et al., 1987; Schönwald et al, 1991; Retsema et al., 1986). The greatest advantages of azithromycin compared to other macrolide antibiotics are its unusual pharmacokinetics: high tissue distribution and metabolic stability. These properties have led in recent years to the widespread use of the azalide scaffold for synthesis of new antibacterial active compounds with advantageous pharmacokinetics.

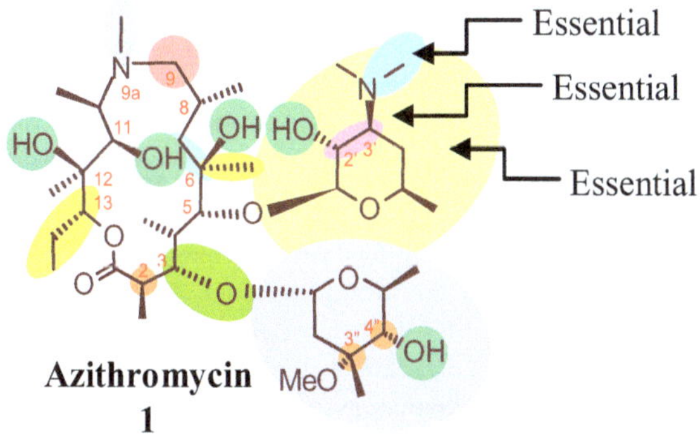

Fig. 1. Azithromycin **(1)** and its position subjected to derivatization

The growing resistance to antibiotics conferred by microorganisms commonly involved in respiratory tract infections has become a serious clinical problem (Prieto et al., 2002). The widespread use of macrolides has contributed to the increase of resistance within *Streptoccoccus pyogenes* and *Streptoccoccus pneumoniae* strains and its level varies worldwide, with an alarming upper rate of 25% in some European countries (Granizo et al., 2000; Szczypa et al., 2000; Nagai 2002 et al.,; Albrich et al., 2004). Gram-positive *S. pyogenes* and *S. pneumonia* is the most common bacterial strains implicated in acute pharyngitis, skin and soft tissue infections and also one of the most problematic respiratory pathogen (Cunningham et al., 2000).

It has been shown that the resistance to macrolide antibiotics in Gram-positive microorganisms can be attributed to two main mechanisms: target site modification and active efflux (Nakajima et al., 1999). It is known that macrolides exert their activity by binding to the large 50S ribosomal subunit. They inhibit bacteria protein synthesis at peptidyl transferase center by blocking the nascent peptide exit tunnel (Poehlsgarrd & Douthwaite, 2003). The modification of specific rRNA bases can prevent macrolides to bind. This may be due to the action of methylases encoded either by *erm*(B) or *erm*(A) genes (Weisblum, 1998). The methylases are responsible for developing macrolide, lincosamide and streptogramin B (MLS_B) resistance; inducible-(iMLS) or constitutive (cMLS). The active drug efflux is another common type of resistance developed by bacteria and is mediated by the membrane-associated pump encoded by the *mef*(A) gene (Sutcliffe et al. 1996). In order to overcome the resistance problems, lots of efforts have been made worldwide to search for novel and more potent agents with all of the desirable features of the earlier generation of macrolides.

The discovery of highly potent representatives of the third-generation of macrolides, like ketolides (Agouridas 1998), acylides (Tanikawa et al. 2001; Tanikawa et al. 2003), anhydrolides (Elliott et al. 1998), etc., was a step forward to tackle the efflux problems (LeMahieu et al. 1974; Pestka & LeMahieu 1974a & 1974b, Pestka et al. 1974; Pestka et al. 1976; Allen. 1977; Van Bambeke et al. 2008)' to (Tanikawa et al., 2001; Tanikawa et al., 2003), anhydrolides (Elliott et al., 1998), etc., was a step forward to tackle the efflux problems (LeMahieu et al., 1974; Pestka & LeMahieu 1974a & 1974b, Pestka et al., 1974; Pestka et al., 1976; Allen. 1977; Van Bambeke et al., 2008).

However, some serious drawbacks have been observed for those compound classes: the emergence of resistance developed shortly after their introduction and rare but serious side effects which lead to restrictions and withdrawal (Bambeke et al., 2008) as seen recently with telithromycin, approved by the United States (USA) Food and Drug Administration (FDA) approved in 2004 by for treatment of mild to moderate community-acquired bacterial pneumonia (CABP) (Cruzan, 2007; Farrell et al., 2010).

Recently, considering azithromycin's beneficial pharmacokinetic properties, our group have led the widespread modification of the azalide scaffold (Fig. 1) in a search for new, to resistant bacterial strains active azalides (Fajdetić et al., 2010; Fajdetić et al., 2011; Hutinec et al., 2010; Kapić et. al, 2010; Kapić et. al, 2011a; Kapić et. al., 2011b; Marušić Ištuk et al., 2011; Matanović Škugor et al., 2010; Palej Jakopović et al., 2010; Pavlović et al., 2010; Pavlović & Mutak, 2011; Štimac et al., 2010).

In this paper, we present the short overview leading to the discovery of novel sulfonylureas, ureas and thioureas of 15-membered azalides as a new class of compounds and their antibacterial activity against some key erythromycin resistant pathogens. Structural features that guided design of novel macrolides included (1) a properly attached aryl/heteroaryl-carbamoyl group for improving activity against MLS_B resistance and (2) cleavage of cladinose sugar and ketolide backbone for improving potency and activity against efflux resistance. It was expected that introduction of unsaturated unit, that is, carbamoyl group, on nitrogen at position 9a of **1** (Fig. 1) will significantly change electronic properties and also steric environment in the 'upper part' of the macrolide. It will also serve as an excellent linker for the attachment of various groups affording preparation of a library of compounds with the goal of identifying novel bacterial inhibitors.

2. Novel sulfonylureas, ureas and thioureas of 15-membered azalides

The first discovered representative of the 15-membered azalides, cyclic amine **2** (Scheme 1) named 9-deoxo-9a-aza-9a-homoerythromycin A, permitted a derivatisation line at the 9a-nitrogen atom (Scheme 1). Its first derivatization was methylation at 9a position and synthesis of 9-deoxo-9a-aza-9a-methyl-9a-homoerythromycin A, azithromycin **(1)**(Kobrehel & Djokić, 1982).

Several *N*-derivatisation lines of azalides skeleton were started in PLIVA in the early 1990s (Schönfeld & Mutak 2002; Mutak 2007), and some of the synthesized compounds showed antibacterial activity. In that respect, the observed activity of initially prepared 9a-*N*-carbamoyl and *N*-thiocarbamoyl derivatives of **2** (Kujundžić et al., 1995) encouraged us to extend our study in this direction.

Thus, a series of new sulfonylurea, urea and thiourea derivatives of 15-membered azalides were prepared in order to study whether antibacterial activity toward resistant strains would be achieved by introduction of aryl-sulfonylcarbamoyl/carbamoyl/thicarbamoyl group into the azalide molecule and how the activity would be affected by nature and position of the substituents in the phenyl ring (Bukvić Krajačić et al., 2005). Of particular interest was to study the influence of the linker between sulfonylcarbamoyl/carbamoyl/thicarbamoyl- group and aglycon moiety on the antibacterial activity. A special attention was paid to achieving the activity against *S. pyogenes* and *S. pneumonia* resistant strains.

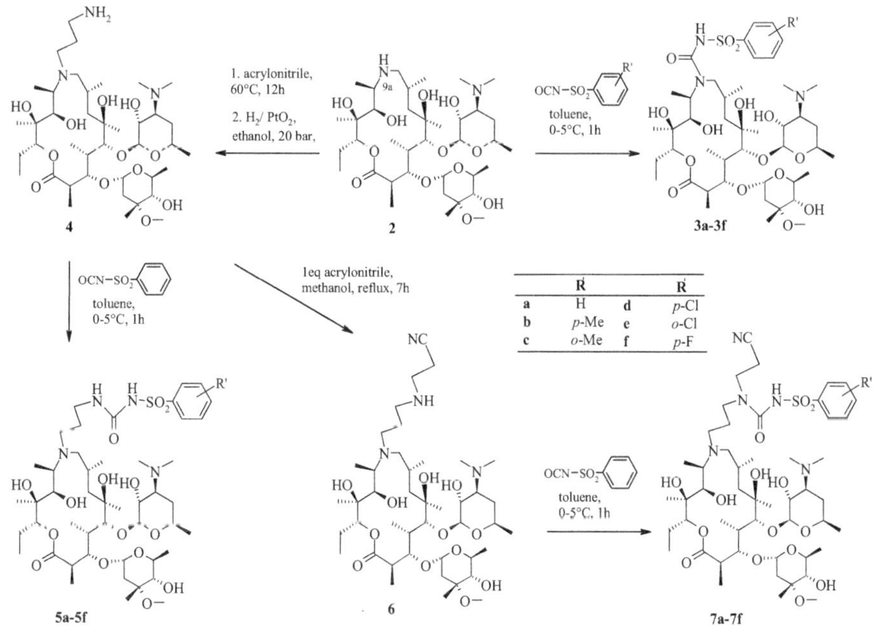

Scheme 1. Synthesis of sulfonylureas **3, 5** and **7**.

2.1 Sulfonylureas

Intermediates **2** (Djokić et al., 1986; Djokić et al., 1988) and **4**, smoothly reacted with substituted benzensulfonyl isocyanates to form 9a-*N*-[*N'*-(aryl)sulfonylcarbamoyl] derivatives, **3a-3f** and **5a-5f** in high yields (Scheme 1). The key intermediate, 9a-*N*-(γ-aminopropyl) derivative **4** was prepared by standard Michael addition of acrylonitrile to the amine **2**, followed by catalytic hydrogenation of obtained 9a-*N*-(β-cyanoethyl) derivative with PtO_2 as a catalyst (Bright et al., 1988). Derivatives **7a-7f**, were prepared by the selective cyanoethylation of amine **4** with equivalent amounts of acrylonitrile, followed by the addition of the substituted benzensulfonyl isocyanates to the intermediate **6**.

For the sulfonylureas directly linked to macrocyclic ring **3a-3f** it was observed that compounds with methyl group and chlorine in *p*- **3b** (MIC 1 μg/ml), **3d** (MIC 1 μg/ml) and *o*- **3c** (MIC 0.5 μg/ml), **3e** (MIC 2 μg/ml) positions and fluorine in *p*-position **3f** (MIC 2 μg/ml) showed significantly improved activity against iMLS resistant *S. pyogenes* strain when compared to azithromycin **1** (MIC 8 μg/ml) and starting amine **2** (MIC 16 μg/ml). Also, these compounds exhibited two level of dilution better activity than **2** (MIC 0.25 μg/ml) and similar activity to **1** (MIC $\leq$0,125 μg/ml) against sensitive *S. pneumonia* (Bukvić Krajačić et al. 2005). However, the activities against Gram-negative bacteria were all lower than those for **1** and **2**. Generally, it was observed that antibacterial activity of the novel arylsulfonylcarbamoyl derivatives **3a-3f**, **5a-5f** and **7a-7f** against all the tested erythromycin susceptible (Ery-S) Gram-positive strains decreased in the series **3a-3f** > **5a-5f** > **7a-7f** by the introduction of a propyl linker and additional cyanoethyl side chain.

2.2 Novel ureas and thioureas & macrolide-sulfonamide conjugate

Various 9a-carbamoyl and thiocarbamoyl derivatives **8** & **9** were prepared (Scheme 2) by reaction of intermediate **2** with corresponding isocyanates or isothiocyanates (Kujundžić et al., 1995). Reactions were usually conducted in toluene to achieve easily crystallisable *N*-alkyl or *N*-aryl substituted ureas. Structures of the *N*-isopropyl- (**8a**) (Kujundžić et al., 1995) and *N*-(4-pyridyl)- (**8g**) (Sheldrick et al., 1995) derivatives were confirmed by single crystal X-ray analysis. In biological testing, only a few derivatives **8** & **9** showed moderate antibacterial activity. Additional halogen-aryl derivatives of **8** & **9** have been synthesized showing moderate activity against resistant strains (Marušić-Ištuk et al., 2000).

Introduction of novel interactive groups into the azalide backbone resulted in further improvements in activity. Strategy which involved macrolide conjugates incorporating antibacterial sulfonamides, such as sulfanilamide, sulfabenz, sulfapyridine and sulfamethoxazole, showed an increased affinity for the ribosome (Bukvić Krajačić et al., 2007). Significant activity against inducible resistant *S. pyogenes* strains was observed by modifications at position 9a of an azalide lacton ring, by the carbamoyl group linked sulfonamides (Scheme 3). Conjugates of 15-membered azalides and sulfonamides **10a-10d** were prepared by the reaction of **2** (Djokić et al. 1986; Djokić et al. 1988) with 4-(chlorosulfonyl)phenylisocyanate. The smoothly formed 9a-(4-chlorosulfonylpheyl)-carbamoyl derivative was transformed without the isolation into the compounds **10a-10d**, by the reaction of ammonia, aniline, 2-aminopyridine and 5-methyl-3-aminoisoxasole, respectively.

Azalide-sulfonamide conjugates **10a** and **10b** possess two to three times better activity against iMLS resistant *S. pyogenes* strain (MIC 2 μg/ml) when compared to both azithromycin **1** (MIC 8 μg/ml) and starting cyclic amine **2** (MIC 16 μg/ml) (Bukvić Krajačić et al., 2007). These activities are comparable to those observed for azalide sulfonylureas **3a-3f** (Bukvić Krajačić et al., 2005). New azithromycin-sulfonamide conjugates **10a** and **10b** exhibit somewhat lower activity than **1** against sensitive *S. pneumonia* and *S. pyogenes* strains. Furthermore, the **10c** and **10d** showed in general lower activity against most of the tested bacterial strains except for sensitive *S. aureus* and *M. catarrhalis* where better activity was observed in comparison with **10a** and **10b** analogs (Bukvić Krajačić et al., 2007).

Further expanding the range of antimicrobial activity, especially against MLS_B and efflux-mediated resistant *S. pyogenes* and *S. pneumoniae* strains was achieved by introduction of carbamoyl and thiocarbamoyl groups attached on propyl linker at the 9a position (Bukvić Krajačić et al., 2009). Novel *N''*-aryl substituted 9a-(*N'*-carbamoyl/thiocarbamoyl-γ-aminopropyl)- **11**, **12** and 9a-[*N'*-(β-cyanoethyl)-*N'*-(carbamoyl/thiocarbamoyl-γ-aminopropyl)]- **13, 14** derivatives were obtained according to efficient procedure described for the preparation of the previous classes of compounds (Scheme 2) (Bukvić Krajačić et al., 2005 & 2007).

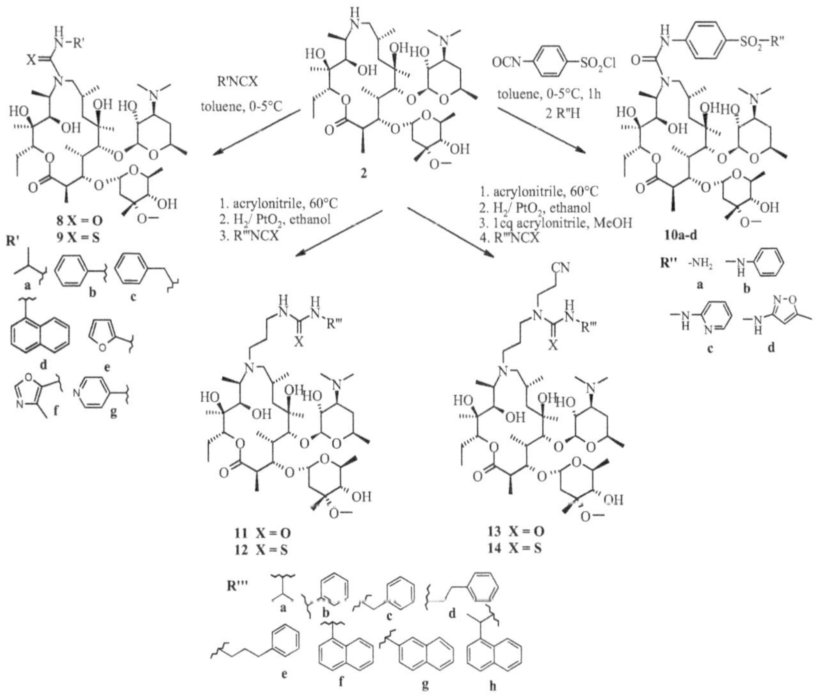

Scheme 2. Synthesis of novel ureas and thioureas of 15-membered azalides and azalide-sulfonamide conjugates

Ureas **11** and **13** and thioureas **12** and **14** (Bukvić Krajačić et al., 2009) showed a significant improvement in antibacterial activity against all tested macrolide-susceptible and resistant bacteria in comparison with carbamoyl/thiocarbamoyl derivatives **8** & **9** (Kujundžić et al. 1995), sulfonylcarbamoyl derivatives **3a-3f** (Bukvić Krajačić et al., 2005) and azithromycin-sulfonamide conjugates **10a-10d** (Bukvić Krajačić et al., 2007). Also, these compounds exhibited a substantially improved *in vitro* antimalarial activity against *P. falciparum* (Bukvić Krajačić et al., 2011b; Hutinec et al., 2011). Several ureas bearing naphthyl supstituents (**11f, 11g, 11h**) were superior *in vitro* to the azithromycin against inducible resistant *S. pyogenes* (MIC 2 μg/ml). Ureas **11f, 11g** and thioureas **12c, 12d, 12e, 12f** possesses good activity against efflux-mediated resistant *S. pyogenes* (MIC 4 μg/ml), comparable to azithromycin (MIC 4 μg/ml).

In general, all tested compounds had high *in vitro* activity against erythromycin susceptible Gram-positive aerobes, *S. pneumoniae* and *S. pyogenes* (MIC ≤ 0.125 μg/ml) (Bukvić Krajačić et al., 2009). Ureas **11** and **13** and thioureas **12** and **14** exhibited excellent activity against susceptible *S. aureus* (MIC 0.25 1 μg/ml), but lacked activity against resistant *S. aureus* strains. Ureas **11f, 11g** and thiourea **12f** also showed *in vitro* activity against efflux-mediated resistant *S. pneumoniae* with MICs 4 μg/ml and their activities were comparable with those observed for azithromycin (MIC 8 μg/ml). Ureas **11g, 11h** and **13h** showed moderate activity against cMLS *S. pneumonia* (MIC 16 μg/ml) (Bukvić Krajačić et al., 2009). *In vitro* activities of ureas **11** and **13**, thioureas **12** and **14** against key community-acquired Gram-negative respiratory pathogens were improved in comparison with sulfonylureas **3a-3f** (Bukvić Krajačić et al., 2005) and azithromycin-sulfonamide conjugates **10a-10d** (Bukvić Krajačić et al., 2007). Ureas **11f, 11g** and **11h** demonstrated high activity against *Moraxella catarrhalis.* Naphthyl substituted ureas **11f, 11g** and **11h** showed better activity against Gram-negative pathogens involved in respiratory tract infections (RTI), *M. catarrhalis* (MIC 0.25 μg/ml) and *H. influenza* (MIC 1 μg/ml) than derivatives with phenyl ring on the alkyl side-chain **11b-11d**. In case of phenylethyl-substituents in **11d** and **12d** the presence of thiocarbamoyl moiety seemed to improve activity against *H. influenzae.* The urea **13** with cyanoethyl chain showed similar antibacterial activity in comparison to the urea **11**. The observed antibacterial activity of ureas and thioureas increased in the series **8** & **9** < **11** & **12** < **13** & **14**, by the introduction of a propyl linker and additional cyanoethyl side-chain (Bukvić Krajačić et al., 2009).

On the basis of excellent *in vitro* antibacterial activity and their structural similarity, several compounds **11f, 11g, 11h, 12c, 12d, 12e, 12f, 13h, 14c, 14d, 14e** were screened for acid stability, cytotoxicity and preliminary pharmacokinetic parametars. In acidic conditions compounds exhibited azithromycin like stability (Bukvić Krajačić et al., 2009). *In vitro* cytotoxicity on Hep G2 and THP-1 cell lines measured for the selected set of compounds revealed that all compounds showed relatively low cytotoxicity *in vitro* (IC_{50}s ≥ 4 μM) (Bukvić Krajačić et al., 2011b). These marked them as potent and selective compounds for further profiling (Steinmeyer, 2006). Metabolic stability of ureas and thioureas were screened *in vitro* using human and mouse liver microsomes and only a few were selected for *in vivo* rat pharmacokinetic studies in order to determine their pharmacokinetic profiles (Table 1) (Bukvić Krajačić et al., 2011b). All compounds demonstrated good *in vitro*, metabolic stability with $t_{1/2}$ greater than 120 min ($t_{1/2}$ = 103 min for compound **14d** in human liver microsomes). As was observed with azithromycin, and in line with the *in vitro* data, these analogs had a low systemic clearance, moderate to high volume of distribution and a very long half-life, however, the oral bioavailability was low (**12c, 12e**) to moderate (Bukvić Krajačić et al., 2011b).

	CL (mL/min/kg)	Vd (L/kg)	$t_{1/2}$ (hr)	Oral F (%)
Azithromycin	11.0	20.0	24.0	33.0
12c	4.0	10.4	30.0	3.4
12e [a]	2.3	2.6	13.4	1.3
14e	24.5	31.7	15.2	21

CL - blood clearance, Vd – apparent volume of distribution at the terminal phase based on drug concentration in blood, $t_{1/2}$ - half life, [a] - IV parameters determined in one rat

Table 1. Pharmacokinetic parameters estimated in blood after intravenous (IV) and oral gavage (PO) administration to Sprague-Dawley rats (10 mg/kg IV and 30 mg/kg PO) (Bukvić Krajačić t al., 2011b).

Preliminary *in vitro* microsomal stability data indicated that these compounds had good metabolic stability, as was confirmed by low clearances *in vivo* for the compounds tested. In comparison to azithromycin, known for its extensive tissue distribution, (Schönfeld & Mutak, 2002) these derivatives had a tendency toward higher volumes of distribution, in line with their increased lipophilic character (approx. 2-3 log units higher than azithromycin, according to calculated logP values, data not shown) due to the presence of strong lipophilic aromatic phenyl and naphtyl rings in the 9a-*N* substituent (Bukvić Krajačić et al., 2011b). Overall, with increased *in vitro* activity and promising *pharmacokinetic* properties, this series of molecules represents a good starting platform for the design of novel antibacterial and antimalarial azalides.

2.3 3-Decladinosyl-derivatives of sulfonylureas, ureas and thioureas

Introduction of unsaturated, sp[2] hybridized, carbamoyl unit at 9a position placed nitrogen atom of **2** significantly change electronic properties and also steric environment in the 'upper part' of the macrolide, what resulted in increased antibacterial activity of the novel sulfonylureas **3,5,7** (Bukvić Krajačić et al., 2005), azalide-sulfonamide conjugates **10** (Bukvić Krajačić et al., 2007), and ureas and thioures **11-14** (Bukvić Krajačić et al., 2009). On the other hand, the selectively achieved cleavage of cladinose sugar, significantly changes the structural behaviour of the 'lower part' of 9a-carbamoyl 15-membered azalides, leading to the 3-*O*-decladinosyl-3-hydroxy ureas and thiouras lacking of any, as expected, antibacterial activity (Bukvić Krajačić et al., 2005; Bukvić Krajačić et al., 2007; Marušić Ištuk et al., 2007).

However, there are some novel highly potent 3-*O*-decladinosyl derivatives of 14-membered macrolides, *e.g.* ketolides (Agouridas et al, 1998), acylides (Tanikawa et al., 2001; Tanikawa et al., 2003), anhydrolides (Elliott et al., 1998), etc. (Schönfeld & Kirst 2002; Pal 2006; Kaneko et al. , 2006; Mutak 2007) (Fig. 2), proved active against resistant bacterial strains.

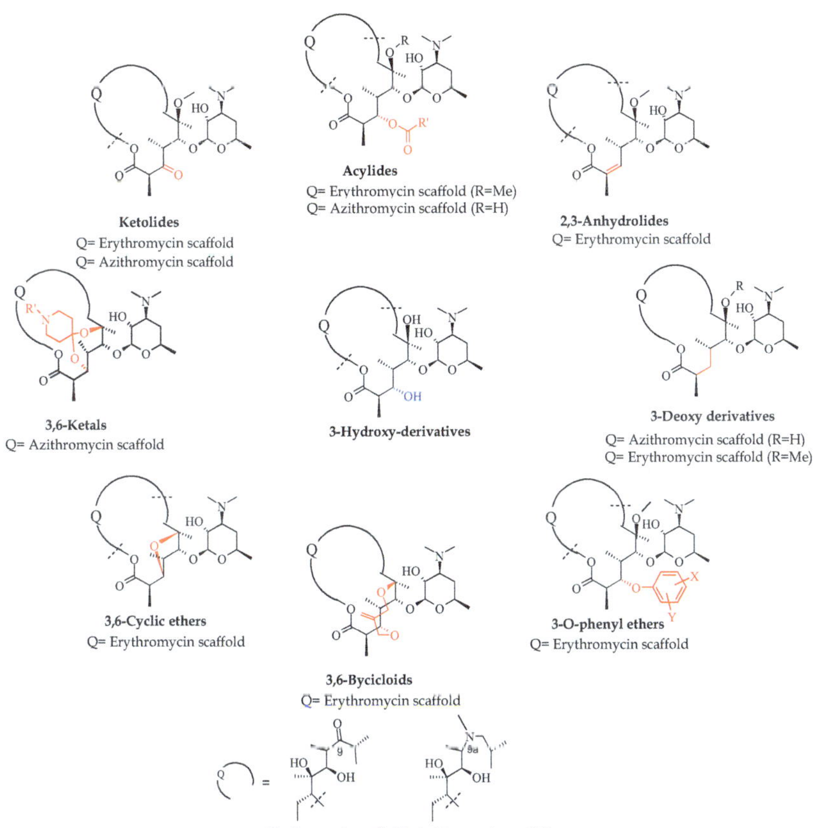

Fig. 2. Novel classes of 3-*O*-decladinosyl derivatives of 14- and 15-membered macrolides

2.3.1 3-Decladinosyl-3-O-substituted derivatives

Isopropyl- and 2,4-dichlorophenyl- derivatives of 9a-carbamoyl-6-hydroxy (**17** & **18**) and 9a-carbamoyl-6-methoxy azalides (**19** & **20**) lacking any antibacterial activity, were selected to study the effects of the 'lower part' of azalide skeleton modifications *via* chemical transformations of hydroxyl group at C-3 position (Scheme 3) (Marušić Ištuk et al., 2007). They afforded formation of the new ketolides **23** and **24**, anhydrolides **27** and **28**, hemiketals **21** and **22**, cyclic ethers **25** and **26**, and acylides **29** and **30** (Scheme 4). In order to perform chemical transformations on the hydroxyl group at position 3, 2'-hydroxyl group which is the most reactive one, was suitably protected. Consequently, reaction of 3-decladinosyl-3-hydroxy- azalides **17**, **18**, **19**, and **20** with acetic anhydride in the presence of a base smoothly afforded 2'-*O*-acetyl-3-decladinosyl-3-hydroxy-6-hydroxy azalides, that under conditions of Pfitzner–Moffat 3-OH group oxidation, followed by subsequent methanolysis of 2'-*O*-acetyl intermediate produces internal 3,6-hemiketal structures **21** and **22**. Under the same reaction conditions 2'-*O*-acetyl-3-decladinosyl-3-hydroxy-6-methoxy derivatives afford 3-keto azalides **23** and **24** (Scheme 3). Introduction of mesyl group at position C-3 of 6-hydroxy-, **17**

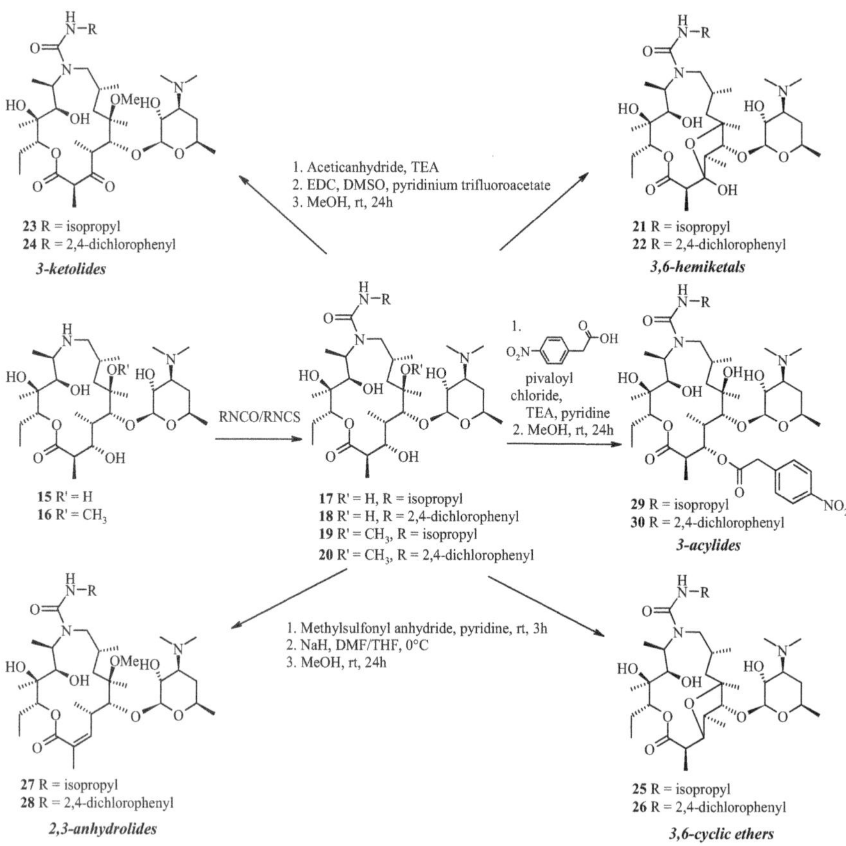

Scheme 3. Synthesis of 3-decladinosyl-3-*O*-substituted azalides

& **18**, and 6-methoxy-, **19** & **20** derivatives and subsequent base-promoted elimination led to the formation of different products. Whereas 6-hydroxy derivatives **17** & **18** produce 3,6-cyclic ethers **25** and **26**, 6-methoxy derivatives **19** & **20** afford 2,3-anhydro azalides **27** and **28**.

Among already known 3-acylides of 14-membered macrolides, 3-*O*-(4-nitrophenyl)acetyl derivative of clarithromycin (TEA-0777) showed the best antibacterial activity (Tanikawa et al., 2001). Accordingly, 9a-carbamoyl acylides having (4-nitrophenyl)acetyl- functionality attached to 3-O position, azalides **29** and **30**, were prepared, to test if antibacterial activity could be enhanced upon attachment of favorite side-arm.

3-Decladinosyl-6-hydroxy and 6-methoxy azalides **15** and **16** and 9a-carbamoyl/9a-thiocarbamoyl derivatives **17, 18, 19** & **20** proved antibacterially inactive against tested strains. Similar situation can be seen with 3,6-hemiketals **21** & **22** and 3,6-cyclic ethers **25** & **26**. However, anhydrolides **27** and **28** as well as ketolides **23** and **24** show good antibacterial activity against efflux resistant *S. pneumonia* but lower in comparison to erythromycin. 9a-Carbamoyl-3-*O*-(4-nitrophenyl)acetyl- acylides **29** and **30** showed the best antibacterial activity against efflux resistant *S. pneumoniae* (MIC 4 μg/ml), and better in comparison to erythromycin (MIC 8 μg/ml). Acylides **29** and **30** also show weak activity against erythromycin-resistant *S. aureus* (Marušić Ištuk et al., 2007).

2.3.2 3-Decladinosyl-3-hydroxy derivatives

As expected, 3-decladinosyl-3-hydroxy- azalides **17** - **20** and **31** - **34** (Fig. 3) lacked any significant antimicrobial activity (Marušić Ištuk et al., 2007; Bukvić Krajačić et al., 2005; Bukvić Krajačić et al., 2007) being consistent with the role cladinose was found to play in antimicrobial activity (LeMahieu et.al., 1974; Kaneko et.al., 2006; Pal, 2006; Tanikawa et.al., 2001; Mutak, 2007).

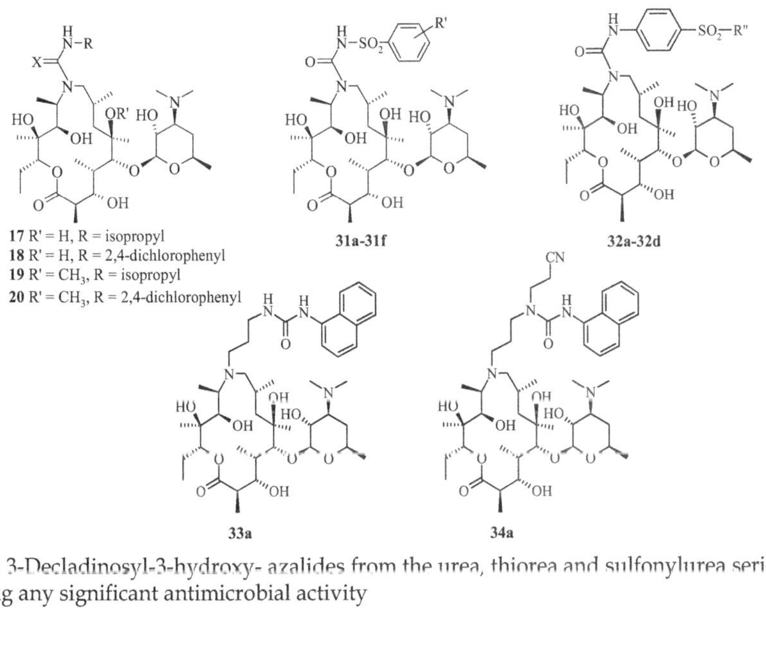

Fig. 3. 3-Decladinosyl-3-hydroxy- azalides from the urea, thiorea and sulfonylurea series, lacking any significant antimicrobial activity

This is supported by recently published NMR binding studies (trNOESY and STD experiments) on 6-*O*-methyl-homoerythromycin derivatives, showing that the absence of cladinose sugar has been found to be the main cause of their inability to bind to their target ribosome (Novak et al., 2009). Stability study of the most active compounds **11f** and **13f** in the artificial gastric juice (Bukvić Krajačić et al., 2009) led to the formation of two decladinosyl derivatives **33a** and **34a** which were tested only against panel of *S. pneumoniae* strains. As was expected decladinosyl urea derivative **34a** did not show activity against tested strains. However, decladinosyl urea derivative **33a** showed significant activity against erythromycin susceptible *S. pneumoniae* strain (1 µg/ml), as well as efflux-mediated *S. pneumoniae* resistant strain (8 µg/ml) comparable to azithromycin. This finding initiated the synthesis of a small library of 3-decladinosyl-3-hydroxy ureas and thioureas of 15-membered azalides termed *"decladinosylides"* (Bukvić Krajačić et al., 2011a).

High reactivity of secondary and primary amino groups of 3-decladinosyl- derivatives **37** and **38** toward isocyanates and isothiocyanates assured highly site-selective introduction of carbamoyl and thiocarbamoyl groups and preparation of ureas **33** & **34** and thioureas **35** & **36** in high yield (Scheme 4). They were found to posses good antibacterial activities against key respiratory Gram-positive and Gram-negative pathogens including efflux-mediated resistant strains.

Among them, most of the synthesized 3-decladinosyl-3-hydroxy derivatives showed moderate to high activity against efflux-mediated resistant *S. pneumoniae* and moderate activity against susceptible *S. pneumoniae* and *S. pyogenes* strains. Against efflux-mediated resistant *S. pneumoniae* compound **35a** (MIC 2 µg/ml) posses better activity compared to azithromycin (**1**) (MIC 8 µg/ml) (Bukvić Krajačić et al., 2011a) and their parent 3-cladinosyl analogues **11** & **13** (MIC 4 to 16 µg/ml) (Bukvić Krajačić et al., 2009), and significantly better in comparison to the 3-decladinosyl-3-hydroxy azithromycin (**16**) (MIC >64 µg/ml).

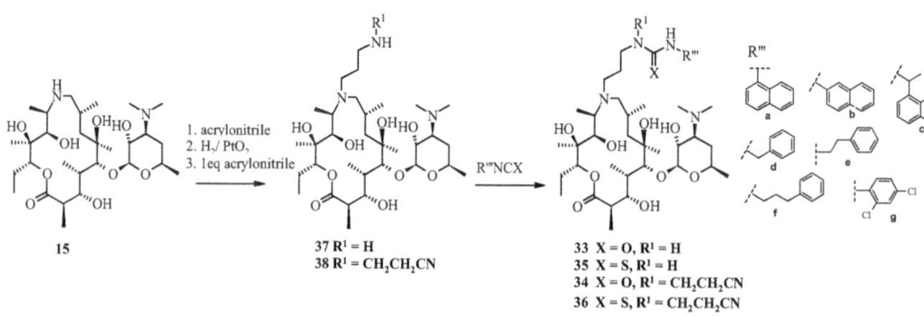

Scheme 4. Synthesis of novel 3-decladinosyl ureas and thioureas of 15-membered azalides.

The racemic urea derivative **33c** showed the highest activity against both, susceptible *S. pneumoniae* and *S. pyogenes* strains, and the same activity as its 3-cladinosyl analogue (±)-**11h** and azithromycin (MIC ≤0.125 µg/ml) (Bukvić Krajačić et al., 2009).

Interestingly, some of discovered 3-decladinosyl-3-hydroxy ureas **33** & **34**, and thioureas **35** & **36**, maintain antibacterial activity against Gram-negative pathogens *H. influenzae* and *M. catarrhalis* (Bukvić Krajačić et al., 2011a) in comparison to their parent 3-cladinosyl derivatives **11, 12, 13** & **14**, (Bukvić Krajačić et al., 2009) and demonstrate large improvement in comparison to the inactive 3-decladinosyl sulfonylureas **31**(Bukvić Krajačić et al., 2005) and 3-decladinosyl azithromycin-sulfonamide conjugates **32** (Bukvić Krajačić et al., 2007). Activity of (±)-**33a** and **35a** against *H. influenzae* is only one dilution lower than the corresponding MIC of azithromycin (MIC 2 μg/ml). Urea (±)-**33c** was more potent (MIC 8 μg/ml) than its 3-cladinosyl analogue (±)-**11h** (MIC 16 μg/ml) against *Enterococcus faecalis* and **33a** showed the same activity against *E. coli* in comparison to its cladinosyl analogue **11f**. (Bukvić Krajačić et al., 2011a).

Thus, it seems that appropriate linked urea or thiourea moiety at 9a-*N* of 3-decladinosyl-3-hydroxy- azalides might interact with particular ribosome binding sites and "substitute" the cladinose sugar interaction. In order to gain more information about that conformational analysis of a compound **35a** was carried out by using systematic conformational search around flexible propyl linker. Analysis of NOE cross peaks in the NOESY spectrum indicated that there is no strong interaction between macrolactone ring and the substituent at 9a-position of **35a,** pointing to the stretched conformations that were also found to be most stable ones in the conformational analysis (Bukvić Krajačić et al., 2011a). Superposed x-ray conformations of ABT-773, (Auerbach et al., 2009), azithromycin (Schlunzen et al., 2003; Hansen et al., 2002), two bound conformations of telithromycin from *Deinococcus radiodurans* (Berisio et al. 2003) and *Haloarcula marismortui* (Hansen et al., 2002) and the lowest conformation for compound **35a** were shown in Fig. 4 (Bukvić Krajačić et al., 2011a).

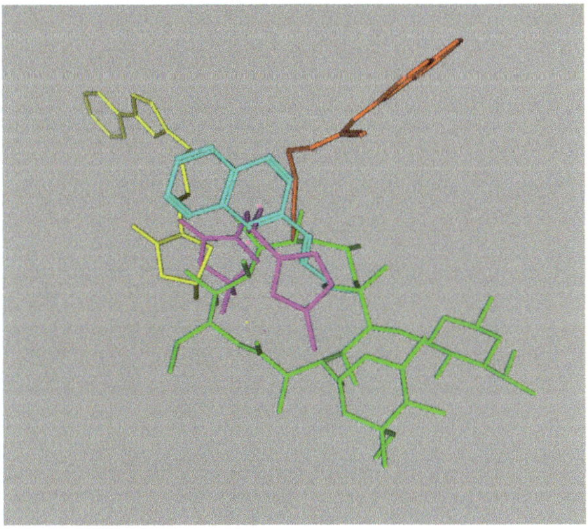

Fig. 4. Superposed x-ray conformations for azithromycin (green) (Hansen et al., 2002), ABT-773 (cyan) (Auerbach et al., 2009), two conformations of telithromycin from *Deinococcus radiodurans* (magenta)(Berisio et al. 2003) and *Haloarcula marismortui* (yellow)(Hansen et al., 2002) complexes and most stable conformation for compound **35a** (red) (Bukvić Krajačić et al., 2011a).

It is clear that substituents at different positions have different spatial arrangements with respect to macrolactone. Until now there is a number of evidence including here mentioned ketolides (Auerbach et al., 2009; Schlunzen et al., 2003; Hansen et al., 2002; Berisio et al., 2003), that high structural diversity is tolerated within the flexible macrolide-binding site of ribosome. In spite of the knowledge gained so far on macrolide binding, (Novak et al., 2006; Novak et al., 2009; Auerbach et al., 2009; Schlunzen et al., 2003; Hansen et al., 2002; Berisio et al., 2003) an understanding of the mode of their interactions with ribosome still remain incomplete with many issues unresolved. Therefore, it can only be speculated about the possible binding mode of the compound **35a** but it is likely that the additional interaction involving 1-naphthyl-propyl- side-chain, attached at the 9a position, might lead to a further stabilization of a complex with ribosome (Bukvić Krajačić et al., 2011a).

3. Concluding remarks

In summary, the coupling of a arylsulfonyl and benzenesulfonamido moiety to the 9a position of 15-membered azalide scaffold *via* carbamoyl linker has indicated improvement in antibacterial activity of novel azalides.

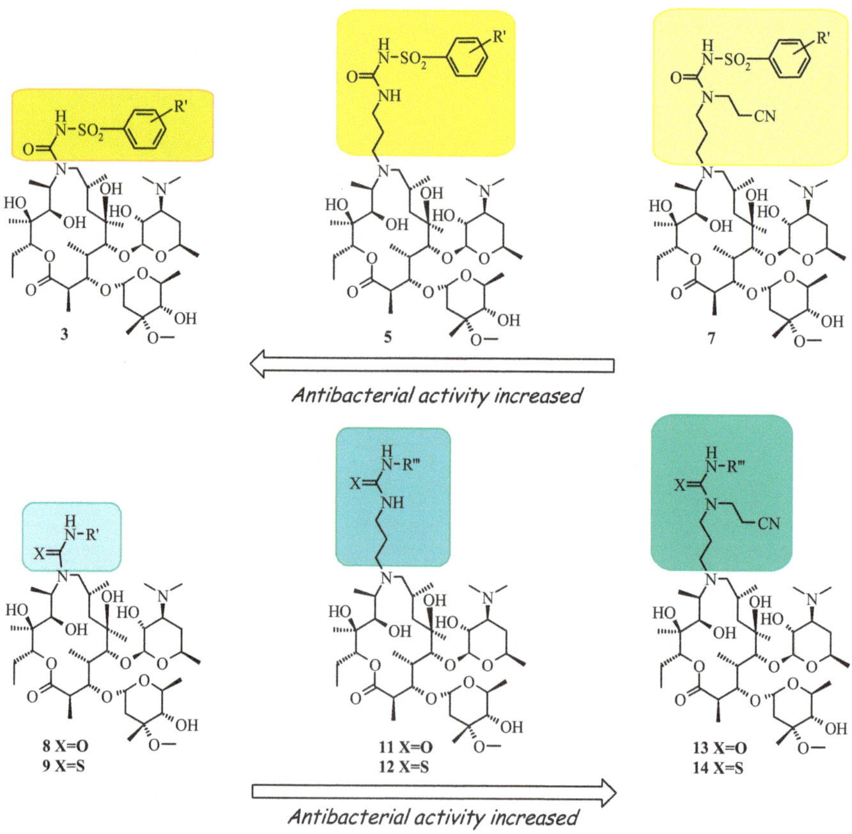

Fig. 5. Antibacterial activities of urea and thiourea derivatives of 15-membered azalides in comparison to sulfonylurea analogues.

Hence, newly synthesised sulfonyl ureas of azalides **3b-3f**, and azalide-sulfonamide conjugates **10a** and **10b** displayed significantly improved activity against inducible resistant *S. pyogenes* strain when compared to azithromycin.

In addition, the introduction of carbamoyl and thiocarbamoyl group at the 9a position of azithromycin like azalide skeleton *via* propyl linker proved to be promising method to tackle the resistance problems.

As a result of a preliminary optimization of an alkyl/aryl moiety attached at the carbamoyl and thiocarbamoyl group all prepared and tested compounds had high *in vitro* activity against erythromycin susceptible Gram-positive aerobes and Gram-negative microorganisms and especially resistant *S. pyogenes* and *S. pneumoniae strains.* It was also, shown here that urea and thiourea derivatives of 3-decladinosyl-3-hydroxy azalides, although lacking a cladinose sugar, showed noticeable antibacterial activity.

Overall mutual comparison of obtained results can be summarized in three items:

- The observed increase of antibacterial activity in the series of ureas and thioureas **11, 12, 13** and **14** (Bukvić Krajačić et al., 2009) in comparison with those of their analogues **8** and **9** (Kujundžić et al., 1995), was opposite to the results obtained for the sulfonylcarbamoyl derivatives **3, 5** and **7** (Bukvić Krajačić et al., 2005) where a decrease of activity was found when sulfonylcarbamoyl moiety was further away from the azalide ring (Fig. 6)

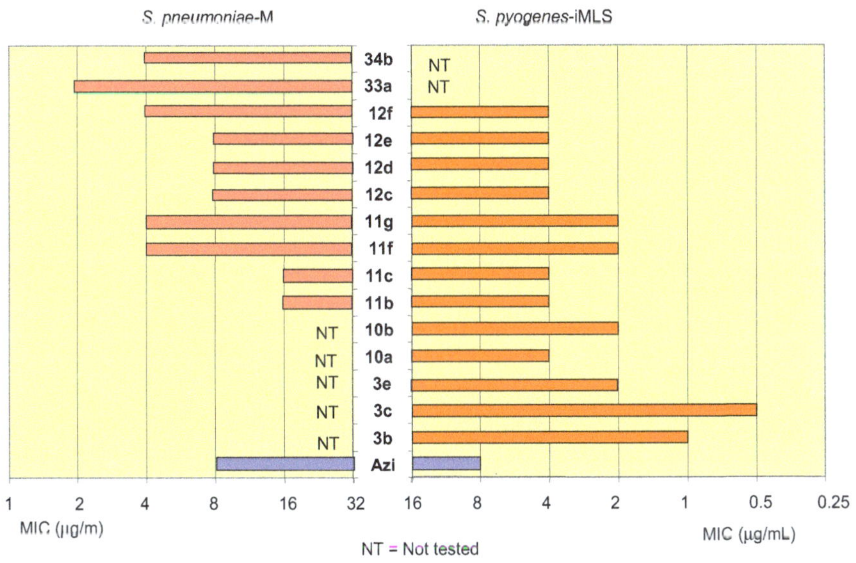

Fig. 6. Antibacterial activity of selected novel sulfonylureas, ureas and thioureas of 15 membered azalides on *S. Pneumoniae efflux-mediated* (Bukvić Krajačić et al., 2009) and *S. pyogenes* iMLS (Bukvić Krajačić et al., 2005) resistant strains in comparison to azithromycin

- Several novel sulfonylureas (Bukvić Krajačić et al., 2005), ureas and thioureas (Bukvić Krajačić et al. 2009) of 15-membered azalides showed same or significantly better activity on *S. pneumoniae efflux-mediated and S. pyogenes* iMLS resistant strains in comparison to azithromycin (Fig 7). Among them, new ureas with naphtyl substituents (**11f, 11g** & **11h**) showed better activity against inducible resistant *S. pyogenes* in comparison to azithromycin. Ureas **11f** & **11g** and thioureas **12c, 12d, 12e** and **12f** possess good activity against efflux-mediated resistant *S. pyogenes*, comparable to azithromycin.

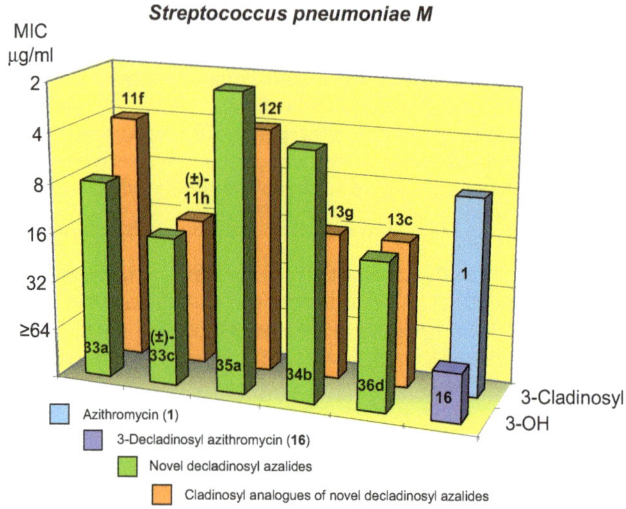

Fig. 7. Antibacterial activity of 3-decladinosyl-3-hydroxy ureas and thioureas on *S. pneumoniae* efflux-mediated resistant strain (Bukvić Krajačić et al., 2011) in comparison to their parent 3-cladinosyl analogues (Bukvić Krajačić et al., 2009) and test standards azithromycin (**1**) and 3-decladinosyl azithromycin (**16**).

- Contrary to the well known fact (LeMahieu, et.al., 1974; Kaneko et.al., 2006; Pal, 2006; Tanikawa, et.al., 2001; Mutak, 2007) and previous results (Bukvić Krajačić et al., 2005, Bukvić Krajačić et al., 2007; Marušić Ištuk et al., 2007), that simple removal of cladinose sugar from macrolides significantly decreases antibacterial activity, unexpectedly, some of the newly discovered 3-decladinosyl-3-hydroxy ureas **33** & **34**, and thioureas **35** & **36** (Bukvić Krajačić et al., 2011) maintain good antibacterial activity against panel of key respiratory Gram-positive and Gram-negative pathogens. Against efflux-mediated resistant *S. pneumoniae* strain they posses comparable or better activity (MIC 2 -16 µg/ml) to their 3-cladinosyl parent analogues **11** & **13** (MIC 4 -16 µg/ml) (Bukvić Krajačić et al., 2009) and azithromycin (**1**) (MIC 8 µg/ml), and significantly better in comparison to the inactive 3-decladinosyl azithromycin (**16**) (MIC >64 µg/ml) (Fig. 7) (Bukvić Krajačić et al., 2011). Also, some 3-decladinosyl-3-hydroxy ureas **33** & **34**, and thioureas **35** & **36**, maintain antibacterial activity against Gram-negative pathogens *H. influenzae* and *M. catarrhalis* in comparison to their parent 3-cladinosyl derivatives (Bukvić Krajačić et al., 2009), and comparable to azithromycin, but demonstrate a large improvement in comparison with inactive 3-decladinosyl azithromycin **16** (Bukvić Krajačić et al., 2011) and other 3-decladinosyl derivatives reported in literature. These small library of 3-decladinosyl-3-hydroxy ureas and thioureas of 15-membered azalides we termed *"decladinosylides."*

In general, novel sulfonylureas, ureas and thioureas of 15-membered azalides and their 3-decladinosyl-3-hydroxy derivatives showed their potential to serve as a good platform for further investigation in order to discover new derivatives having an improved overall biological profile with a special emphasis on resistant bacterial strains.

4. Acknowledgements

The Ministry of Science, Education and Sports of the Republic of Croatia is acknowledged for the financial support (Project No. 006-0000000-3216).

5. References

Agouridas, C.; Denis, A.; Auger, J.; Benedetti, Y.; Bonnefoy, A.; Bretin, F.; Chantot, J. F.; Dussarat, A.; Fromentin, C.; D'Ambrieres, S. G.; Lachaud, S.; Laurin, P.; Martret, O. L.; Loyau, V. & Tessot, N. (1998). Synthesis and Antibacterial Activity of Ketolides (6-*O*-Methyl-3-oxoerythromycin Derivatives): A New Class of Antibacterials Highly Potent Against Macrolide-Resistant and -Susceptible Respiratory Pathogens. *Journal of Medicinal Chemistry*, Vol. 41, No. 21, (September 1998) pp. 4080-4100, ISSN 0022-2623

Albrich, W. C.; Monnet, D. L. & Harbarth, S. (2004). Antibiotic Selection Pressure and Resistance in Streptococcus pneumoniae and Streptococcus pyogenes. *Emerging Infectious Diseases*, Vol. 10, No. 3, pp. 514-517, ISSN 1080-6059

Alihodžić, S.; Fajdetić, A.; Kobrehel, G.; Lazarevski, G.; Mutak, S.; Pavlović, D.; Štimac, V.; Čipčić, H.; Dominis Kramarić, M.; Eraković, V.; Hasenöhrl, A.; Maršić, N. & Schönfeld, W. (2006). Synthesis and Antibacterial Activity of Isomeric 15-Membered Azalides. *Journal of Antibiotics*, Vol. 59, No.12, (December 2006), pp. 753-769, ISSN 0021-8820

Allen, N., (1977). Macrolide Resistance in *Staphylococcus aureus*: Inducers of Macrolide Resistance. *Antimicrobial Agents Chemotherapy*, Vol. 11, (April 1977), pp. 669-674, ISSN 1098-6596.

Andersen, S. L.; Ager, A. L.; McGreevy, P.; Schuster, B. G.; Ellis, W.; Berman, J. (1994). Efficacy of azithromycin as a causal prophylactic agent against murine malaria. *Antimicrobial Agents Chemotheraphy*, Vol. 38, (August 1994). pp. 1862-1863, ISSN 1098-6596

Andersen, S. L.; Ager, A.; McGreevy, P.; Schuster, B. G.; Wesche, D.; Kuschner, R.; Ohrt, C.; Ellis, W.; Rossan, R.; Berman, J. (1995). Activity of azithromycin as a blood schizonticide against rodent and human plasmodia in vivo. *The American Journal Tropical Medicine and Hygiene*, (February 1995). Vol. 52, pp. 159-161, ISSN 0002-9637

Anonymous (2000) Heroes of Chemistry Recipients, American Chemical Society Portal, http://portal.acs.org/portal/acs/corg/content?_nfpb=true&_pageLabel=PP_SUPERARTICLE&node_id=1464&use_sec=false&sec_url_var=region1&__uuid=91e8ce27-b8ba-4450-9088-5835121094b4, Sept. 7, 2011).

Auerbach, T.; Mermershtain, I.; Bashan, A.; Davidovich, C.; Rozenberg, H.; Sherman, D. H.; Yonath, A. (2009). Structural basis for the antibacterial activity of the 12-membered-ring mono-sugar macrolide methymycin *Biotechnologia*, Vol.1, (January 2009), pp. 24-35, ISSN 0860-7796

Bao, K.; Qiao, F.; Liang, L.; Li, H.; Zhu, H.; Zhang, W. & Wu, Y. (2010). Synthesis and antiproliferative activity of novel erythromycin derivatives. *Medicinal Chemistry Communications*, Vol. 1, No. 4, (August 2010). pp. 294-298, ISSN 2040-2503

Berisio, R.; Harms, J.; Schluenzen, F.; Zarivach, R.; Hansen, H.A.S.; Fucini, P. & Yonath, A. (2003). Structural Insight into the Antibiotic Action of Telithromycin against Resistant Mutants. *Journal of Bacteriology*, Vol. 185, No. 14, (May 2003), pp. 4276-4279, ISSN 0021-9193

Bright, G. M. (Pfizer), (1984). Antibacterial N-methyl 11-aza-10-deoxo-10-dihydro-erythromycin A and pharmaceutically acceptable acid addition salts thereof, intermediates therefore, and processes for their preparation. US 4 474 768, Oct. 2, 1984 (US Prior. Nov. 15, 1982).

Bright, G. M.; Nagel, A. A.; Bordner, J.; Watrous, K. A. ; Sciavolino, F. C.; English, A. R.; Retsema, J. A. ; Anderson, M. R. ; Brennan, L. A.; Borovoy, R. J.; Cimochowski, C. R.; Faiella, J. A. ; Girard, A. E.; Girard, D.; Herbert, C.; Manousos, M. & Mason, R. (1988). Synthesis, *in vitro* and *in vivo* activity of novel 9-deoxo-9a-aza-9a-homoerythromycin A derivatives; a new class of macrolide antibiotics, the azalides. *Journal of Antibiotics*, Vol. 41: No. 8, (February 1988), pp. 1029-1047, ISSN 0021-8820

Bukvić Krajačić, M.; Kujundžić, N.; Dumić, M.; Cindrić, M.; Brajša, K.; Metelko, B. & Novak, P. (2005). Synthesis, Characterization and *in vitro* Antimicrobial Activity of Novel Sulfonylureas of 15-Membered Azalides. *Journal of Antibiotics*, Vol. 58, No.6, (June 2005), pp. 380–389, ISSN 0021-8820

Bukvić Krajačić, M.; Novak, P.; Cindrić, M.; Brajša, K.; Dumić, M. & Kujundžić, N. (2007). Azithromycin-sulfonamide conjugates as inhibitors of resistant *Streptococcus pyogenes* strains. *European Journal of Medicinal Chemistry*, Vol. 42 No. 2, (February 2007), pp. 138-145, ISSN 0223-5234

Bukvić Krajačić, M.; Novak, P.; Dumić, M.; Cindrić, M.; Čipčić Paljetak, H. & Kujundžić, N. (2009). Novel ureas and thioureas of 15-membered azalides with antibacterial activity, against key respiratory pathogens. *European Journal of Medicinal Chemistry*, Vol. 44, No. 9, (September 2009), pp. 3459-3470, ISSN 0223-5234

Bukvić Krajačić, M.; Dumić, M.; Novak, P.; Cindrić, M.; Koštrun, S.; Fajdetić, A.; Alihodžić, S.; Brajša, K. & Kujundžić, N. (2011a) Discovery of Novel Ureas and Thioureas of 3-Decladinosyl-3-hydroxy 15-Membered Azalides Active Against Efflux-mediated Resistant *Streptococcus Pneumoniae*. *Bioorganic & Medicinal Chemistry Letters*, Vol. 21 No. 2, (January 2011), pp. 853-856, ISSN 0960-894X

Bukvić Krajačić, M.; Perić, M.; Smith, K. S.; Ivezić Schönfeld, Z.; Žiher, D.; Fajdetić, A.; Kujundžić, N.; Schönfeld, W.; Landek, G. ; Jelić, D.; Ager, A.; Milhous, W. K. ; Ellis, W.; Spaventi, R. & Ohrt , C. (2011b). Synthesis, Structure-Activity Relationship and Antimalarial Activity of Ureas and Thioureas of 15-membered Azalides. *Journal of Medicinal Chemistry*, Vol. 54, No. 10, (April 2011), pp. 3595-3605, ISSN 0022-2623

Čulić, O. ; Bosnar, M.; Marjanovic, N.; Erakovic, V.; Jelic, D. & Verbanac, D. (2006). 9A-Carbamoyl and Thiocarbamoyl azalides with anti-inflammatory activity PCT Int. Appl. WO 2006097849 A1 20060921.

Čulić, O.; Eraković, V. & Parnham, M. (2001). Anti-inflammatory effects of macrolide antibiotics, *European Journal of Pharmacology, Vol. 429, No. 1-3, (October)*, pp.209-229 ISSN: 0014-2999

M. L. Cohen, M. L. (1992). Epidemiology of Drug Resistance: Implications for a Post–Antimicrobial Era, *Science*, Vol. 257, No. 5073 (August 1992), pp. 1050-1055); ISSN: 0036-8075

Cruzan, S. (2007). FDA Announces Label and Indication Changes for the Antibiotic Ketek, February 12, 2007 http://www.fda.gov/NewsEvents/Newsroom/PressAnnouncements/2007/ucm108842.htm (Sept. 8, 2011)

Cunningham, M. W. (2000). Pathogenesis of Group A streptococcal infections. *Clinical Microbiology Review,* Vol. 13, pp. 470-511, ISSN 0983-8512

Djokić, S.; Kobrehel, G.; Lazarevski, G.; Lopotar, N.; Tamburašev, Z.; Kamenar, B.; Nagl, A. & Vicković, I. (1986). Erythromycin series. Part 11. Ring expansion of erythromycin A oxime by the Beckmann rearrangement. *Journal of Chemical Society, Perkin Trans. I* (January 1986) pp. 1881–1990 ISSN 1472-7781

Djokić, S. Kobrehel, G. & Lazarevski, G. (1987). Erythromycin series XII. Antibacterial *in vitro* evaluation of 10-dihydro-10-deoxo-11-azaerythromycin A: synthesis and structure activity relationship of its acyl derivatives. *Journal of Antibiotics,* Vol. 40, pp. 1006-1015; ISSN 0021-8820

Djokić, S; Kobrehel, G.; Lopotar, N.; Kamenar, B.; Nagl, A.& Mrvoš, D. (1988). Erythromycin series. Part 13. Synthesis and structure elucidation of 10-dihydro-10-deoxo-11-methyl-11-azaerythromycin A. *Journal of Chemical Research* (S), pp. 152~153, *ibid.,* Miniprint, pp. 1239-1257, ISSN 0308-2342

Elliott, R. L.; Pireh, D.; Griesgraber, G.; Nilius, A. M.; Ewing, P. J.; Bui, M. H.; Raney, P. M.; Flamm, R. K.; Kim, K.; Henry, R.F.; Chu, D. T. W.; Plattner, J. J. & Or, Y. S.(1998) Anhydrolide Macrolides. 1. Synthesis and Antibacterial Activity of 2,3-Anhydro-6-*O*-methyl 11,12-Carbamate Erythromycin A Analogues. *Journal of Medicinal Chemistry,* Vol. 41, No. 10, (April 1998), pp. 1651-1659, ISSN 0022-2623

Fajdetić, A.; Čipčić Paljetak, H.; Lazarevski, G.; Hutinec, A.; Alihodžić, S.; Đerek, M.; Štimac, V.; Andreotti, D.; Šunjić, V.; Berge, J.M.; Mutak, S.; Dumić, M.; Lociuro, S.; Holmes, D.J.; Maršić, N.; Eraković Haber, V. & Spaventi R., (2010). 4''-*O*-(ω-Quinolylamino-alkylamino)propionyl derivatives of selected macrolides with the activity against the key erythromycin resistant respiratory pathogens, *Bioorganic and Medicinal Chemistry,* Vol. 18, No. 17, (September 2010), pp. 6559-6568, ISSN: 09680896

Fajdetić, A.; Vinter, A.; Čipčić Paljetak, H.; Padovan, J.; Palej Jakopović, I.; Kapić, S.; Alihodžić, S.; Filić, D.; Modrić, M.; Košutić-Hulita, N.; Antolović, R.; Ivezić Schönfeld, Z.; Mutak, S.; Eraković Haber, V. & Spaventi R. Synthesis, activity and pharmacokinetics of novel antibacterial 15-membered ring macrolones, *European Journal of Medicinal Chemistry* Vol.46, No. 8, (August 2011), pp. 3388-3397, ISSN: 0223-5234

Farrell, D. J.; Castanheira, M.; Sader, H. S. & Jones, R. N. (2010).The *in vitro* evaluation of solithromycin (CEM-101) against pathogens isolated in the United States and Europe (2009), *Journal of Infection* Vol. 61, No. 6 (December 2010), pp. 476-483; ISSN 0163-4453

Girard, A. E.; Girard, D.; English, A. R.; Gotz, T. D.; Cimochowski, C. R.; Faiella, J. A.; Haskell, S. L. & Retsema, J. A (1987). Pharmacokinetic and in vivo studies with azithromycin (CP-62,993), a new macrolide with an extended half life and excellent tissue distribution. *Antimicrobial Agents Chemotheraphy,* Vol. 31, (December 1986), pp. 1948-1954, ISSN 1098-6596

Granizo, J.J.; Aguilar, L.; Casal, J.; Dal-Ré, R. & Baquero F. (2000). *Streptococcus pyogenes* resistance to erythromycin in relation to macrolide consumption in Spain (1986-1997). *Journal of Antimicrobial Chemotherapy,* Vol. 46, pp. 959-964, ISSN 1460-2091

Hansen, G. T.; Metzler, K. L.; DeCarolis, E. & Blondeau, J.M.; (2002). The macrolides, *Expert Opin. Investig. Drugs,* Vol. 11, No. 2, (Feb. 2002), pp. 189-215, ISSN 1354-3784, eISSN 1744-7658.

Hansen, J. L.; Ippolito, J. A.; Ban, N.; Nissen, P.; Moore, P. B.; Steitz, T. A. (2002). The Structures of Four Macrolide Antibiotics Bound to the Large Ribosomal Subunit. *Molecular Cell,* Vol. 10, No. 1, (July 2002), pp. 117-128, ISSN 1097-2765

Hutinec, A.; Djerek, M.; Lazarevski, G.; Šunjić, V.; Čipčić Paljetak, H.; Alihodžić, S. Eraković Haber, V.; Dumić, M.; Maršić N. & Mutak S. (2010). Novel 8a-aza-8a-homoerythromycin-4''-(3-substituted-amino)propionates with broad spectrum antibacterial activity, *Bioorganic and Medicinal Chemistry Letters* Vol. 20, No. 11 (June 2010), pp. 3244–3249; ISSN: 0960-894X

Hutinec, A.; Rupčić, R.; Žiher, D.; Smith, K. S.; Milhous, W. ; Ellis, W. ; Ohrt, C. & Ivezić Schönfeld, Z. (2011). An automated, polymer-assisted strategy for the preparation of urea and thiourea derivatives of 15-membered azalides as potential antimalarial chemotherapeutics. *Bioorganic and Medicinal Chemistry,* Vol. 19, No. 5, (March 2011), pp. 1692-1701, ISSN 0968-0896

Kaneko, T., Dougherty, T.J. & Magee, T.V. (2006). Macrolide Antibiotics, In: *Comprehensive Medicinal Chemistry II,* D. Triggle, J. Taylor, J. Plattner, M. C. Desai (Eds.), Vol. 7 pp. 519-566, Therapeutic Areas II, Elsevier, ISBN 0-08-044513-6

Kapić, S.; Čipčić Paljetak, H.; Alihodžić, S.; Antolović, R.; Eraković Haber, V.; Jarvest, R. L.; Holmes, D. J.; Broskey, J. P. & Hunt, E. (2010). 6-Alkylquinolone-3-carboxylic acid tethered to macrolides synthesis and antimicrobial profile, *Bioorganic and Medicinal Chemistry,* Vol. 18, No. 17, (September 2010), pp. 6569-6577, ISSN 0968-0896

Kapić, S.; Fajdetić, A.; Koštrun, S.; Čikoš, A.; Čipčić Paljetak, H.; Antolović, R.; Holmes, D. J. & Alihodžić, S., (2011a). Synthesis and Activity of New Macrolones: Conjugates Between 6(7)-(2′-Aminoethyl)-amino-1-cyclopropyl-3-carboxylic acid (2′-hydroxyethyl) amides and 4″-Propenoyl-azithromycin, *Bioorganic and Medicinal Chemistry, In Press, Accepted Manuscript,* doi: 10.1016/j.bmc.2011.07.011; Accepted Date: 8 July 2011; ISSN 0968-0896

Kapić, S.; Čipčić Paljetak, H.; Palej Jakopović, I.; Fajdetić, A.; Ilijaš, M.; Štimac, V.; Brajša, K.; Holmes, D. J. ; Berge, J. & Alihodžić, S. (2011b). Synthesis of macrolones with central piperazine ring in the linker and its influence on antibacterial activity *Bioorganic and Medicinal Chemistry, In Press, Accepted Manuscript,* doi: 10.1016/j.bmc.2011.07.010; Accepted Date: 8 July 2011; ISSN 0968-0896

Kirst, H. A. (1996a). Expanding the Role of Macrolide Compounds as Terapeutic Agent, In: *Studies in Medicinal Chemistry* Choudhary, M. I. (Ed.), Vol. 1, Harwood Academic Publisher, Amsterdam, pp. 1-47, ISBN: 978-0-444-51572-8

Kirst, H. A. (1996b). Aminoglycoside, Macrolide, Glycopeptide, and Miscellaneous Antibacterial antibiotics, in: Wolf M. E. (Ed.), *Burger's Medicinal Chemistry and Drug Discovery,* Fifth Ed., Vol. 2, Ch. 32, Wiley Interscience, New York, 1996, pp. 463-525; ISBN 0-471 57557-7.

G. Kobrehel, G. & S. Djokić, S. (PLIVA), (1982). Nouveaux derives de l'erythromycine A, procede pour leur preparation et leur utilisation comme substances antibacteriennes, BE 892 357, July 1, 1982, (YU Prior. March 6, 1981)

Kobrehel, G.; Radobolja, G.; Tamburašev, Z.; & Djokić, S. (PLIVA), (1982). 11-Aza-10-deoxo-10-dihydroerythromycin A and derivatives thereof as well a process for their preparation. US 4 328 334 (1982)

Kobrehel, G. & Djokić, S. (PLIVA) (1985). 11-Methyl-11-aza-4-*O*-cladinosyl-6-*O*-desosaminyl-15-ethyl-7,13,14-trihydroxy-3,5,7,9,12,14-hexamethyl-oxacyclopentadecane-2-one and derivatives thereof. US 4 517 359, (May 14, 1985)

Kujundžić, N.; Kobrehel, G.; Banić, Z.; Kelnerić, Z. & Kojić-Prodić, B. (1995) Azalides: Synthesis and antibacterial activity of novel 9a-*N*-(*N'*-substituted carbamoyl and thiocarbamoyl) derivatives of 9-deoxo-9a-aza-9a-homoerythromycin A. *European Journal of Medicinal Chemistry,* Vol. 30, (January 1995), pp. 455–462, ISSN 0223-5234

Kuschner, R. A.; Heppner, D. G.; Andersen, S. L.; Wellde, B. T.; Hall, T.; Schneider, I.; Ballou, W. R.; Foulds, G.; Sadoff, J. C. & Schuster, B. (1994). Azithromycin prophylaxis against a chloroquine-resistant strain of Plasmodium falciparum. *Lancet,* Vol. 343, No. 8910, pp. 1396-1397, ISSN 0140-6736

Labro, M.-T. (2000). Interference of Antibacterial Agents with Phagocyte Functions: Immunomodulation or "Immuno-Fairy Tales"?. *Clinical Microbiology Review,* Vol. 13, (October 2000), pp. 615 - 650, ISSN: 1098-6618.

Labro, M.-T. (2004). Macrolide antibiotics: current and future uses, *Expert Opinion in Pharmacotheraphy.* Vol. 5, No. 3 (March 2004), pp. 541–550, ISSN: 1465-6566

Lee, Y.; Choi, J. Y.; Fu, H.; Harvey, C.; Ravindran, S.; Roush, W. R.; Boothroyd, J. C. & Khosla, C. (2011). Chemistry and Biology of Macrolide Antiparasitic Agents, *Journal of Medicinal Chemistry.* Vol. *54,* No. 8 (April 2011), pp 2792–2804, ISSN 0022-2623

LeMahieu, R. A.; Carson, M.; Kierstead, R. W.; Fern, L. M. & Grunberg E. (1974). Glycoside cleavage reactions on erythromycin A. Preparation of erythronolide A. *Journal of Medicinal Chemistry.* (September 1974), Vol. 17, No. 9, pp. 953-956, ISSN 0022-2623

Marušić-Ištuk, Z.; Kujundžić, N.; Kobrehel, G; Mutak, S & Maršić, N. (2000). Halo derivatives of 9-deoxo-9a-aza-9a-homoerythromycin A. WO 00/66603, November 9 2000

Marušić Ištuk, Z.; Mutak, S.; Kujundžić, N. & Kragol, G. (2007). Novel 9a-carbamoyl- and 9a-thiocarbamoyl-3-decladinosyl-6-hydroxy and 6-methoxy derivatives of 15-membered macrolides. *Bioorganic and Medicinal Chemistry,* (April 2007), Vol. 15, 4498-4510, ISSN 09680896

Marušić Ištuk, Z.; Čikoš, A.; Gembarovski, D.; Lazarevski, G.; Djilović, I.; Matković-Čalogović, D. & Kragol, G. (2011). Novel 9a,11-bridged azalides: One-pot synthesis of N'-substituted 2-imino-1,3-oxazolidines condensed to an azalide aglycone, *Bioorganic and Medicinal Chemistry Vol.* 19, No. 1, (January 2011), pp. 556–566; ISSN 0968-0896

Matanović Škugor, M.; Štimac, V.; Palej, I.; Lugarić, D.; Čipčić Paljetak, H.; Filić, D., Modrić, M.; Đilović, I.; Gembarovski, D.; Mutak, S.; Eraković Haber, V.; Holmes, D. J.; Ivezić-Schönfeld, Z. & Alihodžić, S. (2010). Synthesis and biological activity of 4"-*O*-acyl derivatives of 14- and 15-membered macrolides linked to ω-quinolone-carboxylic unit, *Bioorganic & Medicinal Chemistry,* Vol. 18, No. 17 (September 2010), pp. 6547–6558; ISSN 0968-0896

Mutak, S. (2007). Azalides from Azithromycin to New Azalide Derivatives. *Journal of Antibiotics,* Vol. 60, No. 2, (January 2007), pp. 85–122, ISSN 0021-8820

Mwakwari, S. C.; Guerrant, W.; Patil, V.; Khan, S. I.; Tekwani, B. L.; Gurard-Levin, Z. A.; Mrksich, M. & Oyelere, A. K. (2010). Non-Peptide Macrocyclic Histone Deacetylase Inhibitors Derived from Tricyclic Ketolide Skeleton, *Journal of Medicinal Chemistry,*Vol. *53, No.* 16, (August 2010), pp 6100–6111; ISSN 0022-2623

Nagai, K.; Appelbaum, P. C.; Davies, T. A.; Kelly, L. M. ; Hoellman, D. B. ; Tambic Andrasevic, A.; Drukalska, L.; Hryniewicz, W. ; Jacobs, M. R.; Kolman, J.; Miciuleviciene, J.; Pana, M.; Setchanova, L.; Konkoly Thege, M.; Hupkova, H.; Trupl, J. & Urbaskova, P. (2002). Susceptibility to Telithromycin in 1,011 *Streptococcus pyogenes* Isolates from 10 Central and Eastern European Countries. *Antimicrobial Agents Chemotheraphy,* Vol. 46, No. 2, pp. 546-549, ISSN 1098-6596

Nakajima, Y. (1999). Mechanisms of bacterial resistance to macrolide antibiotics. *Journal Infection and Chemotherapy,* Vol. 5, pp. 61-74, ISSN 1341-321X

Novak, P.; Tatić, I.; Tepeš, P.; Koštrun, S. & Barber, J. (2006). Systematic Approach to Understanding Macrolide-Ribosome Interactions: NMR and Modeling Studies of Oleandomycin and Its Derivatives. *Journal of Physical Chemistry A,* Vol. 110, No. 2, (August 2006), pp. 572-579, ISSN 1089-5639

Novak, P.; Barber, J.; Čikoš, A.; Arsić, B.; Plavec, J.; Lazarevski, G.; Tepeš, P. & Košutić-Hulita, N. (2009). Free and bound state structures of 6-O-methyl homoerythromycins and epitope mapping of their interactions with ribosomes. *Bioorganic & Medicinal Chemistry,* Vol. 17, No. 16, (August 2009), pp. 5857-5867, ISSN 09680896

Ohrt, C.; Willingmyre, G. D.; Lee, P.; Knirsch, C. & Milhous, W. (2002). Assessment of azithromycin in combination with other antimalarial drugs against *Plasmodium falciparum in vitro. Antimicrobial Agents Chemotheraphy,* Vol. 46, (August 2002), pp. 2518-2524, ISSN 1098-6596

Oyelere, A. K.; Chen, P. C.; Guerrant, W.; Mwakwari, S. C.; Hood, R.; Zhang Y. & Fan, Y. (2009). Non-Peptide Macrocyclic Histone Deacetylase Inhibitors, *Journal of Medicinal Chemistry,*Vol. *52, No.* 2, (January 2009), pp 456–468; ISSN 0022-2623

Pal, S. (2006). A journey across the sequential development of macrolides and ketolides related to erythromycin. *Tetrahedron,* Vol. 62, No. 14, (April 2006), pp. 3171–3200, ISSN: 0040-4020

Palej Jakopović, I.; Kragol, G.; Forrest, A. K.; Frydrych, C. S.V.; Štimac, V.; Kapić, S.; Matanović Škugor, M.; Ilijaš, M.; Čipčić Paljetak, H.; Jelić, D.; Holmes, D. J.; Hickey, D. M.B.; Verbanac, D.; Eraković Haber, V. & Alihodžić, S. (2010) Synthesis and properties of macrolones characterized by two ether bonds in the linker. *Bioorganic and Medicinal Chemistry,* Vol. 18, No. 17, (September 2010), pp. *6578-6588,* ISSN: 09680896

Pavlović, D.; Fajdetić, A. & Mutak, S. (2010). Novel hybrids of 15-membered 8a- and 9a-azahomoerythromycin A ketolides and quinolones as potent antibacterials. *Bioorganic and Medicinal Chemistry*, Vol. 18, No. 24, (December 2010), pp. 8566-8582, ISSN: 09680896

Pavlović D. & Mutak , S. (2011). Discovery of 4''-Ether Linked Azithromycin-Quinolone Hybrid Series: Influence of the Central Linker on the Antibacterial Activity, *ACS Med. Chem. Lett.*, Vol. 2 , No. 5 (May 2011), pp 331–336; ISSN: 1948-5875

Pestka, S. & LeMahieu, R. (1974a). Inhibition of [14C]Chloramphenicol Binding to *Escherichia coli* Ribosomes by Erythromycin Derivatives. *Antimicrobial Agents Chemotherapy,* Vol. 6, (July 1974), pp. 39-45, ISSN 1098-6596

Pestka, S. & Lemahieu, R. A. (1974b). Effect of Erythromycin Analogues on Binding of [14C]Erythromycin to *Escherichia coli* Ribosomes *Antimicrobial Agents Chemotherapy,* Vol. 6, (October 1974), pp. 479-488, ISSN 1098-6596.

Pestka, S.; Lemahieu, R. A. & Miller, P. (1974). Correlation of Effects of Erythromycin Analogues on Intact Bacteria and on [14C]Erythromycin Binding to *Escherichia coli* Ribosomes. *Antimicrobial Agents Chemotherapy* Vol. 6, (October 1974), pp. 489-491, ISSN 1098-6596.

Pestka, S.; Vince, R.; LeMahieu, R.; Weiss, F.; Fern, L.; Unowsky, J. (1976). Induction of Erythromycin Resistance in *Staphylococcus aureus* by Erythromycin Derivatives. *Antimicrobial Agents Chemotherapy,* Vol. 9, (January 1976), pp. 128-130, ISSN 1098-6596

Poehlsgarrd, J. & Douthwaite, S. (2003). Macrolide antibiotic interaction and resistance on the bacterial ribosome. *Current Opinion in Investigational Drugs,* Vol. 4, pp. 140-144, ISSN 1472-4472

Prieto, J.; Calvo, A. & Gómez-Lus M. L. (2002). Antimicrobial resistance: a class effect?. *Journal of Antimicrobial Chemotherapy,* Vol. 50 (Suppl. S2), pp. 7-12, ISSN 1460-2091

Retsema, J.; Girard, A.; Schelkly, W.; Manousos, M.; Anderson, M.; Bright, G.; Borovoy, R.; Brenan, L. & Manson R. Spectrum and mode of action of azithromycin (CP-62,993), a new 15-membered-ring macrolide with improved potency against Gram-negative organisms. *Antimicrobial Agents Chemotheraphy,* Vol. 31, (December 1986), pp. 1939-1947, ISSN 1098-6596

Romano, M. F.; Avellino, R.; Petrella, A.; Bisogni, R.; Romano, S. & Venuta, S. (2004). Rapamycin inhibits doxorubicin-induced NF-κB/Rel nuclear activity and enhances the apoptosis of melanoma cells. *European Journal of Cancer,* (December 2004) Vol. 40, No. 16, pp. 28292836, ISSN 0959-8049

Schlunzen, F.; Harms, J. M.; Franceschi, F.; Hansen, H. A.; Bartels, H.; Zarivach, R. & Yonath, A. (2003) Structural Basis for the Antibiotic Activity of Ketolides and Azalides. *Structure,* Vol. 11, No. 3, pp. 329-338, ISSN 0969-2126

Schönfeld W. & Kirst H. A. (Eds.), (2002). *Macrolide Antibiotics,* Birkhäuser Verlag, Basel, ISBN: 978-0-12-526451-8

Schönfeld, W. & Mutak S., (2002). Azithromycin and Novel Azalides In: *Macrolide Antibiotics,* Schönfeld, W.; Kirst H. A. (Eds.), pp. 73-95, Birkhäuser Verlag, Basel, ISBN: 978-0-12-526451-8,

Schönwald, S.; Škerk, V.; Petričević, I.; Cart, V.; Majerus-Mišić, L. & Gunjača, M. (1991). Comparison of three-day and five-day courses of azithromycin in the treatment of atypical pneumonia. *Europen Journal of Clinical Microbiology and Infectious Diseases,* Vol. 10, pp. 877-880, ISSN 0934-9723

Sheldrick, G.M.; Kojić-Prodić; B., Banić; Z., Kobrehel; G. & Kujundžić, N. (1995). Structure of 9-deoxo-9a-*N*-(*N'*-(4'-pyridyl)carbamoyl)-9a-aza-9a-homoerythromycin A and conformational analysis of analogous 9a-aza 15-membered azalides in solid state. *Acta Crystallographica* B51, Part. 3, (June 1995), pp. 358–366, eISSN 1600-5740

Sidhu, A. B.; Sun, Q.; Nkrumah, L. J.; Dunne, M. W.; Sacchettini, J. C. & Fidock, D. A. (2007). In vitro efficacy, resistance selection, and structural modeling studies implicate the malarial parasite apicoplast as the target of azithromycin. *Journal Biological Chemistry,* Vol. 282, (November 2006), pp. 2494-2504, ISSN 0021-9258

Spaventi, R. (2002). R&D Challenges for the Future, PLIVA R & D booklet, PLIVA Zagreb 2002 (http://www.pliva.com/press/news/article/665/RD-Challenges-for-the-Future.html; Sept. 6, 2011)

Steinmeyer, A. (2006). The hit-to-lead process at Schering AG: strategic aspects. *ChemMedChem.,* Vol. 1, pp. 31-36, ISSN 1860-7187

Štimac, V.; Matanović Škugor, M.; Palej Jakopović, I.; Vinter, A.; Ilijaš, M.; Alihodžić S. & Mutak S. (2010).· Initial Scale-Up and Process Improvements for the Preparation of a Lead Antibacterial Macrolone Compound, *Organic Process Resesearch and Development,* Vol. *14,* No. 6, (November 2010), pp 1393–1401 ISSN: 1083-6160

Sunazuka, T.; Omura, S.,.; Iwasaki, S.; Ōmura, S. (2002). Chemical Modification of Macrolides, In *Macrolide Antibiotics, Chemistry, Biology and Practice,* 2nd. Ed., Ōmura S., (Ed.), Academic Press, New York, pp. 99- 180; ISBN 978-0-12-526451-8

Sutcliffe, J.; Tait-Kamradt, A. & Wondrack, L. (1996). *Streptococcus pneumoniae* and *Streptococcus pyogenes* resistant to macrolides but sensitive to clindamycin: a common resistance pattern mediated by an efflux system. *Antimicrobial Agents Chemotheraphy,* Vol. 40, pp. 1817-24, ISSN 1098-6596

Szczypa, K.; Sadowy, E.; Izdebski, R. & Hryniewicz, W. (2004). A rapid increase in macrolide resistance in *Streptococcus pyogenes* isolated in Poland during 1996-2002. *Journal of Antimicrobial Chemotherapy,* Vol. 54, pp. 828~831, ISSN 1460-2091

Takanashi, H. & Cynshi, O. (2009). Motilides: A long and winding road: Lessons from mitemcinal (GM-611) on diabetic gastroparesis, *Regulatory Peptides,*Vol. 155, No. 1-3, (June 2009), pp, 18-23; ISSN: 0167-0115

Tanikawa, T.; Asaka, T.; Kashimura, M.; Misawa, Y.; Suzuki, K.; Sato, M.; Kameo, K.; Morimoto, S. & Nishida, A. (2001). Synthesis and Antibacterial Activity of Acylides (3-*O*-Acyl-erythromycin Derivatives): A Novel Class of Macrolide Antibiotics. *Journal of Medicinal Chemistry,* (October 2001), Vol. 44, No. 24, pp. 4027-4030, ISSN 0022-2623.

Tanikawa, T.; Asaka, T.; Kashimura, M.; Suzuki, K.; Sugiyama, H.; Sato, M.; Kameo, K.; Morimoto, S. & Nishida, A. (2003). Synthesis and Antibacterial Activity of a Novel Series of Acylides: 3-*O*-(3-Pyridyl)acetylerythromycin A Derivatives. *Journal of Medicinal Chemistry,* Vol. 46, No. 13 (May 2003), pp. 2706-2715, ISSN 0022-2623

Travis, J. (1994). Reviving the Antibiotic Miracle? *Science,* Vol. 264, No. 5157 (April 1994), pp. 360-362; ISSN: 0036-8075

Vanaudenaerde, B. M.; Meyts, I.; Vos, R.; Geudens, N. ; De Wever, W.; Verbeken, E.K. ; VanRaemdonck, D.E.; Dupont, L.J. & Verleden, G.M. (2008). A dichotomy in bronchiolitis obliterans syndrome after lung transplantation revealed by azithromycin therapy. *Eururopean Respiratory Journal,* Vol. 32, No. 4, (October 2008), pp 832–843, ISSN: 0903-1936

Van Bambeke, F.; Harms, J. M.; Van Laethem, Y.; Tulkens, P. M. (2008). Ketolides: pharmacological profile and rational positioning in the treatment of respiratory tract infections. *Expert Opinion in Pharmacotherapy* Vol. 9, No. 2, (January 2008), pp. 267-283, ISSN 1465-6566

Weisblum, B. (1998). Macrolide resistance. *Drug Resistance Updates,* Vol. 1, pp. 29-41, ISSN 1368-7646

5

Antimicrobial Activity of Condiments

André Silvério and Maria Lopes
*Department of Microbiology, Faculty of Pharmacy, University of Lisbon
Portugal*

1. Introduction

The phenomenon of antibiosis, life prevents life, observed by Goubert and Pasteur in 1877, gave rise to the use of antibiotics in therapy. In fact, on that date has been found that certain microorganisms were sensitive to the action of products produced by other microorganisms. Unfortunately, many of these products were toxic to the cells of higher animals, and only in 1943, the first antibiotic isolated and studied by Sir Alexander Fleming - penicillin G – was introduced in clinic. Penicillin was discovered in 1929 when Fleming sought potential antibacterial compounds. He noted that a colony of the fungus *Penicillium notatum* had grown up on a plate containing the bacterium *Staphylococcus aureus* and around the fungus had a zone where the bacteria did not grow. The active substance, Fleming called penicillin, but could not isolate it. Several years later, in 1939, Ernst Chain and Howard Florey developed a way to isolate penicillin and used it to treat bacterial infections during the Second World War. The new drug came into use in the clinic in 1946 and had a huge impact on public health. Its discovery and development revolutionized modern medicine and paved the way for the development of many more antibiotics of natural origin.

Antimicrobial activity is understood as the ability of some agents to eliminate microorganisms (aiming at different metabolic or structural targets, as nucleic acid synthesis disruption or peptidoglycan synthesis inhibition) or by inhibiting their growth.

Before the introduction of antibiotics in the 1940s, infections were rare, but rapidly increased in frequency as increased the use of antibiotics. In fact, most antibiotics that were first used in the 1940s and 1950s are no longer used clinically because nowadays the resistance of infectious beings to these antibiotics is very common. Over time they have been developing new antibiotics and with the introduction of each, new drug-resistant bacteria appeared rapidly. Today, we moved the mode of use and prescription of antibiotics in order to try to slow the relentless pace of bacterial evolution, but not yet found a solution to this problem. Microbiologists continue to study how bacteria evolve so that we can predict how they will respond to medical treatment and so we can better manage the evolution of infectious diseases.

This microbiocidal or microbiostatic activity is, on one's mind, usually related with therapeutic objectives or sanitizing activities within the food or pharmaceutical industries. Nevertheless, in our daily routine, and also linked with food microbiology, we are faced with a number of substances, which we use only as culinary additives, that may work as antimicrobial agents or may turn to be a good source of new antimicrobial molecules for industrial application and, therefore, may turn to have an increased economic value. The search for new antibacterial molecules in spices and herbs is particularly important. Multidrug-resistant strains are becoming increasingly common, both in hospitals and community, raising the need for expanding research. Moreover, the effective life duration of classic antibiotics is decreasing, probably due to overconsumption and misuse. The global attention on infectious diseases going epidemic, like human immunodefficiency virus (HIV), raises even more the interest on drugs of non-microbial origin.

In many regions of the world a large variety of plants and herbs are used for their medicinal value, treating various diseases, some of infectious nature. Historically, the use of plants, in particular edible plants, is widely reported since ancient times and is associated with some sort of medicinal effect, and these plants were used (some still are) against bacteria, fungi, viruses and even helmiths (Cowan, 1999). The therapeutic use of such products in some areas is related not only with cultural aspects, traditional medicine, availability of these products, with some plants and herbs endemic to very specific areas, as parts of Latin America, Africa and Asia, but also related with economic issues. Some regions are empoverished and modern medicine and antibiotic-based therapies are not largely available to most people. Most of the very specific plants used in some regions are largely unknown to western medicine and are object of study in the field of ethnopharmacology, especially for research of their antimicrobial properties. Nevertheless, even in some western countries, plant and herb-based treatments are used in "unconventional" therapies, though seen with mistrust by "conventional" medicine.

The use of plants for medicinal purposes involves the use of extracts more or less complex and sometimes it is hard to blame the healing power of a single substance. Although in some parts of the world population is still dependent on ancestral knowledge to alleviate their sufferings, the so-called western medicine world prefers the use of pure substances. The attempt to rationalize the "healing process" by Western medicine led to the study and attempt to isolate the active ingredients of medicinal plants that is to identify the chemical responsible for its healing power.

Many of the plants used in traditional medicine have been well evaluated and several compounds isolated that serve today as "models" to the pharmaceutical industry for drug development. So many of the drugs used today have a story that involves their isolation from plant material, identification in chemical terms, chemical synthesis and evaluation of the pharmacological properties of the pure compound. Often this assessment leads to the need of modifying the chemical structure first identified in the compound extracted from the plant, which is done to improve its pharmacological properties often reducing the adverse effects associated with the initial chemical structure.

This whole process was initiated in the nineteenth century with the investigation of plants used in treating some diseases, and the identification of compounds isolated in terms of its chemical structure was made much later, back in the twentieth century. The first compounds that were isolated were pure morphine (isolated from opium which is obtained from the white poppy capsules) and quinine of *Chinchona* spp. (family of plants used in South America to treat malaria). Both compounds are still used for therapeutic purposes. This process started in the nineteenth century never stopped and is now easier due to improved techniques for the isolation and structural determination of chemical compounds.

Despite the success of conventional medicine, based on the use of pure compounds, it is undeniable the current increased use of "natural medicines" (natural remedies) in Western societies, even though these products are sometimes viewed with suspicion by the professionals linked to the administration health care. One of the problems associated with the use of drugs of plant origin comes from the fact that in most cases, these products are sold without any control. The concentration of the pharmacologically active compounds depends on the season that was harvested, the state of maturation and the conditions under which the plant grew. The lack of regulation could result in the same plant product that was purchased at different times will have different biological activity.

The drug resistance of human and animal pathogens is one of the best documented in biological evolution and a serious problem in both developed and developing countries. The consumption of more than one ton daily antibiotics in some European countries has resulted in resistance to bacterial populations, thus causing a serious public health problem. In view of this scenario, the search for new antimicrobial substances from natural sources, including plants, has gained importance in pharmaceutical companies.

In the past, herbal medicine was taken over by poor people in rural or urban area, due to easy availability and lower costs. Currently, the use of plants as a source of drugs is prevalent in developing countries as an alternative solution to health problems and is well established in some cultures and traditions, especially in Asia, Latin America and Africa. It was through the recognition by man of the healing power of certain plants that was born and developed the pharmacy as we know it today.

All cultures in different parts of the world have developed knowledge of local plants that enabled them to its use for therapeutic purposes. Ancient written sources from Babylon, Egypt, India and China reached us, where the procedures are described for the collection, handling and use of different plant materials for recovery of its healing power.

Herbs, spices, condiments and their essential oils are usually seen merely as a way to season and add flavour or colour to foods, so its chemical complexity is often forgot and, therefore, some of its molecules ignored.

The prediction of specific antimicrobial effects of spices and condiments may be difficult to ascertain, as well as the minimal inhibitory concentration (MIC), not only because the specific mechanism is possibly different in different products, but also because of the amount of spice or condiment, the food to which is added, the cooking process or because the bacterial target, type and concentration, may influence the result, and also differences between *in vitro* (using culture media) and food experiments.

The present chapter intents to show the main results in terms of antimicrobial activity of plants, herbs and condiments, the main techniques envolved and future prospects in this field.

2. History

There are more than 300,000 species of plants, ranging from green algae to seed plants. Only a relatively small amount of these plants has been used since human populations were still collectors. With the beginning of agriculture and the expansion of mankind, the number of plants employed as nourishment or for medicinal purpose increased. The use of plants as a way to ease human ailments dates back to prehistory. In some parts of the World the medicinal practices envolving vegetable products, conventionally called ethnomedicine, may not have changed very dramatically since those ancient times, particularly in tribal areas of South American rain forest, Africa or South East Asia. These areas have a common characteristic - an overwhelming diversity and amount of plant material to be used.

There are many historical records on the use of plants for treating ailments ranging from 4.000 B.C. The first medical record filed in the Pennsylvania Museum is dated 2.100 B.C. and includes a collection of thirty different formulas of drugs of plant origin, animal or mineral. The Egyptian manuscript *Ebers Papirus* (1.500 B.C.), contains 811 prescriptions and 700 drug and the first Chinese text on herbal (500 B.C.) reports names, doses and indications for the use of plants to treat disease. Some of these plants are still used, such as ginseng (*Panax* spp.), *Ephedra* spp., *Cassia* spp. and *Rheum palmatum L.*, including as sources for pharmaceuticals industries.

Early reports, from various civilizations, mentioned several medicinal plants and their effects. The Greek physician Hippochrates (V century B.C.) described 300 to 400 medicinal plants and their effects. Another Greek physician Pedanius Dioscorides (I century A.D.) wrote a catalog of medicinal plants with the Latin title "De Materia Medica", in what is nowadays considered to be one of the world's first pharmacopeias. Even religious documents, as the Christian Bible, indicated some products of vegetable origin with antiseptic properties, namely frankincense and myrrh that were used in Ancient Middle East (including Ancient Egypt) as mouthwashes. In imperial China, we assisted the discovery of tea and other infusions described as having soothing properties and other medicinal characteristics.

As time went by and Man began accumulating more knowledge, critical analysis and observation of results began to follow the true scientific method. The real therapeutic success of many of these plants was mixed. In some cases, cure was achieved or symptoms were truely relieved. Other plants have shown to be only ideal for nutricional purposes. The more dramatic cases were of plants being simply considered source of poisoning.

Since the advent of antibiotics, in the 1920's, following Alexander Fleming's findings, researchers focused in microorganisms to obtain new ways to kill other microorganisms. The development of microbial resistance as well as economic incentives triggered the research and development of new antibiotics in order to maintain a pool of effective drugs in all situations. Although the development of resistant strains is inevitable, the way we manage and use antibiotics has exacerbated the process. The growing emergence of resistance phenomenon led to new classes of antibiotics of synthetic origin. Unfortunately, the rate of new and more efficient antibiotics is not as fast as microorganisms finding new ways to survive. Thus, in the beginning of the 21st century we assist to a race to plants, trying to discover innovative natural weapons to fight infectious diseases and microbial contaminations in food.

Since medicinal plants produce a variety of substances with antimicrobial properties, it is expected that screening programs discover candidate compounds for the development of new antibiotics. However, scientific research to determine the therapeutic potential of plants is limited, there is a lack of scientific studies that confirm the possible experimental antibiotic properties of a large number of these plants. It is expected that compounds that reach targets different from those used by known antibiotics may be active against resistant pathogens.

3. Plants, herbs and condiments

3.1 Conventional products

Worldwide, among the most used and studied spices and condiments known for the proven or supposed antibacterial activity we find aniseed (*Pimpinella anisum*), bay leaf (*Laurus nobilis*), black pepper (*Piper nigrum*), cinnamon (*Cinnamonum verum*), clove (*Syzygium aromaticum*), coriander (*Coriandrum sativum*), garlic (*Allium sativum*), ginger (*Zingiber officinale*), lime (*Citrus aurantifolia*), onion (*Allium cepa*), oregano (*Origanum vulgare*) and thyme (*Thymus vulgaris*). All of these are, generally, widely available in nearly every corner of the world.

Apart from the world areas associated with great vegetable diversity, like tropical regions, densely forested areas of South America, sub-Saharian Africa or Southeast Asia, we also can find a great number of plants/herbs with medicinal use. In an academic study made in 2002, in a Portuguese National Park, with a relatively small area, 346 hectare, 140 different plants were found, with 124 different medicinal uses, 15 aromatic, 16 categorized also as condiments and 20 others, including 2 specimens classified as toxic/poisonous (Rodrigues, 2002).

Table 1 lists a number of well-known plants and herbs, many used daily worldwide, and their most important antimicrobial component.

Common name	Scientific denomination	Antimicrobial component
Alfalfa	*Medicago sativa*	-
Allspice	*Pimenta dioica*	Eugenol
Aloe	*Aloe barbadensis / Aloe vera*	Latex
Apple	*Malus sylvestris*	Phlosetin (flavonoid)
Basil	*Ocimum basilicum*	Terpenoids
Bay	*Laurus nobilis*	Terpenoids
Black pepper	*Piper nigrum*	Piperine
Caraway	*Carum carvi*	Coumarin
Cashew	*Anacardium purshiana*	Polyphenols
Chamomile	*Matricaria chamomilla*	Phenolic acid
Chili peppers	*Capsicum annuum*	Capsaicin
Clove	*Syzygium aromaticum*	Eugenol
Coriander	*Coriadrum sativum*	-
Dill	*Anethum graveolens*	Terpenoids
Eucalyptus	*Eucalyptus globulus*	Tannin
Fava bean	*Vicia faba*	Fabatin
Garlic	*Allium sativum*	Allicin
Olive	*Olea europaea*	Hexanal
Onion	*Allium cepa*	Allicin
Peppermint	*Mentha piperita*	Menthol (terpenoid)
Rosemary	*Rosmarinus officinalis*	Terpenoids
Thyme	*Thymus vulgaris*	Caffeic acid, thymol, tannins
Turmeric	*Curcuma longa*	Curcumin (terpenoid)

Table 1. Plants and herbs and their main antimicrobial components (adapted from Cowan, 1999).

There are some generally accepted conclusions about the antimicrobial abilities of these natural products: spices are less effective in foods than in culture media, probably because of the higher concentration *in vitro* and non-existing co-factors, and Gram-positive bacteria are more sensible than Gram negatives, although some Gram negative strains may be extremely affected as well (Jay, 1982; Zaika *et al.*, 1983), as *Escherichia coli* to varying concentrations of cumin, for example (Allahghadri *et al.*, 2010). Within the Gram positive group, lactic bacteria are considered the less sensitive (Zaika *et al.*, 1983).

Confirming the greater susceptibility to herbs and condiments of Gram positive bacteria when compared with Gram negative, an experiment using forty-six methanolic extracts of dietary spices and medicinal herbs reached results in which *Staphylococcus aureus* was the most sensitive bacteria and *Escherichia coli* the less sensitive bacteria to the extracts tested. The other test species included *Bacillus cereus, Listeria monocytogenes* and *Salmonella anatum*. The experiment also has shown a strong positive correlation between antibacterial activity and the total phenolic content of the herbs (Shan *et al.*, 2007).

Garlic and clove are widely used for culinary purposes due to their strong flavour and aroma. They are also some of the most widely refered condiments in scientific literature when comes to antibacterial activity. Some bacteria that show resistance to conventional antibiotics are susceptible to decoctions or extracts of garlic and clove. Garlic, in particular, was able to inhibit *Staphylococcus epidermidis* and *Salmonella typhi* after one and three hours, respectively. In terms of yeast inhibition, it took one hour to achieve it, and in terms of inhibition diameter, reached larger areas of inhibition for *Candida* than those produced by nystatin. Clove took five hours to completely inhibit yeasts, including *Candida* species (Arora & Kaur, 1999).

There are indications that some spices, or their components may be active not only against resistant strains, but also against clinical isolates (usually studies are carried on academic collection strains). Rahman *et al.*, proved the effectiveness of spice extracts on multi-resistant *Escherichia coli*. In spite the fact each extract, alone, caused no inhibition, the combination of three different aqueous extracts (1:1:1) of ginger, lime and garlic had a synergistic effect, inhibiting the bacteria. The incorporation of 0.3% in culture media was sufficient to inhibit 21 of the 24 Gram positive bacteria tested (Shelef *et al.*, 1980). In a study conducted by Masood et al., using oral isolates as test targets, black pepper decoction shown bacterial toxicity against 75% of the samples, bay leaf was effective against 53% and aniseed against 18%. Coriander did not show any inhibiting activity.

Many herbs and spices also have antifungal activity, which is important to relate, as fungi and its toxins also have a role as origin of food spoilage and food contaminants. Out of 29 spices and herbs studied, clove (genus *Caryophyllus*), star anise (*Illicium anisatum*) and allspice (genus *Pimenta*) completely inhibited the growth of 3 different *Aspergillus* species (*Aspergillus ochraceus, Aspergillus versicolor* and *Aspergillus flavus*) and also inhibited the toxin production. Eugenol extracted from clove and anethol extracted from star anise were incorporated in PDA (Potato Dextrose Agar) medium to test its growth inhibition ability. The concentrations required for total inhibition were 0.4 and 2.0 mg/mL, respectively (Hitokoto *et al.*, 1980).

Dietary and medicinal plants and spices have been constantly studied for their antimicrobial properties, in particular for their antibacterial activity. In a study aimed at finding solutions against diarrhoegenic bacteria, onion, garlic, ginger, black pepper, clove, mint, cumin and turmeric were tested. The microorganisms used in the experiment were *Salmonella typhi, Salmonella typhimurium, Shigella flexneri, Shigella dysenteriae, Escherichia coli* O102 and *Escherichia coli* O157, *Yersinia enterocolitica* and *Campylobacter jejuni*. The most efficient plant was clove, with maximum inhibition diameters for all bacteria, followed by black pepper that showed a high inhibition of *Shigella dysenteriae, Campylobacter jejuni* and both strains of *Escherichia coli*. The less efficient plants were ginger and mint (Vaishnavi *et al.*, 2007).

3.2 Ethnic products

Beyond the more conventional vegetable products known worldwide, there is a great number of plants and herbs that have a great importance in cooking and medicinal practices, especially in Eastern Asian countries. For some plants, the biological properties described include not only antimicrobial activity but also the ability to influence the immune system.

Among these properties, there is the ability to stimulate the production of cytokines, increase the activation of macrophages, lymphocytes and NK cells (Natural killer cells). Chinese traditional medicine often uses plants like *Aloe vera, Angelica* spp., *Astragalus membranaceus, Ganoderma lucidum, Panax ginseng, Scutellaria* spp. and *Zingiber officinale*, some of which, beyond the immunomodulatory activity refered, also show some antimicrobial activity, like toxicity to *Aspergillus candidus* (*Angelica* spp.) and toxicity to MRSA (methicillin-resistant *Staphylococcus aureus*), shown by *Scutellaria* spp. (Tan & Vanitha, 2004).

The purpose of using plants and herbs may not be only a medicinal or therapeutic purpose. The presence of some herbs with antimicrobial activity in some dishes may act as food preservatives. Curry leaf (*Murraya koenigii*) and Vietnamese coriander (*Persicaria odorata*) have shown to be effective against some bacteria isolated from fish. Methanolic extracts of curry leaf and Vietnamese coriander were effective against *Streptococcus agalactiae* (MIC= 0.39 mg/mL) and *Staphylococcus aureus*, respectively (MIC= 3.13 mg/mL) (Najiah et al., 2011).

Asafoetida (*Ferula assafoetida*), a spice used in Indian cuisine, was tested against endemic pathogens in India and shown antibacterial activity against *Salmonella typhi* and *Escherichia coli* O157, leading the authors of the study to conclude that the presence of some spices and condiments acts not only as flavouring agents but also as some sort of protection against gastroentestinal diseases (Vaishnavi *et al.*, 2007).

In Thai cuisine and traditional medicine, galangal (genus *Alpinia*) has a special relevance. Studies have shown that the ryzome of this plant has antimicrobial properties, in particular against *Vibrio paraheamolyticus*. Bacterial inhibition was performed using disks with 10 µL freshly squeezed galangal, although the chloroform extract also shown activity. One of the molecules envolved in the inhibition mechanism was identified as being 1'-acetoxychavicol acetate (Vuddhakul *et al.*, 2006).

Ayurvedic medicinal tradition uses many plants and herbs to treat several diseases, including those of infectious nature. *Ocimum sanctum, Eugenia caryophillata, Achyranthes bidentata* and *Azadirachta indica* are plants used in Nepal and India and were tested for their antibacterial properties against *Escherichia coli, Salmonella typhi, Salmonella paratyphi, Staphylococcus aureus, Klebsiella pneumoniae* and *Pseudomonas aeruginosa* through cup diffusion method. The experimental results have shown that both *Klebsiella pneumoniae* and *Pseudomonas aeruginosa* were resistant to any of the four plant extracts, and *Achyranthes bidentata* extract was ineffective against all bacterial strains. The largest inhibition area was obtained against *Salmonella typhi* by *Eugenia caryophillata* extract (Joshi *et al.*, 2011).

As refered before, the unavailability of conventional antibiotics drives people to search in their own local products solutions for bacterial contamination of food and for infectious diseases. In a study conducted in Algeria, the antibacterial properties of four types of local berries (*Crataegus azarolus, Crataegus monogyna, Ziziphus lotus* and *Eleagnus angustifolia*) and three date (*Phoenix dactylifera*) varieties were analyzed. The targets were seven strains of *Salmonella* isolated from poultry industry. The bacterial strains were shown to be resistant to ticarcillin, amoxicillin, chloramphenicol and co-trimoxazole. Despite local berries extracts were ineffective against the bacteria, the date fruits results have shown moderate inhibition of *Salmonella*. An *Escherichia coli* strain was used as control and its inhibition diameters were smaller than those of *Salmonella* (Ayachi *et al.*, 2009).

Cassia tora, Momordica charantia and *Calendula officinalis* are herbs used by ayurvedic medicine to treat psoriasis and other dermatological episodes. Aqueous and organic extracts of these plants were tested against *Staphylococcus aureus, Bacillus subtilis, Pseudomonas aeruginosa* and *Escherichia coli*. Results have shown that aqueous extracts were more effective than extracts obtained using organic solvents. *Staphylococcus aureus* was the most susceptible bacteria to any of the four herbs tested. However, none of inhibition diameters produced was larger than the diameter produced by the antibiotic used for comparison, streptomycin (Roopashree *et al.*, 2008).

In Brazilian folk medicine, a very large number of plants is used for treatmente of various diseases. This is due not only to ancestral tribal tradition, but mainly to the extreme abundance of vegetable raw materials in tropical environment. One of the plants employed with therapeutic objectives is *Plectranthus ornatus*, one of the many species of *Plectranthus* genus. In a study conducted in Portugal aimed at isolating the antimicrobial components of this plant, MIC were determined by microdilution. Extracts obtained by using different solvents were tested against bacterial strains, Gram positive and Gram negative and *Candida albicans*. The main experimental results show an MIC of 31.25 µg/mL against *Streptococcus faecalis*, using an acetone extract and an MIC of 125 µg/mL against *Staphylococcus aureus*, using a methanol/water extract. Extracts obtained with other organic solvents were devoid of antimicrobial activity (Rijo *et al.*, 2010).

3.3 Others

Beyond the traditional plants and herbs, other "vegetable" edible products are becoming object of attention. Seaweeds are part of oriental food habits for long, like the use of seaweeds in preparation of sushi-like dishes in Japanese cuisine, but the interest in its antimicrobial and other biological activity is recent. Methanolic extracts of six species of edible Irish seaweeds proved to be effective against food pathogenic bacteria like *Listeria monocytogenes, Salmonella abony, Enterococcus faecalis* and *Pseudomonas aeruginosa*, with brown algae more effective than green and red algae (Cox *et al.*, 2010).

4. Molecules involved in antimicrobial activity

Plants, herbs, spices and other products of vegetable origin must be seen as multi ingredient mixtures. Thus, there is a high probability that a product may have different compounds that may act as antimicrobial agents, although present in low concentrations. However, we often relate a plant with a specific molecule. For instance, piperine in pepper, eugenol in clove, allicin in garlic, cinnamic aldehyde in cinnamon stick or thymol in thyme leafs. In other cases, even if the specific molecule is unknown, there seems to be a significant correlation between antibacterial activity and high content of phenolic components (Shan *et al.*, 2007), flavonoids and terpenoids (Cowan, 1999; Rios *et al.*, 1987) which, among other effects, may be associated with membrane disruption.

The membrane disruption, specifically a rupture of the phospholipid bilayer, is the main cause of cell death when natural antimicrobials are concerned. However, cell death can also be precipitated by other factors, including the disruption of enzyme systems. The inhibition of flagellin synthesis in *Escherichia coli* O157:H7, promoted by carvacrol, seems to be of relevance (Tajkarimi *et al.*, 2010).

One of the issues that raises interest, not only scientific but also economic, is the possibility to obtain a source of new anti-retrovirals in the nature. Terpenes, phenols and polysaccharides obtained from several medicinal plants could act as inhibitors of HIV replication, the majority of them targeting HIV reverse transcriptase (Jung *et al.*, 2000).

Some spices and herbs may have the same type of active molecule, and consequently the same bactericidal mechanism. Zaika *et al.* shown that oregano, rosemary, sage and thyme had the same effects. The resistance development observed in their test strains (lactic bacteria) when exposed to one of the herbs, allowed resistance to the other three. The same herbs, nonetheless, were considered to be among the most antimicrobial.

As said previously, plants have a great number of molecules that are responsible for the colour, odour and flavour of vegetable products. Most of these phytochemicals are secondary metabolites, and among those that have antimicrobial activity we find (Cowan, 1999): phenols and polyphenols, terpenoids, essential oils, alkaloids and, finally, lectins and polypeptides.

This list is an atempt to systematise the phytochemicals envolved in antimicrobial activity. From a strictly chemical point of vue, there are phytochemicals that could be put in different groups. As an example of the "confusing" chemical denomination, we have terpenoids, phenols and phenolic terpenoids. However, we chose to follow this list to better organize the available information.

The chemistry envolved in these antimicrobial mechanisms is complex and the diversity of molecules is great. There are other types of natural antimicrobials whose inclusion in any of above mentioned groups is not easy. A group of molecules, obtained from garlic, the thiosulfinates are active against Gram negative strains. Vegetables like broccoli, Brussels sprouts, cabbages but also mustard and horseradish are rich in glucosinolates that have a wide range of antibacterial and antifungal activity.

4.1 Phenols and polyphenols

This group comprises a large number of different molecules like simple phenols, phenolic acids, quinones, flavonoids, flavones, flavonols, tannins and coumarins. They have in common the fact of participating in the aromatic characteristics of plants and are very common.

Phenols like catechol and epicatechin or cinnamic acid (phenolic acid) participate in membrane disruption (Figure 1). Because phenols are very common, the antibacterial activity of plants and herbs is very often related with this phenomenon.

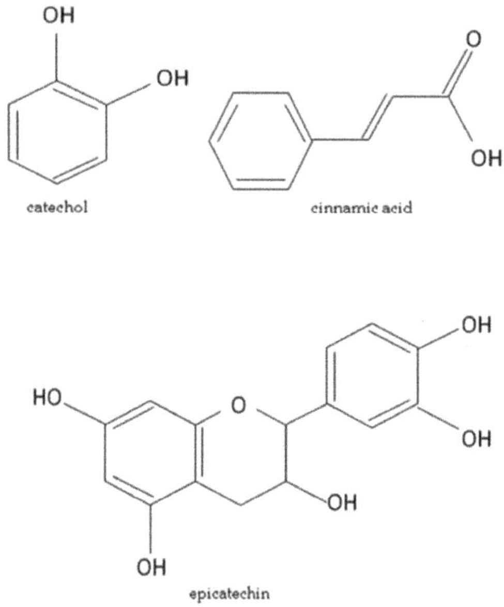

Fig. 1. Structural formulae of some phenols with antimicrobial properties.

The antibacterial activity of quinones, flavonoids, flavones and flavonols seems to be similar. Some examples are hyperacin, chrysin, and abyssinone (Figure 2). Their mechanism of inhibition includes ability to bind to adhesins and specially, enzymatic inhibition.

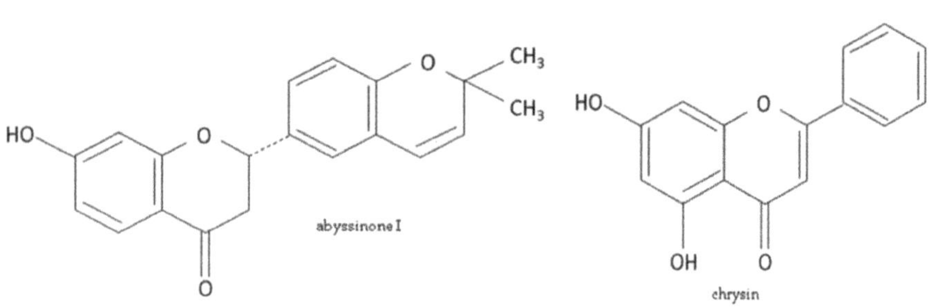

Fig. 2. Chemical structures of abyssinone and chrysin.

Additionally, abyssinone has the ability to inhibit HIV reverse transcriptase, pointing out the therapeutic value that some phytochemicals could have for some infectious diseases (Cowan, 1999). Tannins are one of the most commom chemical groups present in plants and vegetable material. It is easily found in seeds, bark, and other parts of the plant. In terms of organoleptic characteristics, tannins are responsible for astringency. An example of tannins with antimicrobial activity is ellagitannin, and the mechanism of inhibition is related with their ability to bind to proteins, blocking some metabolic pathways. Finally, we have coumarins, like warfarin, whose medicinal/therapeutic use is related to the ability to interact with eucaryotic DNA, which implies some antiviral activity (Figure 3) (Cowan, 1999).

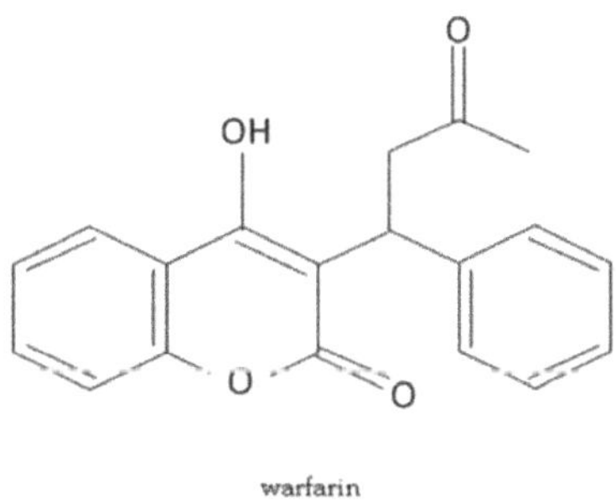

Fig. 3. Chemical structure of a coumarin, warfarin.

4.2 Terpenoids

Like phenols, terpenoids are one of the most common constituents in plants, herbs and spices. As plant metabolites, terpenoids play a role in growth and development but also in the process of resistance against environmental stresses (Figure 4). Their inhibition ability is based on membrane disruption, a mechanism widely refered in scientific literature, but yet not fully understood. Diterpene metabolites like totarol and abietic acid are active against Gram positive bacteria. In fact, diterpenes is one of the largest groups of plant-derived natural products with anti-staphylococcal activity. This is justified by their ability to cross the bacterial cytoplasmatic membrane (due to their amphipathic character).

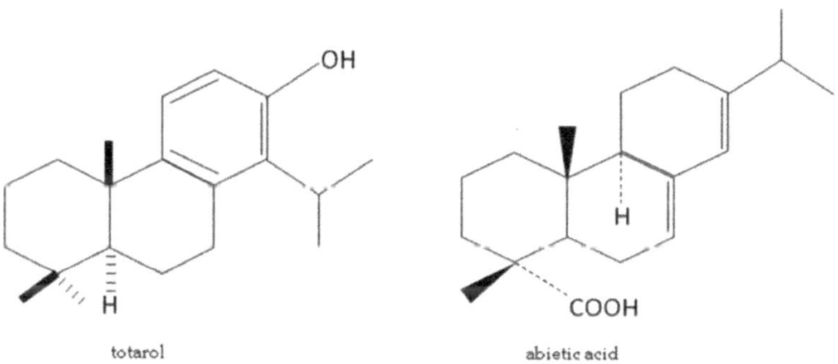

Fig. 4. Chemical structures of totarol and abietic acid.

Totarol also behaves as an efflux pump inhibitor, stopping one of the pathways bacteria can follow to resist antimicrobial molecules (Rijo *et al.*, 2010). Other example of an antimicrobial terpenoid is capsaicin, a phytochemical found in chilli pepper seeds (Cowan, 1999).

4.3 Essential oils

Essential oils do not constitute a separate molecular group. In fact, many of the molecules present in essential oils are terpenoids. However, they are treated separately because scientific literature studies them intensively and they are commercially traded as medicinal products, perfume ingredients or food additives. Essential oils are aromatic oily liquids extracted from plants. As said, essential oils are mixtures, but among the most common molecules present in some essential oils we find carvacrol, thymol, eugenol, perillaldehyde, cinnamaldehyde, cinnamic acid, camphor or linalool (Figure 5). Different plants can be used for the extraction of essential oil, like coriander, cinnamon, oregano, rosemary, sage, clove or thyme, among others. The methods of oil extraction include the traditional steam distillation but also hydrodistillation and more recent supercritical fluid extraction. Some essential oils constituents like carvacrol, thymol, eugenol, perillaldehyde, cinnamaldehyde and cinnamic acid have been shown to have antibacterial activity against such food pathogens like *Listeria monocytogenes, Salmonella typhimurium, Escherichia coli* O157:H7, *Shigella dysenteriae, Bacillus cereus* and *Staphylococcus aureus* with MIC ranging 0.05 µL/mL to 5 µL/mL *in vitro*. In terms of application on foods (as preservative agents) or as constituents in washing solutions for fruits and vegetables, however, MIC of essential oils increases, with values ranging 0.5 to 20 µL/g in first case and 0.1 to 10 µL/mL, in the second (Burt, 2004).

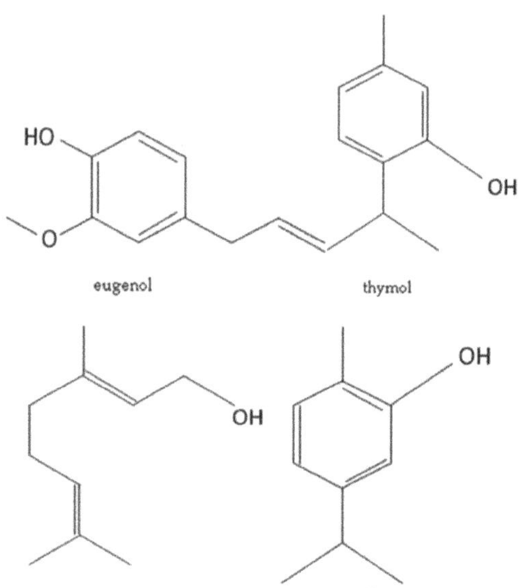

Fig. 5. Chemical structures of some essential oils components.

4.4 Alkaloids

Alkaloids constitute a chemical group that includes many molecules of vegetable origin that are very well known, such as caffein or cocaine. In terms of antimicrobial properties, molecules like berberine and piperine seem have the ability to intercalate into cell wall or DNA (deoxyrribonucleic acid) (Figure 6). Some activity against protozoa is also refered, mainly anti-*Plasmodium* and anti-trypanossome, although *Giardia* and *Entamoeba* infections, common in HIV patients, can also be eliminated through the consumption of some alkaloids. Solamargine, a glycoalkaloid extracted from *Solanum khaniasum* is helpful in HIV infections (Cowan, 1999).

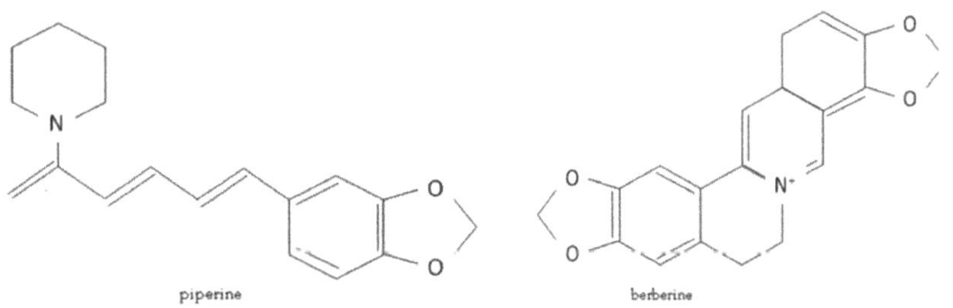

Fig. 6. The piperine and berberine molecules.

4.5 Lectins and polypeptides

Antimicrobial activity of phytochemicals is not only against bacteria, fungi or protozoa. Lectins and polypeptides, whose main characteristic is the ability to form disulfide bridges, are targeted to virus. These molecules are able to block viral fusion or adsorption, probably through competition for cellular binding spots. An example of such phytochemicals is fabatin, found in fava beans (Cowan, 1999). There are vegetables (including potatos) and seeds producing protease inhibitors that are involved in the innate defense response of the host against phytopathogens. This antimicrobial activity could, in the future, be applied in clinical research. Antimicrobial proteins and peptides are produced by various plants and its presence is correlated with plant resistance to some microbial infections. These peptides include lectins, protease inhibitors and antifungal peptides (Kim *et al.*, 2009).

5. Methodologies

Medicinal use of plants is conducted through different ways, according to geographical availability, historic tradition and known efficacy and may include preparation of aqueous infusions and beverages using dried plants, tinctures (plants in alcoholic solutions), inhalation of steam from boiling preparations, ingestion of fresh or cooked parts as ingredients, preparation of topic ointments, essential oils, among others. However, the real scientific and therapeutic value of the plant properties, like antimicrobial potential, needs to be evaluated through proper techniques. The screening of antimicrobial activity may be pursued on two different pathways:

- Analysis and identification of individual components, after extraction;
- Evaluation of inhibition properties on sample microorganisms.

5.1 Analysis and identification of individual components

For the chemical analysis of plants and herbs, one must choose the part of the plant containing the active compounds, and depending on the plant it may be the root (ginseng, for instance), the flowers (lavender, for example), the leaves (like bay leaf and thyme), the bark (cinnamon), the seeds, the fruit or the stem. It is also possible to observe variation of content of antimicrobial molecules in each plant due to different factors as: influence of seasonal harvest, geographic location and altitude and extraction procedures.

Fresh products can be used in order to obtain aqueous mixtures, but before extraction using organic solvents, samples are usually dried and grinded. The samples may be prepared as crude extracts or aqueous and organic solvent extracts. Further operations may include filtration and centrifugation (for clarification). Besides water, extraction is made by use of organic solvents, because most active components are not totally water-soluble. In fact, only a small portion is water-soluble, like polypeptides and polysaccharides (starch). The main organic solvents are ethanol, methanol, chloroform, dichloromethane, diethyl ether, petroleum ether and acetone. The techniques for identification of molecules and description of molecular structure include chromatography (from simple thin-layer chromatography to high-performance liquid chromatography), radioimmunoassay, mass spectrometry, nuclear magnetic resonance and X-ray crystallography.

5.2 Evaluation of inhibition properties

The differences with respect to the techniques employed to investigate the action of plant compounds and a wide variation in the chemical composition of some plant preparations can result in data difficult to compare between surveys. There is also no consensus on acceptable levels of inhibition for plants compounds, when compared with standard antibiotics. The methodologies used for the evaluation of antimicrobial properties of plants, herbs, spices and condiments do not differ significantly from those used in classic clinical microbiology. The inhibitory effects on bacteria and yeasts can be tested by broth dilution assay (evaluation can be performed using optical density or colony viable count), which allows determination and comparison of MIC and susceptibility tests by disk or agar-well diffusion. For classic antibiotics, CLSI (Clinical Laboratories Standards Institute) establishes the exact concentrations to be studied, whereas with spices or herbs there are no such specifications.

A problem that may be encountered when reviewing some scientific literature is the difference between concepts. Although MIC is a well-defined and internationally accepted concept, there are several uses of the term. In her review, Burt (Burt, 2004) gathers a number of possible definitions for MIC, MBC (minimum bactericidal concentration), bacteriostatic concentration and bactericidal concentration. These possible differences in the concepts must be taken into consideration when performing laboratorial assays. Moreover, it is also important when comparing results, in order to know with what values each researcher is comparing his results to. MIC is defined as the lowest concentration resulting in maintenance or reduction of inoculum viability; the lowest concentration required for complete inhibition of test organism up to 48 hours incubation; or as the lowest concentration resulting in a significant decrease in inoculum viability (>90%). MBC is established as being the concentration where 99.9% or more of the initial inoculum is killed or the lowest concentration at which no growth is observed after subculturing into fresh broth. Bacteriostatic concentration is defined as the lowest concentration at which bacteria fail to grow in broth but are cultured when broth is plated onto agar and the bactericidal concentration is considered to be the lowest concentration at which bacteria fail to grow in broth and are not cultured when broth is plated onto agar (Burt, 2004).

For susceptibility tests controls must be performed simultaneously, usually using the antibiotics most suited for the conventional treatment. Tetracycline was used for comparison with thirteen Thai condiments against *Vibrio parahaemolyticus* (Vuddhakul et al., 2007) and fifteen antiobiotics were used when testing the antimicrobial activity of condiments against multidrug resistant *Escherichia coli* isolated from water in Bangladesh (Rahman *et al.*, 2011). Comparison with conventional antibiotics is necessary to categorize the sensibility of a specific microorganism to a plant, herb or condiment as sensible or resistant.

A rigorous evaluation of the individual MIC is sometimes difficult because of the ambiguity of results. Eugenol inhibited 9 out of 14 Gram negative and 12 out of 20 Gram positive bacteria, at a concentration of 493 ppm, by incorporating in Plate Count Agar. But the same paper reported a MIC of 32 ppm for *Candida glabrata* and *Aspergillus niger*, and a MIC of 63 ppm for *Staphylococcus aureus* and *Escherichia coli* (Cowan, 1999).

The variation in concentration of antimicrobial substances is usual and expected. This, coupled with testing different preparations contributes for the difficulty of comparing results from study to study. For instance, allicin in garlic ranges from 0.3 to 0.5%, whereas eugenol in clove ranges from 16 to 18% (Shelef, 1984).

The problem is worsened by the fact each researcher may use different methods for preparing the samples: crude, aqueous extracts, ethanolic or methanolic extracts, chloroform or other solvents, as refered above. The results from testing the inhibitory effect of essential oils is not easy to ascertain, as the hydrophobic nature of such preparations may alter the inhibition areas because of the irregular diffusion, when compared with the more hydrophilic antibiotics. Some researchers add emulsifiers, as Tween 20 or Tween 80, to the oils, but the quantity and nature of the latter must not interfere with the results, like producing false-positive ones. Thus, standardisation of methods becomes difficult to achieve (Nascimento *et al.*, 2006).

There are other methodologies available to use in order to ascertain the effects of antibacterial activity of certain phytochemicals. The rate of inhibition and cell death can be observed through time-kill analysis and survival curves. The physical aspects of antibacterial activity concerning the structural modifications achieved can be observed by the use of scanning electron microscopy (Burt, 2004).

Yeasts susceptibility can be evaluated by techniques similar to those used for bacteria, however the evaluation of antifungal ability of phytochemicals must be performed by other methods. One of these methods is the spore germination assay. Spores are put in contact with the testing compound for a period of time; afterwards they are observed microscopically in a slide (usually fixed with lactophenol cotton blue) and spore germination (or its absence) is observed.

In terms of antiviral ability of plant products, they can be determined by observation of cytopathic effects or plaque formation in cells infected and put in contact with the phytochemicals. Other option is, in the same conditions, to use molecular techniques for detection of products resulting from viral replication, as nucleic acids.

Researchers must have in mind, as mentioned earlier, that different plants may have the same antimicrobial phytochemicals, although they may be in different concentrations, resulting in different MIC for the same molecule. Moreover, the same plant may have more than an antimicrobial molecule, resulting in effects that can not be easily evaluated. An inhibition or decrease in bacterial population may be due to different mechanisms.

6. Herbs, condiments and spices as food preservatives

Safety and high-quality characteristics of food products are some of the attributes growingly demanded by consumers worldwide. Despite technological advances, either by chemical preservatives or mechanical equipment for inactivation or inhibition of microorganisms, there are still problems concerning food spoilage of biological origin. Attention is concentrated on psychrophiles, halophiles and toxigenic foodborne pathogens. Consequently, natural antimicrobial molecules are interesting tools to control microbial food contamination, in addition to their already well-known flavouring properties. The main commercial objective of adding these compounds to foodstuff is extending their shelf-life and increasing, if possible, their nutricional and organoleptic value.

As mentioned earlier, these natural antimicrobials derive from plant products and, historically, are been in use for a long time in areas as China or India. Nowadays the concentrated use of a large number of condiments/spices is mainly performed in hot climate regions. Virtually every group of food raw materials can be added with one or more plants/herbs/spices that work as food preservatives, as shown in Table 2.

Among the species used for food preservation or that have shown to produce inhibition of food contaminants we find: thyme (*Thymus eigii*), ginger (*Zingiber officinalle*), galangal (*Alpinia galanga*), turmeric (*Curcuma longa*) and fingerroot (*Boesenbergia pandurata*). Cinnamon, cloves and cumin also show antimicrobial effects against pathogens, some of which of foodborne origin, like *Staphylococcus aureus, Klebsiella pneumoniae, Pseudomonas aeruginosa, Escherichia coli, Enterococcus faecalis, Mycobacterium smegmatis, Micrococcus luteus* and even *Candida albicans.* We also find condiments as allspice, bay leaf, caraway, coriander, cassia bark and liquorice as a way to eliminate or inhibit foodborne pathogens. In particular, olive tree leaves (*Olea europaea*) shows effects against important species as *Campylobacter jejuni, Helicobacter pylori* and *Staphylococcus aureus.*

The molecules interviening in the antimicrobial process have been object of a specific section within this chapter, but among thje most commom we usually find α-pinene, cineole, limonene, linalool and geranyl acetate.

In terms of use for food preservation, these natural antimicrobial agents may pose problems that must be addressed, namely the existence of antagonism between different agents, degradation of organoleptic profile and the existence of toxic effects for the consumer. These issues have to be considered seriously and the solutions may be in continuing research of the health effects and mainly in finding ways to lower the sensorial perception of some spices/herbs (optimization of food formulation) or by guaranteeing food preservation by combining different methods (conventional techniques plus addition of natural antimicrobials).

Food Group	Plant/spice/herb or active compound	Microbial target
Meat Products	Clove oil, eugenol+coriander, oregano, thyme oils, rosemary oil, clove, tea tree	*Listeria monocytogenes, Aeromonas hydrophila, Escherichia coli* O157:H7
	Oregano+thyme, oregano+marjoram, thyme+sage	*Bacillus cereus, Pseudomonas aeruginosa, Listeria monocytogenes*
	Chinese cinnamon	Pathogenic microorganisms
	Oregano, pimento, oregano+pimento	*Escherichia coli* O157:H7, *Pseudomonas* spp.
	Marjoram oil	Several species
	Eugenol	*Listeria monocytogenes, Aeromonas hydrophila*
	Sage oil	*Bacillus cereus, Staphylococcus aureus, Salmonella typhimurium*
	Mint oil	*Listeria monocytogenes, Salmonella enteritidis*
	Cilantro oil	*Listeria monocytogenes*
	Oregano oil	*Clostridium botulinum* spores
	Rosemary	*Listeria monocytogenes*
Fish	Thyme oil, cinnamaldehyde	*Pseudomonas putida*
	Carvacrol, citral, geraniol	*Salmonella typhimurium*
	Oregano oil	*Photobacterium phophoreum*
	Mint oil	*Salmonella enteritidis*
	Eugenol, linalool, oregano	Increased shelf-life
Dairy	Clove oil, carvacrol	*Listeria monocytogenes*
	Clove, cinnamon, cardamom, peppermint oil	*Streptococcus thermophilus*
	Mint oil	*Salmonella enteritidis*
Vegetables	Thyme oil	*Escherichia coli* O157:H7
	Basil methyl chaviol (BMC)	Natural flora
	Oregano oil	*Escherichia coli* O157:H7
	Cinnamaldehyde	*Escherichia coli* O157:H7
Rice	Carvacrol	Natural flora
	Sage oil	*Bacillus cereus, Staphylococcus aureus, Salmonella typhimurium*
	Basil	Rice storage pests
Fruits	Carvacrol, cinnamic acid	Natural flora

Table 2. List of herbs/spices/condiments or natural antimicrobial molecules used in different groups of foodstuff and their potential targets (adapted from Tajkarimi *et al.*, 2010).

7. Commercial availability and legislation

Some essential oils have been registered by the European Commission as flavouring agents to be used in foodstuff. In terms of legislation related to foodstuff, both the European Union (through European Food Safety Agency and its national branches) and the United States (through Food and Drug Administration) have been continually issuing and updating a number of regulations and list of food additives and supplements that have been authorised and considered safe for human consumption. In particular, some antimicrobial essential oils like cinnamon oil, clove oil, lemon grass oil and their respective active substances (cinnamaldehyde, eugenol and citral) have been generally recognized as safe (GRAS denomination) by the American FDA as food additives.

However, the classification of plant-based products as pharmacologically active substances or medicaments is less clear. They can only be included in foodstuff legislation if not proven as being medicaments. The main obstacle on the legal establishment of these molecules or mixtures originates from potential risks to the consumers health. The risks arise from any toxic effect, unknown to date. Several studies have to be performed on the metabolic effects, physical and chemical characterization of the molecules, microbiological studies, safety assays, and the cost of performing these experiments is high. This financial cost can be an excessive burden to small companies.

Medicaments are molecules with properties of treatment or prevention of human diseases, or with pharmacological, immunological or metabolic action. Plant-based medicaments are regulated, within European Union, by Directive 2004/24/CE. Each member country has to integrate onto their own legislation the contents of this Directive. It comprises not only antimicrobial herbs and plants, but any pharmacologically active vegetable product, in particular those utilized in Chinese traditional medicine and ayurvedic medicine. The European Commission issued it in order to establish concepts and regulate the trade. They define traditional plant-based medicaments as products, of vegetable origin, targeted to treat some illnesses, in use for at least 30 years (including 15 years of use within European Union borders) and that are to be employed without medical supervision and whose administration does not include injection or parenteral use. This usage must be proven by documentation. Some examples of species employed in the production of plant-based medicaments have already been listed along this chapter, as *Calendula officinalis, Echinea purpurea* or *Pimpinella anisum.*

Although being natural products (and sometimes with a long tradition of medicinal use), some of these substances may be harmful to patients and this is why European Union requires specific authorization for these products (which are included in general pharmaceutical legislation) to be placed in the market. The objective is to guarantee quality, safety and efficiency. Neverthless, taking in account the financial burden that some laboratory tests and clinical assays represent, the European Union has introduced a more simplified registration procedure without forgeting the forementioned requirements of quality, safety and efficiency. The companies that produce or trade the plant-based medicaments must present unquestionable documentation proving the innocuity to human health and the established therapeutic use (30 years of use and 15 years within European Union).

8. Conclusion

Spices, condiments and herbs, used fresh or as extracts have a very much reported ability to inhibit some microorganisms. However, analysis of scientific literature shows that researchers must take care when comparing results because experimental standardization has not been achieved yet.

The use of natural medicines has undeniably increased in western societies. The suspicion raised by conventional health care professionals is due to lack of legislation and control. The therapeutic results and the active molecules of these natural products have a variability caused by seasonal conditions, leading consequently to variable biological activity.

In several regions of the world traditional culinary habits and medicinal pratices use plants and herbs in daily routine. Modern conventional medicine is challenged today by the ever growing bacterial resistance to classic antibiotics. More research is necessary to ascertain the real therapeutic value of these products, but these natural resources must not be despised because their clinical and economic value may be greater than has been supposed up to this day.

9. References

Allahghadri, T., Rasooli, I., Owlia, P., Nadooshan, M.J., Ghazanfari, T., Taghizadeh, M. & Astaveh, S.D. (2010). Antimicrobial property, antioxidant capacity and cytotoxicity of essential oil from cumin produced in Iran. *Journal of Food Science,* Volume 75, No 2 (March 2010), pp. (H54-61), ISSN 1750-3841

Arora, D.S. & Kaur, J. (1999), Antimicrobial activity of spices. *International Journal of Antimicrobial Agents,* Volume 12, No 3, (August 1999), pp. (257-262), ISSN 0929-8579

Ayachi, A., Alloui, N., Beneoune, O., Yakhlef, G., Amiour, S., Bouzid, W., Zoughlache, S., Boudjellal, K. & Abdessemed, H. (2009). Antibacterial activity of some fruits, berries and medicinal herb extracts against poultry strains of Salmonella. *American-Eurasian Journal of Agriculture and Environmental Sciences,* Volume 6, No 1, (February 2009), pp. (12-15), ISSN 1818-6769

Burt, S. (2004). Essential oils: their antibacterial properties and potential applications in foods - a review. *International Journal of Food Microbiology.* Volume 94, No 3, (August 2004), pp. (223-253), ISSN 0168-1605

Cowan, M.M. (1999). Plant products as antimicrobial agents. *Clinical Microbiology Reviews,* Volume 12, (October 1999), pp. (564-582), ISSN 1098-6618

Cox, S., Abu Ghannam, N. & Gupta, S. (2010). An assessment of the antioxidant and antimicrobial activity of six species of edible Irish seaweeds. *International Food Research Journal,* Volume 17, No 1, (January 2010), pp. (205-220), ISSN 2231-7546

Hitoko, H., Morozumi, S., Wauke, T., Sakai, S. & Kurata, H. (1980). Inhibitory effects of spices on growth and toxin production of toxigenic fungi. *Applied and Environmental Microbiology,* Volume 39, No 4, (April 1980), pp. (818-822), ISSN: 1098-5336

Jay, J.M. (1982). Effect of diacetyl on food-borne microorganisms. *Journal of Food Science,* Volume 47, No 6, (November 1982), pp. (1829-1831), ISSN 1750-3841

Joshi, B., Sah, G.P., Basnet, B.B., Bhatt, M.R., Sharma, D., Subedi, K., Pandey, J. & Malla, R. (2011). Phytochemical extraction and antimicrobial properties of different medicinal plants: *Ocimum sanctum* (Tulsi), *Eugenia caryophillata* (clove), *Achyranthes bidentata* (Datiwan) and *Azadirachta indica* (Neem). *Journal of Microbiology and Antimicrobials,* Volume 3, No 1, (January 2011), pp. (1-7), ISSN 2141-2308

Jung, M., Lee, S. & Kim, H. (2000). Recent studies on natural products as anti-HIV agents. *Current Medicinal Chemistry,* Volume 7, No 6, (June 2000), pp. (649-661), ISSN 0929-8673

Kim, J.-Y., Park, S.-C., Hwang, I., Cheong, H., Nah, J.-W., Hahm, K.-S. & Park., Y. (2009). Protease inhibitors from plants with antimicrobial activity. *International Journal of Molecular Sciences,* Volume 10, (June 2009), pp. (2860-2872), ISSN 1422-0067

Masood, N., Chaudhry, A. & Tariq, P. (2006). Bactericidal activity of black pepper, bay leaf, aniseed and coriander against oral isolates. *Pakistan Journal of Pharmaceutical Sciences*, Volume 19, No 3, (July 2006), pp. (214-218), ISSN 1011-601X

Najiah, M., Nadirah, M., Arief, Z., Zahrol, S., Tee, L.W., Ranzi, A.D., Amar, A.S., Laith, A.A., Mariam, M., Suzana, S. & Aide, R.J. (2011). Antibacterial activity of Malaysian edible herb extracts on fish pathogenic bacteria. *Research Journal of Medicinal Plants*, Volume 5, No 6, pp. (772-778), ISSN 1819-3455

Nascimento, P.F.C., Nascimento, A., Rodrigues, C.S., Antoniolli, A.R., Santos, P.O., júnior, A.M.B. & Trindade, R.C. (2007). Atividade antimicrobiana dos óleos essenciais: uma abordagem multifatorial dos métodos. *Revista Brasileira de Farmacognosia*, Volume 17, No 1, (Janeiro/Março 2007), pp. (108-113), ISSB 0102-695X

Rahman, S., Parvez, A.K., Islam, R. & Khan, M.H. (2011). Antibacterial activity of natural spices on multiple drug resistant *Escherichia coli* isolated from drinking water, Bangladesh. *Annals of Clinical Microbiology and Antimicrobials*, Volume 10, (March 2011), pp. (1-4), ISSN 1476-0711

Rijo, P. (2010). Phytochemical study and biological activities of diterpenes and derivatives from Plectranthus species. In: *University of Lisbon*, 2011-08-01, Available from: <http://repositorio.ul.pt/handle/10451/2833>

Rios, J.L., Recio, M.C. & Villar, A. (1987). Antimicrobial activity of selected plants employed in the Spanish Mediterranean area. *Journal of Ethnopharmacology*, Volume 21, No 2 (November 1987), pp. (139-152), ISSN 0378-8741

Rodrigues, J.S. (2002). Contributo para o estudo etnobotânico das plantas medicinais e aromáticas na área protegida da Serra do Açor. Instituto da Conservação da Natureza

Roopashree, T.S., Dang, R., Rani, R.H.S. & Narendra, C. (2008). Antibacterial activity of antipsoriatic herbs: Cassia tora, Momordica charantia and Calendula officinalis. *International Journal of Applied Research in Natural Products*, Volume 1, No 3, (September/October 2008), pp. (20-28), ISSN 1940-6223

Shan, B., Cai, Y.Z., Brooks, J.D. & Corke, D. (2007). The *in vitro* antibacterial activity of dietary spices and medicinal herb extracts. *International Journal of Food Microbiology*, Volume 117, No 1, (June 2007), pp. (112-119), ISSN 0168-1605

Shelef, L.A. (1984). Antimicrobial effects of spices. *Journal of Food Safety*, Volume 6, No 1, (March 1984), pp. (29-44), ISSN 1745-4565

Shelef, L.A., Naglik, O.A. & Bogen, D.W. (1980) Sensitivity of some common food-borne bacteria to the spices sage, rosemary and allspice. *Journal of Food Science*, Volume 45, No 4, (July 1980), pp. (1042-1044), ISSN 1750-3841

Tajkarimi, M.M., Ibrahim, S.A. & Cliver, D.O. (2010). Antimicrobial herbs and spice compounds in food. *Food Control*, Volume 21, No 9, (September 2010), pp. 1199-1218, ISSN 0956-7135

Tan, K. & Vanitha, J. (2004). Immunomodulatory and antimicrobial effects of some traditional medicinal herbs: a review. *Current Medicinal Chemistry*, Volume 11, No 11, (June 2004), pp. (1423-1430), ISSN 0929-8673

Vaishnavi, C., Kaur, S. & Kaur, M. (2007). Bactericidal activity of kitchen spices and condiments on enteropathogens. *Natural Product Radiance*, Volume 6, No 1, (Januray/February 2007), pp. (40-45), ISSN 0976-0504

Vuddhakul, V. Bhoopong, P., Hayeebilan, F. & Subhadhirasakul, S. (2007). Inhibitory activity of Thai condiments on pandemic strain of Vibrio parahaemolyticus. *Food Microbiology*, Volume 24, No 4, (June 2007), pp. (413-418), ISSN 0740-0020

Zaika, L.L., Kissinger, J.C. & Wasserman, A.E. (1983). Inhibition of lactic bacteria by herbs. *Journal of Food Science*, Volume 48, No 5, (September 1983), pp. (1455-1459), ISSN 1750-3841

6

The Susceptibility of *Staphylococcus aureus* and *Klebsiella pneumoniae* to Naturally Derived Selected Classes of Flavonoids

Johannes Bodenstein* and Karen Du Toit
Discipline of Pharmaceutical Sciences, University of KwaZulu-Natal (Westville Campus), Durban, South Africa

1. Introduction

The emergence of multi-drug resistant organisms has increasingly become a global public health issue. Rational and appropriate uses of antibiotics as well as strict infection control measurements are recommended in order to reduce the emergence of antibiotic resistant bacteria (Tseng et al., 2011). The complexity in treating multi-drug resistant infections has led to an increase in the search for novel and effective antibiotics, especially structures originating from natural products. Promising molecules could serve as lead compounds to be developed and researched further.

This chapter aims to review the susceptibility of two of the most common micro-organisms that are often implicated in antibiotic resistant infections, namely the Gram-positive *Staphylococcus aureus* and Gram-negative *Klebsiella pneumoniae* against natural products, specifically plants. Numerous researchers have investigated the susceptibility of these bacteria to plant extracts as well as to the individual components thereof. Flavonoids as a group of compounds originating from natural products have been investigated against these bacteria.

Flavonoids are diverse polyphenolic compounds which are widely distributed in the plant kingdom. They are abundantly found in natural sources like fruits, vegetables, seeds, nuts, flowers, tea, wine honey and propolis and therefore form part of the normal diet of humans (Cook & Samman, 1996). Many reports claim the usefulness of flavonoids in medical conditions, including anti-inflammatory, oestrogenic, antimicrobial, antioxidant and chelating, vascular and antitumour activities (Cook & Samman, 1996; Cushnie & Lamb, 2005). Flavonoids consist of a C15 skeleton composed of two phenolic rings, namely the A and B rings linked through a heterocyclic ring, C. They are classified according to their biosynthetic origin into major classes including flavones, flavonols, flavanones, chalcones, flavanols, anthocyanidins, isoflavones and dihydroflavonols. Substitution patterns vary and some flavonoids occur as glycosides which are hydrolysed in the human gut to the aglycones. Flavonoids also occur as monomers, dimers or oligomers (Cook & Samman, 1996; Cushnie & Lamb, 2005).

Many reports exist on the antimicrobial activity of flavonoids (Basile et al., 2010; Du Toit et al., 2009; Tanaka et al., 2011). Extracts as well as isolated compounds were tested against a

* Corresponding Author

comprehensive panel of micro-organisms. Methods of assessing the activity include different diffusion and dilution methods. However, many flavonoids are insoluble in water and will thus have a low rate of diffusion in an aqueous medium such as agar, leading to inaccurate results. Therefore, only results based on dilution methods will be considered and discussed.

Extracts are complex mixtures of many chemical compounds in different ratios and the results of such studies are not contributing to the understanding of the activity of specific flavonoids. Studies that investigated the antibacterial activity of individual flavonoids isolated from natural products will be reviewed instead.

Various parameters have been used to express the antimicrobial activity of flavonoids. The minimum inhibitory concentration (MIC) will be considered and values up to 50 μg/ml will be reported. It must be appreciated that varying laboratory conditions and technical skills will have an influence on published results generated by different research groups and used in this review. The question also arises whether flavonoids exhibit bactericidal or bacteriostatic activity. Although some studies suggest that flavonoids are capable of bactericidal activity, the interpretation of the results remains inconclusive and it has been suggested that bacterial aggregates may be formed, thereby reducing the number of colony forming units in viable counts (Cushnie & Lamb, 2005).

2. *Staphylococcus aureus*

Staphylococcus aureus has long been recognised as an important pathogen in many diseases, for example the toxic shock syndrome, vasculitis and glomerulonephritis. The bacterium is commonly found in the nose and upper respiratory tract, locations that play an important role in the epidemiology and pathogenesis of infection. Therapy of infection has become problematic due to an increasing number of methicillin-resistant strains (MRSA). The difference between MRSA and methicillin-susceptible strains is that MRSA is resistant to β-lactamase stable β-lactam antibiotics. Often this is also associated with resistance to many other antibiotics, which limits the therapeutic options. The prevalence of MRSA has also increased world-wide and new therapeutic agents, optimisation of infection control measures and introduction of new medical devices with a reduced risk of infection are being investigated (Kluytmans et al., 1997).

3. *Klebsiella pneumoniae*

Klebsiella pneumoniae is being considered the most common causative pathogen for infections caused by antibiotic-resistant bacteria. The rate of resistance to carbapenems has increased to more than 25% in the European Union in 2009 (Tseng et al., 2011). The nasopharynx and gastrointestinal tract are commonly colonised by the bacterium and it is well known to cause community-acquired bacterial pneumonia, occurring particularly in chronic alcoholics and showing characteristic radiographic abnormalities due to severe pyogenic infection which has a high fatality rate if untreated. It is an opportunistic pathogen that would most likely attack immunocompromised patients who are hospitalised and suffer from severe underlying diseases such as diabetes mellitus and chronic pulmonary obstructive diseases. The three most common conditions caused by *Klebsiella* spp. are urinary tract infections, septicaemia and wound infections. Septicaemia is particularly problematic in premature infants and patients in intensive care units (Podschun & Ullmann, 1998).

4. Occurrence of flavonoids in plant sources

Several studies have identified flavonoids in natural products. Many flavonoid-containing plants are used therapeutically for the treatment of a variety of non-microbial illnesses as well as microbial infections. Flavonoids were derived from different parts of the plant and tested against *S. aureus* and *K. pneumoniae.* The vast number of identified compounds in studies were limited to cases where antibacterial activity was measured by means of dilution methods and where susceptibility was up to 50 μg/ml, providing a workable approach. At least 44 different compounds were identified according to the criteria, listed in Table 1 and their properties reviewed (Tables 2-7).

Plant/Product	Traditional Use	Part	Compound	Reference
Erythrina costaricensis Micheli (Leguminosae)	Microbial infections	Stems	1	Tanaka et al., 2009
Erythrina costaricensis Micheli (Leguminosae)	Microbial infections	Stems	2	Tanaka et al., 2009
Erythrina poeppigiana (Leguminosae)	Microbial infections	Roots	3	Tanaka et al., 2004
Erythrina poeppigiana (Leguminosae	Microbial infections	Roots	4	Tanaka et al., 2004
Brazilian red propolis	Inflammation, heart disease, diabetes, cancer		5	Oldoni et al., 2011
Erythrina variegata (Leguminosae)	Microbial infections, inflammation	Roots	6	Tanaka et al., 2002
Erythrina variegata (Leguminosae)	Microbial infections, inflammation	Roots	7	Tanaka et al., 2002
Erythrina variegata (Leguminosae)	Microbial infections, inflammation	Roots	8	Tanaka et al., 2002
Erythrina variegata (Leguminosae)	Microbial infections, inflammation	Roots	9	Tanaka et al., 2002
Erythrina variegata (Leguminosae)	Microbial infections, inflammation	Roots	10	Tanaka et al., 2002
Erythrina variegata (Leguminosae)	Microbial infections, inflammation	Roots	11	Tanaka et al., 2002
Erythrina variegata (Leguminosae)	Microbial infections, inflammation	Roots	12	Tanaka et al., 2002
Erythrina variegata (Leguminosae)	Microbial infections, inflammation	Roots	13	Tanaka et al., 2002

Plant/Product	Traditional Use	Part	Compound	Reference
Erythrina variegata (Leguminosae)	Microbial infections, inflammation	Roots	14	Tanaka et al., 2002
Erythrina variegata (Leguminosae)	Microbial infections	Roots	15	Tanaka et al., 2011
Erythrina variegata (Leguminosae)	Microbial infections	Roots	16	Tanaka et al., 2011
Cycas circinalis (Cycadaceae)	Purgative	Leaflets	17	Moawad et al., 2010
Cycas circinalis (Cycadaceae)	Purgative	Leaflets	18	Moawad et al., 2010
Cycas revoluta Thumb (Cycadaceae)	Rheumatic fever, expectorant, astringent, flatulence, vomiting, oestrogen-dependent cancer	Leaflets	19	Moawad et al., 2010
Feijoa sellowiana Berg (Myrtaceae)	Perfume, microbial infections, inflammation, cancer	Fruits	20	Basile et al., 2010
Lonchocarpus minimiflorus (Noctuidae)	Microbial infections	Bark	21	Salvatore et al., 1998
Viscum album ssp. *album* (Loranthaceae)	Hypertension, epilepsy, exhaustion, anxiety, arthritis, vertigo, degenerative inflammation of the joints, cancer	Leaves and stems	22	Orhan et al., 2010
Viscum album ssp. *album* (Loranthaceae)	Hypertension, epilepsy, exhaustion, anxiety, arthritis, vertigo, degenerative inflammation of the joints, cancer	Leaves and stems	23	Orhan et al., 2010
Galium fissurense Ehrend. & Schönb.-Tem. (Rubiaceae)	Diuretic, astringent, gastro-intestinal conditions, gout, epilepsy	Leaves and stems	24	Orhan et al., 2010

Plant/Product	Traditional Use	Part	Compound	Reference
Galium fissurense Ehrend. & Schönb.-Tem. (Rubiaceae)	Diuretic, astringent, gastro-intestinal conditions, gout, epilepsy	Leaves and stems	25	Orhan et al., 2010
Cirsium hypoleucum DC. (Asteraceae)	Haemorrhoids, peptic ulcers, cough, bronchitis	Aerial parts	26	Orhan et al., 2010
Cirsium hypoleucum DC. (Asteraceae)	Haemorrhoids, peptic ulcers, cough, bronchitis	Aerial parts	27	Orhan et al., 2010
Artocarpus sepicanus (Moraceae)	Microbial infections, asthma, tuberculosis, rheumatic fever	Leaves	28	Radwan et al., 2009
Erythrina zeyheri (Leguminosae)	Microbial infections, asthma, tuberculosis, rheumatic fever	Roots	29	Tanaka et al., 2003
Erythrina zeyheri (Leguminosae)	Microbial infections, asthma, tuberculosis, rheumatic fever	Roots	30	Tanaka et al., 2003
Erythrina zeyheri (Leguminosae)	Microbial infections, asthma, tuberculosis, rheumatic fever	Roots	31	Tanaka et al., 2003
Erythrina zeyheri (Leguminosae)	Microbial infections, asthma, tuberculosis, rheumatic fever	Roots	32	Tanaka et al., 2003
Erythrina zeyheri (Leguminosae)	Microbial infections, asthma, tuberculosis, rheumatic fever	Roots	33	Tanaka et al., 2003
Sophora exigua Criab (Leguminosae)	Microbial infections	Roots	34	Tsuchiya et al., 1996
Sophora exigua Criab (Leguminosae)	Microbial infections	Roots	35	Tsuchiya et al., 1996
Sophora exigua Criab (Leguminosae)	Microbial infections	Roots	36	Tsuchiya et al., 1996
Sophora exigua Criab (Leguminosae)	Microbial infections	Roots	37	Tsuchiya et al., 1996
Sophora exigua Criab (Leguminosae)	Microbial infections	Roots	38	Tsuchiya et al., 1996
Sophora exigua Criab (Leguminosae)	Microbial infections	Roots	39	Tsuchiya et al., 1996

Plant/Product	Traditional Use	Part	Compound	Reference
Echinosophora koreensis Nakai (Leguminosae)	Microbial infections	Roots	40	Tsuchiya et al., 1996
Echinosophora koreensis Nakai (Leguminosae)	Microbial infections	Roots	41	Tsuchiya et al., 1996
Echinosophora koreensis Nakai (Leguminosae)	Microbial infections	Roots	42	Tsuchiya et al., 1996
Echinosophora koreensis Nakai (Leguminosae)	Microbial infections	Roots	43	Tsuchiya et al., 1996
Sophora leachiana Peck (Leguminosae)	Microbial infections	Roots	44	Tsuchiya et al., 1996

Table 1. Compounds isolated from different parts of plants/products that occur world-wide and their traditional use. Only compounds tested against *Staphylococcus aureus* and *Klebsiella pneumoniae* by means of dilution methods where the MIC-values were up to 50 μg/ml are reported (refer to Tables 2-7 where the classification, chemistry and biological activity of each compound are explained in more detail).

5. Flavonoids and bacterial susceptibility

The flavonoids identified in different plants/products which were investigated for their antibacterial activity using dilution methods, were divided into 6 structural types and the susceptibility of *S. aureus* and *K. pneumoniae* reviewed. Some of the strains of *S. aureus* were MSRA.

Structural types were used in order to compare similar structures and to determine the influence of substituents on these structures. Susceptibility was also compared where the methods were similar to reduce the presence of too many variables.

Compounds 17-19 (Table 6), which are biflavonoids, exhibited the weakest activity against *S. aureus* in comparison with all the other structures. This may be attributed to the size and stereochemistry of the molecules. The compounds exhibiting the highest activity were compounds 16 (Table 3) and 21 (Table 2), which interestingly share the same substitution pattern at R_1 and R_2 (which were substituted with a γ,γ-dimethylallyl and hydroxyl group respectively). Comparison of compounds 3, 6 and 16 (Table 3), which were all substituted with a γ,γ-dimethylallyl group at R_5, showed that the addition of an extra γ,γ-dimethylallyl group influences activity. Addition at R_3 increases activity and addition at R_1 has an even more pronounced effect in the structural group. Comparison of compounds 30 and 31 (Table 2) showed that substitution at R_5 with a hydroxyl group leads to better activity than substitution with a methoxy group in the specific structural group.

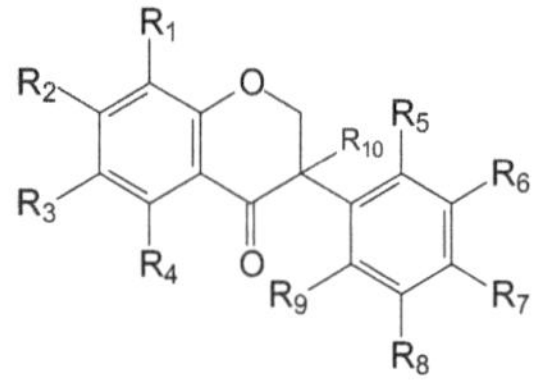

Compound	Structure	Susceptibility (MIC, μg/ml)	
		S. Aureus	*K. Pneumoniae*
1	R_2,R_4,R_6=OH R_3,R_8=γ,γ-dimethylallyl R_7=OCH_3	3.13-6.25*	ND
2	R_2,R_3=2″,2″ dimethylpyran R_4,R_6=OH R_7=OCH_3 R_8=γ,γ-dimethylallyl	12.5- >50*	ND
5	R_2,R_5=OH R_7=OCH_3 (3*S*-enantiomer)	31.2-62.5	ND
8	R_2,R_3=2″,2″ dimethylpyran R_5,R_7=OH (3*R*-enantiomer)	12.5-25*	ND
12	R_1,R_2=2″,2″ dimethylpyran R_3=γ,γ-dimethylallyl R_7,R_9=OH	3.13-12.5*	ND
15	R_1=γ,γ-dimethylallyl R_2,R_3=2″,2″ dimethylpyran R_7,R_9,R_{10}=OH	12.5-25*	ND
21	R_1,R_3=γ,γ-dimethylallyl R_2,R_4,R_6=OH (2*S*-enantiomer)	0.78-1.56*	ND
22	R_2,R_4=OCH_3 R_6=*O*-glc	4	16
23	R_2,R_4=OCH_3 R_6=*O*-[2″-*O*-(5‴-*O*-*trans*-cinnamoyl)-β-*D*-apiofuranosyl]-β-*D*-glucopyranoside	4	16
24	R_2,R_4,R_5=OH R_6=*O*-glc	4	16
25	R_4,R_6=OH R_2=*O*-glc	4	16
28	R_2,R_4,R_6=OH R_3=geranyl (2*S*-enantiomer)	1.23*	ND
29	R_1,R_8=γ,γ-dimethylallyl R_2,R_7,R_9=OH	12.5-25*	ND
30	R_1,R_3=γ,γ-dimethylallyl R_2,R_7=OH R_5=OCH_3 (3*R*-enantiomer)	25- >50	ND
31	R_1,R_3=γ,γ-dimethylallyl R_2,R_5,R_7=OH (3*R*-enantiomer)	3.13-6.25*	ND
32	R_1=γ,γ-dimethylallyl R_2,R_3=2″,2″-dimethylpyran R_5,R_7=OH	6.25-12.5*	ND

Table 2. Isoflavanones of the following structure isolated from plants and propolis (compound 5) and their activities against *Staphylococcus aureus* (*denotes MRSA strains) and *Klebsiella pneumoniae*. ND, not determined.

A study by Du Toit and co-workers reported little activity of the flavonoids luteolin, eriodictyol and quercetin against *S. aureus* and MIC-values could not be determined. These flavonoids are commonly found in propolis (Du Toit et al., 2009). Combinations of flavonoids at different concentrations as well as other components present in the propolis could account for its antimicrobial activity.

Compared to *S. aureus,* it is noteworthy that significantly fewer compounds have been tested against *K. pneumoniae*. Compounds 22-25 (Table 2) and 20, 26-27 (Table 7) were the only compounds tested using dilution methods. Out of the few compounds tested, compound 20 showed the highest activity and it also has the least number of substituents. Future research should investigate the activity of more compounds against *K. pneumoniae*.

New drug targets in the bacterial structure are important. Drugs will be less susceptible to resistance if it has several modes of action. Pharmacokinetic parameters such as bioavailability and plasma protein binding are also important, since successful traditional use indicates that the drug has successfully reached a specific target.

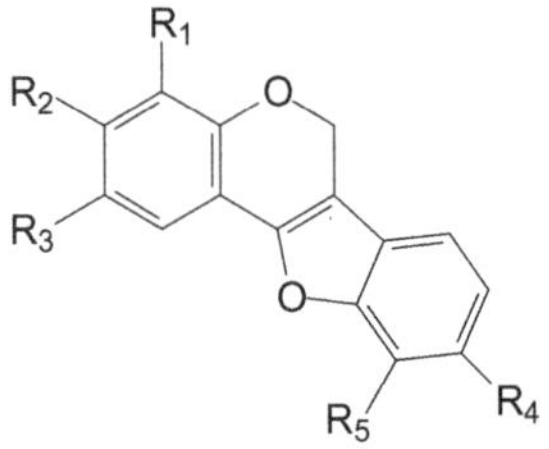

Compound	Structure	Susceptibility (MIC, µg/ml)	
		S. Aureus	*K. Pneumoniae*
3	R_2,R_4=OH R_5=γ,γ-dimethylallyl	12.5*	ND
4	R_2=OH R_4=OCH_3 R_5=γ,γ-dimethylallyl	12.5-25	ND
6	R_2,R_4=OH R_3,R_5=γ,γ-dimethylallyl	3.13-6.25*	ND
9	R_2=OH R_4=OCH_3 R_5=γ,γ-dimethylallyl	12.5-25*	ND
16	R_1,R_5=γ,γ-dimethylallyl R_2,R_4=OH	1.56-3.13*	ND

Table 3. Isoflavonoids of the following structure isolated from plants and their activities against *Staphylococcus aureus* (*denotes MRSA strains) and *Klebsiella pneumoniae*. ND, not determined.

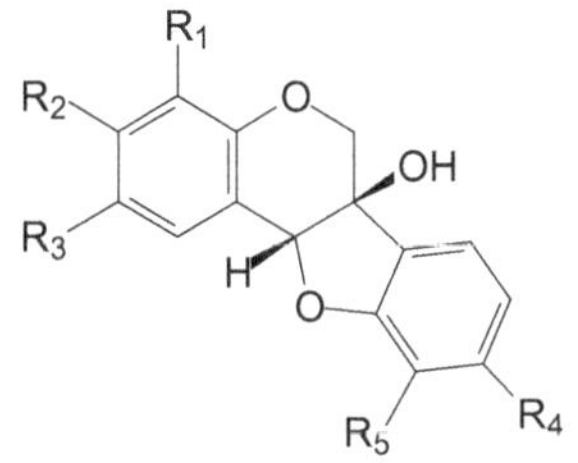

Compound	Structure	Susceptibility (MIC, µg/ml)	
		S. Aureus	*K. Pneumoniae*
7	R_2=OH R_3,R_5=γ,γ-dimethylallyl R_4=OCH_3	12.5-25*	ND
14	R_2,R_4=OH R_3,R_5=γ,γ-dimethylallyl	6.25-12.5*	ND
33	R_1,R_5=γ,γ-dimethylallyl R_2=OH R_4=OCH_3 (6a*S*, 11a*S*-enantiomer)	6.25-25*	ND

Table 4. Isoflavonoids of the following structure isolated from plants and their activities against *Staphylococcus aureus* (*denotes MRSA strains) and *Klebsiella pneumoniae*. ND, not determined.

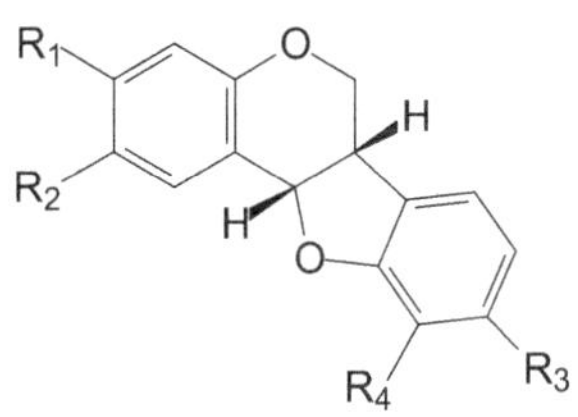

Compound	Structure	Susceptibility (MIC, µg/ml)	
		S. Aureus	*K. Pneumoniae*
10	R_1=OCH_3 R_2=γ,γ-dimethylallyl R_3=OH RR	3.13-6.25*	ND
11	R_1,R_2=2",2"-dimethylpyran R_3=OH R_4=γ,γ-dimethylallyl	6.25-25*	ND
13	R_1=OH R_3,R_4=2",2"-dimethylpyran	25*	ND

Table 5. Isoflavonoids of the following structure isolated from plants and their activities against *Staphylococcus aureus* (*denotes MRSA strains) and *Klebsiella pneumoniae*. ND, not determined.

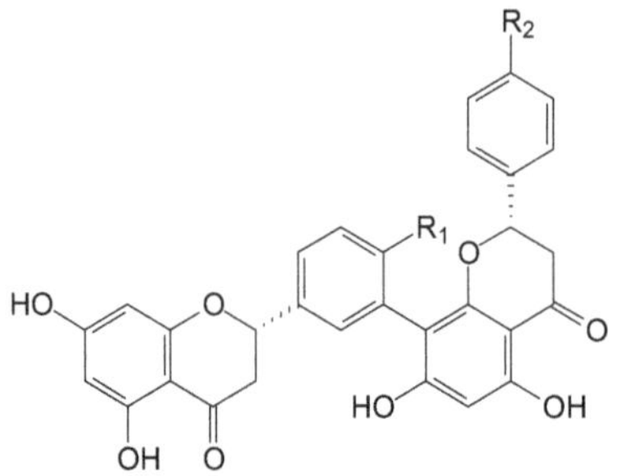

Compound	Structure	Susceptibility (MIC, µg/ml)	
		S. Aureus	*K. Pneumoniae*
17	R_1,R_2=OCH_3 (2*S*, 2″*S*-enantiomer)	17.5*	ND
18	R_1=OCH_3 R_2=OH (2*S*, 2″*S*-enantiomer)	35.9*	ND
19	R_1,R_2=OH (2*S*-enantiomer)	37*	ND

Table 6. Biflavonoids of the following structure isolated from plants and their activities against *Staphylococcus aureus* (*denotes MRSA strains) and *Klebsiella pneumoniae*. ND, not determined.

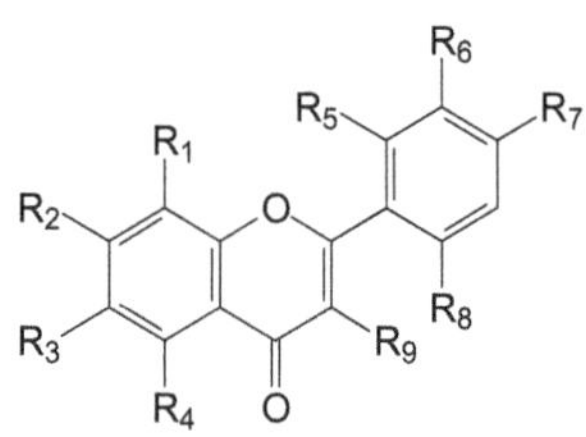

Compound	Structure	Susceptibility (MIC, µg/ml)	
		S. Aureus	*K. Pneumoniae*
20	R_5=OH	7.8	7.8
26	R_2,R_4,R_6,R_7=OH R_9=*O*-glc-rha	4	16
27	R_2,R_4,R_7=OH R_9=*O*-glc-rha	4	16
34	R_1=lavandulyl R_2,R_4,R_7,R_8=OH	3.13-6.25*	ND
35	R_1=lavandulyl R_2,R_4,R_5,R_8=OH R_3=prenyl R_7=OCH_3	3.13-6.25*	ND
36	R_1=prenyl	6.25*	ND

Compound	Structure	Susceptibility (MIC, µg/ml)	
		S. Aureus	*K. Pneumoniae*
	R_2,R_4,R_5,R_8=OH R_7=OCH_3		
37	R_1=lavandulyl R_2,R_4,R_5,R_8=OH	12.5*	ND
38	R_2,R_4,R_5,R_7,R_8=OH R_3=geranyl	12.5*	ND
39	R_1=geranyl R_2,R_4,R_5,R_7,R_8=OH	>25*	ND
40	R_2,R_4,R_7,R_8= OH R_6=geranyl	3.13-12.5*	ND
41	R_2,R_4,R_5,R_7,R_8=OH R_3=lavandulyl	3.13-12.5*	ND
42	R_1=lavandulyl R_2,R_4,R_5,R_7,R_8=OH	6.25-12.5*	ND
43	R_2,R_4,R_7,R_8=OH R_1=prenyl	6.25-12.5*	ND
44	R_1=lavandulyl R_2,R_4,R_8=OH	12.5*	ND

Table 7. Flavones of the following structure isolated from plants and their activities against *Staphylococcus aureus* (*denotes MRSA strains) and *Klebsiella pneumoniae*. ND, not determined.

6. Conclusion

The traditional use of medicinal plants is useful as a guideline in the quest for new drugs. Furthermore plants are a source of novel lead compounds which would generally not have been synthesised. Extraction of these biologically active lead compounds may be expensive and slow and the activity of lead compounds may also not be sufficient to encourage commercialisation. These compounds may also have undesirable side effects, it is therefore important to periodically review the results of research conducted, ruling out unnecessary variation of parameters, to determine the most promising structures. The process of drug design and development could then be accelerated.

7. Acknowledgment

We thank the University of KwaZulu-Natal Competitor Fund for financial support.

8. References

Basile, A.; Conte, B.; Rigano, D.; Senatore, F. & Sorbo, S. (2010). Antibacterial and antifungal properties of acetonic extract of *Feijoa sellowiana* fruits and its effect on *Helicobacter pylori* growth. *Journal of Medicinal Food*, Vol. 13, pp. 189-195.

Cook, N.C. & Samman, S. (1996). Flavonoids – chemistry, metabolism, cardioprotective effects, and dietary sources. *Nutritional Biochemistry*, Vol. 7, pp. 66-76.

Cushnie, T.P. & Lamb, A.J. (2005). Antimicrobial activity of flavonoids. *International Journal of Antimicrobial Agents,* Vol. 26, pp. 343-356.

Du Toit, K.; Buthelezi, S. & Bodenstein, J. (2009). Anti-inflammatory and antibacterial profiles of selected compounds found in South African propolis. *South African Journal of Science,* Vol. 105, pp. 470-472.

Kluytmans, J.; Van Belkum, A. & Verbrugh, H. (1997). Nasal carriage of *Staphylococcus aureus*: Epidemiology, underlying mechanisms, and associated risks. *Clinical Microbiology Reviews,* Vol. 10, pp. 505-520.

Moawad, A.; Hetta, M.; Zjawiony, J.K.; Jacob, M.R.; Hifnawy, M.; Marais, J.P.J. & Ferreira, D. (2010). Phytochemical investigation of *Cycas circinalis* and *Circas revoluta* leaflets: Moderately active antibacterial biflavonoids. *Planta Medica,* vol. 76, pp. 796-802.

Oldoni, T.L.C.; Cabral, I.S.R.; Regitano d'Arce, M.A.B., Rosalen, P.L.; Ikegaki, M.; Nascimento, A.M. & Alencar, S.M. (2011). Isolation and analysis of bioactive isoflavonoids and chalcone from a new type of Brazilian propolis. *Separation and Purification Technology,* Vol. 77, pp. 208-213.

Orhan, D.D.; Özçelik, B.; Özgen, S. & Ergun, F. (2010). Antibacterial, antifungal, and antiviral activities of some flavonoids. *Microbiological Research,* Vol. 165, pp. 496-504.

Podschun, R. & Ullmann, U. (1998). *Klebsiella* spp. as nosocomial pathogens: Epidemiology, taxonomy, typing methods, and pathogenicity factors. *Clinical Microbiology Reviews,* Vol. 11, pp. 589-603.

Radwan, M.M.; Rodriguez-Guzman, R.; Manly, S.P.; Jacob, M. & Ross, S.A. (2009). Sepicanin A – a new geranyl flavanone from Artocarpus sepicanus with activity against methicillin-resistant *Staphylococcus aureus* (MRSA). *Phytochemistry Letters,* Vol. 2, pp. 141-143.

Salvatore, M.J.; King, A.B.; Graham, A.C.; Onishi, H.R.; Bartizal, K.F.; Abruzzo, G.K.; Gill, C.J.; Ramjit, H.G.; Pitzenberger, S.M. & Witherup, K.M. (1998). Antibacterial activity of lonchocarpol A. *Journal of Natural Products,* Vol. 61, pp. 640-642.

Tanaka, H.; Sato, M.; Fujiwara, S.; Hirata, M.; Etoh, H. & Takeuchi, H. (2002). Antibacterial activity of isoflavonoids isolated from *Erythrina variegata* against methicillin-resistant *Staphylococcus aureus*. *Letters in Applied Microbiology,* Vol. 35, pp. 494-498.

Tanaka, H.; Oh-Uchi, T.; Etoh, H.; Sako, M.; Asai, F.; Fukai, T.; Sato, M.; Murata, J. & Tateishi, Y. (2003). Isoflavonoids from roots of *Erythrina zeyheri*. *Phytochemistry,* Vol. 64, pp. 753-758.

Tanaka, H.; Sato, M.; Oh-Uchi, T.; Yamaguchi, R.; Etoh, H.; Shimizu, H.; Sako, M. & Takeuchi, H. (2004). Antibacterial properties of a new isoflavonoid from *Erythrina poeppigiana* against methicillin-resistant *Staphylococcus aureus*. *Phytomedicine,* Vol. 11, pp. 331-337.

Tanaka, H.; Hattori, H.; Oh-Uchi, T.; Sato, M.; Sako, M.; Tateishi, Y. & Rizwani, G.H. (2009). Three new isoflavanones from *Erythrina costaricensis*. *Natural Product Research,* Vol. 23, pp. 1089-1094.

Tanaka, H.; Atsumi, I.; Shirota, O.; Sekita, S.; Sakai, E.; Sato, M.; Murata, H.; Darnaedi, D. & Chen, I-S. (2011). Three new constituents from the roots of *Erythrina variegata* and their antibacterial activity against methicillin-resistant *Staphylococcus aureus*. *Chemistry & Biodiversity,* Vol. 8, pp. 476-482.

Tseng, S-H.; Lee, C-M.; Lin, T-Y.; Chang, S-C. & Chang, F.Y. (2011). Emergence and spread of multi-drug resistant organisms: Think globally and act locally. *Journal of Microbiology, Immunology and Infection,* Vol. 44, pp. 157-165.

Tsuchiya, H.; Sato, M.; Miyazaki, T.; Fujiwara, S.; Tanigaki, S.; Ohyama, M.; Tanaka, T. & Iinuma, M. (1996). Comparative study on the antibacterial activity of phytochemical flavanones against methicillin-resistant *Staphylococcus aureus*. *Journal of Ethnopharmacology,* Vol. 50, pp. 27-34.

7

An Alternative Approaches for the Control of Sorghum Pathogens Using Selected Medicinal Plants Extracts

Varaprasad Bobbarala[1,*] and Chandrasekhar K. Naidu[2]
[1]*Translational Research Institute of Molecular Sciences (TRIMS), Visakhapatnam, AP,*
[2]*Department of Botany, College of Science and Technology, Andhra University, Visakhapatnam*
India

1. Introduction

Sorghum (*Sorghum vulgare* L.) belongs to the tribe Andropogonae of the grass family Poaceae. The genus Sorghum is characterized by spikelet's borne in pairs. Sorghum is treated as an annual, although it is a perennial grass and in the tropics it can be harvested many times. Sorghum crop production has considerably increased in several countries during the past few years. Sorghum is the fifth important cereals after wheat, rice and maize and are significant dietary food for one-third of the world population, these crops are the principal sources of energy, protein, vitamins and minerals for millions of the poorest people in these regions and sustain the lives of the poorest rural people and will continue to do so in the foreseeable future. India is the world's second largest producer of Sorghum. Like all crops, grain Sorghum is subject to infectious diseases which can sometimes limit production. Sorghum is susceptible to fungal and bacterial micro flora under certain environmental conditions. These mycoflora not only threaten plant growth but also affect food quality, causing huge economic losses. Every year, seed and seedling diseases of grain Sorghum are common in India. Grain Sorghum root rot can be a considerable problem in Sorghum production.

Synthetic pesticides are nowadays widely used for the control of plant diseases throughout the world because of their higher effectiveness in controlling disease causing organisms. However, excessive and unsystematic application of these chemicals has created several environmental and health hazards and also some phytopathogens have been developed resistance (Rhouma et al., 2009). Therefore, there is an urgent need to search for effective, safe and biodegradable alternative pesticides. Diseases of cultivated crops remain the major limitation to increased agricultural production. Therefore, protection of plants from pathogens remains a primary concern of agricultural scientists. Despite serious environmental implications associated with the increased use, chemical fungicides remain the first line of defense against bacterial and fungal pathogens.

* Corresponding Author

Natural plant products and their analogues are an important source of new agricultural chemicals (Cardellina, 1988, Gulter, 1988). Medicinal plants as a group comprise approximately 8000 species and account for around 50% of all the higher flowering plant species of India. Over one and a half million practitioners of the Indian System of Medicine use medicinal plants in preventive, promotive and curative applications. In recent years, secondary plant metabolites (Phytochemicals), previously with unknown pharmacological activities, have been extensively investigated as a source of medicinal agents (Krisharaju et al, 2005). Plants have been formed the basis of natural pesticides, that make excellent leads for new pesticide development (Newman et al., 2000). The potential of higher plants as a source of new drugs is still largely unexplored. Hence, last decade witnessed an increase in the investigation on plants as a source of new biomolecules for human disease management (Grierson and Afolayan, 1999). Green plants are found to be an effective reservoir for the bioactive molecules and can provide valuable sources for the discovery of natural pesticides (Akhtar *et al.,* 1997). Therefore in recent years medicinal plant extracts are intensively analyzed with an aim of isolating novel bioactive compounds.

2. Materials and methods

2.1 Plant materials

Fifty medicinal plants (Table-1) were selected in this study based on the information collected from literature (Warrier *et al.,* 1994-1996 and Pullaiah, 2002). All the plant materials were collected in and around Visakhapatnam over the course of the respective growth season during February to April in the year 2005 because of the extracts were generally rich in antibacterial agents after the flowering (sexual) stage and plants from stressful environments (Mitscher *et al.,* 1972). Plant materials were identified with the help of Gamble, "Flora of the Presidency of Madras" and later verified by comparison with the authentic specimens available in the herbariums of NBRI, Lucknow and the Department of Botany, Andhra University, Visakhapatnam. Voucher specimens were deposited in the herbarium of the Botany Department, Andhra University, Visakhapatnam.

2.2 Solvents and chemicals used

All chemicals were purchased from Qualigens fine Chemicals, Mumbai and SD fine chemicals, Mumbai. All culture media components and antibiotics used in this study were procured from Hi Media, Mumbai, India.

2.3 Tested organisms

Based on the disease index of Sorghum (Horne and Frederiksen., 1993) crops in which five phytopathogenic microorganisms were selected to screen the antimicrobial inhibition of the selected plant extracts listed in Table-2. The organisms used were procured from Microbial Type Culture Collection & Gene Bank (MTCC), Chandigarh. The lyophilized form of pure strain is reconstituted in sterile water and produced a suspension of the microbial cells. Inoculation was done with sterile inoculating loop to liquid broth medium. Liquid cultures are then incubated to allow cell replication and adequate growth of the culture, for use in bioassays. Following incubation, liquid cultures are refrigerated to store for further use. Typically, 24 hours will provide sufficient growth to allow visibly thick spread of the microbes as required for bioassay. The bacterial strains are maintained and tested on Nutrient Agar (NA) and Potato Dextrose Agar (PDA) for fungi.

2.4 Preparation of plant extracts

The collected plant materials were chopped into small pieces shade dried and coarsely powdered in Willy mill. The coarsely powdered material weighed and extracted with hexane, chloroform, methanol and water in sequential order of polarity using a soxhlet extractor for five to six hours at temperature not exceeding the boiling point of the solvent. For each gram of dry material 2ml of solvent was used. The extracted solvents were filtered through Whatman no-1 filter paper and subsequently concentrated under reduced pressure (in vacuo at 40°c) using a rotary evaporator. The residue obtained were designated as crude extracts and stored in a freezer at -20°c until assayed.

The dried plant extract residues obtained were redissolved in 0.1% Dimethyl Sulfoxide (DMSO) to get different concentrations (100mg/ml, 300mg/ml and 500mg/ml) of crude extracts and filtration through a 0.45µm membrane filter and stored in sterile brown bottles in a freezer at 20°c until bioassay.

The prepared hexane, chloroform, methanol and water extracts samples were tested for antimicrobial activity against the test organism's the plant pathogens using the agar cup plate method. Streptomycin (5µg) was placed as a positive control in all plates and inoculated with bacteria and for the bacterial cultures used that was incubated at 37°C for 18-24 hours. Bavistin (5µg) was placed as a positive control in all plates inoculated with fungi and for the fungal cultures that were incubated at 26°C for 36-48 h. The microbes were plated in triplicates and average zone diameter was noted.

2.5 Antibacterial activity

The antimicrobial activity of the chloroform, methanol and water extracts of each sample was evaluated by using well diffusion method or cup plate method of Murray *et al.,* (1995) modified by Olurinola, (1996). Which is the most widely used type for identifying the antimicrobial activity, which exploit diffusion of antimicrobial compounds through agar media to demonstrate inhibition of bacteria and fungi.

2.5.1 Composition of nutrient agar medium

Peptone	:	5grams
Meat extract	:	10 grams
Sodium chloride	:	5grams
Agar agar	:	15grams
Distilled water to make	:	1000ml
pH adjusted to	:	7.2 to 7.4

2.5.2 Procedure

This assay performed by two methods agar disc diffusion and agar well diffusion. In these two methods the agar well diffusion essay was used to screen for antimicrobial activity of the hexane, chloroform, methanol and water extracts of different plant species. In agar well diffusion method peptone (0.5 grams), meat extract (1.0 grams), sodium chloride (0.5 grams) and agar (1.5 grams) were dissolved in small quantity of distilled water with the aid of heat on water bath and the volume was made up to 100 ml with purified water. The pH of the nutrient broth was adjusted to 7.2 using 5M sodium hydroxide, and then sterilized in an autoclave maintained at 121°C (15lbs/sq. in.) for 20 minutes.

After sterilization, the medium was inoculated with 3µl aliquots of culture containing approximately 105 CFU/ml of each organism of 24hours slant culture in aseptic condition and transferred into sterile 6 inch diameter petridishes and allowed to set at room temperature for about 10 minutes and then kept in a refrigerator for 30 minutes. After setting a number 3 cup borer (6mm) diameter was properly sterilized by flaming and used to make three to five uniform cups/wells in each petridish. A drop of molten nutrient agar was used to seal the base of each cup. The cups/wells were filled with 50µl of the different extracts of 100mg/ml, 300mg/ml, and 500mg/ml so final drug concentration will be 5mg/well, 15mg/well, and 25mg/well respectively and allow diffusing of plant extract into the medium for about 45 minutes.

Standard drugs Streptomycin (5µg/ml), control (0.1% DMSO) were transferred to the cups of each agar plate by means of sterile pipettes under a laminar flow unit. The solvents used for reconstituting the extracts were similarly analyzed. The plates thus prepared were left for 2 hours in a refrigerator for diffusion and then kept in an incubator at 37°C. After 24 hours, the agar plates were examined for inhibition zones, and the zones were measured in millimeters. The zones of inhibition were measured with antibiotic zone scale in mm and the experiment was carried out in triplicates.

2.6 Antifungal activity

2.6.1 Composition of PDA medium

Potatoes (peeled)	:	200grams
Dextrose	:	20grams
Agar-Agar	:	15grams
Distilled water to make up to	:	1000ml

2.6.2 Procedure

Peeled potatoes (20grams) were cut into small pieces and boiled with 100ml of water for 30 minutes. The pieces are crushed during boiling and the pulp was removed after cooling by filtration through muslin cloth. Dextrose (2grams) and agar (1.5grams) were added and the volume is made up to 100ml. the medium is then distributed in 20ml quantities in two 250ml conical flasks and were sterilized in an autoclave at 121°C (15lbs/sq. in.) for 30min. the medium was inoculated using 4 days cultures of the test organisms in aseptic condition and transferred to sterile 6 inch diameter petri dishes and allowed to set at room temperature for about 10 minutes. Four cups of 6mm diameter bore in medium at equal distance were made in each agar plate by using sterile borer.

Hexane, chloroform, methanol and water extracts in different concentrations (100mg/ml, 300mg/ml, and 500mg/ml) to get the final drug concentration 5mg/well, 15mg/well, and 25mg/well respectively, control (DMSO) and standard (Bavistin 5µg/ml), were transferred to the cups of each agar plate, incubated at room temperature (28°C) and examined for inhibition zones of 36 hours of incubation. The results of different studies provide evidence that some medicinal plants might indeed be potential sources of new antibacterial agents even against some antibiotic-resistant strains (Kone *et al.*, 2004).

2.7 Minimum inhibitory concentration (MIC) assays

Based on the preliminary reports all the medicinal plants were identified to have potent antimicrobial activity and Minimum Inhibitory Concentrations (MIC) of the extracts was determined according to Elizabeth, (2001). A final concentration of 0.5% (v/v) Tween-20 (Sigma) was used to enhance crude extract solubility. A series of two fold dilution of each extract, ranging from 0.2 to 100 mg/ml, was prepared. After sterilization, the medium was inoculated with 3µl aliquots of culture containing approximately 10^5 CFU/ml of each organism of 24 hours slant culture in aseptic condition and transferred into sterile 6 inch diameter petridish and allowed to set at room temperature for about 10 minutes and then kept in a refrigerator for 30 minutes. After the media solidified a number 3-cup borer (6mm) diameter was properly sterilized by flaming and used to make three to five uniform cups/wells in each petridish. A drop of molten nutrient agar was used to seal the base of each cup. Different plant crude extracts ranging from 0.2 to 100mg/ml were added to the cups/wells of each petridish and the control plates without plant extract. Inhibition of organism growth in the plates containing test crude extracts was judged by comparison with growth in blank control plates. The MICs were determined as the lowest concentration of extracts inhibiting visible growth of each organism on the agar plate. Similarly the MICs of methanol extracts were determined against all other microorganisms.

3. Results

Among the 50 plant methanol extracts screened thirteen plant extracts showed antibacterial and antifungal activity by zone of inhibition. These results indicated that the plant extracts showed antibacterial as well as antifungal activity. Hexane, chloroform and aqueous extracts were showed very less activity against all the phytopathogens hence only the methanol extracts reports was analyzed. The methanol extracts activities were increased with increasing concentrations. However, the activity produced by the extract was low when compared with that of the standard. The methanol extracts of fifty medicinal plants (Table-1) showed broad spectrum of antimicrobial activity against the test organisms (Table-2) using agar cup plate method. The plant species were *Adenocalymna allicia, Acacia farnaciana, Avicenia officinales, Bridilia Montana, Coleus forskohlii, Phyllanthus niruri, Grewia arborea, Melia azadirach, Ocimum sanctum, Peltophorum pterocarpum, Scoparia dulcis, Terminalia chebula* and *Withania somnifera*, showed a significant activity against *Macrophomina phaseolina, Rhizoctonia solani* at less than 50mg/ml concentration.

Of all *Terminalia chebula* and *Melia azadirach* showed remarkable largest zones of inhibition against all the phytopathogens tested. Antimicrobial activities are different medicinal plants were represented in Table 3 and 4. Fruit extract of *Terminalia chebula* showed less than 2mg/ml and *Melia azadirach* below 15mg/ml concentrations showed significant activity on all the pathogens tested in this study.

Botanical Name	**Parts used**	**Uses / Ailments treated**
Acacia farnesiana (L.) Willd	Bark, roots	Astringent, Demulcent, Poultice, Stomachic.
Acalypha indica Linn.	Aerial parts	Skin diseases, Ulcers Bronchitis, Head ache, Snake bite
Acanthus ilicifolius Linn.	Leaf extract	Relieve rheumatism
Adenocalymma alliaceum (Lam.)	Leaves	Astringent,
Adhatoda vasica Nees.	Leaves, whole plant	Cough and chronic bronchitis, rheumatism and asthma.
Andrographis paniculata Nees.	Whole plant, leaves	Anti-biotic, anti-viral, anti-parasitic and immune system stimulant.
Avicennia officinalis L.	Seed	Relieving ulcers
Boerhaavia diffusa Linn.	Whole plant	Scabies, myalgia, aphrodisiac
Bridelia montana (Roxb.) Willd	Bark, Root Leaf	Stomach pains, sore eyes and headaches.
Cassia occidentalis Linn.	Whole plant	Boils, Spasm. Hysteria, Whooping cough
Catharanthus roseus Linn.	Leaves and roots	Anti-mitotic and Anti-microtubule agents
Centella asiatica Linn.	Whole Plant	Diuretic, treatment of leprosy, use as brain tonic and stimulates hair growth.
Cleome viscosa Linn.	*Leaves and seeds*	*Anthelmintic, carminative, diaphoretic and rubefacient.*
Coleus forskohlii (Willd.).	Roots	Treat heart and lung diseases, intestinal spasms, insomnia and convulsions. Antispasmodic.
Coriandrum sativum Linn.	Fruits	Colic, Laxative, Blood purifier, Indigestion, sore throat
Derris scandens (Roxb.) Benth	Stem	Arthritis, Anti-inflammatory
Eichhornia crassipes (C.Mart.)	Whole plant	Biomass, soil reclamation
Emblica officinalis Gaertn.	Fruit	Aperient, Carminative, Diuretic, Aphrodasiac, Laxative, Astringent and Refrigerant.
Gmelina arborea Linn.	leaves and roots	Gonorrhea, catarrh of bladder, cough, cleaning the ulcers, insanity, epilepsy, fevers, indigestion, nerve tonic.
Gynandropsis gynandra (L.)	Leaf	Anti-irritant
Hildegardia populifolia (Roxb.)	Stem bark	Dog bite, Malaria.
Holarrhena antidysenterica Foxh.	Bark and seeds	Dysentery, piles, leprosy, colic, dyspepsia, chronic chest complaints, , spleen diseases, jaundice, bilious, calculi
Hiptage benghalensis (L.) Kurz.	Leaves and bark	Insecticidal, cough, inflammation; skin diseases and leprosy
Hyptis suaveolens (L.) Poit.	Leaves	Antispasmodic, antirheumatic and antisoporific
Kyllinga nemaralis Rottb.	Whole Plant	Promotes action of liver, and relief prunitus
Lantana camara Linn.	Whole Plant	Antidote to snake venom, Malaria, wounds cuts ulcers, Eczema, Tumors

Botanical Name	Parts used	Uses / Ailments treated
Melia azedarach L.	Leaves, Seed Flower, Oil,	Vermifuge, Insecticide, Astringent, Antiseptic, antidiabitic, anti bacterial and anti viral
Mimosa pudica Linn.	Whole Plant	Menorrhagia, piles, Skin wounds Diarrhoea, Hydrocele, Whooping caugh and Filiriasis
Moringa heterophylla L.	Roots, Seeds,	Antibiotic Anti-inflammatory and Diabetes
Muntinga calabria Linn.	Leaves	Antiseptic
Marraya Koenigii (L.) Spreng.	Leaves	Skin diseases, Heminthiasis, Hyperdipsia, Pruritus, etc.
Ocimum sanctum Linn.	Leaves, Seeds	Malaria, bronchitis, colds, fevers, absorption, arthritis.
Peltophorum pterocarpum (DC.)	Whole plant	Reclamation
Phyllanthus niruri L.	Leaves or herb	Jaundice, Diabetes
Plumeria rubra Linn.	Leaves	Ulcers, leprosy, inflammations, rubefacient.
Pongamia pinnata (L.) Pierre.	Bark, seeds	Antimalaria, skin disease, rheumatic and leprous sores
Ricinus communis Linn.	Leaves	Jaundice, sores,
Salvadora persic, Linn.	Twigs, roots	Antimicrobial and dental diseases
Scoparia dulcis Linn.	Leaves, bark, roots	Used for upper respiratory problems, congestion, menstrual disorders, fever, wounds and hemorrhoids
Sesbania grandiflora (L.) Pers.	Flowers	Gonorrhoea
Strychnos nux vomica Linn.	Seeds	Cholera, chronic wounds, Ulcers, paralysis, Diabetes
Suaeda maritima (L.) Dumort.	Whole plant	Bioremediation
Tephrosia pumila (Lamk.) *Persoon.*	Root	Rheumatism, fevers, pulmonary problems, bladder disorders, Coughing, hair loss, and reproductive disorders
Tephrosia tinctoria Pers.	Root	Antisyphilitic
Tephrosia villosa (L.) Pers.	Root, Leaves, Bark	Anthelmintic, alexiteric, leprosy, ulcers, antipyretic, cures diseases of liver, spleen, heart, blood, asthma etc.
Terminalia chebula Retz.	Fruit	Antimicrobial, cures digestive problems, mouthwash/ gargle and astringent,
Tinospora cordifolia (Willd.)	Stem	Analgesic and anti-inflammatory.
Tridax procumbens Linn.	Whole plant	Antimicrobial, Anti-oxidant and Anti inflammatory,
Vitex pentaphyllal Linn.	Aerial parts	Foetid discharges, Febrifuge Rheumatism affections, catarrhal
Withania somnifera (L.) Dunal	Leaves	Sore eyes, Febrifuge, ulcers Cure sterility of women sedative

Table 1. List of Medicinal plants

Pathogen	MTCC	Disease
Pseudomonas syringae van Hall	B1604	Bacterial spot
Xanthomonas campestris (Pammel) Dowson	B2286	Bacterial leaf streak
Agrobacterium tumifaciens	B7405	Gall disease
Pantoea agglomerans	B2959	Unnamed disease
Erwinia carotovora	B3609	Stem rot
Aspergillus spp	F4633	Seed rot
Colletotrichum graminicola (Ces.) G.W. Wils.	F2232	Seedling blight and seed rot
Fusarium moniliforme J. Sheld	F156	Fusarium head blight, root and stalk rot
Macrophomina phaseolina	F2165	Charcoal rot
Rhizoctonia solani Kuhn.	F 4633	Rhizoctonia root rot, Sheath blight, stalk rot

Table 2. Pathogen index on *Sorghum vulgare* crop

Most of the methanol plant extracts were active towards pathogens. The plant extracts active against fungi are *T. chebula, Melia azadirach, R. communis, Acanthus ilcifolius, Andrographis paniculata, C. roseus, Derris scandens* and *Tephrosia pumila*. Of the five phytopathogenic fungi tested *Rhizoctonia solani* and *Macrophomina phaseolina* were found sensitive strains and evidenced by most of the methanol extracts showed good zone of inhibition on the agar well diffusion assays and *Colletotrichum graminicola* was found resistant when compared with all the fungi tested.

PLANT NAME	*A. tumefaciens*			*E. caratovara*			*P. agglomerans*			*P. syringae*			*X. campestris*		
	A	B	C	A	B	C	A	B	C	A	B	C	A	B	C
Acacia farnesiana	9	14	18	30	35	36	15	15	20	24	26	28	8	9	12
Acalypha indica	9	9	10	9	11	15	9	11	15	9	11	14	7	8	8
Acanthus ilcifolius	10	11	13	12	14	15	-	-	-	11	13	15	7	10	11
Adenocelima allicia	9	12	14	7	8	12	-	9	10	17	19	21	6	7	9
Adhatoda vasica	10	13	15	-	10	15	7	8	12	9	10	12	-	7	11
Andrographis paniculata	12	10	14	7	10	13	-	-	7	10	13	15	12	13	15
Avicenia officinalis	8	13	14	-	7	9	-	-	8	10	14	15	9	11	13
Boerhavia diffusa	8	7	11	10	12	15	7	8	12	-	-	-	-	-	8
Bridilia montana	16	19	25	24	28	29	11	15	18	21	25	24	23	25	26
Cassia occidentalis	8	11	13	-	7	9	-	-	7	-	-	-	7	7	9
Catharanthus roseus	11	10	10	-	8	9	7	11	15	11	14	16	16	18	23
Centella asiatica	9	10	10	-	-	9	-	7	9	-	7	9	-	10	13
Cleome viscosa	9	10	13	12	11	15	9	10	12	11	10	13	9	10	9
Coleus forskohlii	14	15	18	7	8	10	9	11	14	7	8	11	8	9	11
Coriandrum sativum	-	-	-	9	12	10	-	-	-	12	14	15	11	13	14
Derris scandens	10	12	11	-	8	12	-	-	-	16	17	20	7	7	9
Eichhornia crassipes	9	14	13	10	11	14	7	8	10	7	7	11	12	15	14
Emblica officinales	9	10	11	-	-	7	15	14	18	-	9	11	-	8	12
Grewia arborea	15	17	20	20	21	25	19	21	22	8	9	14	-	8	13
Gyanandropsis gyanandra	10	9	14	8	9	9	9	11	11	-	7	7	7	8	12
Heldigordia populipolia	13	15	15	11	14	15	13	15	16	8	9	9	-	7	9

PLANT NAME	*A. tumefaciens*			*E. caratovara*			*P. agglomerans*			*P. syringae*			*X. campestris*		
	A	B	C	A	B	C	A	B	C	A	B	C	A	B	C
Hoelarrhena antidysenterica	13	14	17	7	8	10	9	10	14	6	7	10	-	-	-
Hyptage bengalenses	-	-	9	-	7	8	-	-	-	9	11	12	7	8	11
Hyptis sueolences	12	11	13	12	13	14	9	10	13	14	15	18	7	10	11
Kyllinga nemoralis	-	-	-	-	7	10	-	-	7	-	8	9	-	9	10
Lantana camara	15	13	13	8	11	13	12	14	15	-	-	7	-	-	7
Melia azedarach	10	15	17	-	-	-	-	9	13	8	10	12	-	-	-
Mimosa pudica	11	12	15	14	13	13	-	-	8	-	-	-	-	-	-
Moringa heterophylla	9	10	12	10	9	12	10	11	14	-	7	8	8	9	11
Muntinga calebria	12	11	10	13	16	21	13	11	15	9	11	15	7	8	8
Murraya koenigii	9	9	11	9	11	12	7	9	9	11	10	15	7	8	10
Ocimum sanctum	9	10	12	-	-	8	13	14	15	14	16	17	22	27	28
Peltophorum pterophorus	21	24	24	19	24	25	20	21	24	9	13	15	18	21	22
Phyllanthus niruri	12	13	15	-	9	12	-	7	10	7	8	11	16	18	19
Plumaria rubrum	-	-	7	-	7	8	-	-	-	15	16	18	-	9	11
Pongamia pinnata	14	13	15	-	-	9	11	13	12	-	-	8	8	9	12
Recinus communis	-	-	-	-	9	9	-	-	-	-	-	9	-	-	9
Salvedara persia	-	-	7	7	8	11	-	-	-	7	10	12	-	7	7
Scoparia dulcic	16	21	20	15	18	17	9	13	14	7	9	11	13	17	19
Sesbanian grandiflora	11	13	16	8	7	10	-	-	-	11	13	14	10	11	15
Strynos nuxvomica	9	10	13	8	11	14	-	-	8	6	10	12	8	9	11
Suaeda maritima	10	9	11	9	12	13	9	10	11	14	15	18	9	8	13
Tephrosia pumila	7	7	9	7	8	10	9	11	13	-	-	-	7	8	8
Tephrosia tinctoria	8	10	11	-	7	7	-	7	10	-	7	8	7	9	10
Tephrosia villosa	14	15	16	-	7	11	-	-	7	-	8	9	6	7	12
Terminalia chebula	19	23	24	26	28	28	11	15	18	22	22	22	28	27	33
Tinospora cordifolia	9	13	14	9	9	11	7	8	10	7	7	9	-	9	10
Tridax procumbens	10	14	12	8	11	14	-	-	9	9	13	16	10	12	15
Vitex negundo	9	11	10	12	10	15	-	9	11	8	9	11	-	7	10
Withania somnifera	17	21	25	18	21	25	-	-	9	13	15	16	9	11	17
Streptomycin (5µg/well)	31			20			25			20			15		

Volume per well: 50µl, A: 100mg/ml=5mg/well, B: 300mg/ml=15mg/well,
C: 500mg/ml= 25mg/well, Borer size used: 6mm
-: no activity, Borer size used: 6mm, Extract /Drug concentration in mg/ml,

Table 3. Antibacterial activity of Medicinal plant crude extracts

PLANT NAME	*A. niger*			*C. graminicola*			*F. moniliformi*			*M. phaseolina*			*R. solani*		
	A	B	C	A	B	C	A	B	C	A	B	C	A	B	C
Acacia farnesiana	-	-	7	-	10	13	18	20	21	17	16	18	-	7	13
Acalypha indica	17	19	25	-	-	-	9	10	14	8	8	10	26	27	29
Acanthus ilcifolius	9	11	13	-	-	9	8	11	14	12	14	15	9	13	15
Adenocelima allicia	10	16	17	9	13	14	16	21	25	15	19	22	11	14	16
Adhatoda vasica	7	9	12	7	8	10	9	11	14	14	15	17	13	14	15
Andrographis paniculata	9	13	15	-	8	12	-	8	8	14	16	16	10	14	15

PLANT NAME	*A. niger*			*C. graminicola*			*F. moniliformi*			*M. phaseolina*			*R. solani*		
	A	B	C	A	B	C	A	B	C	A	B	C	A	B	C
Avicenia officinalis	10	15	17	-	7	7	11	12	15	20	24	27	10	11	14
Boerhavia diffusa	-	7	10	9	10	13	7	9	9	8	10	10	-	-	-
Bridilia montana	7	9	11	8	12	18	8	12	15	15	18	20	7	10	12
Cassia occidentalis	-	7	9	7	10	13	9	-	-	8	10	13			
Catharanthus roseus	-	-	8	7	9	16	12	14	15	17	21	23	9	11	12
Centella asiatica	-	-	7	-	7	10	-	8	13	16	18	21	7	11	14
Cleome viscosa	18	21	24	9	11	15	13	17	23	20	21	25	19	22	26
Coleus forskohlii	15	17	21	8	9	10	12	16	19	16	18	21	15	17	19
Coriandrum sativum	10	14	17	-	9	9	-	-	-	7	9	13	-	-	-
Derris scandens	19	21	24	7	7	9	11	13	17	16	15	19	13	14	17
Eichhornia crassipes	13	13	17	-	-	-	9	10	12	12	14	17	10	11	15
Emblica officinales	-	-	-	-	7	9	-	-	-	7	9	13	-	-	-
Grewia arborea	21	24	28	9	11	11	12	15	20	20	21	25	18	19	24
Gyanandropsis gyanandra	6	7	8	-	-	-	10	10	12	8	8	0	8	9	11
Heldigordia populipolia	-	-	-	8	10	12	7	9	11	8	9	11	7	7	9
Hoelarrhena antidysenterica	7	9	12	7	9	13	14	13	18	6	8	8	8	10	11
Hyptage bengalenses	12	13	16	-	7	8	10	13	16	9	10	12	9	10	11
Hyptis sueolences	-	-	-	9	11	14	7	8	11	20	23	25	12	13	14
Kyllinga nemoralis	7	8	11	-	-	8	-	8	14	11	13	14	7	8	8
Lantana camara	-	-	8	8	7	11	-	-	-	10	11	16	9	12	16
Melia azedarach	21	19	30	12	15	18	20	20	22	7	8	11	35	38	45
Mimosa pudica	9	10	13	-	7	10	8	9	12	10	12	14	-	-	7
Moringa heterophylla	-	-	-	7	9	15	8	8	12	8	10	14	12	15	17
Muntinga calebria	14	17	19	-	8	12	9	12	21	10	9	14	10	10	14
Murraya koenigii	10	13	17	9	11	18	12	15	19	13	15	18	15	16	18
Ocimum sanctum	9	11	12	8	10	14	13	15	16	21	24	28	10	13	14
Peltophorum pterophorus	21	22	29	10	14	19	11	13	17	22	24	27	33	35	40
Phyllanthus niruri	-	10	15	-	-	7	10	7	13	14	19	21	11	13	15
Plumaria rubrum	9	9	13	-	8	8	-	-	9	10	13	13	18	21	25
Pongamia pinnata	-	-	8	-	-	7	8	9	12	13	15	17	7	9	11
Recinus communis	10	14	21	7	10	11	-	-	-	15	18	21	-	-	-
Salvedara persia	12	15	19	-	8	11	-	-	-	19	21	21	12	15	16
Scoparia dulcis	17	21	24	9	11	16	12	16	22	11	14	18	14	19	22
Sesbanian grandiflora	8	8	11	7	8	8	16	19	22	21	25	29	12	15	17
Strynos nuxvomica	-	-	-	-	7	8	-	-	10	17	21	23	-	8	9
Suaeda maritima	12	15	19	-	-	-	10	13	14	13	16	17	14	17	21
Tephrosia pumila	7	7	9	-	-	-	7	9	13	-	-	-	-	-	-
Tephrosia tinctoria	7	7	10	7	10	12	-	-	-	10	12	14	-	-	7
Tephrosia villosa	-	-	8	7	9	16	-	-	7	20	25	26	10	11	15
Terminalia chebula	19	21	25	11	16	20	18	25	29	30	34	35	8	11	14
Tinospora cordifolia	7	9	13				11	15	18	17	18	24	9	8	10
Tridax procumbens	-	-	8	-	8	9	9	10	14	18	20	23	-	7	9
Vitex negundo	-	-	-	-	7	9	7	7	9	13	17	20	8	12	13
Withania somnifera	9	10	14	9	12	14	13	15	17	20	25	26	13	16	21
Bavistin (5µg/well)	32			25			28			20			35		

Volume per well: 50µl, A: 100 mg/ml = 5 mg/well, B: 300 mg/ml =15 mg/well,
C: 500 mg/ml= 25 mg/well, Borer size used: 6mm
na: no activity, Borer size used: 6mm, Extract /Drug concentration in mg/ml,

Table 4. Antifungal activity of Medicinal plant crude extracts

PLANT NAME	*A.tumifaciens*	*E.caratovora*	*P.agglomerans*	*P.syringae*	*X.campestris*	*A.niger*	*C.graminicola*	*F.moniliforme*	*M.phaseolina*	*R.solani*
Acacia farnaciana	75	2	50	100	85	na	100	50	50	300
Acalypha indica	90	90	100	100	100	75	na	100	100	50
Acanthus ilcifolius	na	85	na	75	100	90	na	100	85	100
Adenocelima allicia	90	90	300	90	150	90	75	75	75	90
Adhatoda vasica	90	300	85	100	100	100	100	100	85	85
Andrographis paniculata	85	90	na	100	85	90	na	300	85	90
Avicenia officinales	na	300	na	85	90	90	na	90	75	90
Boerhavia diffusa	100	100	100	100	na	300	28	26	22	18
Bridilia montana	50	25	90	25	25	100	100	100	100	na
Cassia occidentalis	100	100	100	100	100	300	100	100	75	100
Catheranthus roseus	85	100	100	100	75	na	150	100	100	150
Centella asiatica	90	90	85	100	300	na	150	90	75	90
Cleome viscosa	85	85	100	85	90	75	na	300	75	100
Coleus forskohlii	75	90	25	90	100	75	100	90	75	75
Coriandrum sativum	na	90	na	85	85	90	100	85	75	75
Derris scandens	100	300	na	75	100	75	150	na	100	na
Eichhornia crassipes	90	100	100	90	90	85	100	90	75	85
Emblica officinales	85	100	50	100	100	na	na	100	85	75
Grewia arborea	75	25	75	100	300	50	200	na	100	na
Gyanandropsis gyanandra	05	75	05	90	100	300	100	90	2.5	50
Heldigordia populipolia	75	100	75	100	300	na	na	90	100	100
Hoelarrhena antidysenterica	75	85	75	85	100	100	90	100	100	100
Hyptage bengalenses	300	300	na	90	100	85	100	75	300	100
Hyptis suaveolens	75	85	75	100	100	na	150	90	100	90
Kyllinga nemoralis	100	300	na	90	300	100	100	100	50	85
Lantana camara	75	100	85	100	na	na	Na	300	85	100
Melia azedarach	75	na	100	25	na	50	100	na	90	75
Mimosa pudica	85	85	85	85	na	100	75	50	100	75
Moringa heterophylla	90	90	100	100	100	na	150	100	90	na
Muntinga calebria	85	85	85	85	100	75	100	100	100	85
Murraya koenigii	90	100	100	90	100	90	150	100	90	75
Ocimum sanctum	85	85	90	90	75	100	90	85	75	75
Peltophorum pterophorus	50	75	5	75	75	50	100	85	75	90
Phyllanthus niruri	85	100	85	90	90	300	90	90	50	10
Plumaria rubrum	na	300	200	75	300	100	na	90	85	90
Pongamia pinnata	75	na	85	100	100	na	na	na	85	50
Recinus communis	na	300	150	na	na	90	na	100	90	100
Salvedara persia	100	100	na	100	300	85	100	na	75	na
Scoparia dulcis	15	22	12	30	75	45	150	na	75	75
Sesbanian grandiflora	85	100	na	90	85	100	25	20	15	25
Strynos nuxvomica	90	85	85	100	100	na	150	na	75	300
Suaeda maritima	85	90	90	75	90	85	na	90	85	85
Tephrosia pumila	na	100	100	na	100	100	na	100	na	100
Tephrosia tinctoria	100	100	100	na	100	100	100	na	100	na
Tephrosia villosa	85	100	75	90	100	na	100	na	75	90
Terminalia chebula	25	75	2.5	75	50	50	75	50	5	85
Tinospora cordifolia	90	100	100	100	300	100	na	90	75	100
Tridax procumbens	85	100	100	na	100	na	150	100	75	300
Vitex negundo	90	85	100	90	300	na	150	100	85	100
Withania somnifera	50	75	25	85	100	100	90	85	75	75

Volume per well: 50µl, Borer size used: 6mm, na: no activity,
Borer size used: 6mm, Extract / Drug concentration in mg/ml,

Table 5. Antimicrobial activity (MIC) of different plant crude extracts

The methanol extracts of *Terminalia chebula* fruit had potent antimicrobial activity at less than 25mg/ml concentrations. The solvent control of hexane, chloroform, methanol, and DMSO had no effect on microbial growth. And the standard synthetic fungicide Bavistin and antibacterial drugs of Streptomycin and Penicillin had a variety of activity against all the pathogens tested.

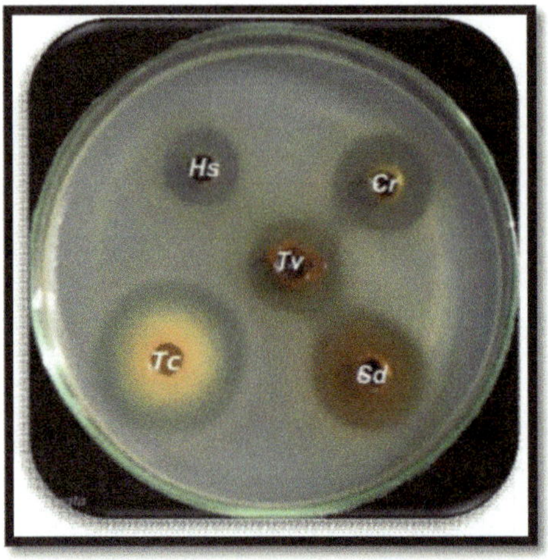

Tc - *T. chebula*, Sd - *S. dulcis*, Hs - *H. sueolences*, Cr - *C. roseus*, Tv - *T. villosa*, Bm - *B. montana*, Eo - *E. officinales*, Pn - *P. niruri*, Av - *A. vasica*, Ap - *A. paniculata*, Aa - *A. allicia*.

Fig. 1. Different plant extracts activity on *M. phaseolina*

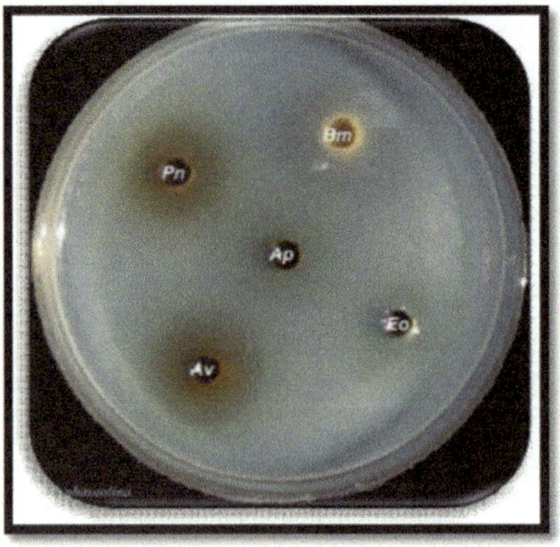

Tc - *T. chebula*, Sd - *S. dulcis*, Hs - *H. sueolences*, Cr - *C. roseus*, Tv - *T. villosa*, Bm - *B. montana*, Eo - *E. officinales*, Pn - *P. niruri*, Av - *A. vasica*, Ap - *A. paniculata*, Aa - *A. allicia*.

Fig. 2. Different plant extracts activity on *M. phaseolina*

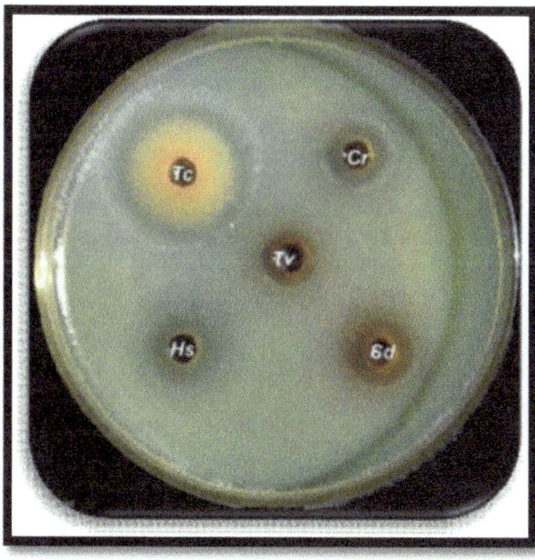

Tc - *T. chebula*, Sd - *S. dulcis*, Hs - *H. sueolences*, Cr - *C. roseus*, Tv - *T. villosa*, Bm - *B. montana*, Eo - *E. officinales*, Pn - *P. niruri*, Av - *A. vasica*, Ap - *A. paniculata*, Aa - *A. allicia*.

Fig. 3. Different plant extracts activity on *R. solani*

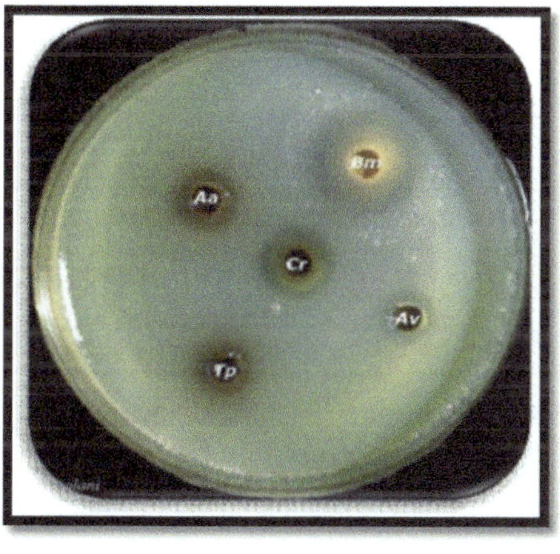

Tc - *T. chebula*, Sd - *S. dulcis*, Hs - *H. sueolences*, Cr - *C. roseus*, Tv - *T. villosa*, Bm - *B. montana*, Eo - *E. officinales*, Pn - *P. niruri*, Av - *A. vasica*, Ap - *A. paniculata*, Aa - *A. allicia*.

Fig. 4. Different plant extracts activity on *R. solani*

4. Discussion

Natural products isolated from higher plants have been providing novel, antimicrobial drugs. Historically, many plant oils and extracts, such as tea tree, clove, Etc. have been used as topical antiseptics, or have been reported to have antimicrobial properties (Hoffman 1987 and Lawless 1995). It is important to investigate scientifically those plants which have been used in traditional medicines as potential sources of novel antimicrobial compounds (Mitscher *et al.*, 1987). Also, the resurgence of interest in natural therapies and increasing consumer demand for effective, safe, natural products means that quantitative data on plant oils and extracts are required.

Majority of studies conducted the search of compounds with antimicrobial properties have targeted plants with a history of ethno botanical uses (Janovska *et al.*, 2003), most of the medicinal plant species screened in this study were previously been surveyed for antimicrobial activities on human pathogens. And very few citations were reported on phytopathogens (Kaushik and Arora, 2003; Jaspal singh and Tripathi, 1993; Krishna kishore and Suresh pande, 2005; Meena and Goplakrishnan, 2005). The observed antimicrobial activity of these plant extracts, and isolated compounds were of highly remarkable.

The present study was designed to obtain information on the antimicrobial effect of 50 Indian medicinal plants on certain plant pathogenic microorganisms. The well diffusion/cup plate method was used in this study since it was found to be better than the disc diffusion method. All the medicinal plant extracts and isolated compounds showed antimicrobial activity against selected pathogens of Sorghum.

Hexane extracts never showed antimicrobial activity. The chloroform and water extracts showed very less antimicrobial activity compared with methanol extracts. This may be due to little diffusion properties of these extracts in the agar or because fresh plants contain active substances which may be affected or disappeared by the steps of extraction methods.

The methanol extracts of all the medicinal plant screened (Table-1) exhibited grater antimicrobial activity. According to Darout *et al.*,(2000) the antimicrobial action of methanol extracts is due to the compounds such as thiocynate, nitrate, chloride and sulphates beside other high polarity soluble compounds which are naturally occurring in most plant materials.

Methanolic extracts of *T. chebula, B. Montana, M. azadirach, W. somnifera, O santum* and *P. pterocarpum* showed greater antimicrobial activity. *Terminalia chebula* possessed 32-40% of tannin content and the antibacterial activity may be indicative of the presence of some metabolic toxins or broad-spectrum antibiotic compounds (Fundter *et al.*, 1992). *M. azadirach* was exhibited good antimicrobial activity against most of the tested pathogens in this study. According to Jacobson, (1995) this activity is due to Nimbidin, extracted from *M. azadirach* demonstrated several biological activities. From this crude principle some tetranortriterpenes, including nimbin, nimbinin, nimbidinin, nimbolide and nimbidic acid have also been showing antimicrobial activities.

The observations reveal that tested medicinal plant methanol extracts activity against all phytopathogenic species. As evidenced, the fungal strains that were sensitive are *M. phaseolina, R. solani* species, *C. graminicola* and *F. moniliforme* found to be resistant strains. Among the tested medicinal plants methanol extracts against the phytopathogenic species, *Terminalia chebula* extracts showed greater antimicrobial activity on all plant pathogens.

In view of the changing agricultural policies throughout the world complete disease control is no longer a target of plant pathologist's reducing the threshold level using cost-effective and eco-friendly management option is the focus of the day. In this context identification of aqueous leaf extract of *T. chebula* and *M. azadirach* methanol extracts as bactericides and fungicides against the pathogens tested are highly significant recommendable. The result of these studies maybe helpful in developing/synthesizing the plant based natural fungicides and insecticides that may be for preventing and curing the common destructive diseases of *Sorghum* crop and other cereal crops. In this context the studied plant extracts is more appropriate and helpful in synthesizing the plant based biofungicides to reduce the pathogen population to lower economic threshold level using cost effective and eco friendly management. This will also offer a great help in facing the emergence spread of antimicrobial resistance.

5. References

Akhtar M.A., M.H. Rahber-Bhatti, M. Aslam, *International Journal of Pest Management*, 1997, 43, 2, 149-153.

Cardellina J. H. (1988): Biologically active Natural Products: Potential Use in Agriculture, 305-311.

Darout, I., Cristy, A., Skaug, N., and P. Egeberg, 2000. Identification and quantification of some potentially antimicrobial anionic components in Miswak extract. *Ind J Pharm*, 32:11-4.

Elizabeth, M., Adrien Szekely, Johnson and David W. Warnock., 2001. *Journal of Clinical Microbiology*, 37(5):1480-1483.

Fundter, J.M., *et al.*, 1992. *Terminalia chebula* Retz. In Lemmens, R.H.M.J. & Wulijarni-Soetjipto, N. (Eds.): Plant Resources of South-East Asia. No. 3: *Dye and tannin-producing plants*, pp 122-125.

Grierson DS, Afolayan AJ (1999). An ethnobotanical study of plants used for the treatment of wounds in the Eastern Cape, South Africa. Ethnopharmacol 67: 327-332.

Gulter H.G. (1988): Natural products and their potential in agriculture. A personal over review., 1-22.

Hoffman, D. L. 1987. *The Herb User's Guide*. Wellingborough, UK: Thorsons Publishing Group.

Horne, C. W., and R. A. Frederiksen, 1993. (http://www.apsnet.org/online/common/names/sorghum.asp).

Jacobson, M., 1995. In the Neem Tree: Source of Unique Natural Products for Integrated Pest Management, Medicine, Industry and other Purposes (ed. Schmutterer, H.), pp. 484-495.

Janovska, D., Kubikova, K., Kokoska, L. 2003. Screening for antimicrobial activity of some medicinal plant species of traditional Chinese medicine. *Czech. J. Food Sci.* 21: 107-111.

Jaspal Singh., and N. N. Tripathi., 1993. *Journal of the Indian Botanical Society*, 72 (1-2) :51-53.

Kaushik, R. D. and Charu Arora, 2002. Fungitoxic activity of methanol extracts of some plants of kamaun, garhwal and tarai regions against fungal pathogens of rice. *Journal of Indian botanical sciences*, 81:327-331.

Kone, W. M., Atindehou, K. K., Terreaux, C., Hosetettman, K., Traore, D., and M. Dosso, 2004. Screening of 50 medicinal plants for antibacterial activity. *Ethnopharmacol Bul,* 93(1):43-49.

Krisharaju A.V. and Rao T. V. N. Sundararaju (2005): Assessment of bioactivity of Indian medicinal plants using Brine shrimp (Alternaria solania) lethality assay. Int. J. Appl. Sci. Engg.,2, 125- 134.

Krishna Kishore, G., and Suresh Pande, 2005. Integrated management of the late leaf spot and rust disease of groundnut with *Prosopis* leaf extract and chlorothalonil. *International journal of pest management,* 51(4):327-334.

Lawless, J., 1995. *The Illustrated Encyclopedia of Essential Oils*. Shaftesbury, UK: Element Books Ltd.

Meena, C., and J. Gopalakrishnan, 2005. Efficacy of plant extracts against bacterial blight. *Annals of plant protection sciences,* 12(2):344-346.

Mitscher, L. A., Drake, S., Gollapudi, S.R. and S. K. Okwute, 1987. A modern look at folkloric use of anti-infective agents. *Journal of Natural Products,* 50:1025–1040.

Mitscher, L. A., R. P. Leu., M. S. Bathala., W. N. Wu., and J. L. Beal, 1972. Antimicrobial agents from higher plants. Introduction, rationale and methodology. Lloydia, 35:157-166.

Murray, S. S., Chappell, J. H., Kenter, A. T., Kraft, R. P., Meehan, G. R., and M. V. Zombeck, 1995. *Proc, SPIE* 3356:974.

Newman D. J., Cragg G. M. and Snader K. M. (2000): The influence of natural products upon drug discovery. Natural Product Research, 17, 215- 234.

Olurinola, P. F., and Ibrahim, Y. K., 1991. Comparative Microbial Contamination Levels in Wet Granulation and Direct Compression Methods of Tablet Production, *Pharm. Acta. Helv,* 66:298-301.

Pullaiah, T., 2002. Medicinal Plants in India, Regency Publications. New Delhi.

Rhouma A, Ben Daoud H, Ghanmi S, Ben Salah H, Romdhane M, Demak M, *Journal of Plant Pathology,* 2009, 91, 2, 339-345.

Warrier P. K., (1994-1996) Indian Medicinal Plants- A compendium of 500 species Vol. 5, p 396.

Antimicrobial Activity of Lectins from Plants

Aphichart Karnchanatat
*The Institute of Biotechnology and Genetic Engineering,
Chulalongkorn University, Bangkok,
Thailand*

1. Introduction

There are at least three reasons for the need in finding out new alternative antimicrobial substances from natural sources. The first reason is that people nowadays concern about toxic of synthetic substances including daily contact chemicals or even drugs used in medical or healthcare purposes (Hafidh et al., 2009). Any synthetic drugs were avoided in order to keep physiological cleans as belief. Thus, natural substances were used increasingly instead as well as any substances used for antimicrobial purposes. The second reason is that new alternative drugs are human hope for better fighting with existed diseases and pathogens. They may replace currently used drugs in points of more efficiency, more abundant, lower side-effect or safer or even lower production cost. It is fact that most alive organisms should have some mechanisms or substances fight with all time contacting pathogens so that they can be survived in nature. Although a plenty of antibiotics were discovered after first time Fleming's declaration, but they were still relatively low amounts compared with overall real natural antimicrobial substances. This mean the natural sources still flourish with novel antimicrobial substances waiting for discovered. Additional small aspect may be raised here. The natural substances are usually good leading compound sources for mostly synthetic drug from the long past due to their diversities are far from human imagination. New chemical structures are always found in natural resources as higher frequency than artificial deducing structures. The final reason is that the mechanism used to synthesize natural substances are available and they are usually can be imitated in small, medium, and even large scale production with present biotechnological knowledge which looks easier than newly designed plants.

Plants are of primary importance in the global ecosystem. They are, together with a small group of bacteria, the only living organisms which are capable of harvesting and storing solar energy by virtue of their photosynthetic apparatus which converts light energy into chemical energy through the reductive assimilation of carbon dioxide. Marine and terrestrial plants are the first link in the global food chain. Virtually all other life on earth depends on the organic molecules they synthesize. Evidently, the fact that the majority of heterotrophic organisms depends on them makes plants favorite targets of a whole variety of parasites and predators. Therefore, plants must defend themselves against their potential enemies. During the past 15 years, a large number of antimicrobial proteins (AMPs) have been identified in different plants (Broekaert et al., 1997). AMPs constitute a heterogenous class of low molecular mass proteins, which are recognized as important components of defense system. They directly interfere with the growth, multiplication and spread of microbial organisms (Lehrer and Ganz, 1999). Different proteins with antibacterial and/or antifungal activity have been isolated from seeds, tubers, and rhizomes, where they accumulate to high levels and may also function as storage proteins. Homologous of the seed proteins have also been identified at very low concentrations in floral and vegetative tissues (Terras et al., 1995; Kheeree et al., 2010; and Charungchitrak et al., 2011). There are several classes of proteins having antimicrobial properties which include thionins, lipid transfer proteins, plant defensins, chitinases, glucanases, 2S albumins, ribosome inactivating proteins and lectin (Ye et al., 2002; and Zhang and Halaweish, 2003).

Lectins are proteins or glycoproteins of a ubiquitous distribution in nature, which have at least one carbohydrate or derivative binding site without catalytic function or immunological characteristics. They have the unique ability to recognize and bind reversibly to specific carbohydrate ligands without any chemical modification; this distinguishes lectins from other carbohydrate binding proteins and enzymes, and makes them invaluable tools in biomedical and glycoconjugate research (Peumans and Van Damme, 1995). Plants were the first discovered source of lectins and, although lectins have since been found to be universally distributed, plants remain the most frequently used source of lectin studies due to both the ease of their extraction and the relatively high yields that can be obtained. Moreover, different families of plants, as well as different tissues within the same plant, can contain different lectins with different bioactivities, including different carbohydrate-binding specificities. It has been suggested that plant lectins may have important roles according to their abundance, including in the immune defence, and also that lectins have been co-opted adapted for several functions during evolution (Sharon and Lis, 2001).

The role of lectins in the defense mechanism of plants may have evolved from the ability to lectins to agglutinate and immobilize microorganisms. The supporting evidence for this proposed role in defense against pathogens falls into two main observed categories, namely (a) the presence of lectins at potential sites of invasion by infectious agents, and (b) the binding of lectins to various fungi and their ability to inhibit fungal growth and germination. A number of studies with respect to the potential defense role of plant lectins have been reported. For example, during the imbibition of dry soybean seeds, lectin is released into the water and the presence of this lectin in the vicinity of germinating seeds hints at possible interactions of lectins with potential pathogens. The developmental pattern of the initial accumulation and final disappearance of lectin can be observed during the seed dormancy, germination and maturation, which may implicate the role of lectins in a defense mechanism necessary for plants in the initial stages of growth. Moreover, some lectins may provide some protection to plants against generalist herbivores (Howard et al., 1995). This chapter is intended to provide exposure for recent papers in details of antimicrobial activity of lectins from plants. This omission can be remedied by reading the more detailed reviews listed in the references.

2. General properties of plant lectins

Lectins are proteins or glycoproteins of non-immune origin derived from plants, animals or microorganisms that have specificity for terminal or subterminal carbohydrate residues. The main characteristic of this class of proteins is their ability to interact with carbohydrates and thus combine with glycocomponents of the cell surface, as well as with cytoplasmatic and nuclear structures and the extracellular matrix of cells and tissues from throughout the animal and plant kingdoms, down to microorganisms (Brooks and Leathem, 1998). The availability of a large number of lectins with distinct carbohydrate specificities has resulted in the use of these proteins as tools in medical and biological research (Singh et al., 1999), and has attracted great interest because of their remarkable effects in a wide range of biological systems, including the purification and characterization of glycoconjugates and the study of cell-surface architecture. The agglutination activity of these highly specific carbohydrate binding molecules is usually inhibited by a specific simple monosaccharide, but for some lectins di-, tri-, and even poly-saccharides are required. They are classified into a small number of sugar specificity groups, such as mannose, galactose, *N*-acetylglucosamine, L-fucose and *N*-acetylneuraminic acid, according to the monosaccharide that is the most effective inhibitor of the lectin-mediated agglutination of erythrocytes (Lis and Sharon, 1986).

The lectins represent a large group of plant proteins. Lectins have been found in less than 500 species, which indicates that only a limited number of higher plants, contain detectable levels of lectins (Van Damme et al., 1998). However, the majority of the studies on lectins have been carried out on legume species (Kocourek, 1986; and Lakhtin, 1994) particularly in their seeds where they comprise up to 15% of the total protein. As a result of these studies, many plant lectins have become a very popular class of proteins because of their obvious potential in aiding researchers in other areas of the life sciences. A variety of lectins are presently envisioned to be involved in one or more at least three roles releasing to plant defense. One such defense role for some lectins may be in the recognition of oligosaccharide signals produced by the breakdown of cell wall components of the plant or pathogen upon contact with the plant. A second type of defense role may involve a direct interaction of a lectin with the infectious agent. A third defense type with a considerable support is that some lectins play role in protecting the plant animal predators (Weis and Drickamer, 1996).

Legumes and monocots are major sources of plant lectins that have been widely studied (Wood et al., 1999). Plant lectins can be classified into four major families of structurally and evolutionary related proteins: legume lectins, type 2 ribosome inactivating proteins, chitin-binding lectins, and monocot mannose-binding lectins. Three other small lectin families (Cucurbitaceae phloem lectins, amaranthins, and jacalin-related lectins) have also been characterized (Van Damme et al., 1999). Legume lectins represent the largest and most thoroughly studied family of plant lectins. They have been isolated from seeds, stem, and bark of legumes (Imberty et al., 2000). The best known legume lectins are phytohemagglutinin (PHA) from red kidney bean, soybean (SBA), jackbean (Concanavalin A), peanut lectin (PNA), and pea (PSL) (Lis and Sharon, 1998). Type 2 ribosome-inactivating proteins consist of the toxic A subunit and Gal/GalNAc binding subunit of B chain. Whereas the A chain has RNA glycosidase activity, the B chain is responsible for binding to the target cell surface and helping in the internalization of the whole protein into cell membrane (Kaku et al., 1996; and Wood et al., 1999). Ricin from seeds of *Ricinus communis*, the first plant lectin, is an example (Sphyris et al., 1995; and Lisgarten et al., 1999). Chitin-binding lectins containing hevein domains have been prevalently found in cereal. Examples are wheat germ agglutinin, pokeweed mitogen, rice, rye, and barley lectins (Lis and Sharon, 1998; and Wood et al., 1999). Monocot mannose-binding lectins were first reported from the snowdrop (*Galanthus nivalis*) (Van Damme et al., 1997). Later several lectins have been extracted and intensively characterized from several monocot families: Alliaceae, Amaryllidaceae, Araceae, Bromeliaceae, Iridaceae, Liliaceae, and Orchidaceae (Wood et al., 1999). For example, *Narcissus pseudonarcissus* (daffodil) and *Scilla campanulata* (bluebell) lectins have been recently reported (Sauerborn et al., 1999; and Wood et al., 1999).

3. History of plant lectins

Lectin, agglutinin, and hemagglutinin are synonym of lectin's names. The first time that Lectin was descript back to 1888 by Stillmark, who study the lectin from the seeds of castor bean (about Ricin A toxic ferment from the seeds of *Ricinus communis* L. and some other Euphorbiaceae Species). He linked the toxicity of castor beans to the occurrence of a hemagglutinaing protein factor. For along time before it was definitely demonstrated that Stillmark's "ricin" was a mixture of a weakly agglutinating protein toxin (still known as ricin) and a nontoxic agglutinin (*Ricinus communis* agglutinin, or RCA). The first evidence for this came from studies by Kabet et al. during World War II. They found by immunochemical methods that the toxic and hemagglutinating properties of "ricin" were due to different substances. Only in 1960 was separation of the two substances achieved by Funatsu, and know that ricin came to the attention of the general public in 1978, following its use as a weapon in the notorious, politically motivated "umbrella murder". The dimensions of the hole, led to the conclusion that ricin was the killing agent, since very few poisons are sufficiently potent to kill a man at such a minute amount. In 1898 Elfstrand introduced for the first time the term "hemagglutinin" as a common name for all plant proteins that cause clumping of cells. The idea that toxicity is an intrinsic property of lectin was abandoned in the beginning of the century after have a report for the first time the present of nontoxic lectin in the legumes *Phaseolus vulgaris* (bean), *Pisum sativum* (pea), *Lens culinaris* (lentil), and *Vicia sativa* (vetch). Following this work more nontoxicity plant hemagglutinin has been found. Eventually, it became Evident that lectin is widespread in the plant kingdom and that toxicity is the exception rather than the rule (Van Damme et al., 1995).

The next milestone in the history of plant lectin was a term. When have been found that some hemagglutinin exhibit a clear preference toward erythrocytes of a particular human blood group within the ABO system (Boyd and Reguera, 1949; and Renkonen, 1948). The term "lectin" originally introduced to emphasize the selective agglutination behavior of some hemagglutinin, it was later applied to all proteins with agglutinating activity. "hemagglutinin" is certainly a more appropriate term than lectin because it refers to the capability of a protein to agglutinate erythrocytes but does not take into account that most lectin can also agglutinate other cells. Hence, the term agglutinin should be preferred. In the absence of a clear consensus, the term lectin is actually most commonly used, but agglutinin and hemagglutinin still persist as synonyms.

The current confusion in the terminology of lectin to a great degree is result in the fact that different names have been introduced before the mechanism causing the macroscopically visible agglutination activity was understood in molecular terms. In 1936 already observed that cane sugar inhibited the agglutination activity of Concanavalin A (Con A) (Summer and Howell, 1936). It was demonstrated in 1952 that the agglutination properties of lectin is base on a specific sugar-binding activity (Watkins and Morgan, 1952). As soon as lectin was recognized as carbohydrate-binding protein they could be distinguished from other proteins on the basis of a well-defined functional criterion. For this reason lectin is now considered initially as carbohydrate-binding proteins rather than as (hem) agglutinin.

4. Occurrence and distribution

Lectins are usually considered as a very large and heterogeneous group of proteins (Goldstein and Poretz, 1986). Although, there is no doubt indeed that numerous plant species of different taxonomic groupings contain lectins. The total number of well-documented cases is about 400. Assuming that all the close relatives of these plants also contain agglutinins and that some new lectins will be discovered in the future, the expected occurrence of lectins is still limited to a small fraction of the plant kingdom. It can be concluded, therefore, that the occurrence of at least the classical agglutinating lectins in plants is the exception rather than the rule. However, in contrast to the relative scarcity of the agglutinating lectins, chimerolectins belonging to the Class I chitinases seem to be present in almost all plant species (Collinge et al., 1993).

Lectins are widely distributed throughout the plant kingdom where they have been found in a variety of tissues of a large number of different plants. In plants, lectins are particularly localized in seeds. Howard et al., 1972, reported that seed lectins are particularly seen in cotyledons where they appear during the later stages of maturation of the seeds. In addition to cotyledons, in some cases appreciable amounts of lectins have been reported in the embryos and small amounts in the seed coats (Pueppke et al., 1978). Immunolocalization studies have revealed that lectins are primarily found in the protein bodies of the cotyledon cells (Herman and Shannon, 1984). During the early seedling growth, Weber and Neumann (1980) noticed the decrease in lectin concentration as the cotyledons are resorbed. A short survey of the occurrence and concentration of lectins in seeds as well as in different types of vegetative tissues reveals striking differences in the location and relative abundance of the individual lectins. Usually, seed lectins are confined to cotyledons (e.g. legumes) or endosperm (e.g. castor bean). Normally lectins account for up to 5% of the total seed proteins. Sometimes, they become predominant protein in the seed representing 50% of the total seed protein (e.g. Phaseolus species). The non-seed lectins are found in all kinds of vegetative tissues such as leaves, stem, bark, bulb, tubers, corns, rhizomes, roots, fruits, flowers, ovaries, phloem sap and even in nectar (Peumans and Van Damme, 1995) and are only minor, quantitatively unimportant proteins. Non-seed lectins may occur in different tissues of the same plant. The snowdrop and daffodil lectins, for instance, have been found in all vegetative tissues, although the lectin is most abundant in the bulbs (Van Damme and Peumans, 1990). Similarly, the potato lectin occurs in tubers, stems, leaves and fruits (Kilpatrick, 1980). There are exceptions also. The ground elder berry lectin is confined to the rhizome only (Peumans et al., 1985). In the case of tulip bulbs, lectins are present in large quantities in the bulb but are almost undetectable in stem and leaves (Van Damme and Peumans, 1995). Some legume lectins are found in seeds as well as in bark tissues. A thorough examination of the genes coding for these lectins revealed that the seed and bark lectins are encoded by different, though highly hommologus, genes (Van Damme et al., 1995).

5. Hemagglutinating activity by plant lectins

Lectins are a group of protein that can bind to carbohydrate (which can be in form of sugar, oligosaccharide, or polysaccharide) specifically. Binding of the lectins is differed from those enzymes, anti-lectin antibodies, and other carbohydrate specific binding protein on that they will never change any bound-carbohydrate properties, not convert such carbohydrate to other substances, not come form immune origin, and being reversible binding. In addition to carbohydrate binding specifically, the lectins can cause cells agglutinated and glycoprotein or carbohydrate precipitated. That is why the lectins are sometimes called "agglutinin" (Sharon and Lis, 2001). Since most lectins have two or more carbohydrate binding sites in their molecules, which can make cross-linkages between cells or carbohydrate containing molecules and form solid network. However, there are also some certain lectins that presented in momovalent binding site, and thus can not agglutinate cells or precipitate carbohydrate.

Some lectins contain more than one type of acting site or one activity in single molecules so that they can bind to carbohydrate and can exhibit other behaviors such as enzymatic activity (which make this lectin called "lectzyme"), mitogenic activity, and transportation activity in the same time. From these phenomena, the lectins can be classified into three types according to their acting sites as "merolecins" (the lectins with only single carbohydrate binding domain, usually small single peptides), "hololectins" (the lectins with two resemble carbohydrate binding domains), "chimerolectins" (the lectins contains both carbohydrate binding domain and other well-defined biological active domains which act dependently of previous domain). Beside this classification, the lectins can also be classified by their ligand specificities in two manners. The first is that by sizes of binding ligand which the lectins can be divided into two group; the lectins that specifically binding to monosaccharides as well as oligosaccharides and the lectins that specifically binding to only oligosaccharides (Peumans and Van Damme, 1995). The second classification manner is relatively old style that was set up during little details of lectin's information known. Thus, they were separated by their legand specificity only in sugar types such as mannose or glucose specific lectins, galactose specific lectins, and sialic acid specific lectins. However, they were recently found that most lectins tended to recognize certain three dimension structure than monosaccharide specificity. Thus, this classification style may not up to date because many of lectins formally grouped in one class are now no longer suitable for such class. Anyways, it may be familiar to some authors and may also found in some present documents.

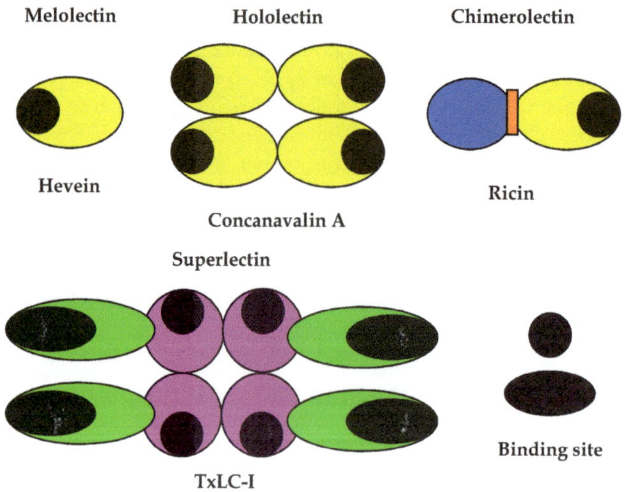

Fig. 1. Schematic representation of the three types of plant lectins: merolectins, hololectins, and chimerolectins. (Peumans and Van Damme, 1995).

Although the lectins have been found in human, animal, plant, and microorganisms, but it looks like that plant lectins were the most investigated for details (Sharon and Lis, 2001; and Chandra et al., 2006). Most lectins are present in seed cotyledons of the plant (but also found in any other parts such as roots, stems, rhizomes, and leaves in lesser amounts). In such tissues, most lectins are located within cytoplasm or protein bodies inside the cells (Moreira et al., 1991). In general, the lectins with the same ligand specificity contain different binding abilities mainly depended on their sources meant different genetic material that produce different lectins with different in three dimension structures. For instances, Tipthara et al., (2007) successfully purified a mannose specific lectin with strong rabbit hemagglutinating activity (0.017 µg of minimum amount that hemagglutination presented) of from *Curcuma Zedoaria*, Thipthara et al., (2008) also purified many lectins with weak activity (0.140 to 0.190 mg minimum amount that hemagglutination presented), Wong et al., (2008) purified mannose/glucose specific lectin with extremely strong activity (83.063 ng minimum amount that hemagglutination presented) from *Castanopsis chinensis*. Most of plant lectins become a set of important tools for glycobiology achievements. They are also applied in detection, isolation, and characterization of glycoconjugated substances mainly in glycoprotein, proteoglycan, and modified polysaccharides (Sharon and Lis, 2001). The lectins are also advantages in immunology, histochemistry, pathology, and physiology areas. One familiar instance which the lectin usage is clearly seen is ABO blood type identification using blood group specific lectin such as Concanavalin A, a lectin derived from jack bean seed (*Canavalia ensiformis*) that can specifically bind to non-reducin α-terminal mannose. This blood groups determination is based on presence or absence of specific glycoprotein on red blood cells that the lectins can bind and make red blood cells agglutination (Moreira et al., 1991) by forming network with red blood cells and then can not be collected as button like form in the U shape bottom well. From this incident, a method widely used for lectin screenings or characterizations mainly involved cells agglutination, especially red blood cells from various animals (Sharon and Lis, 2001). The lectins also have other roles in mammals. There was evidences indicated that the lectins played the important roles in cell differentiation, cell movement and phagocytosis, cell to cell and cells to matrix substances communication, cell organization in tissues, and embryo morphogenesis (Moreira et al., 1991).

On the other hand, consuming of lectins also may cause adverse results in some cases. Several lectins such as Concanavalin A and wheat germ agglutinin (WGA) are toxic to mammalian cells, but relatively low compared with other toxic substances such as approximately 1000 times lower than ricin (an toxic albumin from Caster bean). It is believed that production and accumulation of toxic lectins in some plants are a kind of defending mechanisms which plants develop for protecting them form certain plant eating organisms such as insects and mammals (Peumans and Van Damme, 1995) and plant pathogens. Aside from defense mechanisms, the lectins also have their essential roles in plant-microorganism symbiosis, cell differentiation, pollen recognition, cell wall elongation, and as a reserved protein (Moreira et al., 1991). Interestingly, some plant lectins were found to be well react with viral surface glycoprotein and were hoped to use in controlling many diseases originated from viruses which current methods are still inadequate controllable efficiencies. Balzarini et al., (2004) isolated two mannose-specific lectins from *Galanthus nivalis* (snowdrop) (GNA) and *Hippeastrum* sp. hybrid (Amaryllis) (HHA) and found that they contained *in vitro* anti-HIV virus activities ranged from 0.12 to 1.2 µg/ ml for GNA and from 0.18 to 0.70 µg/ ml for HHA depended on tested viral nature.

6. Plant lectin

Lectins have been found in a wide variety of species almost every major taxonomical classification of flowering plants (Allen and Brilliantine 1969; and Mialonier et al., 1973). Many plants and their individual tissues have been routinely screened for lectins by measuring the ability of their extracts to agglutinate erythrocytes. Although this hemagglutination assay has been of great value in detecting lectins, it is at best semiquantitative; it will not detect inactive or monovalent lectin, nor will it provide accurate estimates of lectin if an endogenous receptor for that lectin is present in the extract. The assay can at times yield false positive results because of nonspecific hemagglutination caused by lipids or by polyphenols such as tannins that are often abundant in plant tissues. It is therefore advisable to verify positive hemagglutination data by inhibiting the activity with specific sugars or by isolating the lectin (Tsivion and Sharon, 1981).

The carbohydrate specificities and structures of lectins from a large variety of plants have been studied in considerable detail. In general, lectins from plants within particular taxonomical groups have distinctive properties that distinguish them from lectins of less closely related plants. It is important to note that the lectins used in these comparisons represent the most abundant and therefore most intensively studied lectins in the plants of these families. These lectins are not all derived from homologous tissues. These differences in origin must be remembered in interpreting these comparisons since, as is discussed below, it is possible that different tissues within the same plant may contain different lectins. This reservation does not apply to comparisons of lectins obtained from homologous tissues of plants within the same family. Homologies within two of these families, the Graminaceae and Leguminoseae, are discussed in further detail below.

Graminaceae: The lectin from monocotyledonous plants is the wheat germ agglutinin, which is a 36,000 molecular weight dimer of identical protein subunits linked by interchain disulfide bonds (Nagata and Burger, 1974; and Rice and Etzler, 1974). The complete amino acid sequence of this lectin has recently been determined (Wright et al., 1984). This lectin has a specificity for oligomers of β (1-4)-*N*-acetyl-o-glucosamine (Allen et al., 1973). Lectins with similar specificities and molecular properties have been isolated from rye (Peumans et al., 1982b) and barley embryos (Mishkind et al.,1983; Peumans et al., 1982b). Indeed, these lectins are so similar that they can undergo subunit exchange to form heterodimers (Peumans et al., 1982a).

Leguminoseae: The seeds of legumes are particularly rich in lectins, and many of these lectins have been characterized extensively (Goldstein and Hayes 1978; Lis and Sharon 1986). As this review was prepared, the complete amino acid sequences of Concanavalin A (Edelman et al. 1972), favin (Cunningham et al., 1979), and lectins from lentil (Foriers et al., 1981), sainfoin (Kouchalakos et al., 1984), *Phaseolus vulgaris* (Hoffman et al., 1982), soybean (Hemperly et al., 1983), and pea (Higgins et al., 1983) have been determined. In addition, the NH_2 terminal amino acid sequences of at least 15 other legume lectins are available. Comparisons of these sequences have shown extensive homologies, particularly among those lectins from plants within the same tribes. It is clear that these lectins have been conserved during evolution of the legumes and that the homologies in their NH_2 terminal amino acid sequences reflect the taxonomical relationships of the plants in this family (Foriers et al., 1977; and Foriers et al., 1979).

7. Sugar binding activity and specificity of plant lectins

Broadly reveal, lectins can be divided into those that bind monosaccharides as well as oligosaccharides, and those that recognize oligosaccharides only (Wu et al., 2001). It is noteworthy that almost all saccharides recognized by lectins are typical constituents of animal cell surfaces. This is perhaps a reflection of the method commonly used for lectin detection (Tsivion and Sharon, 1981), as a result of which lectins recognizing sugars not present on erythrocytes might have been overlooked.

7.1 Mannose/glucose

A lectin with specificity for mannose and glucose residues has been isolated in crystalline form the fava bean (*Vicia laba*) by a procedure which included absorption to Sephadex. It has a molecular weight of 50,000 Da and appears to be a tetramer made of two subunits of 18,000 Da and two subunits of 9,000 Da. These studies determine amino acid sequence and three-dimensional structure of lectin were similar with structural features of Concanavalin A (Irvin, 1976).

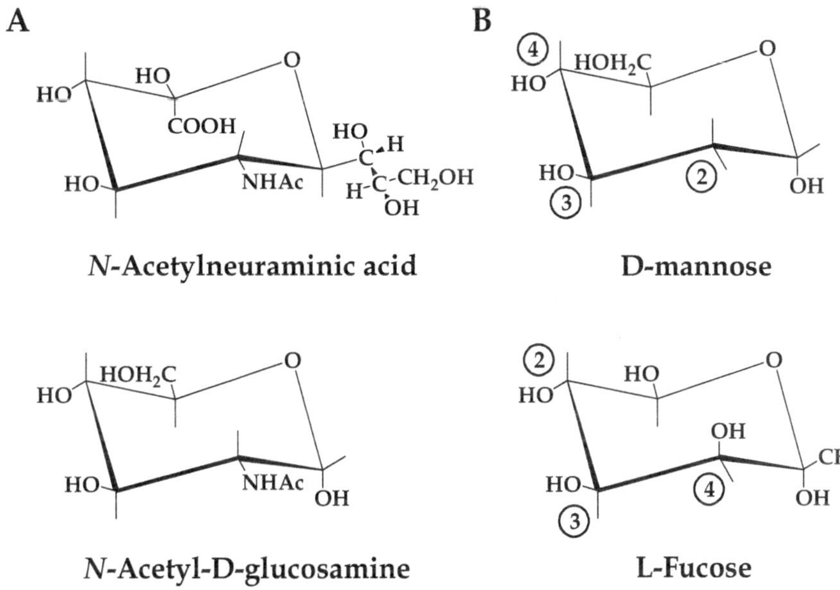

Fig. 2. Common structural features of *N*-acetylneuraminic acid and *N*-acetylglucosamine (A) and of mannose and fucose (B). Similarity of *N*-acetylglucosamine and *N*-acetylneuraminic acid at positions C-2 (acetamido) and C-3 (hydroxyl) of the pyranose ring is observed when the sialic acid molecule is suitably rotated. Rotation of the fucose molecule by 180 Å allows superimposition of its ring oxygen, 4-OH, 3-OH and 2-OH with the ring oxygen, 2-OH, 3-OH and 4-OH of mannose, respectively. Groups that thus occupy the same positions in space are underlined. (Sharon, 1993).

7.2 Galactose/*N*-acetylgalactosamine

As mentioned, lectin interacts with galactose or *N*-acetylgalactosamine such as the lectin from the corn coleoptyle. It is a glycoprotein had molecular mass under non-denaturing conditions was 88.7 kDa And had carbohydrates that constituted 12% of the total weight comprised galactose, mannose, and *N*-acetyl-D-glucosamine (Martinez-Cruz et al., 2001). In 2003 Konozy et al. were found *Erythrina speciosa* seeds can be specific with D-galactose and had two identical subunits of molecular mass was 27.6 kDa include the lectin was a neutral carbohydrate content of 5.5% (Konozy et al., 2003). *N*-acetyl-D-galactosamine-specific lectin isolation from *Glycine max* L. Merrill SA88 them were found the soybean lectin consists of four subunits it had molecular weight of each 30,000 Da in one-step purification with high purity and high yield (about 90% recovery from the crude extract) by use Poly (hydroxypropyl methacrylate-glycidyl methacrylate) beads were as an affinity matrix and *N*-acetyl-D-galactosamine (GalNAc) was as an affinity ligand (Percin et al., 2009).

7.3 Fucose

Aleuria aurantia lectin (AAL) is a commercially available lectin that is known for its high affinity for α-1, 6-fucosylated oligosaccharides and it is widely used to estimate the extent of α-1,6-fucosylation on glycoproteins and to fractionate glycoproteins. For research a novel probe for core fucose from *Aspergillus oryzae* L-fucose-specific lectin (AOL) has strongest preference for the alpha 1,6-fucosylated chain among α-1,2-, α-1,3-, α-1,4-, and α-1,6-fucosylated pyridylaminated (PA)-sugar chains. These results suggest that AOL is a novel probe for detecting core fucose in glycoproteins on the surface of animal cells (Matsumura et al., 2007). Furthermore, *Lotus tetragonolobus* lectin is a fucose-specific legume lectin. It is a homotetramer composed of four legume lectin domains was 27,800 Da (Moreno et al., 2008).

7.4 Sialic acids

Most of Sialic acid-specific lectins was found in invertebrates such as those from the Indian horseshoe crab (Mohan et al., 1982), marine crab *Scylla serrata* (Mercy and Ravindranath, 1992), lobster, tunicalase, fungus *Hericium arinaceum* (Kawagishi et al., 1994) and leaves of mulberry (Ratanapo et al., 1998). A lectin from the white shrimp *Litopenaeus setiferus* (LsL) hemolymph is a heterotetramer of two 80 kDa and two 52 kDa subunits, *N*-acetylated sugars, such as GlcNAc, GalNAc, and NeuAc, were the most effective inhibitors of the LsL hemagglutinating activity. Desialylation of erythrocytes or inhibitory glycoproteins abolished their capacity to bind LsL, confirming the relevance of sialic acid in LsL-ligand interactions (Alpuche et al., 2005). In 2009 the *Phaseolus coccineus* lectin (PCL) specificity towards sialic acid showed the molecular mass of 30 kDa consisting of homodimer subunits. Moreover the purified PCL was devoid of antifungal activity against *Candida albicans* and Penicillium *italicum,* but markedly inhibited the growth of *Hericium maydis, Rhizoctonia solani*, Gibberella *sanbinetti,* and Sclerotinia *sclerotiorum* while the same concentration of PCL decrease the 50% hemagglutinating activity was inhibited by sialic acid it suggesting a significant correlation between sialic acid-specific site and its bi-functional bioactivities (Chen et al., 2009).

8. Structure of plant lectin

Different lectin families are in general structurally unrelated. And even in those cases where a common fold is recruited, convergent evolution is the most likely explanation. Some lectin families such as the galectins recognize only one specific oligosaccharide, and consequently have a very conserved recognition site. On the other extreme, members of the C type lectin family span a wide variety of specificities. Consequently, their recognition sites are highly variable, and different specificities can easily be engineered by site directed mutagenesis (Iobst and Drickamer, 1994; and Kolatkar and Weiss, 2009). A general feature of binding sites of all lectins seems to be that they consist of a primary binding site that is capable of recognizing in a specific way a single monosaccharide residue, usually with a low affinity (in the millimolar range). Very often, but not always, there are further subsites that can be occupied by sugar residues connected to the one bound in the primary site. This allows for a modest increase in affinity. Folding in common between plant and animal lectins are β-sandwich fold, β-Trefoil folds and Hevein domains. The legume lectin-like β-sandwich fold found in Galectins that conserved family of β-galactosyl binding lectins that occur in both vertebrates and invertebrates (Hirabayashi et al., 2009). Except for the legume lectins, galectins and pentraxins, it is observed in a number of carbohydrate processing and other enzymes such as β-glucanase and asparagine amidase (Keitel et al., 1993; and Kuhn et al., 1994).

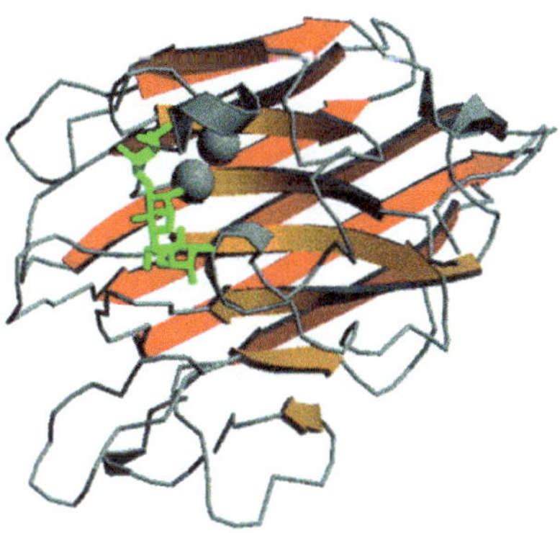

Concanavalin A

Fig. 3. The legume lectin-like β-sandwich folds illustrated by a member of the legume lectins (Concanavalin A in complex with the trisaccharide [Man(α-1, 3)]Man(α-1, 6)Man). In each case, only a single monomer of the multimeric protein is shown. Bound carbohydrate is shown in ball-and-stick. Metal ions are shown as grey spheres, bound ligands are shown in green ball-and-stick representation (Loris, 2002).

The β-trefoil fold was first identified as a carbohydrate recognition domain in ricin (Montfort et al., 1987). Later, it was also found to be the fold of amaranthin. The β-trefoil fold is another fairly common fold, first identified in soybean trypsin inhibitor (Sweet et al. 1974). It consists of a repeat of three subdomains, each consisting of a fourstranded antiparallel β-sheet.

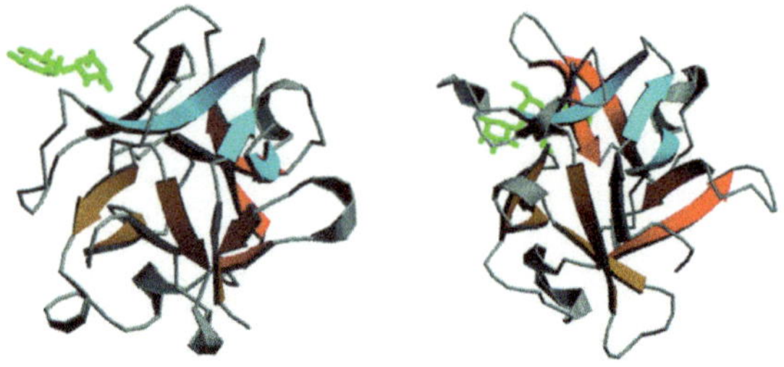

Fig. 4. The β-trefoil folds illustrated by the first domain of the subunit ricin (in complex with lactose), the first domain of amaranthin (in complex with the T-antigen) In each case, for clarity, only a single β-trefoil domain is shown in an identical orientation, although each protein is a multidomain as well as a multimeric protein. Bound carbohydrate is shown in green ball-and-stick (Loris, 2002).

Lectins comprise a structurally very diverse class of proteins characterized by their ability to bind carbohydrates with considerable specificity. Although lectins bind monosaccharides rather weakly, they employ common strategies for enhancing both the affinity and specificity of their interactions for more complex carbohydrate ligands. Members of the legume lectin family show considerable sequence and structural homology, but differences in their carbohydrate-binding specificity. The legume lectin monomer has a molecular weight of 25,000 and is composed primarily of a six- and a seven-stranded antiparallel-sheet. Concanavalin A (Con A), *Lathyrus ochrus* isolectin I (LOL I), and pea lectin all show mannose and glucose-binding specificity, and the X-ray crystal structures of their carbohydrate complexes show a monosaccharide binding- site geometry very similar to that of the LOL I-α-methyl-o-mannopyranoside complex.

The first lectin structures to be determined derived from two phylogenetically conserved families, the *Leguminoseae* (Sharon and Lis 2001; and Young and Oomen, 1992) and the *Gramineae* (Raikhel et al., 1993). Over the past ten years, major advances in X-ray crystallographic technology and the relative ease of isolation and crystallization of plant lectins have led to a rapid increase in crystal structures. The leguminous lectins clearly have dominated the field with some ten structures known today. Four of these, peanut lectin, soybean lectin, lentil lectin and hemagglutinin L, have been determined within the past three years. These lectins display diverse sugar-binding specificitiesistructures.

Lectins of the *Amaryllidaceae, Orchidaceae, Alliaceae, Araceae* and *Liliaceae* families are in the class of the mannosespecific *Liliatae* and constitute the third major structurally characterized plant lectin superfamily (Van Damme et al., 1994). They are nonseed lectins of multigene families isolated from plant bulbs (Van Damme et al., 1994) and function either as dimers or tetramers, as do the legume lectins. Their strict and exclusive specificity solely for mannose has imparted some unusual biological properties *in vitro* to this lectin family including their antiviral properties against retroviruses (e.g. HIV) (Hammaar et al., 2006). Snowdrop lectin (GNA) is a tetrameric lectin (M_r =50,000 Da) and is the first member of the *Amaryllidaceae* family crystallographically investigated.

9. Physicochemical properties of plant lectin

9.1 Composition

There are no structural features common to all lectins. Many of these proteins are relatively rich in aspartic acid, serine and threonine, which comprise as much as 30% of their amino acid content and are low in sulfur-containing amino acids. Such a pattern of amino acids is characteristic of plant proteins. In contrast, lectins such as those from wheat germ, potato and pokeweed are rich in cysteine with 20, 11.5 and 18% of the total amino acid residues respectively, most or all of which are in the form of cysteine. The high content of disulfide bonds in wheat germ agglutinin endows the protein with stability to heat (Aub et al., 1963), to proteolytic enzymes and to denaturing agents such as detergents, urea, alkali and acids (Nagata and Burger, 1972; and Rice and Etzler, 1974). The potato and *Datura stramonium* lectins are rich in hydroxyproline (Lamport, 1969). A few lectins, such as Concanavalin A, wheat germ and peanut agglutinins are devoid of covalently bound sugars. Most lectins, however, are glycoproteins with carbohydrate contents that can be as high as 50%, e.g., potato lectin. The table shown below (Table 1) is on the sugar contents of certain important glycoprotein lectins. The sugar constituents in animal glycoproteins are the same as those found in other plant glycoproteins, with the exception of L-arabinose.

Lectin	Mannose	Galactose	L-Fucose	L-Arabinose	GlcNAc	Xylose	C-P linkage	Reference
Bandeiraea simplicifolia	5.8		1		2.6	1		Lescar et al., 2007
Datura stramonium				2.8	4.5			Kilpatrick, 1978
Glycine max	4.5				1.2		GlcNAc-Asn	Lis et al., 1973
Phaseolus lunatus	3.2	3.7	0.5		1.3		GlcNAc-Asn	Mach et al., 1991
Phaseolus vulgaris	7.3				2.8		GlcNAc-Asn	Ohtani, K., and Misaki, A. (1980)
Solanum tuberosum		3		47			Ara-Hyp, Gal-ser	Matsumoto et al., 1983
Wistaria floribunda	0.77	1.63			0.65		GlcNAc-Asn	Kurokawa et al., 1976

Table 1. Well-characterized glycoprotein lectins

The molecular weight of lectins in plants ranges from 36,000 Da for wheat germ agglutinin (Nagata and Burger, 1972; and Rice and Etzler, 1974) to 265,000 for lima bean lectin (Galbraith and Goldstein, 1970). The lower limit of MW of animal lectins is found to be 14 kDa (Lis and Sharon, 1998). Some lectins exhibit a pronounced tendency to aggregate. Thus, the MW of Concanavalin A at pH below 6 is 51,000 Da and at physiological pH it is 12,000 Da (Mc Cubbin and Kay, 1971; and Wang et al., 1971). Upon storage at room temperature, soybean agglutinin and peanut agglutinin also possibly undergo irreversible self-association to high molecular weight aggregates (Lotan et al., 1975). The subunits are identical in most lectins. But lectins comprising of non-identical subunits are known as seen in soyabean agglutinin (Lotan et al., 1975) and the lectin from *Dolichos biflorus* (Carter and Etzler, 1975) which are tetramers, consisting of two types of subunits (Wright et al., 1996). A different type of subunit heterogeneity was first demonstrated in Concanavalin A (Abe et al., 1971; and Wang et al., 1971). The anti-B lectin from *Bandeiraea simplicifolia* consists of a family of five closely related proteins, each of which is a tetramer of one or two types of subunits. One of the subunits is specific for *N*-acetyl galactosamine, whereas the specificity of the other is confined to α-galactose (Goldstein and Hayes, 1978). The structure of *Bandeiraea simplicifolia* isolectins is analogous to that of PHA isolectins. They have five tetrameric proteins comprising of varying proportions of two classes of subunits (Miller et al., 1973; Rasanen et al., 1973; and Leavitt et al., 1977). These subunits show difference in properties. It is assumed that it is due to their difference in the primary structure of subunits (Miller et al., 1973).

9.2 Metal ion requirements

With a few exceptions, all lectins examined contain metal ions and in some cases evidence has been presented for the requirement of Mn^{2+} or Ca^{2+} (Emmerich et al., 1994) for activity (Table 2). Treatment with ethylene-diamine tetra acetic acid (EDTA) at neutral pH did not remove the metal ions from Concanavalin A (Doyle et al., 1984), soybean agglutinin (Jaffe et al., 1974) or lima bean lectin (Galbraith and Goldstein, 1970). Reversible removal of metal

Lectin	Metal content (atom / mole)				References
	Mn^{2+}	Ca^{2+}	Zn^{2+}	Metal	
Bandeiraea simplicifolia I	1.2	2.0		Ca^{2+}	Lescar et al., 2002
Canavalia ensiformis	4.0	4.0		Mn^{2+}	Magnuson et al., 1983
Datura stramonium	<0.2		<0.2		Kilpatrick, 1978
Dolichos biflorus	1.6	5.4	2.0		Etzler et al., 1970
Euonymus europeus		8.0	0.7		Petryniak et al., 1977
Glycine max	1.0-1.7	3.5-4.1	0.28	Mn^{2+}	Lis and Sharon, 1973
Lens culinaris	0.64	3.8		Mn^{2+}	Westbrook et al., 1984
Marasrous oreades			0.7		Winter et al., 2002
Ononis hircina	1.0		1.0		Horejsr et al., 1978
Pisum sativum	1.0	2.5		Ca^{2+}	Reeke et al., 1986
Phaseolus coccineus	0.15	4.8	1.0		Perez-Campos et al., 1997
Phaseolus lunatus	1.0	4.0		Mn^{2+}	Mach et al., 1991
Phaseolus vulgaris	0.24	6.2		Mn^{2+}	Andrews, 1974
Ricinus communis	<0.1	<0.1	<0.1		Mandal et al.,1989
Sarothamnus scoparius	1.5		0.8		Gurtler, 1978
Ulex europeus I	0.42	2.0	0.82		Sugii and Kabat, 1982
Vicia cracca	0.9		2.4		Sitohy et al., 2007

Table 2. Metal content and metal requirements for activity of lectins

ions can be achieved under acidic conditions. The Mn^{2+} in lectins can be replaced by a variety of transition-metal ions without loss of biological activity as demonstrated for Concanavalin A (Agrawal and Goldstein, 1968; and Shoham et al., 1973). Ca^{2+} in Concanavalin A could be replaced by Cd^{2+}, but not by Ba^{2+} (Shoham et al., 1973). The metal ions confer a high degree of structural stability to Concanavalin A, protecting the lectin against heat inactivation and hydrolysis by proteolytic enzymes (Thomasson and Doyle, 1975). Ni^{2+} alone protects Concanavalin A against proteolysis at pH 7.0 but not at pH 8.2. Some lectins require metal ions for the saccharide-binding activity (Sumner and Howell, 1936). Extensive studies by NMR have revealed a complicated set of interlocking equilibrium involving the apoprotein and various complexes with metal ions and the saccharides (Brewer et al., 1983).

10. Isolate and purification of lectin

Purified lectins are essential for establish their molecular properties and are highly desirable for their many applications. In the past, lectins have been obtained solely from native sources, but they can now be produced also by recombinant techniques. Isolation of a lectin begins commonly with extraction of the tissue or organ in which it is present. This is simple in the case of plants, especially their seeds (Goldstein and Poretz, 1986; and Rudiger, 1993). The seeds are ground and the meal obtained is extracted with a neutral buffer. Often it is advisable to pre-extract the dry meal with an organic solvent, such as petroleum ether, to remove colored materials derived from the seed coat and lipids that may be present in large amounts. Animal tissues are either homogenized directly in the extraction buffer or the tissue is extracted first with acetone to remove water and lipids. The extraction buffer should preferably contain protease inhibitors to prevent degradation of the lectin during purification, and, in the case of membrane bound lectins, a detergent as well. Preliminary fractionation of the crude extract (e.g., by ammonium sulfate precipitation) is often done to obtain a protein fraction devoid of other constituents (e.g., polysaccharides in the case of plants). Final purification is achieved by affinity chromatography on a suitable adsorbent. A wide variety of affinity adsorbents, to suit any taste or purse, have been described in the literature and many of them can be purchased ready-made These include polysaccharides such as Sephadex, a polymer of glucose employed for the purification of Concanavalin A and pea lectin agarose (or Sepharose), a polymer of galactose, for the purification of the lectins from castor bean; acid-treated Sepharose for the purification of SBA; and chitin, a polymer of *N*-acetylglucosamine, for the purification of WGA. In the absence of readily available polysaccharides, use can be made of adsorbents consisting of carbohydrates or glycoproteins as such, or in the form of a synthetic derivative, that are covalently attached to an insoluble carrier. For instance, lactose coupled to Sepharose is the reagent of choice the purification of the lectins from peanut, eel electric organ or calf heartmuscle. *N*-acetylglucosamine bound to the same support serves for the purification of potato lectin and WGA, whereas immobilized porcine AH blood type substance is employed for the purification of the blood type A specific DBL and HPA. When working with lectins of an uncommon specificity, adsorbents have to be tailor made, as for example Sepharose bound asialoglycophorin for the purification of the blood type *N*-specific for lectin from *Vicia graminea*.

The lectin was purified from crude extract of mixer solution, commonly use chromatography technique such as, affinity chromatography, ion exchange chromatography, and gel filtration chromatography. In 2004 had a research that used affinity chromatography to purify the lectin from human serum proteins by Concanavalin A sepharose column coupled to two-dimensional gel electrophoresis. The purified sample had 2 fractions before use this technique (Rodriguez-Pineiro et al., 2004). Next year, a lectin from the marine red alga *Gracilaria ornata* (*Gracilariaceae, Rodophyta*); GOL was purified by 2 steps chromatography technique consist of ion exchange chromatography on DEAE-cellulose and affinity chromatography on mucin-Sepharose 4B. The GOL significantly affected the development of *Callosobruchus maculatus* larvae, indicating the possibility of using this lectin in a biotechnological strategy for insect management of stored cowpea seeds. (Leite et al., 2005). In 2007 Shi et al. study lectin from raw and canned red kidney bean (*Phaseolus vulgaris*). They used gel filtration technique to purify. Use Affi-gel Blue gel sepharose compare to thyroglobulin-Sepharose to purify the lectin from red kidney bean. Found that the lectin from thyroglobulin more purify than Affi-gel Blue gel (Shi et al., 2007).

An alternative approach for the preparation of lectins has been made possible by the advent of recombinant DNA technology. It is based on the isolation of the cDNA or genomic DNA of the lectin, its insertion into a suitable vector and expression in an appropriate host cell. Isolation of the cDNA requires knowledge of at least part of the primary sequence of the lectin itself or of a structurally similar one. By this technique, several plant lectins, among them of pea (Stubbs et. al., 1986; and Van Eijsden et al., 1992), *Erythrina corallodendron* (Arango et al., 1993), peanut (Sharma and Surolia, 1994) and *Griffonia simplicifolia* (Zhu et al., 1996) have been expressed in *Escherichia coli*. Expression of plant lectins was also achieved in other systems, e.g. WGA in *Saccharomyces cerevisiae* (Nagahora et al., 1992), PHA and GNA in *Pichia pastoris* (Raemaekers et al., 1999), PNA in insect cells (Kumar et al., 1999) and SBA in monkey cells (Adar et al., 1997); (for a more complete listing of recombinant plant lectins) (Streicher and Sharon, 2003).

11. Lectins in edible plants

Many lectin-containing plants are common constituents of the diet of humans and farm animals. Since lectins are known to act on cells in a variety of ways, such as agglutination, mitogenic stimulation and killing, and they are often resistant to heat and proteolytic enzymes, including those of intestinal bacteria, the effects of consumption of these proteins deserve special consideration. For many years it has been known that they occur in legumes such as soybeans, kidney beans, lima beans, mung beans, lentils, garden peas and peanuts that are a major food source for humans and animals in one part of the world. Although lectin containing foods are frequently consumed in cooked or otherwise processed form, such treatments may not always be adequate to completely inactivate the lectins present. Thus, lectins have been detected in roasted peanuts (Wang et al., 1999). Slow cooking of beans, without boiling, does not always eliminate lectin activity as observed with kidney beans cooked for 11 hr at 82 °C or for 5 hr at 91 °C. The stability of plant lectins in the stomach is evidenced, for example, by the finding that when Concanavalin A, PHA or WGA were intragastrically administered into rats between 50 and 90% of the lectin was recovered after 1 hr from the stomach by homogenizing the tissue in phosphate-buffered saline containing the appropriate specific sugar. Moreover, in the few experiments with humans that ate lectin-containing foods, namely tomatoes (Kilpatrick et al., 1985), red kidney beans (Pusztai et al., 1989) or peanuts, either raw or roasted (Wang et al., 1999) the lectins have not only withstood the acidity and the proteolytic enzymes of the intestinal tract, but a significant proportion of the amount ingested has reached the circulatory system with unimpaired hemagglutinating and immunological activities. In rodents, a diet containing lectins provoked intestinal and systemic immune responses to these proteins (Gomez et al., 1995). Furthermore, human serum was found to contain antibodies to the lectins of peanut, soybean and wheat germ (Tchernychev and Wilchek 1996).

12. Biological role

Lectins are present abundantly in many plants. Despite this abundance, their precise biological roles in the plants to which they belong, are not well understood. The available evidences suggest two main roles for them.

12.1 Mediation of symbiotic relationship between nitrogen fixing microorganisms, primarily, rhizobia and leguminous plants

Lectins localized at the root hairs are the entry sites for rhizobia. The lectins then aggregate the rhizobia in the root nodules and make them immobile (Hamblin and Kent, 1973; Bohlool and Schmidt, 1974; Diaz et al., 1989; Brewin and Kardailsky, 1997; and Hirsch, 1995). Type specificity of host-parasite interactions between leguminous plants and particular strains of rhizobia infecting them is determined by lectins. The expression of the pea lectin gene in white clover roots enabled them to be nodulated by a rhizobium strain specific for the pea plant (Van Eijsden et al., 1995).

12.2 Protection of plants from predatory animals and phytopathogens

Abrin, a type-II ribosome-inactivating protein (RIP), was the first lectin to be recognized as a defence protein (Peumans and Van Damme, 1995). Soon afterwards ricin also came to be recognized as a defence protein (Olsnes, 2004). Type-II RIPs which belong to the plant lectin family with β-trefoil fold are known to be toxic to animals and insects (Hartley and Lord, 2004; and Stirpe, 2004). Lectins from *Phaselous vulgaris* (PHA), *Robinia pseudocacia* and *Sambuscus nigra* have been reported to be toxic to higher animals (Peumans and Van Damme, 1995). Lectins from many plants, when ingested by animals, have resulted in toxic effects (Lis and Sharon, 1998), fungal growth in *Trichoderma viride* is inhibited by wheat germ aggiutinin (WGA) (Mirelman el al., 1975). Brambl and Gade (1985) have shown that eleven purified lectins, representing a wide spectrum of sugar specificity, inhibited the growth of fungal species *Neurospora crassa, Aspergilius amsteldomi* and *Botryodiplodia theobromae.* Known antifungal lectins include those which bind chitin (Peumans and Van Damme, 1995; Hirsch et al., 1995; Eijsden et al., 1995; Kijne, 1997; and Selitrennikoff, 2001). The anti-insect activity of many plants has been attributed to the presence of lectins in them. For example PHA (Chrispeels and Raikhel, 1991) pea nut agglutinin (PNA), WGA, *Maclura pomifera* agglutinin (MPA) and lectins from potato, thorn apple and osage orange show anti-insect activity against cowpea weevil. WGA and *Bauhinea purpurea* agglutinm arc toxic to *Ootrinia nubilalio* larvae. Snow drop and garlic lectin show toxic effects on cowpea weevil and tobacco hornworm (Hilder et al., 1995, and Peumans and Van Damme, 1995).

13. Application to antimicrobial activity

The cell wall of bacteria not only precludes any interaction between the glycoconjugates on their membrane and carbohydrate-binding proteins but also prevents these proteins from penetrating the cytoplasm. Therefore, plant lectins cannot alter the structure and/or permeability of the membrane or disturb the normal intracellular processes of invading microbes. Therefore, if lectins play a role in the plant's defense against bacteria, it must be through an indirect mechanism that is based on interactions with cell wall carbohydrates or extracellular glycans.

In 1936, a using lectin in clinical microbiology began when Summer and Howell (Summer and Howell, 1936) had a report that Concanavalin A can agglutinated various *Mycobacterium* spp. The interactions between plant lectin and microorganisms have been applied for typing of bacteria, fungi, and protozoa. It is useful for characterizing bacterial cell components and for detecting bacteriophage receptors. (Etzler, 1983; Lis and Sharon, 1986; and Nicolson, 1974). The unique property of lectin to bind non-covalently to simple sugars and polysaccharides has attracted interest in microbial taxonomy. Lectin has a role in the clinical laboratory identification and taxonomic classification of many microorganisms. Because lectins are generally monoclonal proteins and because they possess a spectrum of specificities and molecular weights, they are substantial tools for diagnostic microbiology applications. Recent observations with regard to the binding of plant lectins to components of the bacterial cell wall peptidoglycans (such as muramic acid, *N*-acetylmuramic acid, *N*-acetylglucosamine and muramyl dipeptides) revealed that seed lectins from several legume species strongly interact with these bacterial surface carbohydrates (Ajouba et al., 1994). Evidently, the observation that legume seed lectins can recognize and bind to the bacterial cell wall does not imply that such an interaction occurs *in vivo* and certainly does not prove that these lectins are involved in the protection of the seedlings against bacteria.

Lectin has been used for investigating virulence factors, surface structures, and identification of gram-positive bacteria. For example; lectin from *Dolichos biflorus* was used to confirm its specificity for identifying group C streptococci. In another test, its crude extract was coupled to polystyrene particles with a spacer arm to yield an effective lectin-latex reagent that agglutinated group C streptococcal antigens prepared as nitrous acid, autoclave,or enzyme extracts. (Slifkin and Gil, 1984) Group C streptococcal isolates from horses and cattle agglutinated with lectin from *Dolichos biflorus* and *Helix pomatia*. (Schalla et al., 1986). Concanavalin A could be precipitated various bacterial polysaccharides, with interacts specifically with bacterial cell walls containing glycosidic residues associated with teichoic acid. Accordingly, bacteria teichoic acids from cell wall containing α-glucopyranisyl residues,such as *Lactobacillus plantarum*, *Staphylococcus aureus*, and *Bacillus subtilis*. (Archibald and Coapes, 1971; Doyle et al., 1982; and Reeder and Ekstedt, 1971). Lectins from soy bean have been used to assay for detecting *Bacillus anthracis* (Cole et al., 1984). The use of soybean agglutinin (SBA) to detect very low numbers of buffered suspention of *Bacillus anthracis* vegetative cells and spores has been reported (Graham et al., 1984). The strategy was to bind the cells or spores to polystyrene plates and to detect the bound forms with horseradish peroxidase labeled soybean agglutinin (called the lectinosorbent assay).

The contrast of gram-negative bacteria and gram-positive bacteria is the cell wall of gram-negative bacteria contains to lipid but cell wall of gram-positive bacteria does not have the lipid. In 1968, Doyle et al., provided evidence that Concanavalin A reacts with macromolecules that are devoid of terminal glucopyranose or mannopyranose residues (Doyle et al., 1968). Their investigations demonstrated that Concanavalin. A precipitates lipopolysaccharide preparation derived from various strains of *Escherichia coli* as well as from *Shigella flexneri* and *Salmonella abortivoequina*. In 1970, other investigators demonstrated that Concanavalin A can be used to detect lipopolysaccharides of various Salmonella strains as determined by gel diffusion. (Goldstein and Staub, 1970).

In 2010, Petnual et al. reported the antimicrobial activity of *Curcuma longa* lectin, expressed as the minimal inhibitory concentration (MIC), was found to inhibit the growth of all five microbial species tested, the four bacteria, *Bacillus subtilis, Staphylococcus aureus, Escherichia coli,* and *Pseudomonas aeruginosa,* plus the yeast *Candida albicans,* at MIC values of ≥ 0.011, 0.005, 0.092, 0.002 and 0.0046 mg/ml, respectively (Petnual et al. 2010). These results demonstrate that the *Curcuma longa* rhizome lectin is likely to be at least one of the, if not the, candidate molecule responsible for the antibacterial action observed in rhizome extracts from this plant. An outstanding feature of the antibacterial activity of the isolated lectin is it is somewhat nonselective against this fairly diverse selection of bacteria. The potentially broad effect of the *Curcuma longa* rhizome lectin on the growth inhibition of several diverse bacterial strains, confirms the important interaction between the lectin and all the strains under consideration. From the tested strains, *Pseudomonas aeruginosa* (lowest MIC) seemed to be most sensitive to the presence of lectin. Previouse studies of the binding of plant lectins to bacterial cell wall peptidoglycans indicate that several lectins of different carbohydrate specificities can recognize most of the components of the bacterial cell wall, such as muramic acid, *N*-acetylglucosamine, *N*-acetylmuramic acid and muramyl dipeptide (Ajouba et al., 1994).

Archidendron jiringa seed lectin was selected to test for antimicrobial activity with *Escherichia* coli, Pseudomonas auroginosa, Bacillus subtilis, Staphylococcus aurous, and Candida albican (Charungchitrak et al., 2011). The MIC of Archidendron jiringa seed lectin with Candida albican equal in S. aurous to be 0.0567 mg /ml and in Bacillus subtilis to be 0.2266 mg/ ml. But the MIC with *Escherichia* coli and Pseudomonas auroginosa is not detected, demonstrating stronger antimicrobial activity against gram-positive than gram-negative bacteria. Accordingly, the binding of lectins to muramic acid and N-acetylmuramic acid, carbohydrates present in the bacterial cell wall (mainly in gram-positive bacteria), has been reported (Ajouba et al., 1994). These data suggest that lectins probably play a role in plant defense, not only against phytopathogenic invertebrates, herbivores or fungi, but also against bacteria. The carbohydrate-binding site probably plays a key role in this activity, being responsible for the recognition of bacteria. Almost all microorganisms express surface-exposed carbohydrates. These carbohydrates may be covalently bound, as in glycosylated teichoic acids to peptidoglycan, or non-covalently bound, as in capsular polysaccharides (Hirmo, et al., 1997; and Caldeon, et al., 1997). Every surface-exposed carbohydrate is a potential lectin-reactive site. The ability of lectins to form complexes with microbial glycoconjugates has made it to be employed as probes and sorbents for whole cells, mutants, and numerous cellular constituents and metabolites.

The lectin from *Curcuma amarissima* inhibited 4 microbial growth consist of *Bacillus subtilis, Candida albicans, Escherichia coli,* and *Staphylococcus aureus* at concentration ≥ 0.446, 0.446, 0.223, and 0.892 mg/ml respectively. But can not inhibite *Pseudomonas auroginasa* growth because at the surface of *Pseudomonas auroginosa* cell does not have polysaccharide ligands which can interact with *Curcuma amarissima* lectin. (Kheeree et al., 2011) Similar to Legume lectin from *Trinella foenumgraecum, Trifolium alexandrium, Bauhinia variegata,* and *Delonix regia* had a research that these lectins from sephadex G-150 can agglutinated both gram negative and gram positive bacteria (*Mycobacterium rhodochrous, Bacillus cercur, Bacillus megaterium,*

Bacillus sphaericus, Escherichia coli, Seratia marcescens, Corynebacterium xerosis, and *Staphylococcus aureus)* (Reda et al., 1992). Inaddition β-galactoside-binding lectin was extracted from the skin of amphibian, *Bufo arenarum*. It had an antimicrobial activity against Gram negative bacteria (*Escherichia coli* K12 4100 and wild strains of *Escherichia coli* and *Proteus morganii*) and Gram positive bacteria (*Enterococcus faecalis*) (Alicia *et al*., 2003).

Several investigators have concluded that lectins are useful reagents for the study of fungal cell surfaces and may also be of value as important aids in the classification of fungi (Barkai and Sharon, 1978). The major components of fungal cell wall is Chitin, a polymer of β-(1, 4)-*N*-acetyl-D-glucosamine (Barkai and Sharon, 1978; and Ebisu et al., 1977). The report of lecin interaction to fungal, such as fluorescein-conjugated wheat germ agglutinin has been shown to be an effective probe to detect chitin on hypha surfaces. (Barkai and Sharon, 1978; Galun et al., 1976; Galun et al., 1981; Mirelman et al., 1975; Molano et al., 1980; Tkacz and Lampson, 1972; Tracz et al., 1971; Tropchin et al., 1981). In 1975 Mirelman et al. was found wheat germ agglutinin (WGA) can be inhibits spore germination and hyphal growth of *Trichoderma viride* and interferes with the synthesis of chitin (Mirelman et al., 1975). A novel mannose-binding lectin was purified from rhizomes of *Ophiopogon japonicus* was showed antifugal activity in three phytopathogenic fungi namely *Gibberella saubinetii* and *Rhizoctonia solani* (Tian et al., 2008).

In 2010, Petnual et al. purified *Curcuma longa* lectin at a dose of 47 μg and 94 μg/0.3 cm² disc showed antifungal activity against the three tested phytopathogenic fungal species, *Exserohilum turicicum, Fusarium oxysporum* and *Colectrotrichum cassiicola* (Fig. 5). While the lectin dose of 47 μg/0.3 cm² disc slightly inhibited the growth of these three fungi, that at 94 μg/0.3 cm² disc showed a higher and significant degree of antifungal activity on all three isolates (Petnual et al. 2010). This effective lectin dose of around 100 μg/ 0.3 cm² disc is in accord with that reported for the lectin from *Annona muricata* seeds against the growth of *Fusarium oxysporum, Fusarium solani* and *Colletotrichum musae* (Damico, et al., 2003), and for the lectin from *Astragalus mongholicus* against *Fusarium oxysporum, Colletorichum* sp. and Drechslera *turcia* (Yan, et al., 2005). Other lectins, such as those from potato (Gomez, et al., 1995) and red kidney beans (Ye, et al. 2001), have also been reported to exhibit antifungal activity. However, novel non-lectin proteins with antifungal activity in plant rhizomes are also known, such as the 32 kDa protein in ginger rhizomes which exhibits antifungal activity toward *Fusarium oxysporum* at a dose of 32-160 μg/ 0.3 cm² disc of ginger rhizome (Wang and Ng, 2005).

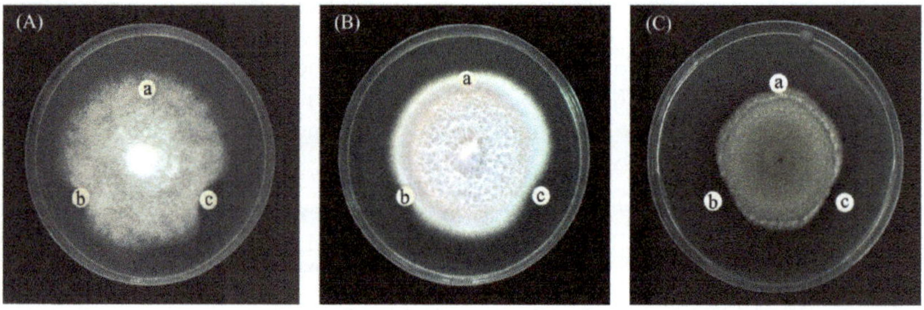

Fig. 5. Inhibitory affect of *Curcuma longa* lectin on antifungal protein toward *Exserohilum turicicum* (A), *Fusarium oxysporum* (B) and *Colectrotrichum cassiicola* (C). The negative control is 10 μl of 20 mM Tris-HCl buffer pH 7.4 (a), 47 μg *Curcuma longa* lectin. (b) and 94 μg *Curcuma longa* lectin (c) (Petnual et al., 2010).

In 2011, Kheeree et al. purified *Curcuma amarissima* lectin showed *in vitro* antifungal activity against three plant pathogenic fungal species, *Colectrotrichum cassiicola, Exserohilum turicicum,* and *Fusarium oxysporum.* It strongly inhibited the growth of *Colectrotrichum cassiicola* at 17.5 μg for *Fusarium oxysporum* and *Exserohilum turicicum,* which were strongly inhibited at the higher concentration of 35 μg (Fig. 6). Antifungal activity has been observed in other lectins where, for example *Astragalus mongholicus* root lectin revealed antifungal activity against various species of phytopathogenic fungi (Yan et al., 2005). Similarly with lectin from *Talisia esculenta* seeds inhibited the growth of *Fusarium oxysporum, Colectrotrichum lindemuthianum,* and *Saccharomyces cerevisiae.*(Freire et al., 2002) *In vitro* studies demonstrated that two novel chitin-binding lectins seeds of *Artocarpus integrifolia* inhibited the growth of *Fusarium moniliforme* and *Saccharomyces cerevisae* (Trindade et al., 2006). Many studies of plant lectins have assumed that they are implicated in host defense mechanism as antifungal proteins. However, to date only a small number of lectins have been reported to have actual antifungal activity such as lectin from the rhizomes of *Ophiopogon japonicus* showed antifungal activity against *Gibberella saubinetii* and *Rhizoctonia solani* (Tian et al., 2008). The purified *Phaseolus coccineus* Lectin (PCL) was devoid of antifungal activity against *Candida albicans* and Penicillium *italicum* (Chen et al., 2009).

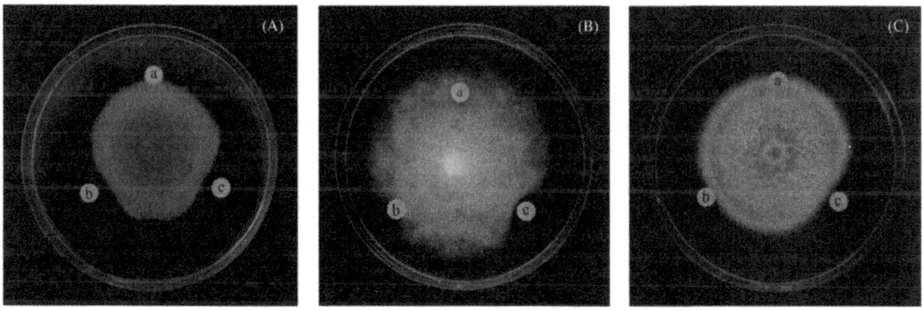

Fig. 6. Inhibitory effect of purified *Curcuma amarissima* lectin on the *in vitro* growth on PDA plates (as an antifungal activity bioassay) of; (A) *Colectrotrichum cassiicola,* (B) *Fusarium oxysporum* and (C) *Exserohilum turicicum.* For each plate, 0.625 cm diameter discs were seeded with 10 μl of TBS (a) alone as the negative control, or containing either (b) 17.5 μg/ ml or (c) 35 μg/ ml purified *Curcuma amarissima* lectin (Kheeree et al., 2011).

A large body of data exists on the interaction of lectins with a relatively broad spectrum of parasites ranging from the protozoa through the metazoa. Although Concanavalin A was used by many investigators as a lectin probe for these organisms, many other lectins have been shown to be of value in the study of cell surfaces and the identification and differentiation of the parasites. In some instances virulence of parasitic protozoa appears to be related to their surface properties, as revealed by interactions with lectins. Thus, several investigators have deemed important the comparison of surface saccharides of parasites known to differ in their virulence traits. It has been conjectured that the virulence of the trophozoite form of *Entamoeba histolytica* may depend, in part, on its surface properties. Data have been presented indicating that only strains isolated from cases of amoebic dysentery agglutinate with Concanavalin A (Martinez-Palomo et al., 1973) strains isolated from asymptomatic cases of amoebic dysentery, however, do not agglutinate with this lectin.

The unique property of lectins to bind noncovalently to simple sugars and therefore to polysaccharides and glycoconjugates has attracted the interest of virologists. In virology, lectins have been used for detection of viral glycoproteins in purified and infected cells, as well as for viral purification. Lectin studies have revealed information about the structure of viral glycoproteins, structures important in their pathogenicity. A significant contribution of lectin use in virology has been in the development of unique diagnostic methods that yield specific identification of viral agents. Purified influenza virus yields macroscopically visible flocculation when mixed with Concanavalin A. (Klenk et al., 1984) When influenza virus is treated with a proteolytic enzyme, the glycoprotein spikes of the virus are released. These treated viral particles no longer agglutinate with this lectin, but will flocculate in the presence of *N*-acetylgalactosamine-associated lectins, such as *Dolichos biflorus* or *Helix pomatia*. Other viruses, including arboviruses, vesicular stomatitis virus, paramyxoviruses, leukoviruses, and hepatitis B virus, also agglutinate with Concanavalin A. Concanavalin A was shown to block specifically adsorption of the bacteriophage binding sites of *Bacillus subtilis* possessing α-glucosylated teichoic acids in the cell walls associated with teichoic acids. It was suggested that the application of this lectin might be useful as a means to correlated bacteriophage and serologic typing of staphylococci. (Archibald and Coapes, 1972).

14. Conclusion

Biochemical and molecular studies of numerous lectins eventually demonstrated that only a limited number of carbohydrate-binding motifs evolved in plants (Peumans et al. 2000). Since the specificity of these binding motifs is primarily directed against foreign glycans, it is generally accepted now that many plant lectins are involved in the recognition and binding of glycans from foreign organisms, and accordingly play a role in plant defense (Peumans and Van Damme 1995; and Van Damme et al. 1998). Most plant lectins are probably involved in the plant's defense. Whereas direct interference with viruses and microorganisms are rather exceptional, the deleterious effects of plant lectins on predatory invertebrates and higher animals are obvious. Considering the abundance of lectins in storage organs and their storage protein-like behavior, we believe that plants accumulate part of their nitrogen reserve in the form of carbohydrate-binding proteins, which can be used as passive-defense proteins. Although low antimicrobial activity could be obtained from plant lectins, the information was still promising important for future research because nowadays extraction of bioactive compounds directly from their natural source is not the only way for the investigation. If the structure of the bioactive compound was elucidated, using knowledge on recombinant DNA technology could possibly produce a synthetic compound. And since antimicrobial-resistant organisms have been the major problem in medical treatment, searching for new antimicrobial compounds are still is interested.

15. Acknowledgement

The authors thank the Chulalongkorn University Graduate School thesis grant, the 90th Anniversary of Chulalongkorn University fund, the Thailand Research Fund, through the TRF-MAG window II, the National Research University Project of CHE, the Ratchadaphiseksomphot Endowment Fund (AM1019A, and AS613A), and the Thai Government Stimulus Package 2 (TKK2555), for financial support of this research, as well as the Institute of Biotechnology and Genetic Engineering for support and facilities.

16. References

Abe, Y., Iwabuchi, M., and Ishii, S.I. (1971). Multiple forms in the subunit structure of Concanavalin A. Biochemical and Biophysical Research Communications, 45, 1271-1278.

Adar, R., Streicher, H., Rozenblatt, S., and Sharon, N. (1997). Synthesis of soybean agglutinin in bacterial and mammalian cells. *European Journal of Biochemistry*, 249, 684-689.

Agrawal, B.B., and Goldstein, I.J. (1968). Protein-carbohydrate interactin. XV. The role of bivalent cations in Concanavalin A-polysaccharide interaction. Canadian Journal of Biochemistry, 46, 1147-1150.

Ajouba, A., Causse, H., Van Damme, E.J.M., Peumans, W.J., Cambillau, C., and Rouge, P. (1994). Interactions of plant lectins with the components of the bacterial cell wall peptidoglycan. *Biochemical Systematics and Ecology*, 22, 153-159.

Alicia S.R., Adriana, D., Adriana, G., Susana, G., Manuel, A., and Sara, S. (2003). Antibacterial activity of lactose-binding lectins from *Bufo arenarum* skin. *Biocell*, *27*, 37-46.

Alpuche, J., Pereyra, A., Agundis, C., Rosas, C., Pascual, C., Slomianny, M.C., Vazquez, L., and Zenteno, E. (2005). Purification and characterization of a lectin from the white shrimp *Litopenaeus setiferus* (Crustacea decapoda) hemolymph. *Biochimica et Biophysica Acta*, 1724, 86-93.

Allen, N.K and Brilliantine, L. (1969). A survey of hemagglutinins in various seeds. *Journal of Immunology*, 102, 1295-1299.

Allen, A.K., Neuberger, A. and Sharon, N. (1973). The purification, composition and specificity of wheat-germ agglutinin. *Journal of Biochemistry*, 131, 155-162.

Andrews, A.T. (1974). Navy (Haricot)-bean (*Phaseolus vulgaris*) lectin. Isolation and characterization of two components from a toxic agglutinating extract. *Biochemical Journal*, 139, 421-429.

Arango, R., Rodriguez-Arango, E., Adar, R., Belenky, D., Loontiens, F.G., Rozenblatt, S., and Sharon, N. (1993). Modification by site directed mutagenesis of the specificity of *Erythrina corallodendron* lectin for galactose derivatives with bulky substituens at C-2. *FEBS Letters*, 330, 133-136.

Archibald, A.R., and Coapes, E.H. (1971). The interaction of Concanavalin A with teichoic acids and bacterial cell walls. *Biochemical Journal*, 123, 665-667.

Archibald, A.R., and Coapes, E.H. (1972). Blocking of bacteriophage receptor sites by Concanavalin A. *Journal of General Microbiology*, 73, 581-585.

Abe, Y., Iwabuchi, M., and Ishii, S.I. (1971). Multiple forms in the subunit structure of Concanavalin A, Biochemical and Biophysical Research Communications, 45, 1271-1278.

Balzarini, J., Hatse, S., Vermeire, K., Princen, K., Aquaro, S., Perno, C., Clereq, E., Egberink, H., Mooter, G.V., Peumans, W., Damme, E.V., and Schols, D. (2004). Mannose-specific plant lectins from the *Amaryllidaceae* family qualify as efficient microbicides for prevention of human immunodeficiency virus infection. *Antimicrobial Agents and Chemotherapy*, 48, 3858-3870.

Barkai, G.R., and Sharon, N. (1978). Lectin as a tool for the study of yeast cell walls. *Experimental Mycology*, 2, 110-113.

Bohlool, B.B., and Schmidt, E.L. (1974). Lectins: A possible basis for specificity in the rhizobium-legume root nodule symbiosis. *Science*, 185, 269-271.

Boyd, W.C., and Reguera, R.M. (1949). Studies on hemagglutinins present in seeds of some representatives of the family Leguminoseae. *Journal of Immunology*, 62, 333-339.

Brambl, R., and Gade, W. (1985). Plant seed lectins disrupt growth of germinating fungal spores. *Physiologia Plantarum*, 64, 402-408.

Brewer, H.B.Jr., Fairwell, T., Kay, L., Meng, M., Ronan, R., Law, S., and Light, J.A. (1983). Human plasma proapoA-I: isolation and amino-terminal sequence. Biochemical and Biophysical Research Communications, 113, 626-632.

Brewin, N.J., and Kardailsky, I.V. (1997). Legume lectins and nodulation by rhizobium. *Trends in Plant Science*, 2, 92-98.

Broekaert, W.F., Cammue, B.P.A., De Bolle, M.F.C., Thevissen, K., De Samblanx, G.W., and Osborn, R.W. (1997). Antimicrobial peptides from plants. *Critical Reviews in Plant Sciences*, 16, 297-323.

Brooks, S.A., and Leathem, A.J. (1998). Expression of *N*-acetyl galactosaminylated and sialylated glycans by metastases arising from primary breast cancer, *Invasion Metastasis*, 18, 115-121.

Chandra, N.R., Kumar, N., Jeyakani, J., Singh, D.D., Gowda, S.B., and Prathima M.N. (2006). Lectindb: a plant lectin database. *Glycobiology Advance*, 16, 938-946

Charungchitrak, C., Petsom, A., Sangvanich, P., and Karnchanatat, A. (2011). Antifungal and antibacterial activities of lectin from the seeds of *Archidendron jiringa* Nielsen. *Food Chemistry*, 126, 1025-1032.

Chen, J., Liu, B., Ji, N., Zhou, J., Bian, H., and Li, C. (2009). A novel sialic acid-specific lectin from *Phaseolus coccineus* seeds with potent antineoplastic and antifungal activities. *Phytomedicine*, 16, 352-360.

Chrispeels, M.J., and Raikhel, N.V. (1991). Lectins, lectin genes, and their role in plant defense. *Plant Cell*, 3, 1-9.

Caldeon, A.M., Buck, G., and Doyle, R.J. (1997). Lectin-microorganism complexes. *The Electronic Lectin Journal: Lectins, Biology, Biochemistry, Clinical Biochemistry*, 12, 87-984583-0-2.

Carter, W.G., and Etzler, M.E. (1975). Isolation, characterization, and subunit structures of multiple forms of *Dolichos biflorus* lectin, *Journal of Biological Chemistry*, 250, 2756-2762.

Cole, H.B., Ezzell, W.J., Keller, F.K., and Doyle, J.R. (1984). Differentiation of *Bacillus anthracis* and other Bacillus species by use of lectins. *Journal of Clinical Microbiology*, 19, 48-53.

Collinge, D.B., Kragh, K.M., Mikkelsen., J.D., Nielsen, K.K., Rasmussen, U., and Vad, K. (1993). Plant chitinases. *Plant Journal*, 3, 31-40.

Cunningham, B.A., Hemperly, J.J., Hopp, T.P., and Edelman, G.M. (1979). Favin versus Concanavalin A: circularly permuted amino acid sequences. *Proceedings of the National Academy of Sciences*, 76, 3218-3222.

Damico, D.C., Freire, M.G., Gomes, V.M., Toyama, M.H., Marangoni, S., Novello, J.C. and Macedo, M.L. (2003). Isolation and characterization of a lectin from *Annona muricata* seeds. *Journal of Protein Chemistry* 22, 655-661.

Diaz, C.L., Melchers, L.S., Hooykaas, P.J.J., Lugtenberg, B.J.J., and Kijne, J.W. (1989). Root lectin as a determinant of host-plant specificity in the rhizobium-legume symbiosis. *Nature*, 338, 579-581.

Doyle, R.J., Nedjat-Haiem, F., Keller, K.F., and Frasch, C.E. (1984). Diagnostic value of interactions between members of the family Neisseriaceae and lectins. *Journal of Clinical Microbiology*, 19, 383-387.

Doyle, R.J., Nedjat-Haiem, F., Miller, R.D., and Keller, K.F. (1982). Interaction between plant agglutinins and Legionella species. *Journal of Clinical Microbiology*, 15, 973-975.

Doyle, R.J., Woodside, E.E., and Fishel, W.C. (1968). Protein-polyelectrolyte interactions. The Concanavalin A precipitin reaction with polyelectrolytes and polysaccharide derivatives. *Biochemical Journal*, 106, 35-40.

Ebisu, S., Lonngren, J., and Goldstein, I.J. (1977). Interaction of pneumococcal S-14 polysaccharide with lectins from *Ricinus communes,Triticum vulgaris* and *Bandeiraea simplicifolia*. *Carbohydrate Research*, 58, 187-191.

Edelman, G.M., Cunningham, B.A., Reeke, G.N.Jr., Becker, J.W., Waxdal, M.J., and Wang, J.L. (1972). The covalent and three-dimensional structure of Concanavalin A. *Proceedings of the National Academy of Science*, 69, 2580-2584.

Eijsden, R.R., Diaz, C.L., Pater, B.S., and Kijne, J.W. (1995). Sugar-binding activity of pea (*Pisum sativum*) lectin is essential for heterologous infection of transgenic white clover hairy roots by *Rhizobium leguminosarum* biovar viciae. *Plant Molecular Biology*, 29, 431-439.

Emmerich, C., Helliwell, J.R., Redshaw, M., Naismith, J.H., Harrop, S.J., Raftery, J., Kalb, A.J., Yariv, J., Dauter, Z., and Wilson, K.S. (1994). High-resolution structures of single-metal-substituted Concanavalin A: the Co, Ca-protein at 1.6 Å and the Ni, Ca-protein at 2.0 Å, Acta Crystallographica Section D: Biological Crystallography, 50, 749-756.

Etzler, M.E. (1983). Distribution and properties of the *Dolichos biflorus* lectins: a model system for exploring the role of lectins in plants. *Progess in Clinical and Biological Research*, 138, 197-207.

Etzler, M.E., Anderson, B., Beychok, S., Gruezo, F., Lloyd, K.O., Richardson, N.G., and Kabat, E.A. (1970). Immunochemical studies on blood groups. XLVI. Oligosaccharides isolated after hydrolysis of hog gastric mucin blood group A + H substance previously treated with the blood group de-N-acetylating enzyme. *Archives of Biochemistry and Biophysics*, 141, 588-601.

Freire, M.D.G., Gomes, V.M., Corsini, R.E., Machado, O.L.T., De Simone, S.G., and Novello, J.C. (2002). Isolation and partial characterization of a novel lectin from *Talisia esculenta* seeds that interferes with fungal growth. *Plant Physiology and Biochemistry*, 40, 61-68.

Foriers, A., Wuilmart, C., Sharon, N., and Strosberg, A.D. (1977). Extensive sequence homologies among lectins from leguminous plants. *Biochemical and Biophysical Research Communications*, 75, 980-986.

Foriers, A., DeNeve, R., and Strosberg, A.D. (1979). Lectin sequences as a tool for chemotaxonomical classification. *Physiologie Vegtale*, 17, 597-606.

Foriers, A., Lebrun, E., Van Rappenbusch, R., DeNeve, R., and Strosberg, A.D. (1981). The structure of the lentil (*Lens eulinaris*) lectin. Amino acid sequence determination and prediction of the secondary structure. *Journal of Biological Chemistry*, 256, 5550-5560.

Galbraith, W., and Goldstein, I.J. (1970). Phytohemagglutinins: A new class of metalloproteins. Isolation, purification, and some properties of the lectin from *Phaseolus lunatus*. *FEBS Letters*, 9, 197-201.

Galun, M., Braun, A., Frendorf, A., and Galun, E. (1976). Hyphal walls of isolated lichen fungi: autoradiographic localization of precursor incorporation and binding of fluoresceinconjugated lectins. *Archives of Microbiology*, 108, 9-16.

Galun, M., Malki, D., and Galun, E. (1981). Visualization of chitin-wall formation in hyphal tips and anastomases of *Diplodia natalensis* by fluorescein conjugated wheat-germ agglutinin and [^{3}H] *N*-acetyl-D glucosamine. *Archives of Microbiology*, 130, 105-110.

Goldstein, I.J., and Staub, M.A. (1970). Interaction of Concanavalin A with polysaccharides of Salmonellae. *Immonochemistry*, 7, 315-319.

Goldstein, I.J., and Hayes, C.E. (1978). The lectins: carbohydrate-binding proteins of plants and animals. *Advances in Carbohydrate Chemistry and Biochemistry*, 35, 127-340.

Goldstein, I.J., and Poretz, R.D. (1986). Isolation, Physicochemical Characterization and Carbohydrate-Binding Specificity of Lectins. In: *The Lectins: Properties, Functions and Applications in Biology and Medicine*. Liener, I.E., Sharon, N., and Goldstein, I.J. (eds.), pp. 35-247, Academic Press, Orlando, Florida.

Gomez, E., Ortiz, V., Ventura, J., Campos, R. and Bourges, H. (1995). Intestinal and systemic immune responses in rats to dietary lectins. *Advances in Experimental Medicine and Biology*, 371A, 533-536.

Graham, K., Keller, K., Ezzell, W.J., and Doyle, J.R. (1984). Enzyme-linked lectinosorbent assay (ELLA) for *Bacillus anthracis*. *European Journal of Clinical Microbiology and Infectious Diseases*, 3, 210-212.

Gurtler, L.G. (1978) The fucosyl specific lectins of *Ulex europaeus* and *Sarothamnus scoparius*. Biochemical characteristics and binding properties to human B-lymphocytes *Biochimica et Biophysica Acta*, 544, 593-604.

Hafidh, R.R., Abas, F., Abdulamir, A.S., Jahanashiri, F., Bakar, F.A., and Sekawi, Z. (2009). A review: cancer research of natural products in Asia. *International Journal of Cancer Research*, 5, 69-82.

Hamblin, J., and Kent, S.P. (1973). Possible role of phytohaemagglutinin in *Phaseolus vulgaris* L. *Nature New Biology*, 245, 28-30.

Hammaar, L., Hissch, I., Machado, A., De Mareuil, J., Baillon, J., and Chermann, J.C. (2009). Lectin effects on HIV-1 infectivity. *Annals of the New York Academy of Sciences*, 724, 166-169.

Hartley, M.R., and Lord, J.M. (2004). Cytotoxic ribosome-inactivating lectins from plants. *Biochimica et Biophysica Acta*, 1701, 1-14.

Hemperly, J.J. (1983). Circular permutation of amino acid sequences among legume lectins. *Trends in Biochemical Sciences*, 8, 100-102.

Herman, E.M., and Shannon, L.M. (1984). Immunocytochemical localization of Concanavalin A in developing jack-bean cotyledons. *Planta*, 161, 97-104.

Higgins, T.J.Y., Chandler, P.M., Zurawski, G., Button, S.C., and Spencer, D. (1983). The biosynthesis and primary structure of pea seed lectin. *Journal of Biological Chemistry*, 258, 9544-9549.

Hilder, V.A., Powell, K.S., Gatehouse, A.M.R., Gatehouse, J.A., Gatehouse, L.N., Shi, Y., Hamilton, W.D.O., Merryweather, A., Newell, C.A., Timans, J.C., Peumans, W.J., Van Damme, E., and Boulter, D. (1995). Expression of snowdrop lectin in transgenic tobacco plants results in added protection against aphids. *Transgenic Research*, 4, 18-25.

Hirabayashi, J., Hashidate, T., Nishi, N., Nakamura, T., Hirashima, M., Urasima, T., Oka T., Futai, M., Muller, W.E.G., Yagi, F., and Kasai, K. (2009). How galectins have evolved oligosaccharide specificity. *Biochimica et Biophysica Acta*, 1572, 263-273.

Hirmo, S., Utt, M., Wadström, T. (1997) Sialylglycoconjugate and proteoglycan-binding microbial lectins. *The Electronic Lectin Journal: Lectins, Biology, Biochemistry, Clinical Biochemistry*, 12, 87-984583-0-2.

Hirsch, A.M., Brill, L.M., Lim, P.O., Scambray, J., and Van Rhijn, P. (1995). Steps toward defining the role of lectins in nodule development in legumes. *Symbiosis*, 19, 155-173.

Hoffman, L.M., Ma, Y., and Barker, R.F. (1982). Molecular cloning of *Phaseolus vulgaris* lectin mRNA and use of cDNA as a probe to estimate lectin transcript levels in various tissues. *Nucleic Acids Research*, 10, 7819-7828.

Horejsr, V., Chaloupecka, O., and Kocourek, J. (1978). Studies on lectins. XLIII. Isolation and characterization of the lectin from restharrow roots (*Ononis hircina* Jacq.). *Biochimica et Biophysica Acta*, 539, 287-293.

Howard, I.K., Sage, H.J., and Horton, C.B. (1972). Studies on the appearance and location of hemagglutinins from a common lentil during the life cycle of the plant. *Archives of Biochemistry and Biophysics*, 149, 323-326.

Imberty, A., Gautier, C., Lescar, J., Perez, S., Wyns, L., and Loris, R. (2000). An unusual carbohydrate binding site revealed by the structures of two *Maackia amurensis* lectins complexed with sialic acid-containing oligosaccharides. *Journal of Biological Chemistry*, 275, 17541-17548.

Iobst, S.T. and Drickamer, K. (1994). Binding of sugar ligands to Ca^{2+}-dependent animal lectins. II. Generation of high-affinity galactose binding by site-directed mutagenesis. *Journal of Biological Chemistry*, 269, 15512-15519.

Irvin, E.L. (1976). Phytohemagglutinins (Phytolectins). *Annual Review of Plant Physiology*, 27, 291-319.

Jaffe, L.F., Robinson, K.R., and Nuccitelli, R. (1974). Local cation entry and self-electrophoresis as an intracellular localization mechanism. *Annals of the New York Academy of Sciences*, 238, 372-389.

Kaku, H., Tanaka, Y., Tazaki, K., Minami, E., Mizuno, H., and Shibuya, N. (1996). Sialylated oligosaccharide-specific plant lectin from Japanese elderberry (*Sambucus sieboiliana*) bark tissue has homologous structure to type II ribosome-inactivating protein, ricin and abrin. *Journal of Biological Chemistry*, 271, 1480-1485.

Kawagishi, M., Mori, H., Uno, A., Kimura, A., and Chiba, S., (1994). A sialic acid-binding lectin from the mushroom *Hericium erinaceum*. *FEBS Letters*, 340, 56-58.

Keitel, U., Simon, O., Borriss, R., and Heinemann, U. (1993). Molecular and activesite structure of a Bacillus 1,3-1,4-β-glucanase. *Proceedings of the National Academy of Sciences of the United States of America*, 90, 5287-5291.

Kijne, J.W., Bauchrowitz, M.A., and Diaz, C.L. (1997). Root lectins and rhizobia. *Plant Physiology*, 115, 869-873.

Kilpatrick, D.C., Pusztai, A., Grant, G., Graham, C., and Ewen, S.W.B. (1985). Tomato lectin resists digestion in the mammalian alimentary tract and binds to intestinal villi without deleterious effects. *FEBS Letters*, 185, 299-305.

Kilpatrick, D.C., and Yeoman, M.M. (1978). Purification of the lectin from *Datura stramonium*. *Biochemical Journal*, 175, 1151-1153.

Kheeree, N., Sangvanich, P., and Karnchanatat, A. (2011). Antifungal and Antiproliferative Activities of Lectin from the Rhizomes of *Curcuma amarissima* Roscoe. *Applied Biochemistry and Biotechnology*, 162, 912-925.

Klenk, H.D., Becht, H., and Rott, R. (1984). Reaction of viruses and virus-infected cells with heterophile agglutinins. *Annals of the New York Academy of Sciences*, 234, 355-367.

Kocourek, J. (1986). Historical Background. In: *The Lectin: Properties, Functions, and Application in Biology and Medicine*, Liner, I.E., Sharon N. and Goldstein, I.J. (eds.), pp. 1-32, Academic Press Inc, New York.

Kolatkar, A.R. and Weiss, W.I. (2009). Structural basis of galactose recognition by C-type animal lectins. *Journal of Biological Chemistry*, 271, 6679-6685.

Konozy, E.H., Bernardes, E.S., Rosa, C., Faca, V., Greene, L.J., and Ward, R.J. (2003). Isolation, purification, and physicochemical characterization of a D-galactose-binding lectin from seeds of *Erythrina speciosa*. *Archives of Biochemistry and Biophysics*, 410, 222-229.

Kouchalakos, R.N., Bates, O.J., Bradshaw, R.A., and Hapner, K.D. (1984). Lectin from sainfoin (*Onobrychis viciifolia* Scop.) Complete amino acid sequence. *Biochemistry*, 23, 1824-1830.

Kuhn, P., Tarentino, A.L., Plummer, T.H. and Roey Van, P. (1994). Crystal structure of peptide-N(4)-(N-acetyl-β-D-glucosaminyl) asparagine amidase at 2.2 Å resolution. *Biochemistry*, 33, 11699-11706.

Kumar, M., Behera, A.K., Kumar, S., Srinivas, V.R., Das, H.R., Surolia, A., and Das, R.H. (1999). Expression, purification and characterization of peanut (*Arachis hypogaea*) agglutinin (PNA) from baculovirus infected insect cells. *Bioscience Reports*, 19, 227-234.

Kurokawa, T., Tsuda, M., and Sugino, Y. (1976). Purification and characterization of a lectin from *Wistaria floribunda* seeds. *Journal of Biological Chemistry*, 251: 5686-5699.

Lakhtin, V.M. (1994). Molecular organization of lectins (A review). *Molecular Biology (Moscow, Russian Federation, English Edition)*, 28, 157-177.

Lamport, D.T. (1969). The isolation and partial characterization of hydroxyproline-rich glycopeptides obtained by enzymic degradation of primary cell walls. *Biochemistry*, 8, 1155-1163.

Leavitt, R.D., Felsted, R.L., Egorin, M.J., and Bachur, N.R. (1977). Recombinations of subunits of *Phaseolus vulgaris* isolectins. *Journal of Biological Chemistry*, 252, 2967-2971.

Lehrer, R.I., and Ganz, T. (1999). Antimicrobial peptides in mammalian and insect host defence. *Current Opinion in Immunology*, 11, 23-27.

Leite, Y.F.M.M., Silva, L.M.C.M., Amorim, R.C.D.N., Freire, E.A., de Melo Jorge, D.M., and Grangeiro, T.B. (2005). Purification of a lectin from the marine red alga *Gracilaria ornata* and its effect on the development of the cowpea weevil *Callosobruchus maculatus* (Coleoptera: Bruchidae). *Biochimica et Biophysica Acta (BBA) - General Subjects*, 1724, 137-145.

Lescar, J., Loris, R., Mitchell, E., Gautier, C., Chazalet, V., Cox, V., Wyns, L., Perez, S., Breton, C., and Imberty, A. (2002). Isolectins I-A and I-B of *Griffonia* (Bandeiraea) *simplicifolia*. Crystal structure of metal-free Gs I-B(4) and molecular basis for metal binding and monosaccharide specificity. *Journal of Biological Chemistry*, 277, 6608.

Lescar, J., Sanchez, J.F., Audfray, A., Coll, J.L., Breton, C., Mitchell, E.P., and Imberty, A. (2007). Structural basis for recognition of breast and colon cancer epitopes Tn antigen and Forssman disaccharide by *Helix pomatia* lectin. *Glycobiology*, 17, 1077-1083.

Lis, H., and Sharon, N. (1973). The biochemistry of plant lectins (phytohemagglutinins). *Annual Review of Biochemistry*, 42, 541-574.

Lis, H., and Sharon, N. (1986). Applications of lectins. In: *Properties, Functions and Applications in Biology and Medicine*, Leiner, I.F., Sharon, N., Goldstein, I.J. (eds.), pp. 294-357, Academic Press, New York.

Lis, H., and Sharon, N. (1998). Lectins: carbohydrate-specific proteins that mediate cellular recognition. *Chemical Reviews*, 98, 637-674.

Lisgarten, J.N,, Chattopadhyay, T.K., Pitts, J.E., Palmer, R.A., Reynolds, C.D., Dao-Thi, M.H., Van Driessche, E., and Beeckmans, S. (1999). Crystallization of *Helix pomatia* agglutinin (HPA), a protein from the edible snail. *Acta Crystallographica Section D-Biological Crystallography*, D55, 1903-1905.

Loris, R. (2002). Principles of structures of animal and plant lectins. *Biochimica et Biophysica Acta*, 1572, 198-208.

Lotan, R., Skutelsky, E., Danon, D. and Sharon, N. (1975). The purification, composition, and specificity of the anti-T lectin from peanut (*Arachis hypogaea*). *Journal of Biological Chemistry*, 250, 8518-8523.

Mach, L., Scherf, W., Ammann, M., Poetsch, J., Bertsch, W., Marz, L., and Glossl, J. (1991). Purification and partial characterization of a novel lectinb from elder (*Sambucus nigra* L.) fruit. *Biochemical Journal*, 278, 667-671.

Magnuson, J., Alter, G., Appel, D., Christie, D., Munske, G., and Pandolfino, E. (1983). Metal ion binding to Concanavalin A. *Journal of Biosciences*, 5, 9-17.

Mandal, C., and Basu, S. (1989). Physiochemical studies on achatininH, a novel sialic acid-bindinglectin. *Biochemical Journal*, 257, 65-71.

Martinez-Cruz, M., Zenteno, E., and Cordoba, F. (2001). Purification and characterization of a galactose-specific lectin from corn (*Zea mays*) coleoptyle. *Biochimica et Biophysica Acta*, 1568, 37-44.

Martinez-Palomo, A., Gonzales-Robles, A., and De la Torre, M. (1973). Selective agglutination of pathogenic strains of *Entamoeba histolytica* induced by Concanavalin A. *Nature*, 245, 186-187.

Matsumoto, I., Jimbo, A., Mizuno, Y., Seno, N., and Jeanloz, R. W. (1983). Purification and characterization of potato lectin. *Journal of Biological Chemistry*, 258, 2886-2891.

Matsumura, K., Higashida, K., Ishida, H., Hata, Y., Yamamoto, K., Shigeta, M., Mizuno-Horikawa, Y., Wang, X.C., Miyoshi, E., Gu, J.G., and Taniguchi, N. (2007). Carbohydrate binding specificity of a fucose-specific lectin from *aspergillus oryzae* - A novel probe for core fucose. *Journal of Biological Chemistry*, 282, 15700-15708.

Mc Cubbin, W.D., and Kay, C.M. (1971). Molecular weight studies on Concanavalin A. Biochemical and Biophysical Research Communications, 44, 101-109.

Mercy, P.D., and Ravindranath, M.H. (1992). An agglutinin with unique specificity for *N*-glycolyl sialic acid residues of thyroglobulin in the hemolymph of a marine crab, *Scylla serrata* (Forskal). *Experientia*, 48, 498-500.

Mialonier, G., Privat, J.P., Monsigny, M., Kahlen, G. and Durand, R. (1973). Isolement, proprietes physico-chimiques et localisation in vivo d'une phytohemagglutine (lectine) de *Phaseolus vulgaris* L. (var. rouge). *Physiologie Vegetale*, 2, 519-537.

Miller, J.B., Noyes, C., Heinrikson, R., Kingdon, H.S., and Yachnin, S. (1973). Phytohemagglutinin mitogenic proteins. Structural evidence for a family of isomitogenic proteins. *Journal of Experimental Medicine*, 138, 939-951.

Mirelman, D., Galun, E., Sharon, N., and Lotan, R. (1975). Inhibition of fungal growth by wheat germ agglutinin. *Nature*, 256, 414-416.

Mishkind, M.L, Palevitz, B.A., and Raikhel, N.V. (1983). Localization of wheat germ agglutinin-like lectins in various species of the Gramineae. *Science*, 220, 1290-1292.

Mohan, S., Dorai, D.T., Srimal, S., and Bachhawat, B.K. (1982). Binding studies of a sialic acid-specific lectin from the horseshoe crab *Carcinoscorpius rotunda caudata* with various sialoglycoproteins. *Biochemical Journal*, 203, 253-261.

Molano, J., Bowers, B., and Cabib, E. (1980). Distribution of chitin in the yeast cell wall. An ultrastructural and chemical study. *The Journal of Cell Biology*, 85, 199-212.

Montfort, W., Villafranca, J.E., Monzingo, A.F., Ernst, S.R., Katzin, B., Rutenber, E., Xuong, N.H., Hamlin, R., and Robertus, J.D. (1987). The three-dimensional structure of ricin at 2.8 Å. *Journal of Biological Chemistry*, 262, 5398-5403.

Moreno, F.B.M.B., De Oliveira, T.M., Martil, D.E., Vicoti, M.M., Bezerra, G.A., Abrego, J.R.B., Cavada, B.S., and De Azevedo, W.F. (2008). Identification of a new quaternary association for legume lectins. *Journal of Structural Biology*, 161, 133-143.

Moreira, R.A., Ainouz, I.L., Oliveira, J.T.A., and Cavada, B.S. (1991). Plant lectins, chemical and biological aspects. *Memórias do Instituto Oswaldo Cruz*, 86 supplement 11, 211-218.

Nagahora, H., Ishikawa, K., Niwa, Y., Muraki, M., and Jigami, Y. (1992). Expression and secretion of wheat germ agglutinin by *Saccharomyces cerevisiae*. *European Journal of Biochemistry*, 210, 989-997.

Nagata, Y., and Burger, M. (1974). Molecular characteristics and specificity for sugar binding. *Journal of Biological Chemistry*, 249, 3116-3122.

Nicolson, G.L. (1974). The interactions of lectins with animal cell surfaces. *International Review of Cytology*, 39, 89-190.

Ohtani, K., and Misaki, A. (1980). The structure of the glycan moiety of tora-bean (*Phaseolus vulgaris*) lectin. *Carbohydrate Research*, 87, 275-285.

Olsnes, S. (2004). The history of ricin, abrin and related toxins. *Toxicon*, 44: 361-370.

Pusztai, A., Greer, F., and Grant, G. (1989). Specific uptake of dietary lectins into the systemic circulation of rats. *Biochemical Society transactions*, 17, 481-482.

Percin, I., Yavuz, H., Aksoz, E., and Denizli, A. (2009). *N*-Acetyl-D-galactosamine-Specific Lectin Isolation from Soyflour with Poly(HPMA-GMA) Beads. *Journal of Applied Polymer Science*, 111, 148-154.

Perez-Campos, E., Lascurain, R., Sierra, C., Espinosa, B., Debray, H., Bouquelet, S., and Zenteno, E. (1997). Erythroagglutinin from *Phaseolus coccineus* Var. Alubia: Chemical characterization, sugar specificity, and effect on blood coagulation factors. *Journal of Agricultural and Food Chemistry*, 45, 3747-3752.

Petnual, P., Sangvanich, P., and Karnchanatat, A. (2010). A lectin from the rhizomes of turmeric (*Curcuma longa* L.) and its antifungal, antibacterial and alpha-glucosidase inhibitory activities. *Food Science and Biotechnology*, 19, 907-916.

Petryniak, J., Pereira, M.E., and Kabat, E.A. (1977). The lectin of *Euonymus europeus*: purification, characterization, and an immunochemical study of its combining site. *Archives of Biochemistry and Biophysics*, 178, 118-134.

Peumans, W.J., de Ley, M., Stinissen, H.M., and Broekaert, W.F. (1985). Isolation and partial characterization of a new lectin from seeds of the greater celandine (*Chelidonium majus*). *Plant Physiology*, 78, 379-383.

Peumans, W.J., Stinissen, H.M., and Carlier, A.R. (1982a). Subunit exchange between lectins from different cereal species. *Planta*, 154, 568-572.

Peumans, W.J, Stinissen, H.M., and Carlier, A.R. (1982b). Isolation and partial characterization of WGA-like lectins from rye (*Secale cereale*) and barley (*Hordeum vulgare*) embryos. *Biochemical Journal*, 203, 239-243.

Pueppke, S.G., Bauer, W.D., Keegstra, K., and Ferguson, A.L. (1978). Role of lectins in plant-microorganism interactions II. Distribution of soybean lectin in tissues of *Glycine max* Merr. *Plant Physiology*, 61, 779-784.

Peumans, W.J., and Van Damme, E.J.M. (1995). Lectins as plant defense proteins. *Plant Physiology*, 109, 347-352.

Ratanapo, S., Ngamjunyaporn, W., and Chulavatnatol, M. (1998). Sialic acid binding lectins from leaf of mulberry (*Morus alba*). *Plant Science*, 139, 141-148.

Raemaekers, R.J., De Muro, L., Gatehouse, J.A., and Fordham-Skelton, A.P. (1999). Functional phytohemagglutinin (PHA) and *Galanthus nivalis* agglutinin (GNA) expressed in *Pichia pastoris*: correct N-terminal processing and secretion of heterologous proteins expressed using the PHA-E signal peptide. *European Journal of Biochemistry*, 265, 394-403.

Raikhel, N.V., Lee, H.I., and Broekaer, W.F. (1993). Structure and function of chitin-binding proteins. *Annual Review of Plant Physiology and Plant Molecular Biology*, 44, 591-615.

Rasanen, V., Weber, T.H., and Grasbeck, R. (1973). Crystalline kidney-bean leucoagglutinin, European Journal of Biochemistry, 38: 193-200.

Reda, H.S., and Abd-El-Raheem, R., and El-Shanshoury. (1992). Antimicrobial activity of legume seed proteins. *Botany Bulletin of Academia Sinica*, 33, 185-190.

Reeder, N.J., and Ekstedt, D.R. (1971). Study of the interaction of Concanavalin A with staphylococcal teichoic acids. *Journal of Immunology*, 106, 334-340.

Reeke, G.Jr., and Becker, J. (1986). Three-dimensional structure of favin: saccharide binding-cyclic permutation in leguminous lectins. *Science*, 234, 1108-1111.

Renkonen, K.O. (1948). Studies on hemagglutinins present in seeds of some representatives of leguminoseae. *Annales Medicinae Experimentalis et Biologiae Fenniae*, 26, 66-72.

Rice, R.H., and Etzler, M.E. (1974). Subunit structure of wheat germ agglutinin. *Biochemical and Biophysical Research Communications*, 59, 414-419.

Rodriguez-Pineiro, A.M., Ayude, D., Rodriguez-Berrocal, F.J., and Paez, de la Cadena, M. (2004). Concanavalin A chromatography coupled to two-dimensional gel electrophoresis improves protein expression studies of the serum proteome. *Journal of Chromatography B*, 803, 337-343.

Rudiger, H. (1993). Purification of Plant Lectins. In: *Lectins and Glycobiology*, Gabius, H.J. and Gabius, S. (eds.), pp. 31-46. Springer, Berlin.

Sauerborn, M.K., Wright, L.M., Reynolds, C.D., Grossmann, J., and Rizkallah, P.J. (1999). Insights into carbohydrate recognition by *Narcissus pseudonarcissus* lectin: The crystal structure at 2 Å resolution in complex with α-1, 3 mannobiose. *Journal of Molecular Biology*, 290, 185-199.

Schalla, W.D., Whittington, L.W., Rice, J.R., and Larson, A.S. (1986). Epidemiological characterization of *Neisseria gonorrhoeae* by lectins. *Journal of Clinical Microbiology,* 22, 379-382.

Selitrennikoff, C.P. (2001). Antifungal proteins. Applied and Environmental Microbiology, 67, 2883-2894.

Sharma, V., and Surolia, A. (1994). Cloning by genomic PCR and production of peanut agglutinin in *Escherichia coli.*, Gene, 148, 299-304.

Sharon, N. (1993). Lectin-carbohydrate complexes of plants and animals: an atomic view. *Trends in Biochemical Sciences,* 18, 221-226.

Sharon, N., and Lis, N. (2001). The structural basis for carbohydrate recognition by lectins. *Advances in Experimental Medicine and Biology,* 491, 1-16.

Shi, J., Xue, S.J., Kakuda, Y., Ilic, S., and Kim, D. (2007). Isolation and characterization of lectins from kidney beans (*Phaseolus vulgaris*). *Process Biochemistry,* 42, 1436-1442.

Shoham, M., Kalb, A.J., and Pecht, I. (1973). Specificity of metal ion interaction with Concanavalin A. *Biochemistry,* 12: 1914-1917.

Singh, R.S., Tiwary, A.K., and Kennedy, J.F. (1999). Lectins: sources, activities and applications. Critical Reviews in Biotechnology, 19, 145-178.

Sitohy, M., Doheim, M., and Badr, H. (2007). Isolation and characterization of a lectin with antifungal activity from Egyptian *Pisum sativum* seeds. *Food Chemistry,* 104, 971-979.

Slifkin, M., and Gil, G.M. (1984). Identification of group C streptococcal antigen extracts with lectin-bound polystyrene particals. *Journal of Clinical Microbiology,* 19, 83-84.

Sphyris, N., Lord, J.M., Wales, R., and Roberts, L.M. (1995). Mutational analysis of ricinus lectin B-chains. *Journal of Biological Chemistry,* 270, 20292-20297.

Stirpe, F. (2004). Ribosome-inactivating proteins. *Toxicon,* 44, 371-383.

Streicher, H., and Sharon, N. (2003). Recombinant plant lectins and their mutants. *Methods in Enzymology,* 363, 47-77.

Stubbs, M.E., Carver, J.P., and Dunn, R.J. (1986). Production of pea lectin in *Escherichia coli. Journal of Biological Chemistry,* 261, 6141-6144.

Sugii, S., and Kabat, E.A. (1982) Further immunochemical studies on the combining sites of *Lotus tetragonolobus* and *Ulex europaeus* I and II lectins. *Carbohydrate Research,* 99, 99-101.

Summer, J.B. and Howell, S.F. (1936). The identification of the hemagglutinin of the Jack bean with Concanavalin A. *Journal of Bacteriology,* 32, 227-237.

Sweet, R.M., Wright, H.T., Janin, J., and Chothia, C. (1974). Crystal structure of the complex of porcine trypsin with soybean trypsin inhibitor (Kunitz) at 2.6- Å resolution. *Biochemistry,* 13, 4212-4228.

Tchernychev, B., and Wilchek, M. 1996. Natural human antibodies to dietary lectins. *FEBS Letters,* 397, 139-142.

Tian, Q., Wang, W., Miao, C., Peng, H., Liu, B., Leng, F. (2008). Purification, characterization and molecular cloning of a novel mannose-binding lectin from rhizomes of *Ophiopogon japonicus* with antiviral and antifungal activities. *Plant Science,* 175, 877-884.

Terras, F.R.G., Eggermont, K., Kovaleva, V., Raikhel, N.V., Osborn, R.W., Kester, A., Rees, S.B., Torrekens, S., Van Leuven, F., Vanderleyden, J., Cammue, B.P.A., Broekaert, W.F. (1995). Small cysteine-rich antifungal proteins from radish: their role in host defense. *Plant Cell,* 7, 573-588.

Tipthara, P., Sangvanich, P., Macth, M., and Petsom, A. (2007). Mannose-binding lectin from *Curcuma zedoaria* Rosc. *Journal of Plant Biology*, 50, 163-173.

Thipthara, P., Petsom, A., Roengsumran, S., and Sangvanish, P. (2008). Hemagglutinating activity and corresponding putative sequence identity from *Curcuma aromatica* rhizome. *Journal of the Science of Food and Agriculture*, 88, 1025-1034.

Thomasson, D.L., and Doyle, R.J. (1975). Monovalent Concanavalin A. Biochemical and Biophysical Research Communications, 67, 1545-1552.

Tkacz, J.S. and Lampson, O.J. (1972). Wall replication in Saccharomyces species: use of fluorescein-conjugated Concanavalin A to reveal the site of mannan insertion. *Journal of General Microbiology*, 72, 243-247.

Tracz, J.S., Cybolska, B.E., and Lampson, O.J. (1971). Specific staining of wall mannan in yeast cells with fluorescein-conjugated Concanavalin A. *Journal of Bacteriology*, 105, 1-5.

Tropchin, G., Poulian, D., Herbaut, J., and Biguet, J. (1981). Cytochemical and ultrastructural studies of Candida albicans.II. Evidence for a cell wall coat using Concanavalin A. *Journal of Ultrastructure Research*, 75, 50-59.

Tsivion, Y. and Sharon, N. (1981). Lipid mediated hemagglutination and its relevance to lectin-mediated agglutination. *Biochimica et Biophysica Acta*, 642, 336-344.

Van Damme, E.J., Barre, A., Mazard, A.M., Verhaert, P., Horman, A., Debray, H., Rouge, P., Peumans, W.J. (1999). Characterization and molecular cloning of the lectin from *Helianthus tuberosus*. *European Journal of Biochemistry*, 259, 135-142.

Van Damme, E.J., Barre, A., Rouge, P., Van Leuven, F., and Peumans, W.J. (1995). The seed lectins of black locust (*Robinia pseudoacacia*) are encoded by two genes which differ from the bark lectin genes. *Plant Molecular Biology* 29, 1197-1210.

Van Damme, E.J.M., and Peumans, W.J. (1990) Developmental changes and tissue distribution of lectin in *Galanthus nivalis* L. and *Narcissus* cv. Carlton. *Planta*, 182, 605-609.

Van Damme, E.J.M., Peumans, W.J., Barre A., and Rougé, P. (1998). Plant lectins: A composite of several distinct families of structurally and evolutionary related proteins with diverse biological roles. *Critical Reviews in Plant Sciences*, 17, 645-662.

Van Damme, E.J.M., Peumans, W.J., Pusztai, A., and Bardocz, S. (1997). *Handbook of Plant Lectins: Properties and Biomedical Applications*. Chichester, John Wiley & Sons.

Van Damme, E.G., Smeets, K., Torrekens, S., Van Leuven, F., and Peumans, W.J. (1994). Characterization and molecular cloning of mannose-binding lectins of the *Orchidaceae* species *Listera ovate, Epipactis belleborine* and *Cymbidium hybrid. European Journal of Biochemistry*, 93, 769-777.

Van Eijsden, R.R. (1995). Sugar-binding activity of pea (*Pisum sativum*) lectin is essential for heterologous infection of transgenic white clover hairy roots by *Rhizobium leguminosarum* biovar viciae. *Plant Molecular Biology*, 29, 431-439

Van Eijsden, R.R., Hodmaker, F.J., Diaz, C.L., Lugtenberg, B.J.J., De Pater, S., and Kijne, J.W. (1992). Mutational analysis of pea lectin. Substitution of Asn135 for Asp in the monosaccharide-binding site eliminates mannose/glucose binding activity. *Plant molecular biology*, 20, 1049-1058.

Wang, Q., Lu-Gang, Y., Campbell, B.J., Milton, J.D., and Rhodes, J.M. (1999). Identification of intact peanut lectin in peripheral venous blood. *Lancet*, 352, 1831-1832.

Wang, J.L., Cunningham, B.A., and Edelman, G.M. (1971). Unusual fragments in the subunit structure of Concanavalin A. Proceedings of the National Academy of Sciences of the United States of America, 68, 1130-1134.

Wang, H., and Ng, T.B. (2005). An antifungal protein from ginger rhizomes. *Biochemical and Biophysical Research Communications*, 336, 100-104.

Watkins, W.M. and Morgan, W.T.J. (1952). Neutralization of anti-H agglutinin in eel by simple sugar. *Nature*, 169, 825-826.

Weber, E., and Neumann, D. (1980). Protein bodies, storage organelles in plant seeds. Biochemie und Physiologie der Pflanzen, 175, 279-306.

Weis, W.I., and Drickamer, K. (1996). Structural basis of the lectin-carbohydrate recognition. *Annual Review of Biochemistry*, 65, 441-473.

Westbrook, C.A., Gasson, J.C., Gerber, S.E., Selsted, M.E., and Golde, D.W. (1984). Purification and characterization of human T-lymphocyte-derived erythroid-potentiating activity. *Journal of Biological Chemistry*, 259, 9992-9996.

Winter, H.C., Mostafapour, K., and Goldstein, I.J. (2002). The Mushroom Marasmius oreades lectin is a blood group type B agglutinin that recognizes the Gal 1,3 Gal and Gal 1,3 Gal 1,4 GlcNAc porcine xenotransplantation epitopes with high affinity, *Journal of Biological Chemistry*, 277, 14996-15001.

Wong, J.H., Chan, H.Y., and Ng, T.B. (2008). A Mannose/glucose-specific lectin from chinese evergreen chinkapin (*Castanopsis chinensis*). *Biochimica et Biophysica Acta*, 1780, 1017-1022.

Wood, S.D., Wright, L.M., Reynolds, C.D., Rizkallah, P.J., Allen, A.K., Peumans, W.J., and Van Damme, E.J. (1999). Structure of the native (unligated) mannose-specific bulb lectin from *Scilla campanulata* (bluebell) at 1.7 Å resolution. *Acta Crystallographica Section D-Biological Crystallography*, 55, 1264-1272.

Wright, C.S., Gavilanes, F. and Peterson, D.L. (1984). Primary structure of wheat germ agglutinin isolectin 2. Peptide order deduced from X-ray structure. *Biochemistry*, 23, 280-287.

Wright, C.S., and Hester, G. (1996). The 2.0 Å structure of a cross-linked complex between snowdrop lectin and a branched mannopentose: evidence for two unique binding modes. *Structure*, 4, 1339-1352.

Wu, A.M., Wu, J.H., Tsai, M.S., Kaltner, H., and Gabius, H.J. (2001). Carbohydrate specificity of a galectin from chicken liver (CG-16). *Biochemical Journal*, 358, 529-538.

Yan, Q., Jiang, Z., Yang, S., Deng, W. and Han, L. (2005). A novel homodimeric lectin from *Astragalus mongholicus* with antifungal activity. *Archives of Biochemistry and Biophysics*, 442, 72-81.

Ye, X.Y., Ng, T.B., Tsang, P.W., and Wang, J. (2001). Isolation of a homodimeric lectin with antifungal and antiviral activities from red kidney bean (*Phaseolus vulgaris*) seeds. *Journal of Protein Chemistry*, 20, 367-375.

Ye, X.Y., Ng, T.B., Rao, P.F. (2002). Cicerin and arietin, novel chickpea peptides with different antifungal potencies. *Peptides*, 23, 817-822.

Young, N.M., and Oomen, R.P. (1992). Analysis of sequence variation among legume lectins. A ring of hypervariable residues forms the perimeter of the carbohydrate binding site. *Journal of Molecular Biology*, 228, 924-934.

Zhang, D., and Halaweish, F.T. (2003). Isolation and identification of foetidissimin: a novel ribosome-inactivating protein from *Cucurbita foetidissima*. *Plant Science*, 164: 387-393.

Zhu, K., Bressan, R.A., Hasegawa, P.M., and Murdock, L.L. (1996). Identification of Nacetylglucosamine binding residues in *Griffonia simplicifolia* lectin II. *FEBS Letters*, 390, 271-274.

9

Mechanisms Determining Bacterial Biofilm Resistance to Antimicrobial Factors

Kamila Myszka and Katarzyna Czaczyk
Poznań University of Life Sciences
Poland

1. Introduction

In most natural environments, the process of bacterial surface association is prevailing cells lifestyle. The tendency of bacteria to colonize solid materials is advantageous from an ecological standpoint. This mechanism allows bacteria the colonization of a nutritionally favorable new niche and encouraging symbiotic relationships between the cells. Sessile mode of growth provides also some level of protection from external stresses (Costerton et al., 1995; Dunne, 2002; Russell, 2002). Anchored bacteria are being linked to common human diseases ranging from tooth decay and paradontose to nosocomial infections and both biliary tract and kidney infections (Costerton et al., 1999; Potera, 1999). According to Russell (1999) and Wood et al. (2011) 80% of bacterial chronic inflammatory and infectious human diseases involve biofilm. In industrial environments surface-bound bacteria are the potential source of contamination of processed material that in consequence may lead to spoilage or transmission of pathogens (Bower et al., 1996; Gunduz & Tuncel, 2006; Myszka & Czaczyk, 2011).

Attached bacteria to organic or inorganic surfaces form thin layer called biofilm or biological layer. Biofilms consist of a single microbial species or multiple microbial species (O'Toole et al., 2000). However mixed-species biological layers predominate in most environments, single-species biofilms occur in a variety of infections and on the abiotic surface exploited in medicine and industry practice (Adal & Farr, 1996; Donlan, 2002). Despite of difference of ecosystems in which biofilms can develop, in each case the component microbial cells reach homeostasis and are optimally organized to convert all available nutrients to usefulness products for cells (O'Toole et al., 2000; Sutherland, 2001; Myszka & Czaczyk, 2009).

Biofilm-associated bacteria perform chemically diverse biocide-resistance phenotype (Mah & O'Toole, 2001; White & McDermott, 2001). It has been estimated that biofilms can tolerate antimicrobial agents (disinfectants, antibiotics, surphactants) at concentrations of 10-1000-times that needed to inactivate genetically equivalent planktonic bacteria (Jefferson, 2004). It is worth point out that almost all clinically and industrially approved antimicrobial agents are being less active against sessile bacteria. So far selection of antimicrobial agents for industry and medical properties based on their activity against planktonic bacteria (estimation the indexes of the minimal inhibitory concentration (MIC) and the minimal bactericidal concentration (MBC) for different antimicrobial agents).

The problem of high resistance of biofilm to antimicrobials has not been dissolved yet. In the United States annual cost of eradication of biofilms in hospital conditions exceeded $ 1 billion per year (Costerton et al., 1995; Archibald & Gaynes, 1997; Potera, 1999). Recent study demonstrated that biofilm resistance has a multifactorial character (Izano et al., 2009; Simões et al., 2009). Analysis of all described data can enable control of detrimental biofilms.

2. Structure of biofilm

Tolker-Nielsen & Molin (2000) stated that biofilms communities in natural environments have unique architecture although some structural features can be considered universal. Application of scanning confocal laser microscopy performed that biofilms formed on solid surfaces and exposed to a continuous flow of nutrients, are highly hydrated layers composed of microcolonies embedded in an organic polymer matrix of microbial origins (Lawrence et al., 1991; Gilbert et al. 2002a; Czaczyk & Myszka, 2007). Microcolonies are separated by water channels that allow the fluids to flow throughout the biofilm, making the distribution of nutrients and oxygen easer (Lindsay & von Holy, 2006; Shafahi & Vafai, 2009). Moreover, the water channels between the microcolonies provide a means of removing metabolic end products (Davey et al., 2003; Lindsay & von Holy, 2006). This system of nutrients and metabolic end products distribution functions only in periphery regions of biofilms. The cells within biofilms are more tightly packed and have worse access to nutrients and oxygens. Differences in nutrients and oxygen availability within the biofilm structure affect in differences in metabolic activity among the cells. In addition, the cells within biofilms secrete signal molecules that control formation of microcolonies of complicated architecture and diverse function (Parsek & Greenberg, 2005). Structural heterogeneity of biofilm provides an effective barrier that limit penetration of antimicrobial agents throughout the biological layer (Nobile & Mitchell, 2007; Roeder et al., 2010). Kinetic diffusion of antimicrobial compound of relative molecular weight of 100kDa through mature biofilm might be reduced to 60-80% as compared with its action against planktonic cells (DeBeer et al., 1994; Stewart, 1996). Moreover, suspended cells are directly exposure to toxic compounds. Biofilm-associated bacteria are much less permeable to the biocides. DeBeer et al. (1994) observed this phenomenon investigating the rate of penetration of chlorine into *Pseudomonas aeruginosa/Klebsiella pneumoniae* biofilm matrix. Also Suci et al. (1994) noticed transport limitation of ciprofloxacin through *Pseudomonas aeruginosa* biofilm. In this study, during the 21-min exposure, the presence of the antibiotic in periphery region of tested biofilm reached only 20% of ciprofloxacin concentration in the bulk medium (Suci et al., 1994). Gilbert et al. (1989) used perfused biofilm fermentors, in combine with continuous culture and observed that much of resistance of Gram-positive and Gram-negative biofilms was associated with the presence of nutrient-starved microocolonies.

Darouiche et al. (1994) noticed that although the presence of vancomycin in a *Staphylococcus epidermidis* biofilm exceeded bactericidal concentration, it was not sufficient to kill surface-bound bacteria. These authors support the notion that vancomycin resistance of *Staphylococcus epidermidis* biofilm, was not due to limited diffusion of the compound through biological layer, but rather to a reduction in the antimicrobial effect of the drug (Darouiche et al., 1994). Anderl et al. (2000) observed similar effect during investigation of rate of penetration of ampicillin and ciprofloxacin through *Klebsiella pneumoniae* biofilm. In this work, the inability of transport of ampicillin through biofilm was affected by the production of the drug degrading enzyme β-lactamase. Ampicillin was able to penetrate biological layer formed by a β-lactamase-deficient mutant without difficulty. In contrast, ciprofloxacin diffused through *Klebsiella pneumoniae* biofilm without delay. Differences in the effect of penetration of both ciprofloxacin and ampicillin through *Klebsiella pneumoniae* wild-type and β-lactamase-deficient mutant biofilms, suggesting that biofilm resistance is multifactorial (Anderl et al., 2000).

3. Glycocalyx

Costerton et al. (1978) termed glycocalyx as the integral part of the biofilms of Gram-positive and Gram-negative bacteria. Glycocalyx known as either as slime or capsule may provide the forces responsible for cohesion and adhesion to the solid surfaces (Flemming, 1995; Mayer et al., 1999). This is performed by the weak interaction such as electrostatic interactions, hydrogen bonds and van der Waals forces (Flemming, 1995; Dunne, 2002). During biofilm maturation process, slime cementing and immobilizing the cells (Sutherland, 2001). Glycocalyx in biofilm structure varies in its thickness from 0.2 to 1.0μm (Flemming et al., 1992; Flemming & Wingender, 2001; Branda et al., 2005). Its composition is remarkably flexible and is control by the nature of the biofilm growth environment (Brown & Williams, 1985; Costerton, 1988; Anwar et al., 1990). The fibrous polysaccharides and globular glycoproteins components of the capsule are influenced by the condition applied upon cultivation. Brown & Williams (1985) and Costerton (1988) demonstrated that for the bacterial biofilm it is pivotal importance to maintain plasticity in the composition of its envelope to respond to changes in the growth environment. Such mechanisms enable the pathogenic bacteria surviving an extremely hostile environment when they enter the host (Anwar et al., 1990).

Recent reports suggest that slimes are responsible for the microbial biofilm resistance (Drenkard, 2003; Leid et al., 2005). Glycocalyx may cause alterations in the gaining access of antibacterial molecules to its targets located inside the cells (Anwar et al., 1990; Beech et al., 2005). According to Lewis (2001) glycocalyx matrix provides effective resistance for biofilm bacteria against large molecules such as antimicrobial proteins and their components. This physiological barrier is also effective against smaller peptides-defensins and their analogs (Lewis, 2001). Studies from a number of laboratories have concluded that the glycocalyx acting as a barrier, trapping antibacterial molecules from external environment and isolating the enclose cells from fluctuations in the surrounding environments (Gilbert et al., 1990; Flemming, 1995). The slime changes the charge and the free energy on bacterial surfaces, thereby limiting biocides transport (Hogt et al., 1986). Molecules binding capacity based on estimated number of available carboxyl and hydroxyl groups. The diffusion barrier's role of glycocalyx may also vary according to its soluble state (Siegrist & Gujer, 1985; Hoyle et al., 1992). Glycocalyx have been shown to accumulate antibacterial molecules up to 25% of their weight (Jang et al., 1990; Drenkard, 2003). Extracellular alginate, a slime produced by *Pseudomonas aeruginosa* has been studied for its ability to trap antimicrobial agents. This ability appears to be related to anionic nature of the exopolymer. Cationic substances can thus be retained within the matrix and prevented from acting upon the biofilm bacteria. Alginate has also been shown to bind positively-charged biocides and inhibit their activity (Suci et al., 1994). Also Hentzer et al. (2001) observed that alginate overproduction affects *Pseudomonas aeruginosa* biofilms resistance to antibiotic tobramycin treatment. On the other hand, Dunne et al. (1993) and Yasuda et al. (1994) noticed that rifampicin, vancomycin, cefotiam and ofloxacin penetrated *Staphylococcus epidermidis* biofilms that formed on the dialysis membrane upon long-term exposure to antibiotics. These results support the notion that limitation of diffusion by glycocalyx matrix cannot always define resistance to antibacterial compounds. Transport limitations of biocides by glycocalyx depends on the present of the adsorption sites in the matrix (Carlson & Silverstein, 1998). After long-term exposure to antibiotics, saturating all possible binding sites in the glycocalyx matrix by the drugs enabled delivering and killing *Staphylococcus epidermidis* and *Staphylococcus aureus* biofilm (Dunne et al., 1993; Boles & Horswill, 2011).

In addition, adsorption sites within glycocalyx may also serve to anchor exoenzymes from external environments. Such immobilized enzymes are capable to impede the penetration and action of susceptible drugs (Hoyle et al., 1990). Giwercman et al. (1991) found that β-lactamases may accumulate in the glycocalyx of *Pseudomonas aeruginosa* giving the whole biofilm population the potential for decreased β-lactam susceptibility. In addition, in mixed-species biological layers, the synthesis of neutralizing enzymes by one member of the community may confer protection for whole tested sessile populations (Stewart et al., 2000). Exoenzymes trapped within the biofilm matrix, may not only protect the sessile population from the antimicrobial activity of particular agents but also serve as a source of substrates scavaging the metabolites of biocides degradation and elimination (Morton et al., 1998).

Another form of biocides quenching by glycocalyx matrix has been demonstrated by Characklis (1989). The author found that chlorine react with extracellular polysaccharides in the mature biofilms and that this results in disruption of the structure of biological layer. The effect of this process may cause problems especially in industry practice by release of biofilm fragments of pathogenic microorganisms into water phase (Characklis, 1989). On the other hand, under particular circumstances, released biofilm fragments are more sensitive to biocides treatment. Gaylarde and Videla (1994) reported that eradication of biofilm from The North Sea pipelines by biocides caused initially increasing of the sulphate reducing bacterial count in the liquid from $2x10^2$CFU/ml to $3.1x10^3$CFU/ml. Interestingly, 2 hours later, the amount of the sulphate reducing bacterial amount fell to the value of $5{,}0x10^1$CFU/ml. The study of Gaylarde and Videla (1994) indicated that liberated sessile bacteria are susceptible to antimicrobials agents.

4. Metabolic and growth rate heterogeneity

Differences in nutrients and oxygen availability within biofilm affect in differences in growth rate and metabolic activity of bacteria. Wentland et al. (1996) and Xu et al. (1998) used fluorescent probes and reporter genes to visualized patterns of bacterial growth and cells metabolic activities in biofilm. Different concentrations of the key metabolic substrates and products within biofilm proved that surface-bound communities contain cells at all phases of bacterial growth and cells at the different activity levels (Stewart, 2002). This leads to microbial population heterogeneity. The problem occurs both in single-species and mixed-species bacterial biofilms (Xu et al., 2000). Better access to nutrients and oxygen in the periphery region of biofilm promotes metabolic activity of cells. In this part of biological layer the bacteria are able to proliferate. In contrast, in the deeper part of biofilm the metabolic potential of bacteria is limited by the worse diffusion process of nutrients (Senior, 2004). Chapman et al. (1993), Wentland et al. (1996) and Xu et al. (1998) identified slow-growing or stationary-phase cells inside biofilm matrix. It was characterized by the decreased level of RNA (tRNA and rRNA) synthesis and accumulation of a guanine nucleotide-guanosine 3',5'-bis-pyro-phosphate (ppGpp). The authors demonstrated these effects in *in vitro* experiments by changing a conditions of biofilm maturation process from a nutrient-rich to a minimal ones (Chapman et al., 1993; Wentland et al., 1996; Xu et al. 1998).

Similar information concerning the metabolic and growth rate heterogeneity of cells within biofilms has come from studies of cellular enzyme synthesis (Poulsen et al., 1993; Wimpenny et al., 2000). Mitchison (1969) performed that level of enzyme synthesis is influenced by a series of sequenced changes in the particular stage of the bacteria growth cycle. For instant in periphery sphere of bacterial communities where cells are able to proliferate, part of the cellular enzymes are continuously active, and part of them only double at specific point to allow equality in the daughter cells (Mitchison, 1969). Mitchison (1969) also demonstrated that during division stage cellular enzymes may be proportional to cell mass. In slow-growing or stationary-phase bacteria, cellular enzymes synthesis is arrested (Sternberg et al., 1999).

Because most of biocides killing metabolically active bacteria, it has been proposed that bacteria at the dormant growth phase in the deeper region of biofilm are less susceptible to antimicrobial agents (Evans, et al., 1989; Toumanen, et al., 1989; Lewis, 2001; Stewart, 2002; Gilbert et al., 2002b; Bulter et al., 2010). These effects were observed in amino acid-starved communities where the cells were able to produce ppGpp (Pissbaro et al., 1990). Evans et al. (1989), Toumanen et al. (1989) and Duguid et al. (1992) investigated growth-rate-related effects upon laboratory conditions for biofilms of *Pseudomonas aeruginosa, Escherichia coli* and *Staphyloccocus epidermidis*. The authors stated that the sensitivities of biofilms cells to penicillin, tobramycin and ciprofloxacin increased with the increasing growth rate of examined bacteria. These results suggest that the dormant phase of bacteria biofilm protects the cells from antimicrobial action of antibiotics (Evans et al., 1989; Toumanen et al., 1989; Duguid et al., 1992). The slow growth rate plays also an important role in mediating resistance of *Pseudomonas aeruginosa* biofilm to β-lactams (Tanaka et al., 1999; Alvarez-Ortega et al., 2010). According to Betzner et al. (1990) *Escherichia coli* at the dormant growth phase, activates the RelA-dependent synthesis of ppGpp that limits anabolic processes in cells. The presence of ppGpp suppressed the activity of a major *Escherichia coli* autolysin, SLT that makes the bacteria in non-growing zones of biofilm more tolerant to antibiotic treatment (Betzner et al., 1990). In addition, a mutation in *relA*, a gene coding ppGpp synthase, did not effect the growth rate. The population of *relA* mutants was more sensitive to killing by antibiotics. Rodionov and Ishiguro (1995) stated that ppGpp inhibits peptidoglycans production, that would explain the reduced levels of activity of the bacteria cell wall inhibitors. From a practical standpoint, it would be interesting to examine whether *relA* mutants become also eliminating by other antimicrobial agents that do not target the cell wall.

In contrast, the Tanaka et al. (1999) researchers also demonstrated that growth rate heterogeneity in *Pseudomonas aeruginosa* biofilm did not limited bactericidal action of fluoroquinolones (Tanaka et al., 1999). In addition, Brooun et al. (2000) observed that *Pseudomonas aeruginosa* in non-growing zones of biofilms are resistant only to part of commercially available antibiotics. For instant, slow growth rate increased resistance of *Pseudomonas aeruginosa* to tetracycline, but did not influence on the resistance of examined bacteria to tobramycin. In this experiment the susceptibility of majority of *Pseudomonas aeruginosa* cells within biofilms were not much different from what is stated for planktonic bacteria. The greater parts of *Pseudomonas aeruginosa* biofilm were killed by clinically achievable range of antibiotics concentrations (about 5μg/mg) (Brooun et al., 2000). Brooun et al. (2000) also reported that after biofilm maturation, further increase in the antibiotic concentration had no effect on killing of *Pseudomonas aeruginosa* biofilm. The results of Tanaka et al. (1999) and Brooun et al. (2000) reinforced the idea that under the particular circumstances metabolic and growth rate heterogeneity may only contribute to increasing tolerant of bacterial biofilms to antimicrobials agents. Brooun et al. (2000) also stated that only a small fractions of bacteria are responsible for the very high level of resistance of *Pseudomonas aeruginosa* biofilms. According to Lewis (2000) the greater number of bacteria in biofilms are usually not more resistance to killing than free-floating cells and die more rapidly after treatment with a lethal dose of antibiotics. Under particular circumstances bacteria in non-growing zones of biofilms are preserved by the presence of biocides that only inhibits their growth (Lewis, 2000; Singh et al., 2006).

In biofilms metabolic activities of bacteria are controlled by oxygen availability. Biofilms of *Pseudomonas aeruginosa* grow in a gaseous environment of pure oxygen were killed by ciprofloxacin and tobramycin antibiotics (Walters et al., 2003). In contrast, Tresse et al. (1995) reported that reduction of oxygen availability enhanced of antibiotic resistance of agar-entrapped *Escherichia coli*. Also Hill et al. (2005) observed that anaerobically biofilm-grown isolates of *Pseudomonas aeruginosa* were significantly less susceptible for meropenem, tobramycin and ciprofloxacin treatments. According to Yoon et al. (2002) under strict anaerobic conditions, bacteria form robust biofilm, and that specific gene products were essential to develop such anaerobic biofilms. Metabolic and phenotypic changes under anaerobic conditions lead to increased levels of biocide resistance of bacterial biofilms. Sauer et al. (2002) based on analysis of protein patterns of *Pseudomonas aeruginosa* mature biofilm, demonstrated that a large part of biological layer is exposure to oxygen limitation.

5. Persister phenomena

Bacterial biofilms include persisters, cells that neither grow nor die during exposure to bactericidal agents, thus exhibit multidrug tolerance (MDT) (Lewis, 2005; Cheng & Hardwick, 2007; Lewis, 2008). While measuring a dose-response of a *Pseudomonas aeruginosa* biofilm to ofloxacin, Brooun et al. (2000) observed that a fraction of persister cells was not killed even by very high doses of the antibiotics. These cells appeared invulnerable in contrast to fairly sensitive *Pseudomonas aeruginosa* biofilm (Brooun, et al., 2000). Also in *Escherichia coli*, increasing concentration of ciprofloxacin or imipenem leaded to an initial 100- to 1000-fold reduce of live cells of a biofilm, remaining small population insensitive persisters to further increases in drug concentration (Ashby et al., 1994). These data suggest that most of the cells in the biofilm are as susceptible to bactericidal agents as planktonic bacteria. Only the persister fraction is responsible for survival of the whole sessile population (Ashby et al., 1994; Brooun et al., 2000). Also Spoering & Lewis (2001) noticed that stationary phase planktonic and sessile bacteria were tolerant to anitimicrobials at similar level and that resistance of stationary phase and biofilm bacteria was dependent on the persister fraction. In addition, the increased resistance to killing of biofilm is due to high level of persisters produced by stationary phase bacteria inside biofilm (Spoering & Lewis,

2001). It is also important to emphasize that persisters are not simply non-growing cells in stationary culture. Keren et al. (2004b) noticed that fluoroquinolones and mitomycin C eliminated the bulk of *Escherichia coli* biofilm and left 1-10% intact persisters. From a medical perspective, the presence of persisters in biofilm is problematic. In planktonic population, a fraction of persisters that survive antibiotic action, is eliminate by the immune system (Hoyle et al., 1990; del Pozo & Patel, 2007). Biofilm persisters are protected from the immune system by glycocalyx matrix. In sessile bacterial population persisters are responsible for biofilm regrowth when the antibiotics concentration decrease or when the treatment is discontinued (Hoyle et al., 1990; Lewis, 2000).

The formation of persisters is dependent on the bacteria growth state (Lewis, 2007). Keren et al. (2004b) performed a test for measuring a rate of persisters after adding spent stationary medium to early log cells of *Escherichia coli* and *Pseudomonas aeruginosa*. Authors noticed that spent medium did not increase presisters of examined bacteria. In addition, persisters are rapidly lost if a stationary population is diluted (Keren et al., 2004b). The work of Keren et al. (2004b) demonstrated that formation of persisters dependent on the level of bacterial metabolic activity.

Falla & Chopra (1998) suggested that presisters are not mutant, but rather dormant variant of the wild type cells. Keren et al (2004a) observed that repeated reinoculation maintaining the cells in an log phase affects to a complete loss of persisters in *Escherichia coli* population. The work of Keren et al. (2004a) suggest that persisters are not formed in response to bactericidal agents exposure. According to Lewis (2005) persisters representing specialized survival cells whose formation is controlled by the growth stage of the bacterial culture. Moreover persisters are the cells with forfeiting rapid propagation system which ensures survival of cells in presence of lethal doses of antimicrobial factors (Lewis, 2005).

The tolerance of persisters to antibiotics works, not by preventing bactericidal binding, but by interfering with the lethal action of the compounds. Lewis (2007) postulated that persisters produce multidrug resistance protein (MDR protein) that shut down the antibiotic targets. It is worth point out that bactericidal properties of antibiotics occur by corrupting the target function of cells, rather than by inhibiting it. For instant, erythromycin blocks protein synthesis (Menninger & Otto, 1982). Streptomycin leads translational misreading, that produces truncated toxic peptides, causing the cell death. Shutting down the ribosome in a persister cells would produce tolerance to bactericidal aminoglycosides (Kornder, 2002; Lewis, 2005). According to Lewis (2005) persister protein can shut down most of antibiotics targets, formatting the resistant, dormant persister cells.

The phenomenon of tolerance of persisters to antimicrobial agents has also been linked with programmed cell death (PCD) system (Webb et al., 2003; Lewis, 2005; Lewis, 2007). Lewis (2000) suggests that actions of antimicrobial compounds are not responsible for cell death, but that they lead to cell damage that indirectly trigger PCD. The most common observation of PCD in bacterial biofilm is autolysis of cells. Autolysis is a self-digestion of the cell wall by peptidoglycan hydrolases termed autolysin (Shockman et al., 1996). Both production and hydrolysis of peptidoglycan are essential for creating the cell wall, therefore some autolysisns are the part of normal bacteria growth activity in biofilm (Lewis, 2000). Because a bactericidal compound that diffuses throughout biofilm would not able to eliminate whole sessile population, Lewis (2005) proposed that persisters have a defective PCD mechanism.

The work of Moyed & Bertrand (1983) supported this statement. Moyed & Bertrand (1983) discovered in *Escherichia coli* a toxin-antitoxin system (*hipAB* locus) that has a potential of both killing the cells and improving survival after exposure to lethal doses of antimicrobial factors. The inactivation of the toxin-antitoxin systems by insertional elements or by mutation, induced defects in PCD system in *Escherichia coli* and made the bacteria more susceptible to antimicrobial agents (Han et al., 2011).

6. *Quorum sensing*

A mechanism which cannot be overlooked when discussing bacterial biofilm resistance to antimicrobial factors is *quorum sensing*. Within biofilm, bacteria are able to sense an increase of the cell population density and respond to it by the induction of particular set of genes (Whitehead et al., 2001; Shirtliff, et al., 2002; González & Keshavan, 2006; Turovskiy et al., 2007). *Quorum sensing* termed also cell-to-cell signaling system, includes in gram-negative bacteria the production and secretion of an acyl homoserine lactones (AHL), which diffuse through the cell wall, from the cell to the medium (Eberl, 1999; Williams et al., 2007). *Quorum sensing* mechanism in gram-positive bacteria typically use secreted peptides as signal compounds and a two-component regulatory system (composed of a membrane-bound histidine kinase receptor and an intracellular response regulator) to detect the peptide and trigger the required changes in gene expression (Kleerebezem et al., 1997; Suntharalingam & Cvitkovitch, 2005). A third examined form of *quorum sensing* mechanism employes a family of related molecules termed autoinducers-2. This system was found in both gram-negative and gram-positive bacteria (Platt & Fuqua, 2010).

According to Whitehead et al. (2001) and González & Keshavan (2006) several important biofilm features are likely to affect signal molecules production. The number of active cells in the biological layer, which is influenced by the bacteria growth and the synthesis of both of glycocalyx matrix and degradative enzymes, may affects signal molecules production (Chopp, 2003; Mentag et al., 2003; Newton & Fray, 2004; Sakuragi & Kolter, 2007). Moré et al. (1996), Schaefer et al. (1996) and Parsek et al. (1999) observed that metabolic activity of gram-negative bacteria will likely affect the availability of cellular substrates pools for signal molecules production, *S*-adenosylmethionine and acyl-carrier protein, thereby increasing signal molecules production. For gram-negative bacteria, *S*-adenosylmethionine is the amino acid substrate necessary for the synthesis of *quorum sensing* signal compounds, whereas acyl carried protein is the donor of fatty acid chain in the biosynthesis of signal molecules of *Vibrio fischerii* (Eberhard et al., 1991).

Quorum sensing mechanism controls also the biofilm maturation process (Davies et al., 1998; Costerton, 1999; Watnick & Kolter, 2000). The work of Kjelleberg & Molin (2002) and Williams et al. (2007) demonstrated that the diffusion process of signal molecules within biofilm is unlimited. Inside biological layers there are shorter-distance migration of signal molecules and therefore the contact between the cells and reaction to signal molecules by the cells is more probable (Whitehead et al., 2001). The role of signal molecules-mediated *quorum sensing* in biofilm formation has been examined for *Brukholderia cenocepacia, Aeromonas hydrophila, Pseudomonas aeruginosa, Pseudomonas putida* and *Serratia marcescens* (Davies et al., 1998; Huber et al., 2001; Lynch et al., 2002; Steidla et al., 2002; Labbate et al., 2007). Davies et al. (1998) demonstrated that cell-to-cell signal *N*-(3-oxododecanoyl)-L-homoserine lactone (3-oxo-C12-HSL) is needed for the development of *Pseudomonas aeruginosa* biofilm with a wild-type structure: loosely packed biomass with a mushroom appearance with notable amount of extracellular polysaccharides and water channel traversing the entire the biological layer. Whereas, signal molecules-negative mutants of *Pseudomonas aeruginosa*, *Brukholderia cenocepacia* and *Aeromonas hydrophila* showed defects in the late stages of biofilm maturation and thus were unable to form biofilms with the wild-type architecture (Huber et al., 2001; Lynch et al., 2002; Steidla et al., 2002; Labbate et al., 2007).

Because heterogonous architecture of biofilms and the synthesis of degradative enzymes deactivate biocides, it seems reasonable to speculate that biofilm antimicrobial agents resistance could also be influenced by *quorum sensing* system. Moreover, coordinated expression of *quorum sensing*-mediated phenotypes is crucial in cells migration to a more suitable environment/better nutrient supply and in adaptation to a new modes of growth, which may afford protection from deleterious environment (Whitehead et al., 2001; Abee et al., 2011). However, to date *quorum sensing* system as factor decreasing the biofilm susceptibility to antimicrobial agents has been studied in a limited number of strains. Davies et al. (1998) and Hassett et al. (1999) reported that exposure of *quorum sensing*-negative mutant biofilms to the antimicrobial agents SDS and hydrogen peroxide caused detachment and dispersion of surface-anchored bacteria. In addition, Hassett et al. (1999) have reported that cell-to-cell signaling mechanism in *Pseudomonas aeruginosa* controls the expression of the catalase and superoxide dismutase genes and mediates biofilms resistance to hydrogen peroxide. According Shih & Hoang (2002) *quorum sensing*-deficient mutant biofilms susceptibility to kanamycin correlated with thinner biofilm formation and lower EPS production. Above results provide evidences that biofilm respond directly or indirectly to environmental stress via a *quorum sensing* system.

Interestingly, resent reports have also demonstrated chelating properties of cell-to-cell signals (Schertzer, et al. 2009). Such non-signaling features were stated for *Pseudomonas aeruginosa quorum sensing* molecules. Weinberg (2008) examined multiple meaning of *quorum sensing* system in mixed-species bacterial population. The author performed that *Pseudomonas aeruginosa* may kills competing bacteria in the growth environment by hijacking the bacteria's iron stores using 2-heptyl-3-hydroxy-4-quinolone signal. According to Weinberg (2008) *Pseudomonas* quinolone signal is a high affinity iron chelator. The ability of signal molecules to trap external positive-charged compounds is similar to antimicrobial action of glycocalyx matrix (Schertzer, et al, 2009). However, this role of cell-to-cell signal molecules to biofilm resistance properties needs to be examined in more detail.

7. General stress response

A general stress response is characterized by numerous changes in bacteria physiology and morphology that increasing cellular stress resistance (Hengge-Aronis, 1999; Lee et al., 2009). The formation of cell envelope and synthesis of thin aggregative fimbriae in *Escherichia coli* and *Salmonella enteritis* serovar *Typhimurium* are both under control of general stress response. These features affect cell to cell contact (Atlung & Brøndsted, 1994; Römling et al., 1998). Moreover, the study of Hengge-Aronis et al. (1993) performed that under extreme conditions, the general stress response functions as a factor preventing cellular damage rather than repaired it. This mechanism induced by many different stresses including nutrients deprivation (which results in stationary phase of bacteria growth cycle), high or low temperature, high osmolarity and acidic pH (Lange & Hengge-Aronis, 1991; Lee et al., 1995; Xu et al., 2001). Some evidences suggest also that biofilm development process leads to an early general stress response (Brown & Barker, 1999).

Exposure of *Escherichia coli* to adverse environments can induce RpoS, a sigma subunit of RNA polymerase, that acts as a central regulator. In *Escherichia coli* above 50 sigma factor-controlled genes determine stress tolerance of cells, whereas others mediate the physiological rearrangement or redirect the metabolism of bacteria upon stress condition (Hengge-Aronis, 1999; Whiteley et al., 2000). Analysis of the molecular reactions in dense population of *Escherichia coli* revealed the influence of sigma factor-controlled genes on production of trehalose (Liu et al., 2000). Trehalose is the stress protectant in bacteria. In *Escherichia coli*, this molecule acts as osmoprotectant and is essential for bacteria desiccation tolerance (Strøm & Kaasen, 1993; Welsh & Herbert, 1999). Trehalose also plays an important role in thermotolerane of *Escherichia coli* (Hengge-Aronis et al., 1991). *rpoS* mutants that devoided of the typical features associated with the general stress response were unable to accumulate trehalose and they died off rapidly in stationary phase (Hengge-Aronis et al., 1991; Lange & Hengge-Aronis, 1991; McCann et al., 1991).

In bacterial populations, RpoS-controlled promoter regions include multiple binding sites for additional regulators such as cAMP-CRP or the histone-like proteins H-NS, leucine-responsive regulatory protein (Lrp), integration host factor (IHF) and FIS (Barth et al., 1995; Marschall et al., 1998). These regulators determining RpoS specificity (Marschall, et al. 1998).

As focused in literature, the general stress response acts both as a rapid emergency response and as a long-term mechanism, that enables the cell adaptation to nutrient deprivation and other environmental stresses that cause changes in cellular metabolism (Gentry et al., 1993; Hengge-Aronis, 1999). Activation of the general stress response in the cells, immobilized in biofilm matrix, may results in increasing resistance to biocides action (Drenkard, 2003). However, this mechanism needs to be examined in more detail. Drenkard (2003) demonstrated that the general stress response maintain cell viability upon stationary phase when nutrients availability is limited. It is highly probable that environments within biofilm would promote the expression of the RpoS. This process affecting the physiological changes that mediate protection of biofilms to environmental stresses (Drenkard, 2003). Adams & McLean (1999) observed that *Escherichia coli* that lack *rpoS* are unable to form biofilm of wild type architecture. The study of Cochran et al. (2000) demonstrate that thin biofilms formed by *Pseudomonas aeruginosa* mutants of *rpoS* are susceptible to hydrogen peroxide.

8. Efflux pumps

Efflux pumps can affect both intrinsic and acquired resistance to antimicrobial agents by applying the energy to limit the cytoplasmic compound concentration to subtoxic level (Nikaido, 1992; Hogan & Kolter, 2002; Liaw, et al., 2010). Efflux system was first described as a mechanism of negatively impact to tetracycline susceptibility in *Escherichia coli* population. It was the plasmid-encoded single component Tet protein export of tetracycline throughout the cytoplasmic membrane (Ball et al., 1980).

A set of efflux systems facilitates bacteria to survive in extreme environments. Bacterial efflux pumps are involved in the multidrug resistance (MDR) phenotype combined with other more specific resistance systems including target mutation and enzymatic modification of antimicrobial agents (Zgurskaya & Nikaido, 2000; Davin-Regli et al., 2008; Bolla et al., 2011). The mechanism of efflux pumps in *Escherichia coli*, *Enterobacter aerogenes* and *Klebsiella pneumoniae* may also serve down regulation of porin production that slow down the penetration of hydrophilic solutes, and decrease the transmembrane diffusion of lipophilic solutes (Nikaido & Vaara, 1985; Plésiat & Nikaido, 1992; Li & Nikaido, 2004; Pagés et al., 2008). However, under particular circumstances, the outer membrane barrier cannot be the whole explanation of the bacteria resistance to inhibitors (Nikaido 1996). In fact, the equilibration across the outer membrane is reached very quickly, in the part of the surface-to-volume ratio that is very large to compare with bacterial cell size. Thus, the periplasmic concentration of many antibiotics may achieve 50% of their external value (Nikaido, 1989).

In the literature, numerous plasmid and chromosome-encoded efflux systems, both agent- or class-specific and multidrug have been performed in a various of microorganisms where they are the major determinant in the intrinsic resistance of the bacteria to action of dyes, detergents and different classes of antibiotic including β-lactams (Nikaido, 1989; Nikaido, 1994; Markham & Neyfakh, 2001; Butaye et al., 2003). Bacterial efflux pumps compose of five classes of systems including: the major facilitator superfamily (MF), the ATP-binding cassette family (ABC), the resistance-nodulation-division family (RND), the small multidrug resistance family (SMR), and the multidrug and toxic compound extrusion family (MATE) (Putman et al., 2000; Kumar & Schweizer, 2005; Poole & Lomovskaya, 2006). To drive antimicrobial agents efflux, the ABC family system hydrolyses ATP, whereas the MF family, the RND family and the MATE family function as secondary transporters, catalysing drug-ion antiport (H^+ or Na^+) (Poole, 2005).

The RND family transporters are most commonly found in bacteria cells (Poole, 2001). In gram-negative bacteria this system operates as a part of a tripartite mechanism that includes: a membrane fusion protein that is associated with the cytoplasmic membrane, a transporter protein that export substrates throughout the inner membrane, and an outer membrane factor (OMF) that enables the passage of the substrate throughout the outer membrane (Poole, 2005). The RND family transporters are the first line of bacterial defense that can promote the acquisition of additional resistance mechanisms such as target mutations or drug modification (Davin-Regli et al., 2008; Li & Nikaido, 2009). Pagés et al. (2008) and Pagés et al. (2010) performed that the expression of RND efflux pumps is an important prerequisite for the selection of fluoroquinolone resistant strains carrying the target mutation. According to Stover et al. (2000), *Pseudomonas aeruginosa* encode 12 efflux systems of the class of the RND family. However, to date only MexAB-OprM, MexCD-OprJ, MexEF-OprN, MexGHI-OmpD, MexJK and MexXY have been detailed characterized (Poole & Srikumar, 2001; Chuanchuen et al., 2002; Blair & Piddock, 2009; Breidenstein, et al., 2011).

Molecular analysis of efflux pumps assesses the role of this mechanism in biofilm resistance to antimicrobial agents. Exposure the bacterial biofilms to insufficient dose of antibiotics, such as tetracycline and chloramphenicol, and to xenobiotics, such as salicylate and chlorinated phenols, induces the expression of multi-drug resistance operons and efflux pumps (Levy, 1992; Ma et al., 1993). Also DNA microarray analysis of mature *Pseudomonas aeruginosa* PA01 biofilm demonstrated that none of genes encoding the RND efflux system were induced in sessile bacterial population grown in antibiotic-free environments (Whiteley et al., 2001).

Numerous of works have focused on the identification of genes that could contribute efflux system-mediate resistance of bacterial biofilms. Maira-Litran et al. (2000) examined the systems of *mar* and *acrAB* that confer on *Escherichia coli* biofilm the multidrug resistance phenotype. The *mar* operon is a regulator controlling the expression of various genes in *Escherichia coli* cells constituting the *mar* regulon. Upregulation of *mar* in planktonic bacteria effects a resistance phenotype to antimicrobial agents such as antibiotics (penicillins, cephalosporins, rifampicin, nalidixic acid and fluoroquinolones), oxidative stress agents and organic solvents (Alekshun & Levy, 1997). *mar* can be induced by sub-lethal doses of commonly used therapeutics such as tetracycline, chloramphenicol, salicylate and paracetamol (Cohen et al., 1993; Seoane & Levy, 1995). The *acrAB* efflux pump is upregulated in *mar* mutants and determined the multidrug resistant phenotype of *mar* mutant isolates (Ma et al., 1995; Ma et al., 1996). According to Maira-Litran et al. (2000) the constitutive expression of *acrAB* efflux pump effects lower susceptibility of *Escherichia coli* biofilm to sub-lethal doses of ciprofloxacin. In addition, the expression of *mar* and its target genes is related to stationary phase of bacteria growth. Authors observed the highest level of *mar* expression within the depth of *Escherichia coli* biofilm, where the metabolic activity of examined bacteria were the most suppressed (Maira-Litran et al., 2000).

Brooun et al. (2000) and De Kievit et al. (2001) examined the expression of the genes associated with efflux pumps (MexAB-OprM and MexCD-OprJ) in developing biofilms of *Pseudomonas aeruginosa*. Brooun et al. (2000) underscored the importance of these pumps in the resistance to ofloxacin. Authors demonstrated that at low concentration of ofloxacin *Pseudomonas aeruginosa* mature biofilm with lacking MexAB-OprM was less resistant to antibiotic than mature biofilm that overexpressed the pump (Brooun et al. 2000). De Kievit et al. (2001) found that expression of the genes that encode MexAB-OprM and MexCD-OprJ, are decreased over time during biofilm maturation. In addition, authors, using the overexpressing and efflux pumps mutants of *Pseudomonas aeruginosa* revealed that none of efflux pumps analyzed plays a significant role at decreasing susceptibility of *Pseudomonas aeruginosa* biofilm to antibiotics (De Kievit, et al., 2001). Therefore to assess the true function of efflux pump in bacterial biofilm resistance to antimicrobial agents, further experiments of additional not yet characterized loci with homology to efflux system are needed.

9. Conclusion

Survival of bacterial after disinfection and antibiotic treatment represents a problem for the modern medicine and industry practice. Commonly applied antibiotics and disinfectants are able to eliminate planktonic bacteria released from the biofilm but often are unable to treat biofilm-embedded cells. This may cause difficult to eradicate infectious.

Biofilm resistance to bactericidal agents is usually multifactorial and may vary from one microorganism to another. Environmental heterogeneity that exists inside the biofilm might promote the formation heterogeneous communities of bacteria, such that different levels of resistance can be employed throughout the entire population. For instant, the bacteria at periphery region of biofilm might be protected by the glycocalyx matrix, by the efflux systems and by the enzymes that inactivate certain antimicrobial compounds. The cells in the intermediate position of biofilm became starved for a particular nutrient, and they slow their growth. Transition from exponential to slow or no growth/persisters phenomena is also be accompanied by the increased in resistance of bacteria biofilm to bactericidal agents.

Upon the extreme conditions setting the general stress response mechanism by surface-bound bacteria may prevents cellular damage.

Whatever new biocides/antibiotics are developed, the high number of bacteria within biofilms will combine to overcome their action and lead to resistance formation. The only way to avoid or to slow the speed of excess resistance formation is systematic and in-depth investigation of resistant bacteria isolated from naturally occurred biofilms. The information derived from lab investigations can provide insight strategies to subvert both biocide and antibiotic resistance of surface-bound bacteria.

10. References

Abee, T., Kovács, Á.T., Kuipers, O.P. & van der Veen, S. (2011). Biofilm formation and dispersal in Gram-positive bacteria. *Current Opinion in Biotechnology*, Vol. 22, pp. 172-179, ISSN 0958-1669

Adal, K.A. & Farr, B.M. (1996). Central venous catheter-related infections: a review. *Nutrition*. Vol. 12, No. 3, pp. 208-213, ISSN 0899-9007

Adams, J.L. & McLean, R.J. (1999). Impact of *rpoS* deletion on *Escherichia coli* biofilms. *Applied and Environmental Microbiology*, Vol. 65, No. 9, pp. 4285-4287, ISSN 0099-2240

Alekshun, M.N. & Levy, S.B. (1997). Regulation of chromosomally mediated multiple antibiotic resistance: the *mar* regulon . *Antimicrobial Agents and Chemotherapy*, Vol. 44, No. 10, pp. 2067-2075, ISSN 0066-4804

Alvarez-Ortega, C., Wiegand, I., Olivares, J., Hancock, R.E.W. & Martinez, J.L. (2010). Genetic determinants involved in the susceptibility of *Pseudomonas aeruginosa* to β-lactam antibiotics. *Antimicrobial Agents and ChemotherapyAntimicrobial Agents and Chemotherapy*, Vol. 54, No. 10, pp. 4159-4167, ISSN 0066-4804

Anderl, J.N., Franklin, M.J. & Stewart, P.S. (2000). Role of antibiotic penetration limitation in *Klebsiella pneumoniae* biofilm resistance to ampicillin and ciprofloxacin. *Antimicrobial Agents and Chemotherapy*, Vol. 44, No. 7, pp. 1818-1824, ISSN 0066-4804

Anwar, H., Dasgupta, M.K & Costerton, J.W. (1990). Testing the susceptibility of bacteria in biofilms to antibacterial agents. *Antimicrobial Agents and Chemotherapy*, Vol. 34, No. 11, pp. 2043-2046, ISSN 0066-4804

Archibald, L.K. & Gaynes, R.P. (1997). Hospital acquired infections in the United States: the importance of interhospital comparisions. *National Nosocomial Infections*, Vol. 11, pp. 245-255, ISSN 0147-443X

Ashby, M.J., Neale, J.E., Knott, S.J. & Critchley, I.A. (1994). Effect of antibiotics on non-growing planktonic cells and biofilms of *Escherichia coli*. *Journal of Antimicrobial Chemotheraphy*, Vol. 33, No. 3, pp. 443-452, ISSN 0305-7453

Atlung, T. & Brøndsted, L. 1994. Role of the transcriptional activator AppY in regulation of the *cyx appA* operon of *Escherichia coli* by anaerobiosis, phosphate starvation and growth phase. *Journal of Bacteriology*, Vol. 176, No. 17, pp. 5414-5422, ISSN 0021-9193

Ball, P.R., Shales, S.W. & Chopra I. (1980). Plasmid-mediated tetracycline resistance in *Escherichia coli* involves increased efflux of the antibiotic. *Biochemical and Biophysical Research Communications*, Vol. 93, pp. 74-81, ISSN 0006-291X

Barth, M., Marschall, C., Muffler, A., Fischer, D. & Hengge-Aronis, R. (1995). A role for the histone-like protein H-NS in growth phase-dependent and osmotic regulation of α^s and many α^s-dependent genes in *Escherichia coli*. *Journal of Bacteriology*, Vol. 177, No. 12, pp. 3455-3464, ISSN 0021-9193

Beech, I.B., Sunner, I.A. & Hiraoka, K. (2005). Microbe-surface interactions in biofouling and biocorrosion processes. *International Microbiology*, Vol. 8, no. 3, pp. 157-168, ISSN 1139-6709

Betzner, A.S., Ferreira, L.C., Holtje, J.V. & Keck, W. (1990). Control of the activity of the soluble lytic transglycosylase by the stringent response in *Escherichia coli*. *FEMS Microbiology Letters*, Vol. 55, pp. 161-164, ISSN 1574-6968

Blair, J.M.A. & Piddock, L.J.V. (2009). Structure, function and inhibition of RND efflux pumps in Gram-negative bacteria: an update. *Current Opinion in Microbiology*, Vol. 12, pp. 512-519, ISSN 1369-5274

Boles, B.R. & Horswill, A.R. (2011). Staphylococcal biofilm disassembly. *TRENDS in Microbiology*, Vol. 19, No. 9, pp. 499-455, ISSN 0966-842X

Branda, S.S., Vik, A., Friedman, L. & Kolter, R. (2005). Biofilm: the matrix revisited. *TRENDS in Microbiology*, Vol. 13, pp. 20-26, ISSN 0966-842X

Breidenstein, E.B.M., De la Fuente-Núñez, C. & Hancock, R.E.W. (2011). *Pseudomonas aeruginosa*: all roads lead to resistance. *TRENDS in Microbiology*, Vol. 19, No. 8, pp. 419-426, ISSN 0966-842X

Brooun, A., Liu, S. & Lewis, K. (2000). A dose-response study of antibiotic resistance in *Pseudomonas aeruginosa, Antimicrobial Agents and Chemotherapy*, Vol. 44, No. 3, pp. 640-646, ISSN 0066-4804

Brown, M.R. & Barker, J. (1999). Unexplored reservoirs pathogenic bacteria: protozoa and biofilms. *TRENDS in Microbiology*, Vol. 7, No. 1, pp. 46-50, ISSN 0966-842X

Brown, M.R.W. & Williams, P. (1985). The influence of environment on envelope properties affecting survival of bacteria in infections. *Annual Review of Microbiology*, Vol. 39, pp. 527-556, ISSN 0066-4227

Bolla, J.-M., Alibert-Franco, S., Handzlik, J., Chevalier, J., Mahamoud, A., Boyer, G., Kieć-Kononowicz, K. & Pagés, J.-M. (2011). Strategies for bypassing the membrane barrier in multidrug resistant gram-negative bacteria. *Federation of European Biochemical Societes Letters*, Vol. 585, pp. 1682-1690, DOI 10. 1016

Bower, C.K., McGuire J. & Daeschel, M.A. (1996). The adhesion and detachment of bacteria and spores on food-contact surfaces. *Trends in Food Sciences and Technology*, Vol. 7, pp. 152-157, ISSN 0924-2244

Bulter, M.T., Wang, Q. & Harshey, R.M. (2010). Cell density and mobility protect swarming bacteria against antibiotics. *Proceedings of the National Academy of Sciences USA*, Vol.107, No. 8, pp. 3776-3781, ISSN 0027-8424

Carlson, G. & Silverstein, J. (1998). Effect of molecular size and charge on biofilm sorption of organic matter. *Water Research*, Vol. 32, No. 5, pp. 1580-1592, ISSN 0043-1354

Cloete, T.E. (2003). Resistance mechanisms of bacteria to antimicrobial compounds. *International Biodeterioration & Biodegradation*, Vol. 51, pp. 277-282, ISSN 0964-8305

Chapman, J.S., Diehl, M.A. & Lyman, R.C. (1993). Biocide susceptibility and intracellular gluthatione in *Escherichia coli*. *Journal of Industrial Microbiology*, Vol. 12, pp. 403-407, ISSN 1476-5535

Characklis, W.G. 1989. Bioengineering report, fouling biofilm development: a process analysis. *Biotechnology and Bioengineering*. Vol. 23, pp. 1923-1960, ISSN 1097-0290

Cheng, W.-C. & Hardwick, J.M. (2007). A quorum of bacterial programmed cell death. *Molecular Cell*, Vol. 30, pp. 515-517, ISSN 1097-2765

Chopp, D.L. (2003). The dependence of *quorum sensing* on the depth of a growing biofilm. *Bulletin of Mathematical Biology*, Vol. 65, pp. 1053-1079, ISSN 1522-9602

Chuanchuen, R., Narasaki, C.T. & Schweizer, H.P. (2002). The MexJK efflux pump of *Pseudomonas aeruginosa* requires OprM for antibiotic efflux but not for efflux of triclosan. *Journal of Bacteriology*, Vol. 184, No. 18, pp. 5036-5044, ISSN 0021-9193

Cochran, W.L., Suh, S.-J., McFeters, G.A. & Stewart, P.S. (2000). Role of RpoS and AlgT in *Pseudomonas aeruginosa* biofilm resistance to hydrogen peroxide and monochloramine. *Journal of Applied Microbiology*, Vol. 88, No. 3, pp. 546-553, ISSN 1365-2672

Cohen, S.P., Levy, S.B., Foulds, J. & Rosner, J.L. (1993). Salicylate induction of antibiotic resistance in *Escherichia coli*: activation of the *mar* operon and *mar*-independent pathway. *Journal of Bacteriology*, Vol. 175, No. 24, pp. 7856-7862, ISSN 0021-9193

Costerton, J. W. (1988). Structure and plasticity at various organization levels in the bacterial cells. *Canadian Journal of Microbiology*, Vol. 34, pp. 513-521, ISSN 0008-4166

Costerton, J.W., Lewadowski, D.E., Caldwell, D.R., Korber, D.R. & Lappin-Scott, H.M. (1995). Microbial biofilms. *Annual Review of Microbiology*, Vol. 49, pp. 711-745, ISSN 0066-4227

Costerton, J.W. (1999). Introduction to biofilm. *International Journal of Antimicrobial Agents*, Vol. 11, No.3-4, pp. 237-239, ISSN 0924-8579

Costerton, J.W., Stewart, P.S. & Greenberg, E.P. (1999). Bacterial biofilms: A common cause of persistent infections. *Science*, Vol. 284, pp. 1318-1322, ISSN 1095-9203

Czaczyk, K. & Myszka, K. (2007). Biosynthesis of extracellular polymeric substances (EPS) and its role in microbial biofilm formation. *Polish Journal of Environmental Studies*, Vol. 16, No. 6, pp. 799-806, ISSN 1230-1485

Darouiche, R.O., Dhir, A., Miller, A.J., Landon, G.C., Raad, I.I. & Musher, D.M. (1994). Vancomycin penetration into biofilm covering infected prostheses and effect on bacteria. *The Journal of Infectious Disease*, Vol. 170, pp. 720-723, ISSN 0022-1899

Davey, M.E., Caiazza, N.C. & O'Toole, G.A. (2003). Rhamnolipid surfactant production affects biofilm architecture in *Pseudomonas aeruginosa* PAO1. *Journal of Bacteriology*, Vol. 185, No. 3, pp. 1027-1036, ISSN 0021-9193

Davies, G.D., Parsek, M.R., Pearson, J.P., Iglewski, B.H., Costerton, J.W. & Greenberg, E.P. (1998). The involvement of cell-to-cell signals in the development of a bacterial biofilm. *Science*, Vol. 280, pp. 295-298, ISSN 1095-9203

Davin-Regli, A., Bolla, J.M., James, C.E., Lavigne, J.P., Chevalier, J., Garnotel, E., Molitor, A. & Pagés, J. M. (2008). Membrane permeability and regulation of drug "influx and efflux" in enterobacterial pathogens. *Current Drug Targets*, Vol. 9, pp. 750-759, ISSN 1389-4501

DeBeer, D., Srinivasan, R. & Stewart, P.S. (1994). Direct measurement of chlorine penetration into biofilms during disinfection. *Applied and Environmental Microbiology*, Vol. 60, No. 12, pp. 4339-4344, ISSN 0099-2240

De Kievit, T.R., Parkins, M.D., Gillis, R.J., Srikumar, R., Ceri, H., Poole, K., Iglewski, B.H. & Storey, D.G. (2001). Multidrug efflux pumps: expression patterns and contribution to antibiotic resistance in *Pseudomonas aeruginosa* biofilms. *Antimicrobial Agents and Chemotherapy*, Vol.45, No. 6, pp. 1761-1770, ISSN 0066-4804

del Pozo, J.L. & Patel, R. (2007). The challenge of treating biofilm-associated bacterial infections. *Clinical Pharmacology & Therapeutics*, Vol. 82, pp. 204-209, ISSN 0009-9236

Donlan, R.M. (2002). Biofilms: Microbial life on surfaces. *Emerging Infectious Disease*, Vol. 8, No. 9, pp. 881-890, ISSN 1080-6059

Drenkard, E. (2003). Antimicrobial resistance of *Pseudomonas aeruginosa* biofilms. *Microbes and Infections*, Vol. 5, pp. 1213-1219, ISSN 1286-4579

Duguid, I.G., Evans, E., Brown, M.R.W. & Gilbert, P. (1992). Growth-rate-independent killing by ciprofloxacin of biofilm-derived *Staphylococcs epidermidis* evidence for cell-cycle dependency. *Journal of Antimicrobial Chemotherapy*, Vol. 30, No. 6, pp. 791-802, ISSN 1460-2091

Dunne, W.M., Mason, E.O. & Kaplan, S.L. (1993). Diffusion of rifampin and vancomycin through a *Staphylococcus epidermidis* biofilm. *Antimicrobial Agents and Chemotherapy*, Vol. 37, No. 12, pp. 2522-2526, ISSN 0066-4804

Dunne, W.M. (2002). Bacterial adhesion: seen any good biofilms lately?. *Clinical Microbiology Reviwes*, Vol. 15, No. 2, pp. 155-166, ISSN 0893-8512

Eberhard, A., Longin, T., Widrig, C.A. & Stranick, S.J. (1991). Synthesis of the *lux* gene autoinducer in *Vibrio fischeri* is positively autoregulated. *Archives of Microbiology*, Vol. 155, No. 3, pp. 294-297, ISSN 1432-072X

Eberl, L. (1999). *N*-acyl homoserine lactone-mediated gene regulation in gram-negative bacteria. *Systematic and Applied Microbiology*, Vol. 22., pp. 1-9, ISSN 0723-2020

Evans, D.J., Brown, M.R.W., Allison, D.G. & Gilbert, P. (1989). Susceptibility of bacterial biofilms to tobramycin: role of specific growth rate and phase in the division cycle. *Journal of Antimicrobial Chemotheraphy*, Vol. 25, No. 4, pp. 585-591, ISSN 1460-2091

Falla, T.J. & Chopra, I. (1998). Joint tolerance to beta-lactam and fluoroquinolone antibiotics in *Escherichia coli* results from overexpression of *hipA*. *Antimicrobial Agents and Chemotheraphy*, Vol. 42No. 12, pp. 3282-3284, ISSN 0066-4804

Flemming, H.C. (1995). Sorption sites in biofilms. *Water Sciences and Technology*. Vol. 32, No. 8, pp. 27-33, ISSN 0273-1223

Flemming, H.C. & Wingender, J. (2001). Relevance of microbial extracellular polymeric substances (EPSs) - Part I: Structural and ecological aspects. *Water Sciences and Technology*, Vol.43, pp. 1-8, ISSN 0273-1223

Gaylarde, C. & Videla, H.A. (1994). The control of corrosive biofilms by biocides. *Corrosion Reviews*, Vol. 2, pp. 85-94, ISSN 0048-7538

Gentry, D.R., Hernandez, V.J., Nguyen, L.H., Jensen, D.B. & Cashel, M. (1993). Synthesis of the stationary-phase sigma factor is positively regulated by ppGpp. *Journal of Bacteriology*, Vol. 175, No. 24, pp. 7982-7989, ISSN 0021-9193

Gilbert, P., Allison, D.G., Evans, D.J., Handley, P.S. & Brown, M.R.W. (1989). Growth rate control of adherent bacterial populations. *Applied and Environmental Microbiology*, Vol. 55, pp. 1308-1311, ISSN 0099-2240

Gilbert, P., Collier, P.J. & Brown, M.R. (1990). Influence of growth rate on susceptibility to antimicrobial agents: biofilms, cell cycle, dormancy, and stringent response. *Antimicrobial Agents and Chemotherapy*, Vol. 34, No. 10, pp. 1865-1868, ISSN 0066-4804

Gilbert, P., Allison, D.G. & McBain, A.J. (2002a). Biofilms *in vitro* and *in vivo*: do singular mechanisms imply cross-resistance? *Journal of Applied Microbiology*, Vol. 92, pp.98S-110S, ISSN 1364-5072

Gilbert, P., Maira-Litran, T., McBain, A.J., Rickard, A.H. & Whyte F.W. (2002b). The physiology and collective recalcitrance of microbial biofilm communities. *Advances in Microbial Physiology*, Vol. 46, pp. 202-256, ISSN 0065-2911

González, J.E. & Keshavan, N.D. (2006). Messing with bacterial *quorum sensing*. *Microbiology and Molecular Biology Reviwes*, Vol. 70, No. 4, pp. 859-875, ISSN 1098-5557

Gunduz, G.T. & Tuncel G. (2006). Biofilm formation in an ice cream plant. *Antonie van Leeuwenhoek International Journal of General and Molecular Microbiology*, Vol. 89, pp. 329-336, ISSN 0003-6072

Han, X., Geng, G., Zhang, L. & Lu. T. (2011). The role of *Escherichia coli* YrbB in the lethal action of quinolones. *Journal of Antimicrobial Chemotheraphy*, Vol. 66, No. 2, pp. 323-331, ISSN 0305-7453

Hassett, D.J., Ma, J-F., Elkins, J.G., McDermott, T.R., Ochsner, U.A., West, S.E.H., Huang, Ch-T., Fredericks, J., Burnett, S., Stewart, P.S., McFeters, G., Passador, L. & Iglewski, B.H. (1999). Quorum sensing in *Pseudomonas aeruginosa* controls expression of catalase and superoxide dismutase genes and mediates biofilm susceptibility to hydrogen peroxide. *Molecular Microbiology*, Vol. 34, No. 5, pp. 1082-1093, ISSN 1365-2958

Hengge-Aronis, R., Klein, W., Lange, R., Rimmele, M. & Boos, W. (1991). Trehalose synthesis genes are controlled by the putative sigma factors encoded by *rpoS* and are involved in stationary phase thermotolerance in *Escherichia coli*. *Journal of Bacteriology*, Vol. 173, No. 24, pp. 7918-7924, ISSN 0021-9193

Hengge-Aronis, R., Lange, R., Henneberg, N. & Fischer, D. (1993). Osmotic regulation of *rpoS*-dependent genes in *Escherichia coli*. *Journal of Bacteriology*, Vol. 175, No. 1, pp. 259-265, ISSN 0021-9193

Hengge-Aronis, R. (1999). Interplay of global regulators in the general stress response of *Escherichia coli*. *Current Opinion of Microbiology*, Vol. 2, pp. 148-152, ISSN 1369-5274

Hentzer, M., Teitzel, G.M., Balzer, G.J., Heydorn, A., Molin, S., Givskov, M. & Parsek, M.R. (2001). Alginate overproduction affects *Pseudomonas aeruginosa* biofilm structure and function. *Journal of Bacteriology*, Vol. 183, No. 18, pp. 5395-5401, ISSN 0021-9193

Hill, D., Rose, B., Pajkos, A., Robinson, M., Bye, P., Bell, S., Elkins, M., Thompson, B., MacLeod, C., Aaron, S.D. & Harbour, C. (2005). Antibiotic susceptibilities of

Pseudomonas aeruginosa isolates derived from patients with cystic fibrosis under aerobic, anaerobic, and biofilm conditions. *Journal of Clinical Microbiology*, Vol. 43, no. 10, pp. 5085-5090, ISSN 1098- 660X

Hogan, D. & Kolter, R. (2002). Why are bacteria refractory to antimicrobials? *Current Opinion in Microbiology*, Vol. 5, pp. 472-477, ISSN 1369-5274

Hogt, A.H., Dankert, J., Hulstaert, C.E. & Feijen, J. (1986). Cell surface characteristics of coagulase-negative staphylococci and their adherence to fluorinated poly(ethylene propylene). *Infection and Immunity*, Vol. 51, pp. 294-301, ISSN 0019-9567

Hoyle, B.D., Jass, J. & Costerton, J.W. (1990). The biofilm glycocalyx as a resistance factor. *Journal of Antimicrobial Chemotherapy*, Vol. 26, No. 1, pp. 1-2, ISSN 0305-7453

Hoyle, B.D., Alcantara, J. & Costerton, J.W. (1992). *Pseudomonas aeruginosa* biofilm as a diffusion barrier to piperacillin. *Antimicrobial Agents and Chemotheraphy*, Vol. 36, No. 9, pp. 2054-2056, ISSN 0066-4804

Huber, B., Riedel, K., Hentzer, M., Heydorn, A., Gotschlich, A., Givskov, M., Molin, S. & Eberl, L. (2001). The *cep quorum-sensing* system of *Brukholderia cepacia* H111 controls biofilm formation and swarming motility. *Microbiology*, Vol. 147, pp. 2517-2528, ISSN 1465-2080

Izano, E.A., Shah, S.M. & Kaplan, J.B. (2009). Intercellular adhesion and biocide resistance in nontypeable *Haemophilus influenzae* biofilms. *Microbial Pathogenesis*, Vol. 46, pp. 207-213, ISSN 0882-4010

Jang, L.K., Geesey, G.G., Lopez, S.L., Eastman, S.L. & Wichlacz, P.L. (1990). Use of a gel-forming biopolymer directly dispensed into a loop fluidized bed reactor dissolved copper. *Water Research*, Vol. 26, pp. 1085-1092, ISSN 0043-1354

Jefferson, K.K. (2004). What drives bacteria to produce biofilm?. *FEMS Microbiology Letters*, Vol. 236, pp. 163-173, ISSN 0378-1097

Keren, I., Kaldalu, N., Spoering, A., Wang, Y. & Lewis, K. (2004a). Persister cell and tolerance to antimicrobials. *FEMS Microbiology Letters*, Vol. 230, pp. 13-18, ISSN 1574-6968

Keren, I., Shah, D., Spoering, A., Kaldalu, N. & Lewis, K. (2004b). Specialized persister cells and the mechanism of multidrug tolerance in *Escherichia coli*. *Journal of Bacteriology*, Vol. 186, No. 24, pp. 8172-8180, ISSN 0021-9193

Kjelleberg, S. & Molin, S. (2002). Is a role for quorum sensing signals in bacterial biofilms? *Current Opinion in Microbiology*, Vol. 5, pp. 254-258, ISSN 1369-5274

Kleerebezem, M., Quadri, L.E.N., Kuipers, O.P. & De Vos, W.M. (1997). *Quorum sensing* by peptide pheromones and two-component signal-transduction systems in gram-positive bacteria. *Molecular Microbiology*, Vol. 24, No. 5, pp.895-904, ISSN 1365-2958

Kordner, J.D. (2002). Streptomycin revisted: molecular action in the microbial cell. *Medical Hypotheses*. Vol. 58, No. 1, pp. 34-46, ISSN 0306-9877

Kumar, A. & Schweizer, H.P. (2005). Bacterial resistance to antibiotics: active efflux and reduced uptake. *Advanced Drug Delivery Reviews*, Vol. 57, pp. 1486-1513, ISSN 0169-409X

Labbate, M., Zhu, H., Thung, L., Bandara, R., Larsen, M., Willcox, M., Givskov, M., Rice, S. & Kjelleberg, S. (2007). Quorum sensing regulation of adhesion in *Serratia marcescens*

MG1 is surface dependent. *Journal of Bacteriology*, Vol. 189, No. 7, pp. 2702-2711, ISSN 0021-9193

Lange, R. & Hengge-Aronis, R. (1991). Growth phase-regulated expression of *bolA* and morphology of stationary phase *Escherichia coli* cells is controlled by the novel sigma factor (*rpoS*). *Journal of Bacteriology*, Vol. 173, No. 14, pp. 4474-4481, ISSN 0021-9193

Lawrence, J.R., Korber, D.R., Hoyle, B. D., Costerton, J.W. & Caldwell, D.E. (1991). Optical sectioning of microbial biofilms. *Journal of Bacteriology*, Vol. 173, pp. 6558-6567, ISSN 0021-9193

Lee, I., Lin, J., Hall, H.K., Bearson, B. & Foster, J.W. (1995). The stationary-phase sigma factor (RpoS) is required for a sustained acid tolerance response in virulent *Salmonella typhimurium*. *Molecular Microbiology*, Vol. 17, No. 1, pp. 155-167, ISSN 1365-2958

Lee, S., Hinz, A., Bauerle, E., Angermeyer, A., Juhaszova, K., Kaneko, Y., Singh, P.K. & Manoil, C. (2009). Targeting a bacterial stress response to enhance antibiotic action. *Proceedings of the National Academy of Sciences USA*, Vol. 106, No. 34, pp. 14570-14575, ISSN 0027-8424

Leid, F.G., Willson, C.J., Shritliff, M.E., Hassett, D.J., Parsek, M.R. & Jeffers, A.K. (2005). The exopolysaccharide alginate protects *Pseudomonas aeruginosa* biofilm bacteria from IFN-γ-mediated macrophage killing. *The Journal of Immunology*. Vol. 175, pp. 7512-7518, ISSN 0022-1767

Lewis, K. (2000). Programmed death in bacteria. *Microbiology and Molecular Biology Reviews*, Vol. 64, No. 3, pp. 503-514, ISSN 1098-5557

Lewis, K. (2001). Riddle of biofilm resistance. *Antimicrobial Agents and Chemotheraphy*, Vol. 45, pp. 999-1007, ISSN 0066-4804

Lewis, K. (2005). Persister cells and the riddle of biofilm survival. *Biochemistry*, Vol. 70, No. 2, pp. 327-336, ISSN 0006-2979

Lewis, K. (2007). Persister cells, dormancy, and infectious disease. *Nature*, Vol. 5, pp. 48-56, DOI: 10.1038

Lewis, K. (2008). Multidrug tolerance of biofilms and persister cells. *Current Topics in Microbiology and Immunology*, Vol. 322, pp. 107-131, ISSN 0070-217X

Levy, S.B. (1992). Active efflux mechanisms for antimicrobial resistance. *Antimicrobial Agents and Chemotherapy*, Vol. 36, No. 4, pp. 695-703, ISSN 0066-4804

Li, X.Z. & Nikaido, H. (2004). Efflux-mediated drug resistance in bacteria. *Drugs*, Vol. 69, pp. 159-204, ISSN 0012-6667

Li, X.Z. & Nikaido, H. (2009). Efflux-mediated drug resistance in bacteria: an update. *Drugs*, Vol. 69, pp. 1555-1623, ISSN 0012-6667

Liaw, S.-J., Lee, Y.-L. & Hsueh, P.-R. (2010). Multidrug resistance in clinical isolates of *Stenotrophomonas maltophilia*: roles of integrons, efflux pumps, phosphoglucomutase (SpgM), and melanin and biofilm formation. *International Journal of Antimicrobial Agents*, Vol. 35, pp. 126-130, ISSN 0924-8579

Lindsay, D. & von Holy, A. (2006). Bacterial biofilms within the clinical setting: what healthcare professionals should know. *Journal of Hospital Infection*, Vol. 64, pp. 313-325, ISSN 0195-6701

Liu, X., Ng, C. & Ferenci, T. (2000). Global adaptations resulting from high population densities in *Escherichia coli* cultures. *Journal of Bacteriology*, Vol. 182, No. 15, pp. 4158-4164, ISSN 0021-9193

Lynch, N.J., Swift, S., Kirke, D.F., Keevil, C., Dodd, C.E. & Williams, P. (2002). The regulation of biofilm development by *quorum-sensing* in *Aeromonas hydrophila*. *Environmental Microbiology*, Vol. 4, No. 1, pp. 18-28, ISSN 1462-2920

Ma, D., Cook, D.N., Alberti, M., Pong, N.G., Nikaido, H., & Hearst, J.E. (1993). Molecular cloning and characterisation of *arcAB* and *acrE* genes of *Escherichia coli Journal of Bacteriology*, Vol. 175, pp. 6299-6313, ISSN 0021-9193

Ma, D., Cook, D.N., Alberti, M., Pon, N.G., Nikaido, H. & Hearst, J.E. (1995). Genes *acrA* and *acrB* encode a stress-induced efflux system of *Eschericha coli*. *Molecular Microbiology*, Vol. 16, No. 1, pp. 45-55, ISSN 1365-2958

Ma, D., Alberti, M., Lynch, C., Nikaido, H. & Hearst, J.E. (1996). The local repressor *AcrR* plays a modulation role in the regulation of *acrAB* genes of *Escherichia coli* by global stress signals. *Molecular Microbiology*, Vol. 19, No. 1, pp. 101-112, ISSN 1365-2958

Maira-Litran, T., Allison, D.G. & Gilbert, P. (2000). An evaluation of the potential of the multiple antibiotic resistance operon (*mar*) and the multidrug efflux pump *acrAB* to moderate resistance towards ciprofloxacin in *Escherichia coli* biofilms. *Journal of Antimicrobial Chemotherapy*, Vol. 45, No. 6, pp. 789-795, ISSN 1460-2091

Markham, P.N. & Neyfakh, A.A. (2001). Efflux-mediated drug resistance in gram-positive bacteria. *Current Opinion in Microbiology*, Vol. 4, pp. 509-514, ISSN 1369-5274

Marschall, C., Labrousse, V., Kreimer, M., Weichart, D., Kolb, A. & Hengge-Aronis, R. (1998). Molecular analysis of the regulation of *csiD*, a carbon starvation inducible gene in *Escherichia coli* that is exclusively dependent α^s and requires activation by cAMP-CRP. *Journal of Molecular Biology*, Vol 276, pp. 339-353, ISSN 0022-2836

Mayer, C., Moritz, R, Kirschner, C., Borchard, W., Maibaum, R., Wingender, J. & Flemming, H.-C. (1999). The role of intermolecular interactions: studies on model systems for bacterial biofilms. *International Journal of Biological Macromolecules*, Vol. 26, pp. 3-16, ISSN 0141-8130

McCann, M.P., Kidwell, J.P. & Matin, A. (1991). The putative α factor KatF has a central role in development of starvation-mediated general resistance in *Escherichia coli*. *Journal of Bacteriology*, Vol. 173, No. 13, pp. 4188-4194, ISSN 0021-9193

Menninger, J.R. & Otto, D.P. (1982). Erythromycin, carbomycin, and spiramycin inhibit protein synthesis by stimulating the dissociation of peptidyl-tRNA from ribosomes. *Antimicrobial Agents and Chemotheraphy*, Vol. 21, No. 5, pp. 811-818, ISSN 0066-4804

Mentag, R., Luckevich, M., Morency, M.-J. & Séguin, A. (2003). Bacterial disease resistance of transgenic hybrid poplar expressing the synthetic antimicrobial peptide D4E1. *Tree Physiology*, Vol. 23, No. 6, pp. 405-411, ISSN 0829-318X

Mitchison, J.M. (1969). Enzyme synthesis in synchronous cultures. *Science*, Vol. 165, pp. 657-663, ISSN 1095-9203

Moré, M.I., Finger, L.D., Stryker, J.L., Fuqua, C., Eberhard, A. & Winans, S.C. (1996). Enzymatic synthesis of a *quorum sensing* autoinducer through use of defined substrates. *Sciences*, Vol. 272, No. 5268, pp. 1655-1658, ISSN 1095-9203

Morton, L.H.G., Greenway, D.L.A., Gaylarde, C.C. & Surman, S.B. (1998). Consideration of some implications of the resistance of biofilms to biocides. *International Biodeterioration & Biodegradation*, Vol. 41, pp. 247-259, ISSN 0964-8305

Moyed, H.S. & Bertrand, K.P. (1983). hipA, a newly recognized gene of *Escherichia coli* K-12 that affects frequency of persistence after inhibition of murein synthesis. *Journal of Bacteriology*, Vol. 155, No. 2, pp. 768-775, ISSN 0021-9193

Myszka, K. & Czaczyk, K. (2009). Characterization of adhesive exopolysaccharide (EPS) produced by *Pseudomonas aeruginosa* under starvation conditions. *Current Microbiology*, Vol. 58, pp.541-546, ISSN 1432-0991

Myszka, K. & Czaczyk, K. (2011). Bacterial biofilms on food contact surfaces - a review. *Polish Journal of Food Sciences and Nutrition*, Vol. 61, No. 3, pp. 173-180, ISSN 1230-0322

Newton, J.A. & Fray, R.G. (2004). Integration of environmental and host-derived signals with quorum sensing during plant microbe interactions. *Cellular Microbiology*, Vol. 6, No. 3, pp. 213-224, ISSN 1462-5822

Nikaido, H. & Vaara, M. (1985). Molecular basis of bacterial outer membrane permeability. *Microbiological Reviews*, Vol. 49, No. 1, pp. 1-32, ISSN 0146-0749

Nikaido, H. (1989). Outer membrane barrier as a mechanism of antibacterial resistance. *Antimicrobial Agents and Chemotheraphy*, Vol. 33, No. 11, pp. 1831-1836, ISSN 0066-4804

Nikaido, H. (1992). Porins and specific channels of bacterial outer membranes. *Molecular Microbiology*, Vol. 6, No. 4, pp. 435-442, ISSN 1365-2958

Nikaido, H. (1996). Multidrug efflux pumps of gram-negative bacteria. *Journal of Bacteriology*, Vol. 178, No. 20, pp. 5853-5859, ISSN 0021-9193

Nobile, C.J. & Mitchell, A.P. (2007). Microbial biofilms: e pluribus unum. *Current Biology*, Vol. 17, pp. R349-R353, ISSN 0960-9822

O'Toole, G., Kaplan, H.B. & Kolter, R. (2000). Biofilm formation as microbial development. *Annual Review of Microbiology*, Vol. 54, pp. 49-79, ISSN 0066-4227

Pagés, J.-M., James, C.E. & Winterhalter, M. (2008). The porin and the permeating antibiotic: a selective diffusion barrier in gram-negative bacteria. *Nature Reviews Microbiology*, Vol. 6, pp. 893-903, ISSN 1740-1526

Pagés, J.-M., Alibert-Franco, S., Mahamoud, A., Bolla, J.M., Davin-Regli, A., Chevalier, J. & Garnotel, E. (2010). Efflux pumps of gram-negative bacteria, a new target for new molecules. *Current Topics of Medicinal Chemistry*, Vol. 8, pp. 1848-1857, ISSN 1568-0266

Parsek, M.R., Val., D.L., Hanzelka, B.L., Cronan, J.E. & Greenberg, E.P. (1999). Acyl homoserine-lactone quorum-sensing signal generation. *Proceedings of the National Academy of Sciences USA*, Vol. 96, No. 8, pp. 4360-4365, ISSN 0027-8424

Parsek, M.R. & Greenberg, E.P. (2005). Sociomicrobiology: the connections between quorum sensing and biofilms. *TRENDS in Microbiology*, Vol. 13, No. 1, pp. 27-33, ISSN 0966-842X

Pisbarro, A.G., De Petro, M.A. & Ishiguro, E.E. (1990). Dissociation of the ampicilin-induced lysis of amino acid-deprived *Escherichia coli* into two stages. *Journal of Bacteriology*, Vol. 172, No. 4, pp. 2187-2190, ISSN 0021-9193

Platt, T.G & Fuqua, C. (2010). What's in a name? The semantics of *quorum sensing*. *TRENDS in Microbiology*, Vol. 18, No. 9, pp. 383-387, ISSN 0966-842X

Plésiat, P. & Nikaido, H. (1992). Outer membranes of gram-negative bacteria are permeable to steroid probes. *Molecular Microbiology*, Vol. 6, No. 10, pp. 1323-1333, ISSN 1365-2958

Poole, K. (2001). Multidrug resistance in Gram-negative bacteria. *Current Opinion in Microbiology*, Vol. 4, pp. 500-508, ISSN 1369-5274

Poole, K. & Srikumar, R. (2001). Multidrug efflux in *Pseudomonas aeruginosa*: components, mechanisms and clinical significance. *Current Topics in Medicinal Chemistry*, Vol. 1, pp. 59-71, ISSN 1862-2461

Poole, K. (2005). Efflux-mediated antimicrobial resistance. *Journal of Antimicrobial Chemotherapy*, Vol. 56, pp. 20-51, ISSN 1460-2091

Potera, C. (1999) Forging a link between biofilms and disease. *Science*, Vol. 283, pp. 1837-1839, ISSN 10950-9203

Poulsen, L.K., Ballard, G. & Stahl, D.A. (1993). Use of rRNA fluorescence in situ hybridization for measuring the activity of single cells in young and established biofilms. *Applied and Environmental Microbiology*, Vol. 59, No. 5, pp. 1354-1360, ISSN 0099-2240

Rodionov, D.G. & Ishiguro, E.E. (1995). Direct correlation between overproduction of guanosine 3',5'-bispyrophosphate (ppGpp) and penicillin tolerance in *Escherichia coli*. *Journal of Bacteriology*, Vol. 177, No. 15, pp. 4224-4229, ISSN 0021-9193

Roeder, R.S., Lenz, J., Tarne, P., Gebel, J., Exner, M. & Szewzyk, U. (2010). Long-term effects of disinfectants on the community composition of drinking water biofilms. *International Journal of Hygiene and Environmental Health*, Vol. 213, pp. 183-189, ISSN 1438-4639

Römling,U., Sierralta, W.D., Eriksson, K. & Normark, S. (1998). Multicellular and aggregative behaviour of *Salmonella typhimurium* strains is controlled by mutations in the *agfD* promoter. *Molecular Microbiology*, Vol. 28, pp. 249-264, ISSN 0950-382X

Russell, A.D. (1999). Bacterial resistance to disinfectants: present knowledge and future problems. *Journal of Hospital Infectious*, Vol. 43, pp. S57-S68, ISSN 0195-6701

Russell, A.D. (2002). Antibiotic and biocide resistance in bacteria: introduction. *Journal of Applied Microbiology*, Vol. 92, pp. 1S-3S, ISSN 1364-5072

Sakuragi, Y. & Kolter, R. (2007). *Quorum sensing* regulation of the biofilm matrix genes (*pel*) of *Pseudomonas aeruginosa*. *Journal of Bacteriology*, Vol. 189, No. 14, pp. 5383-5386, ISSN 0021-9193

Sauer, K., Camper, A.K., Ehrlich, G.D., Costerton, J.W. & Davies, D.G. (2002). *Pseudomonas aeruginosa* displays mulrtiple phenotypes during development as a biofilm. *Journal of Bacteriology*, Vol. 184, No. 4, pp. 1140-1154, ISSN 0021-9193

Schaefer, A.L., Val, D.L., Hanzelka, B.L., Cronan, J.E. & Greenberg, E.P. (1996). Generation of cell-to-cell signals in *quorum sensing*: acyl homoserine lactone synthase activity of a purified *Vibrio fischeri* LuxI protein. *Proceedings of the National Academy of Sciences USA*, Vol. 93, No. 18, pp. 9505-9509, ISSN 0027-8424

Schertzer, J.W., Boulette, M.L. & Whiteley, M. (2009). More than a signal: non-signaling properties of quorum sensing molecules. *TRENDS in Microbiology*, Vol. 17, No. 5, pp. 189-195, ISSN 0966-842X

Schockman, G.D., Daneo-Moore, L., Kariyama, R. & Massidda, O. (1996). Bacterial walls, peptydoglycan hydrolases, and autolysin. *Microbial Drug Resistance*, Vol. 2, pp.95-98, ISSN 1931-8448

Senior, K. (2004). Navigating the hidden depths of biofilms. *The Lancet Infectious Diseases*, Vol. 4, pp. 196

Seoane, A.S. & Levy, S.B. (1995). Characterization of MarR, the repressor of the multiple antibiotic resistance (*mar*) operon in *Escherichia coli*. *Journal of Bacteriology*, Vol. 177, No. 12, pp. 3414-3419, ISSN 0021-9193

Shafahi, M. & Vafai, K. (2009). Biofilm affected characteristics of porous structures. *International Journal of Heat and Mass Transfer*, Vol. 52, pp. 574-581, ISSN 0017-9310

Shih, P.-C. & Huang, C.-T. (2002). Effects of quorum sensing deficiency on *Pseudomonas aeruginosa* biofilm formation and antibiotic resistance. *Journal of Antimicrobial Chemotheraphy*, Vol. 49, pp. 309-314, ISSN 1460-2091

Shirtliff, M.E., Mader, J.T. & Camper, A.K. (2002). Molecular interactions in biofilms. *Chemistry & Biology*, Vol. 9, pp. 859-871, ISSN 1074-5521

Siegrist, H. & Gujer, W. (1985). Mass transfer mechanisms in a heterotrophic biofilm. *Water Research*, Vol. 19, pp. 1369-1378

Simões, M., Simões, L.C. & Vieira, M.J. (2009). Species association increases biofilm resistance to chemical and mechanical treatments. *Water Research*, Vol. 43, pp. 229-237, ISSN 0043-1354

Singh, R., Paul, D. & Jain, R.K. (2006). Biofilms: implications in bioremediation. *TRENDS in Microbiology*, Vol. 14, No. 9, pp. 389-397, ISSN 0966-842X

Spoering, A.L. & Lewis, K. (2001). Biofilm and planktonic cells of *Pseudomonas aeruginosa* have similar resistance to killing by antimicrobials. *Journal of Bacteriology*, Vol. 183, No. 23, pp. 6746-6751, ISSN 0021-9193

Steidla, A., Allesen-Holm, M., Riedel, K., Berg, G., Givskov, M., Molin, S. & Eberl, L. (2002). Identification and characterization of N-acylhomoserine lactone-dependent quorum-sensing system in *Pseudomonas putida* strain IsoF. *Applied and Environmental Microbiology*, Vol. 68, No. 12, pp. 6371-6382, ISSN 1098-5336

Stewart, P.S. (1996). Theoretical aspects of antibiotic diffusion into microbial biofilms. *Antimicrobial Agents and Chemotheraphy*, Vol. 40, No. 11, pp. 2517-2522, ISSN 0066-4804

Stewart, P.S., Roe, F., Rayner, J., Elkins, J.G., Lewandowski, Z, Ochsner, U.A. & Hassett, D.J. (2000). Effect of catalase on hydrogen peroxide penetration into *Pseudomonas aeruginosa* biofilms. *Applied and Environmental Microbiology*, Vol. 66, No. 2, pp. 836-838, ISSN 0099-2240

Stewart, P.S. (2003). Diffusion in biofilms. *Journal of Bacteriology*, Vol. 185, No. 5, pp. 1485-1491, ISSN 0021-9193

Sternberg, C., Christensen, B.B., Johansen, T.,Nielsen, A.T., Andersen, J.B., Givskov, M. & Molin, S. (1999). Distribution of bacterial growth activity in flow-chamber biofilms.

Applied and Environmental Microbiology, Vol., 65, No. 9, pp. 4108-4117, ISSN 0099-2240

Stover, C.K., Pham, X.Q., Erwin, A.L., Mizoguchi, S.D., Warrener, P., Hickey, M.J., Brinkman, F.S., Hufnagle, W.O., Kowalik, D.J., Lagrou, M., Garber, R.L., Goltry, L., Tolentino, E., Westbrock-Wadman, Y., Yuan, Y., Brody, L.L., Coulter, S.N., Folger, K.R., Kas, A., Larbig, R., Lim, R., Smith, K., Spencer, D., Wong, G.K., Wu, Z., Paulsen I.T., Reizer, J., Saier, M.H., Hancock, R.E., Lory, S. & Olson, M.V. (2000). Complete genome sequence of *Pseudomonas aeruginosa* PA01, an opportunistic pathogen. *Nature*, Vol. 406, pp. 959-964, ISSN 0028-0836

Strøm, A.R. & Kaasen, I. (1993). Trehalose metabolism in *Escherichia coli*: stress protection and stress regulation of gene expression. *Molecular Microbiology*, Vol. 8, pp. 205-210, ISSN 1365-2958

Suci, P.A., Mittelman, M.W., Yu, F.P. & Geesey, G.G. (1994). Investigation of ciprofloxacin penetration into *Pseudomonas aeruginosa* biofilms. *Antimicrobial Agents and Chemotherapy*, Vol. 38, No. 9., pp. 2125-2133, ISSN 0066-4804

Suntharalingam, P. & Cvitkovitch, D.G. (2005). *Quorum sensing* in streptococcal biofilm formation. *TRENDS in Microbiology*, Vol. 13, No. 1, pp. 3-6, ISSN 0966-842X

Sutherland, I.W. (2001). The biofilm matrix - an immobilized but dynamic microbial environment. *TRENDS in Microbiology*, Vol. 9, No. 5, pp. 222-227, ISSN 0966-842X

Tanaka, G., Shigeta, M., Komatsuzawa, H., Sugai, M., Suginaka, H. & Usui, T. (1999). Effect of the growth rate of *Pseudomonas aeruginosa* biofilms on the susceptibility to antimicrobial agents: beta-lactams and fluoroquinolones. *Chemotherapy*, Vol. 45, pp. 28-36, ISSN 0009-3157

Tolker-Nielsen,T. & Molin, S. (2000). Spatial organization of microbial biofilm communities. *Microbial Ecology*, Vol. 40, pp. 75-84, ISSN 0095-3628

Toumanen, E., Cozens, R., Tosch, W., Zak, O. & Tomasz, A. (1989). The rate of killing of *Escherichia coli* by beta-lactam antibiotics is strictly proportional to the rate of bacterial growth. *Journal of General Microbiology*, Vol. 132, pp. 1297-1304, ISSN 1350-0872

Tresse, O., Jouenne, T. & Junter, G.-A. (1995). The role of oxygen limitation in the resistance of agar-entrapped, sessile-like *Escherichia coli* to aminoglycoside and β-lactam antibiotics. *Journal of Antimicrobial Chemotheraphy*, Vol. 35, pp. 521-526, ISSN 1460-2091

Turovsky, Y., Kashtanov, D., Paskhover, B. & Chikindas, M.L. (2007). *Quorum sensing*: fact, fiction and everything in between. *Advences in Applied Microbiology*, Vol. 62, pp. 191-234, ISSN 0065-2164

Yasuda, H., Ajiki, Y., Koga, T. & Yokota T. (1994). Interaction between clarithromycin and biofilms fordem by *Staphylococcus epidermidis*. *Antimicrobial Agents and Chemotherapy*, Vol. 38, No. 9., pp. 2138-2141, ISSN 0066-4804

Yoon, S.S., Hennigan, R.F., Hilliard, G.M., Ochsner, U.A., Parvatiyar, K., Kamani, M.C., Allen, H.L., DeKievit, T.R., Gardner, P.R., Schwab, U., Rowe, J.J., Iglewski, B.H., McDermott, T.R., Mason, R.P., Wozniak, D.J., Hancock, R.E., Parsek, M.R., Noah, T.L., Boucher R.C. & Hassett. (2002). *Pseudomonas aeruginosa* anaerobic respiration in biofilms: relationships to cystic fibrosis pathogenesis. *Developmental Cell*, Vol. 3, pp.593-603, ISSN 1534-5807

Walters III, M.C., Roe, F., Bugnicourt, A., Franklin, M.J. & Stewart, P.S. (2003). Contributions of antibiotic penetration, oxygen limitation, and low metabolic activity to tolerance of *Pseudomonas aeruginosa* biofilms to ciprofloxacin and tobramycin. *Antimicrobial Agents and Chemotherapy*, Vol. 47, No. 1, pp. 317-323, ISSN 0066-4804

Watnick, P. & Kolter, R. (2000). Biofilm, city of microbes. *Journal of Bacteriology*, Vol. 182, No. 10, pp. 2675-2679, ISSN 0021-9193

Webb, J.S., Thompson, L.S., James, S., Charlton, T., Tolker-Nielsen, T., Koch, B., Givskov, M. & Kjelleberg, S. (2003). Cell death in *Pseudomonas aeruginosa* biofilm development. *Journal of Bacteriology*, Vol. 185, No. 15, pp. 4585-4592, ISSN 0021-9193

Weinberg, E.D. (2008). Iron availability and infections. *Biochimica et Biophysica Acta*, DOI: 10.10.16/j.bbagen.2008.07.002

Welsh, D.T. & Herbert, R.A. (1999). Osmotically induced intracellular trehalose, but not glycine betaine accumulation promotes desiccation tolerance in *Escherichia coli*. *FEMS Microbiology Letters*, Vol. 174, No. 1, pp. 57-63, ISSN 1574-6968

Wentland, E.J., Stewart, P.S., Huang, C.-T. & McFeters, G.A. (1996). Spartial variations in growth rate within *Klebsiella pneumoniae* colonies and biofilm. *Biotechnology Progress*, Vol. 12, pp. 316-321, ISSN 1520-6033

White, D.G. & McDermott, P.F. (2001). Biocides, drug resistance and microbial evolution. *Current Opinion in Microbiology*, Vol. 4, No. 3, pp. 313-317, ISSN 1369-5274

Whitehead,N.A., Barnard, A.M.L., Slater H., Simpson, N.J.L. & Salmond, G.P.C. (2001). *Quorum sensing* in gram-negative bacteria. *FEMS Microbiology Reviews*, Vol. 25, pp. 365-404, ISSN 1574-6976

Whiteley, M., Parsek, M.R. & Greenberg, E.P. (2000). Regulation of quorum sensing by RpoS in *Pseudomonas aeruginosa*. *Journal of Bacteriology*, Vol. 182, No. 15, pp. 4356-4360, ISSN 0021-9193

Whiteley, M., Bangera, M.G., Bumgarner, R.E., Parsek, G.M., Teitzel, G.M., Lory, S. & Greenberg, E.P. (2001). Gene expression in *Pseudomonas aeruginosa* biofilm. *Nature*, Vol. 413, pp. 860-864, ISSN 0028-0836

Williams, P., Winzer, K., Chan, W.C. & Cámara, M. (2007). Look who's talking: communication and *quorum sensing* in the bacterial world. *Philosophical Transactions of the Royal Society B: Biological Sciences*, Vol. 262, No. 1483, pp. 1119-1134, DOI: 10.1098/rstb.2007.2039

Wimpenny, J., Manz, W. & Szewzyk, U. (2000). Heterogeneity in biofilms. *FEMS Microbiology Reviews*, Vol. 24, pp. 661-671, ISSN 1574-6976

Wood, T.K., Hong, S.H. & Ma, Q. (2011). Engineering biofilm formation and dispersal. *TRENDS in Biotechnology*, Vol. 29, No. 2, pp. 87-94, ISSN 0167-7799

Xu, K.D., Stewart, P.S., Xia, F., Huang, C.-T. & McFeters, G.A. (1998). Spatial physiological heterogeneity in *Pseudomonas aeruginosa* biofilms is determined by oxygen availability. *Applied and Environmental Microbiology*, Vol. 64, No. 10, pp. 4035-4039, ISSN 0099-2240

Xu, K.D., McFeters, G.A. & Stewart, P.S. (2000). Biofilm resistance to antimicrobial agents. *Microbiology*, Vol. 146, pp. 547-549, ISSN 1465-2080

Xu, K.D., Franklin, M.J., Park, C.H., McFeters, G.A. & Stewart, P.S. (2001). Gene expression and protein levels of the stationary phase sigma factor, RpoS, in continuously-fed *Pseudomonas aeruginosa* biofilms. *FEMS Microbiology Letters*, Vol. 199, No. 1, pp. 67-71, ISSN 1574-6968

Zgurskaya, H.I. & Nikaido, H. (2000). Multidrug resistance mechanism: drug efflux across two membranes. *Molecular Microbiology*, Vol. 37, No. 2, pp. 219-225

10

Antimicrobial Activity of Endophytes from Brazilian Medicinal Plants

Chirlei Glienke[1,*], Fabiana Tonial[2], Josiane Gomes-Figueiredo[1,2], Daiani Savi[2], Vania Aparecida Vicente[2], Beatriz H. L. N. Sales Maia[3] and Yvelise Maria Possiede[4]

[1]*Department of Genetics, Federal University of Parana (UFPR), Setor de Ciências Biológicas, Centro Politécnico, Curitiba, Paraná,*
[2]*Department of Basic Pathology, Federal University of Parana (UFPR), Setor de Ciências Biológicas, Centro Politécnico, Curitiba, Paraná,*
[3]*Department of Chemistry, Federal University of Parana (UFPR), Setor de Ciências Exatas, Centro Politécnico, Curitiba, Paraná,*
[4]*Department of Biology, Federal University of Mato Grosso do Sul, Campo Grande, Mato Grosso do Sul*
Brazil

1. Introduction

The increased use of antibiotics has become the bacteria resistant. Currently, there are increasing problems worldwide with multiresistant bacteria. Examples of the resistance problems on a global scale are the methicillin-resistant *Staphylococcus aureus* (MRSA), vancomycin-resistant enterococci and *Enterobacteriaceae* producing beta-lactamases. A study of the *World Health Organization (WHO)* revealed that 90% of the bacteria strains are resistant to drugs of first choice. Bioprospecting studies of endophytic microorganisms for pharmaceutical and biotechnological purposes are fundamental for the discovery of new substances for human therapeutics including antibiotics, antimalarials, and anticarcinogenics (Strobel & Long 1998; Strobel 2002; Strobel & Daisy 2003). Endophytic fungi of medicinal plants are currently being widely studied in the search for new potentially useful secondary metabolites. The production of bioactive secondary metabolites by medicinal plants and by the endophytes provided countless drugs selected as important therapeutic options for innumerable disease. The endophytes still have wide potential to be explored what could expand even more the phenomenal contribution to health and well being. Aware of the reality of multi-resistant pathogenic microorganisms and the producing capacity of antimicrobial compounds by endophytes it is indispensable the search of antibiotic substances with new mechanisms of action, less toxic effect and/or medication enhance through this apparently inexhaustible bioactive metabolites source (Demain &

* Corresponding Author

Sanchez, 2009). Some studies show a relation between the endophyte secondary metabolites producing and the plant where it is found increasing the interest in endophytic microbiota of medicinal plants. Gene transference from the plant to the endophyte and the other way around is said to happen allowing common secondary metabolites production (Peixoto Neto et al., 2004). The classical example was the isolation of the fungi *Taxomyces andreanae* from the plant *Taxus brevifolia*, both taxol producers, making possible the use of this antitumor and the preservation of the medicinal plant (Stierle et al., 1993).

Recent and promising reports of the some brazilian medicinal plant and endophytes fungi as a source of important bioactive compounds and novel structures (Table 1). Endophytic fungi from *Lippia sidoides* demonstrate pharmaceutical potential and can be seen as an attractive source of biologically active compounds (Souza-Motta et al., 2011). One isolate of *Penicillium janthinellum*, endophytic from fruits of *Melia azedarach* (Meliaceae) producers of polyketides citrinin, emodin, 1,6,8-trihydroxy-3-hydroxymethylanthraquinone, and a new modified anthraquinone, named janthinone. The authors reported citrinin inhibited 100% of *Leishmania* growth after 48h at a concentration of 40 mg mL^{-1} (Marinho et al., 2005). Oliveira et al. (2010), in study with metabolites produced by the fungus *Pestalotiopsis guepinii* isolated from *Virola michelii* reported a new anthraquinone derivative, named guepinone, along with the known substances isosulochrin and chloroisosulochrin. *In vitro* quantitative and qualitative information obtained in study with endophytic fungi isolated from comfrey (*Symphytum officinale* L.) leaves indicates potential against the phytopathogenic fungus *S. sclerotiorum* (Rocha et al., 2009). Therefore, the use of bioactive products from the endophytic strains and/or the biological control with *S. sclerotiorum* needs investigation. Two novel benzopyrans have been isolated from *Curvularia* sp., an endophytic fungus from *Ocotea corymbosa* showed weak in vitro antifungal activity against *Cladosporium sphaerospermum* and *C. cladosporioides* (Teles et al., 2006). Endophytic fungi recovered from leaves of the bioactive Brazilian plant species *Ageratum myriadenia, Palicourea tetraphylla, Piptadenia adiantoides* and *Trixis vauthieri* could be a promising source of antitumoral, leishmanicidal and trypanocidal secondary metabolites, which could be used for the development of new drugs (Rosa et al., 2010). Dendryol E and dendryol F, two novel anthraquinone derivatives, have also been isolated from *Phoma sorghina*, endophyte found in association with the medicinal plant *Tithonia diversifolia* (Borges & Pupo, 2006). *Chaetomium globosum* was isolated as an endophytic fungus from the healthy leaves of *Viguiera robusta* (Momesso et al., 2008) and were identified genera *Alternaria, Cochliobolus, Diaporthe, Epicoccum, Guignardia, Phoma,* and *Phomopsis* from *Luehea divaricata*, known popularly in Brazil as açoita-cavalo (Bernardi-Wenzel et al., 2010). Crude extracts of endophytic fungi isolated from *Smallanthus sonchifolius* also showed antimicrobial effectiveness (Ramos et al., 2010) The antibacterial activity of the azaphylones, citrinin and citrinin H-1, were identified in *Penicillium* species isolated as endophytic fungi from *Melia azedarach* and *Murraya paniculata* (Pastre et al., 2007). *Xylaria* sp., an endophytic fungus from *Piper aduncum* were evaluated against the fungi *C. cladosporioides* and *C. sphaerospermum* and cytotoxicity *in vitro* against HeLA and CHO cells lines were investigated, the cytochalasins showed a strong activity against HeLA (Silva et al., 2010). Oliveira et al. (2009) isolated as endophytes two strains of *Penicillium* sp. from *Alibertia macrophylla* (Rubiaceae), producers of orcinol and 4-

hydroxymellein, which exhibited detection limits of 5.00 and 10.0 μg against *Cladosporium cladosporioides* and *C. sphaerospermum*. Silva et al. (2005 and 2006) reported a isolate of *Phomopsis cassiae* endophytic from *Cassia spectabilis* (Fabaceae) producer of ethyl 2,4-dihydroxy-5,6-dimethylbenzoate and phomopsilactone. Both displayed strong antifungal activity against the phytopatogenic fungi *Cladosporium cladosporioides* and *C. sphaerospermum*, as well as cytotoxicity against human cervical tumor cell line (HeLa), in *in vitro* assays. *Bacillus pumilus* was isolated from cassava (*Manihot esculenta*) cultivated by Brazilian Amazon Indian tribes, which produces other metabolite with antifungal activity, the pumilacidin (Melo et al., 2009).

Medicinal plant	Endophytes fungi	References
Ageratum myriadenia	*Alternaria arborescens, Bipolaris* sp., *Penicillium citrinum and Penicillium griseofulvum*	Rosa et al., 2010
Cassia spectabilis	*Phomopsis cassiae*	Silva et al., 2005 and 2006
Lippia sidoides	*Colletotrichum gloeosporioides, Alternaria alternata, Guignardia bidwelli and Phomopsis archeri*	Souza-Motta et al., 2011
Luehea divaricata	*Alternaria,Cochliobolus, Diaporthe, Epicoccum, Guignardia, Phoma and Phomopsis*	Bernardi-Wenzel et al., 2010
Maytenus ilicifolia	*Pestalotipsis sp., Pestalotiopis vismae and Pestalotiopsis microspora*	Figueiredo et al., 2007
Melia azedarach L.	*Penicillium* sp. and *P. janthinellum*	Marinho et. al., 2005
Murraya paniculata	*Penicillium* sp.	Pastre et al., 2007
Ocotea corymbosa	*Curvalaria* sp	Teles et al., 2006
Palicourea tetraphylla	*Arthrium* sp. , *Fusarium oxysporum, Penicillium griseofulvum and Penicillium citrinum*	Rosa et al., 2010
Piper aduncum	*Xylaria* sp.	Silva et al., 2010
Piptadenia adiantoides	*Arthrium* sp. *Gibberella* sp.	Rosa et al., 2010
Smallanthus sonchifolius	*Papulaspora immersa and Arthrinium arundinis*	Ramos et al., 2010
Spondias mombin	*Guignardia* sp.	Rodrigues-Heerklotz et al., 2001
Symphytumofficinale L	*Trichophyton* sp., *Chrysosporium* sp., *Candida pseudotropicalis and Candida tropicalis*	Rocha et al., 2009
Tithonia diversifolia	*Phoma sorghina*	Borges & Pupo, 2006
Trixis vauthieri	*Arthrium* sp. and *Xylaria* sp.	Rosa et al., 2010
Viguiera robusta,	*Chaetomium globosum*	Momesso et al., 2008
Virola michelii	*Pestalotiopsis guepinii*	Oliveira et al., 2011

Table 1. Some Brazilian medicinal plants and endophytic fungi associated

An important medicinal plant in this context is *Maytenus ilicifolia*, commonly known as espinheira santa. *M. ilicifolia* is native to South America, being most commonly found in southern Brazil, and is widely used in the treatment of stomach ulcers and other gastric problems. The heavy exploitation of this plant because of its medicinal properties led it to be included in the current list of endangered species (SEMA, 1995; Bittencourt, 2000). *Schinus terebinthifolius* Raddi (peppertree) is other important medicinal plant in Argentina, Brazil and Paraguay (Mytinger & Williamson, 1987). In Brazil the bark, leaves and fruits have been used in popular medicine due to their medicinal properties (Guerra et al., 2000; Lorenzi, 2002; Dgáspari et al., 2005; Ribas et al., 2006). Actions anti-inflammatory and antiseptic for treatment of wounds, urinary and respiratory infections are listed as medicinal properties popularly known (Lima et al., 2006). Studies showed antimicrobial (Degáspari et al., 2005; Schmourlo et al., 2005; Fenner et al., 2006; Ribas et al., 2006; Johann et al., 2007; Soares et al., 2007) and antitumor activities (Queires et al., 2006). *Vochysia divergens*, popularly known as cambará, is a tree commonly found in wet soils of "Pantanal Matogrossense" in Brazil. This tree has great economic importance for the local population, especially in the production of wood. Despite the economic interest and broad popular medicinal usage of the *V. divergens*, there are very few reports on the chemical composition and biological activity of this plant. In respect to the biological activities related to this species, it was verified that the etanolic extract of *V. divergens* barks presented bactericide activity against *Staphylococcus aureus* and antinociceptive activity. Leaves and barks are used in popular medicine against respiratory and gastrointestinal problems (Hess et al., 1995).

Looking forward to find a solution for the advance of multi-resistant bacteria the present study made a comparison between the composts with antimicrobial activity produced by the leaves of the medicinal plants *S. terebinthifolius* and from its endophytes and from the plants *M. ilicifolia* and *V. divergens*. The antimicrobial activity and the chemical composition of the crude extract and fractions of the *S. terebenthifolius* leaves, were analyzed. Parallel with it, endophytes from the same tree were isolated and selected in order to extract its active secondary metabolites. Those extracts with positive result were also chemist evaluated and compared with the extract and fractions from the leaves. Endophytes were isolated from these 3 medicinal plants and selected in order to extract their active compounds. Similarities and differences between active compounds produced by S. terebinthifolius leaves and some of their endophytes were analised.

2. Methods

2.1 Plant material

The peppertree (*S. terebinthifolius*) leaves were collected from a tree found at the latitude - 25°26.827S, longitude - 49°13.997O. The botanical identification has been made at the herbarium of the Botanical Department of Federal University of Parana (UFPR - UPCB), where a specimen of the plant can be found under the registration: UPCB-30848. *M. ilicifolia* leaves were collected from Centro Nacional de Pesquisa de Floresta (CNPF) of EMBRAPA (Empresa Brasileira de Pesquisa Agropecuária), Paraná, Brazil (latitude -25.369227, longitude -49.189301). The *V. divergens* leaves were collected from 10 tree from Pantanal, Brazil (latitude -19.254108, longitude -57.030029).

2.2 Isolation of endophytes from plant

To the endophytic isolation, preference was given to leaves with no marks, scratches or wounds, according to methodology described by Petrini (1991). The leaves were washed in running water. The petioles were paraffin-embedded and went through this battery of solutions: sterile distilled water for 1 minute, ethanol 70% for 1 minute, sodium hypochlorite 3% for 4 minutes, ethanol 70% for 30 seconds and sterile distilled water for 6 minutes. The leaves were cut in fragments that were later cultivated for 20 days at 28°C in a potato-dextrose-agar medium or selective agar for actinomycete (AC) (Küster & Williams, 1964). To eliminate the epiphytic microorganisms of V. divergens leaves we used the purification protocol of six steps (Bettiol, 2008), in medium AC added of Tetracycline (100 µg/mL) and Cycloheximide (50 µg/mL). The living cultures were deposited in the LabGeM collection, Federal University of Paraná, Curitiba, Paraná, Brazil (http://www.labgem.ufpr.br/).

2.3 Endophytes identification

An analysis based on a polyphasic approach integrating taxonomic information, morphological traits and the sequencing of the ITS1-5.8S-ITS2 of the rDNA or 16S was used, as described by Gomes-Figueiredo et al. (2007). Isolates were initially identified based on their microscopic and macroscopic characteristics including their morphology and characteristics when grown on the following culture media: PDA, oatmeal agar (OA) (20 g l^{-1} oat, 20 g l^{-1} glucose, 15 g l^{-1} agar), malt extract agar (MEA), and complete medium (CM) (Pontecorvo et al., 1953). Isolates were incubated for 7 days at 22 or 28°C and a 12 h light: 12 h dark photoperiod. The experimental design was completely randomized with 3 replicates. Colonies were analyzed with respect to their average diameter (cm), the aspect of their borders, the aspect and coloration of the mycelium, sporulation, mycelium characteristics, the production of acervuli, the coloration of the reverse of the Petri dish, the viscosity and coloration of the medium, and the size and coloration of the conidia. A total of 20 conidia from each culture medium were observed under light microscopy (x 1000 magnification) after being grown for 7, 14, and 21 days. Conidia were assessed with respect to their width and length and the length of the apical appendages. The coloration of the median cells was also recorded. For actinomycetes identification, characteristics of colonies were used, after growth in AC medium. The isolates Gram-stained were observed under light microscopy (x 1000 magnification).

The fungi isolates were randomly selected as morphotypes according to Arnold et al. (2000), and the endophytes that presented at least one of the extracts with antimicrobial activity were submitted to identification using ITS sequences of the rDNA. DNA extraction followed method described by Raeder & Broda (1985), modified by Glienke-Blanco et al. (2002). For the fungi, the primers V9G (De Hoog et al., 2003) and ITS4 (White et al., 1990) were used to amplify the ITS1-5.8S-ITS2 of the nuclear ribosomal RNA, in the following reaction mixture (50 µl): 0,2 mM of each dNTP, 1X Tris/HCl, 1.5 mM $MgCl_2$, 1.5 U Taq polymerase, 0.06 µM each primer and 50ng of DNA; the PCR was processed in a Mastercycler Gradient (Eppendorf®) with the following program: 94 °C for 2 min at the start followed by 35 cycles of 94 °C for 30 s, 55 °C for 1 min and 72 °C for 1 min and a final extension of 72 °C for 3 min. For the actinomycete the primers Sm6F

(5'GGTGGCGAAGGCGGA 3') and Sm5R (5' GAACTGAGACCGGCTTTTTGA 3') were used to amplify the 16S rDNA. Amplification conditions followed Arzanlou et al. (2008) for the fungi and Monciardini et al. (2002) for the actinomycete. Amplicons were sequenced using both PCR primers and DYEnamic ET Dye Terminator Cycle Sequencing Kit for MegaBACE (Amersham Biosciences). Sequences were manually aligned using Mega v. 5 software (Kumar et al., 2004) by inserting gaps. The obtained sequences were aligned according to existing sequences at the data base NCBI though the BLASTn program. Phylogenetic analyses of the aligned sequence data were performed with PAUP (Phylogenetic Analysis Using Parsimony) v. 4.0b10 (Swofford, 1998).

2.4 Endophytes extracts

Endophytes were selected for the extraction of active metabolites by fermentation. After the growth in potato-dextrose-agar medium in Petri dishes for 7-14 days at 28°C, fragments of the endophytes with a diameter of 10mm were removed and sowed in Erlenmeyers with 50mL and 100mL of the liquid medium Czapeck (Silva et al., 2004), MPE (Hamada et al., 1974) and malt extract broth (20 g l^1 malt extract, 1 g l^1 peptone, 20 g l^1 glucose), and were incubated at 28°C at 120rpm. The 50mL cultures were incubated for 24 hours, while the ones with 100mL of medium were cultivated for 7 days. After the predetermined period the mycelium was separated of the metabolic medium by paper Whatman n°4 vacuum filtration and then stored. Either compounds from the culture and the ones retained on the cell structures were extracted with ethyl acetate p. a. (EtOAc; Merck). Solvent evaporation was carried out using a rotaevaporator at 45°C. The final extract was weighed and diluted in methanol, methanolic extracts (ME) at a concentration of 10 mg/mL (Corrado & Rodrigues, 2004). The fermentative liquid was lyophilized, weighed and also diluted in ultrapure sterilized water, aqueous extracts (AE) at concentration of 10 mg/mL.

2.5 Antimicrobial activity of endophytes extracts

For the evaluation of the antimicrobial activity of the secondary metabolites obtained from the culture of the endophytes was used bioautographic TLC agar overlay assay (Corrado & Rodrigues, 2004). To evaluate the activity of the extracts obtained through the maceration of the endophytic cell mass, an adaptation of a manual patterned by Clinical and Laboratory Standards Institute (2003*a*) was used. The results were collected through the measurement of the growth inhibition halo formed around the well. The microorganisms used on the tests were: *Staphylococcus aureus* (ATCC 27213 and ATCC 25923), *Escherichia coli* (ATCC 25922), *Pseudomonas aeruginosa* (ATCC 27853), *Enterococcus faecalis* (ATCC 29212), *Klebsiella pneumonia* (ATCC 700603), *Micrococcus luteus* (ATCC 9314), methicillin-resistant *Staphylococcus aureus* (MRSA) and *Candida albicans* (ATCC 10231). Test organisms were grown overnight in a Müeller-Hinton broth (MH , Merck) at 37 °C and were diluted until reaching the concentration of 10^6 cells/mL. As positive control chloranphenicol 1mg/mL for bacterial strains and nystatin 100000UI/mL for *C. albicans* were used. Methanol was applied as solvent control and saline solution was used as negative control.

2.6 Peppertree crude methanolic extract and fractions

The dried leaves were put in contact with petroleum ether for six days, having the solvent freshened when saturated. After removing the filtrated with petroleum ether the leaves were exposed to methanol for nine days having the solvent freshened when necessary (Harbone, 1998). The concentrated crude methanolic extract was partitioned using the following gradient elution: petroleum ether, petroleum ether: dichloromethane 1:1, dichloromethane, dichloromethane: ethyl acetate 1:1, ethyl acetate, ethyl acetate: methanol 1:1 and methanol.

2.7 Antimicrobial activity of peppertree crude methanolic extract and fractions

For this evaluation an adaptation from the macrodilution method (Clinical and Laboratory Standards Institute 2003*b*) has been used. In a test tube with Müller-Hinton broth already with the extract/fraction in a known concentration, the microorganism to be combated *(Staphylococcus aureus, Pseudomonas aeruginosa or Candida albicans)* was inoculated. To isolate the solvent influence (dimethyl sulfoxide) at the activity of the extract/fraction used, controls having different solvent concentration were prepared. The test tubes were incubated and after that the turbidity standard was analyzed. For an exact analysis of the results an aliquot of 100µL of each test tube was sowed in a Petri dish with Müller-Hinton agar and incubated at 35°C for 24 hours for posterior growth analysis by colonies counting. For the yeast the incubation period was 48 hours at 35°C. The test was carried out in duplicate.

2.8 Chemical comparison

The bioactive extracts obtained from peppertree endophytes were compared with the compounds present in the crude methanolic extract of the leaves and fractions active by thin-layer chromatography. The revealing substances used were: Dragendorff reactive, potassium hydroxide, sulfuric vanillin, ferric chloride - 1.5%, anisaldehyde and ninhydrin (Ordóñez et al., 2006; Rodrigues et al., 2009).

3. Results

3.1 Isolation and identification of endophytes

One hundred thirty-one endophytes were isolated from peppertree leaves. Nine endophytes active metabolites producers were identified. These, 2 were identified as *Alternaria* sp., 3 as *Phomopsis* sp., 1 as *Penicillium roseopurpureum*, 1 as a basidiomycete, and 1 as *Streptomyces* sp. One hundred ninety-one endophytes were isolated from leaf fragments of *M. ilicifolia*, belonging to 6 genera of fungi: *Alternaria, Phyllosticta, Xylaria, Phomopsis, Pestalotiopsis* and *Colletotrichum*. Eighteen actinomycetes were isolated from 4000 samples *Vochysia divergens*, with isolation rates of 0.47%, of these 61.1% (11) were isolated from petiole and 38.9% (07) leaves. Three taxa were identified: *Microbispora* sp. (10 isolates), *Micromonospora* sp. (2 isolates) and *Streptomyces sampsonii* (2 isolates).

3.2 Antimicrobial activity

Antibacterial activity of the methanolic extracts from endophytes of *S. terebinthifolius*_was evaluated (Table 2). From the twenty isolates selected to fermentation, three released bioactive compounds in the medium culture: *Phomopsis* sp. (LGMF655) and *Alternaria* sp. (LGMF692) released active metabolites against *S. aureus;* and *Streptomyces* sp. (LGMF696) released active metabolites against *C. albicans.* Eight isolates had secondary metabolites with antimicrobial activity on their cell structures (Table 3). Thirteen endophytic *Pestalotiopsis* spp. Isolates obtained from *M. ilicifolia* were used for evaluation of the antimicrobial activity. *Pestalotiopsis* sp. (14JES) was effective in inhibiting MRSA, *K. pneumoniae, M. luteus, S. aureus,* and *E. coli;* and the isolate *Pestalotiopsis microspora* showed similar results, except that it was unable to inhibit *K. pneumonia. P. vismae* showed traces of inhibition against *S. aureus* and *E. coli;* and 2 isolates of *Pestalotiopsis* sp. (10JAES and 11JAES) showed inhibition against *S. aureus* and *M. luteus,* respectively (Table 2).

The extract of endophytic actinomycetes isolated from *V. divergens* showed activity against pathogenic bacteria (Table 2). The *Microbispora* genus isolates showed activity against several clinical strains. The isolate (N4P61) inhibited *P. aeruginosa* while the isolate N34C1 had activity against *S. aureus* and *E. coli.* The isolate N5P3 was effective in inhibiting *S.aureus* MRSA, *E. coli, P. aeruginosa* including *C. albicans.* Besides that two isolates identified as *Microbispora* sp. (N43B2 e N4P61) and two isolates of *Streptomyces sampsonii* (A3F5 e A1P10) showed activity against *C. albicans.*

The crude extract from all the plants studied presented antimicrobial activity. So far, we have got detailed data of the *Schinus* plant's extract fractionation, and the minimum inhibitory concentration (MIC) of the crude extract from leaves and the fractions were evaluated (Table 4).

		E. faecalis		MRSA	*K.pneumonia*		*P. aeruginosa*		*M. luteus*		*S. aureus*	*E. coli*		*C. albicans*
		ME	ME	AE	ME	ME	AE	ME	ME	AE	ME	AE	ME	AE
M. ilicifolia	*Pestalotiopsis sp.* (10JAES)	0	0	nt	0	0	nt	0	Tr	nt	0	nt	0	nt
	Pestalotiopsis sp. (11JAES)	0	0	nt	0	0	nt	Tr	0	nt	0	nt	0	nt
	Pestalotiopsis sp. (14JAES)	0	+	nt	+	0	nt	+	+	nt	+	nt	0	nt
	P. microspora	0	+	nt	0	0	nt	+	+	nt	+	nt	0	nt
	P. vismae	0	Tr	nt	0	0	nt	0	0	nt	Tr	nt	0	nt

		E. faecalis		MRSA		*K.pneumonia*	*P. aeruginosa*		*M. luteus*	*S. aureus*		*E. coli*		*C. albicans*
		ME	ME	AE	ME	ME	AE	ME	ME	AE	ME	AE	ME	AE
S. terebinthifolius	*Phomopsis* sp.	0	0	nt	0	0	nt	0	+	nt	0	nt	0	nt
	Alternaria sp.	0	0	nt	0	0	nt	0	+	nt	0	nt	0	nt
	Streptomyces sp.	0	0	nt	0	0	nt	0	0	nt	0	nt	+	nt
V. divergens	N43B2	nt	0	0	nt	0	0	nt	0	0	0	0	+	0
	N2P10	nt	0	0	nt	0	0	nt	0	0	0	0	0	+
	N4P61	nt	0	0	nt	+	0	nt	0	0	0	0	+	0
	A3F5	nt	0	0	nt	0	0	nt	0	0	0	0	+	+
	A1F10	nt	0	0	nt	0	0	nt	0	0	0	0	+	0
	N34C1	nt	0	0	nt	0	0	nt	0	+	0	+	0	0
	N5P3	nt	0	+	nt	0	+	nt	0	+	0	+	0	+

NOTE: **O**: no inhibition; **Tr**: traces of inhibition; + inhibition zone between 4 – 5 mm in diameter. Nt: not tested

Table 2. Antibacterial activity of the methanolic (ME) and aqueous (AE) extracts

	S. aureus	*C. albicans*	*P. aeruginosa*
Alternaria **sp. (LGMF626)**	X		
Alternaria **sp. (LGMF692)**	X		
Basideomycete (LGMF713)	X		
Penicillium roseopurpureum **(LGMF698)**	X	X	
Phomopsis **sp. (LGMF627)**		X	
Phomopsis **sp. (LGMF694)**	X		X
Streptomyces **sp. (LGMF696)**	X	X	
Not identify (LGMF673)	X	X	

X = represent the pathogen that was inhibited by the extract

Table 3. Endophytes with active metabolites on their cell structures

3.3 Chemical comparison of active compounds

Results of the TLC suggest the presence of phenolic and anthraquinone compounds at the crude extract of the leaves of peppertree and active fractions. Yet, according to the present results, the crude extract and the ethyl acetate fraction had alkaloids and terpenoids.

The chemical analysis of the compounds with antimicrobial activity extracted from the endophytes of the peppertree leaves suggest the presence of alkaloids in all the tested extracts. Two microorganisms (*Alternaria* sp. - LGMF692 and *Streptomyces* sp. - LGMF696) also produced anthraquinones while one of them (*Phomopsis* sp. - LGMF655) produced terpenoids.

4. Discussion

Resistance to antimicrobial drugs today, remains a major problem in modern health care, about the impact on treatment options, mortality, infection control and economic issues. All identified taxon in this study, *Alternaria* (Kjer et al., 2009), *Phomopsis* (Du et al., 2008), *Penicillium* (Bertinetti et al., 2009), *Pestalotiopsis* (Liu, 2011), basidiomycete (Suay et al., 2000) and *Streptomyces* (Maruna et al., 2010) had already been described as producers of metabolite with antimicrobial activity. Although the TLC method is only qualitative, it is a simple and relatively cheap technique to recognize the inhibitory activity of a large quantity of organic extracts. However, our study has shown that fungal endophytes isolated from Brazilian native plant species have chemical and biochemical properties potentially useful. In the Table 1 there is a list of other Brazilian medicinal plant and endophytes fungi with antimicrobial activity. Further investigation may yield novel compounds with practical applications in a variety of biotechnological areas, with countless useful drugs as important therapeutics options for innumerable disease. The mechanical removal of cell metabolites from the inside part of their structure amplified the action spectrum of the extracted compounds besides revealing a higher number of endophytes producing active substances in relation to the attempt on releasing bioactive compounds on the culture medium. Apparently the microorganisms store these compounds for a future competition situation. The pursuit of cell release of these substances by different fermentation means would provide better biotechnological conditions for production of these compounds in higher amount for a more detailed study to be carried out.

The results of the bioautographic TLC agar overlay assay are at present only qualitative; however, it indicates that the endophytic extracts have antimicrobial potential, suggesting the need for further investigations to elucidate the chemical structure of the secondary metabolites that provide the antimicrobial properties to these endophytic isolates. Owing to the high genetic variability among *Pestalotiops* species found in the present study, new isolation efforts of "espinheira santa" endophytes should be carried out with the goal of bioprospecting, given the importance of the genus *Pestalotiopsis* in the biotechnological study of secondary metabolites, in particular, the inhibition of the activity of cells in gastric tumors (Lee et al. 1996; Strobel et al. 1998).

In the present study, isolates 6JAES and 29JES, which showed antimicrobial activity and were suggested as belonging to the species *P. microspora,* are of special importance, given that this species has become important in the past few years in the production of taxol and other secondary metabolites of antifungical, anticarcinogenic, and antioxidant properties (Strobel 2002; Strobel & Daisy 2003).

Despite the economic interest and broad popular medicinal usage of the *Vochysia divergens* plant there are very few reports on the chemical composition and biological activity of this plant. In respect to the biological activities related to this species, it was verified that the ethanolic extract of *V. divergens* barks presented bactericide activity against *Staphylococcus aureus* and antinociceptive activity (Hess et al., 1995). The endophytic actinomycetes of the V. divergens plant showed activity against *C. albicans, S. aureus, E. coli, P. aeruginosa* and MRSA, suggesting a higher potential to the antimicrobial activity than the one found on the plant by Hess (1995). Bioprospecting studies of endophytic actinomycetes for pharmaceutical and biotechnological purposes are fundamental for the discovery of new substances for human therapeutics including antibiotics, antimicotic, and anticarcinogenics (Bi et al. 2011).

The peppertree crude methanolic extract present higher activity against *C. albicans* followed by *S. aureus*, and less active against *P. aeruginosa*. The fractions dichloromethane: ethyl acetate and ethyl acetate were more active against the Gram positive microorganism followed by the Gram negative and with less action against the yeast tested. There is a difference between the antimicrobial activities found to the crude extract of the plant in relation to their fractions, probably due to the existence of an interaction of compounds on the crude extract, what would enhance the activity against *C. albicans*. Therefore, when the extract is fractionated these compounds are put apart, reducing their potential to act. According to another study about peppertree antimicrobial activity it was verified that the aqueous extract when fractionated would lose activity against *C. albicans* (Schmourlo et al., 2005), confirming the importance of synergism in this case. Apparently compound interactions that help crude extract activity in relation to fractions against yeast do not show the same effect to the bacteria tested. It indicates a higher concentration of active compounds against these microorganisms or an elimination or decrease of compounds interfering, mainly the in the dichloromethane: ethyl acetate fraction.

It is suggested that most the active extracts of endophytes studied are compound by alkaloids. Other compound classes were also revealed in these extracts, however less frequent, two endophytes, an isolate from *Alternaria* sp. and another from de *Streptomyces* sp. had produced anthraquinones and an isolate from *Phomopsis* sp. had produced terpenoids. Results of TLC reveal there are strong evidences that phenolic compounds present on peppertree, found either on the crude extracts as well as the two active fractions, were responsible for the antimicrobial activity of the plant. Other authors also address the activity of the plant to a group of phenolic compounds, the polifenoles (Ceruks et al., 2008; Degáspari et al., 2005; Queires & Rodrigues, 1998).

Yet, the crude extract and active fractions of the plant also presented anthraquinones (Table 4), creating a new hypothesis that the antimicrobial substances linked to the peppertree could be connected to this group of compounds. Another study had identified anthraquinones, fenoles and triterpenes in the extract with antimicrobial activity of *S. terebinthifolius* bark, however not in the leaves extract (Lima et al., 2006).

With data obtained it was not found direct connection between the secondary metabolites with antimicrobial activity produced by the plant with the ones produced by the studied endophytes, once none endophytic chemical profiles studied showed the presence of phenolic compounds. This fact shows the enormous diversity of secondary metabolites present on nature and the importance of looking for active substances in medicinal plants and their endophytes.

	S. aureus	*C. albicans*	*P. aeruginosa*
Crude Extract (methanolic)	2300μg/mL	2000μg/mL	>3600μg/mL*
Dichloromethane:Ethyl Acetate Fraction	500μg/mL	>2300μg/mL*	1700μg/mL
Ethyl Acetate Fraction	1000μg/mL	>2300μg/mL*	2200μg/mL

* In these cases it was observed a reduction on the colonies number indicating activity. To prevent the interference of the solvent used on the results the extract/fraction volumes should not be over 250μL.

Table 4. Minimum inhibitory concentration (MIC) of the crude extract from leaves and fractions

5. References

Arnold, A.E.; Maynard, Z.; Gilbert, G.S.; Coley, P.D.; Kursar, T.A. (2000). Are tropical fungal endophytes hyperdiverse? *Ecology Letters.* Vol. 3, pp. 267-274.

Arzanlou, M.; Groenewald, J.Z.; Fullerton, R.A.; Abeln, E.C.A.; Carlier, J.; Zapater, M.F., Buddenhagen, I.W.; Viljoen, A.; Crous, P.W. (2008). Multiple gene genealogies and phenotypic characters differentiate several novel species of *Mycosphaerella* and related anamorphs on banana. *Persoonia,* Vol. 20, pp. 19-37.

Bertinetti, B.V.; Peña, N.I.; Cabrera, G.M. (2009). An antifungal tetrapeptide from the culture of *Penicillium canescens. Chem and Biod.* Vol. 6, pp. 1178-1184.

Bernardi-Wenzel, J. et al. (2010). Evaluation of foliar fungal endophyte diversity and colonization of medicinal plant *Luehea divaricata* (Martius et Zuccarini). *Biol. Res.* Vol.43, n.4, pp. 375-384.

Bettiol, W. (2008). *Controle biológico de doenças de plantas.* p. 388. 1th Ed. Embrapa: Jaguaraúna.

Bi, S.F.; Li, F.; Song, Y.C.; Tan, R. X. (2011). New acrylamide and oxazolidin derivatives from a termite-associated Streptomyces sp. *Nat. Prod. Commun.* 6: 353-355

Corrado, M., & Rodrigues, K.F. (2004). Antimicrobial evaluation of fungal extracts produced by endophytic strains of *Phomopsis* sp. *J Basic Microbiol.* Vol. 44, pp. 157-160.

Ceruks, M.; Romoff, P.; Fávero, A.O.; Lago, J.H.G. (2007). Constituintes fenólicos polares de *Schinus terebentifolius* Raddi (*Anacardiaceae*). *Quim Nova,* Vol. 30, pp. 507-599.

Clinical and Laboratory Standards Institute (2003a). Performance Standards for Antimicrobial Disk Susceptibility Tests; approved standard - 8th edn. Clinical and Laboratory Standards Institute document M2-A8. Clinical and Laboratory Standards Institute, Wayne, PA.

Clinical and Laboratory Standards Institute (2003b). Methods for Dilution Antimicrobial Susceptibility Tests for Bacteria That Grow Aerobically; approved standard - 8th edn. Clinical and Laboratory Standards Institute document M7-A6. Clinical and Laboratory Standards Institute, Wayne, PA.

Borges, W. S. & Pupo, M. T. (2006). Novel Anthraquinone Derivatives Produced by *Phoma sorghina,* an Endophyte Found in Association with the Medicinal Plant *Tithonia diversifolia* (Asteraceae). *J. Braz. Chem. Soc.* Vol. 17, pp.929-934.

Gomes-Figueiredo, J.; Pimentel, I.C.; Vicente, V.A.; Pie, M. P.; Kava-Cordeiro,V.; Galli-Terasawa, L.; Pereira,J.O.; Souza,A.Q.L.; Glienke, C. (2007). Bioprospecting highly diverse endophytic *Pestalotiopsis* spp. with antibacterial properties from *Maytenus ilicifolia*, a medicinal plant from Brazil. *Canadian Journal of Microbiology*. Vol, 53, pp.1123-1132.

De Hoog G.S.; Vicente V.; Caligiorne, R.B.; Kantargliocu, S.;Tintelnot, K.; Gerrits van den Ende, A.H.G.; Haase, G. (2003). Species diversity and polymorphism in the *Exophiala spinifera* clade containing opportunistic black yeast-like fungi. *Journal of Clinical Microbiology*. Vol. 41, pp. 4767-4778.

Degáspari, C.H.; Waszczynskyj, N.; Pardo, M.R.M. (2005). Atividade antimicrobiana de *Schinus terebentifolius* Raddi. *Ciênc. agrotec.*, Vol. 29, n.3, pp.617-622.

Demain AL, Sanchez S (2009) Microbial drug discovery: 80 years of progress. *The Journal of Antib.* Vol. 62, pp. 5-16.

Du, X.; Lu C.; Li Y et al. (2008) Three new antimicrobial metabolites of *Phomopsis* sp. *The Journal of Antib.* Vol. 61, pp. 250-253.

Fenner R. *et al.* (2006). Plantas utilizadas na medicina popular brasileira com potencial atividade antifúngica. *Rev. Brás. Cienc. Farm.* Vol. 42, n°3, pp. 369-394.

Glienke-Blanco, C.; Aguilar-Vildoso, C. I; Vieira, M. L. C.; Barroso, P. A. V.; Azevedo, J. L. (2002). Genetic variability in the endophytic fungus *Guignardia citricarpa* isolated from *citrus*. *Genetic and Molecular Biology*. Vol. 25, n.2, pp.251-255.

Guerra, M.J.M.; Barreiro, M.L.; Rodriguez, Z.M.; Rubalcaba, Y. (2000). Actividad antimicrobiana de um extracto fluido al 80% de *Schinus terebenthifolius* Raddi (copal). *Rev. Cubana Plant. Med.* Vol.5, n.1, pp.23-25.

Hamada, M.; Kondo, S.; Yokoyama, T. et al. (1974) Minosaminomycin, a new antibiotic containing myo-inosamine. *The Journal of Antib.* Vol. 27, pp. 81-83.

Harborne, J.B. (1998). *Phytochemical methods. A guide to modern techniques of plant analysis.* 3th edn. London, Chapman & Hall.

Hess. S. C., Brum, R. L., Honda, N. K., Cruz, A. B., Moretto, E., Cruz, R. B. and Yunes, R. A. 1995. Antibacterial activity and phytochemical analysis of *Vochysia divergens* (*Vochysiaceae*). *Journal of Ethnopharmacology*. Vol.47, pp. 97-100.

Johann, S.; Pizzolatti, M.G; Donnici, C.L.; Resende, M.A. (2007). Atividade antifúngica de plantas utilizadas na medicina tradicional brasileira contra fungos de relevância clínica. *Brazilian Journal of Microbiology*. Vol.38, n.4, pp.632-637.

Kjer, J.; Wray, V.; Edrada-Ebel, R.; et al. (2009) Xanalteric acids I and II and related phenolic compounds from an endophytic *Alternaria* sp. isolated from the mangrove plant *Sonneratia alba*. Journ of Nat Prod. Vol. 72, pp. 2053-2057.

Kumar, S., Tamura, K., Nei, M., (2004). MEGA3: Integrated software for Molecular Evolutionary Genetics Analysis and sequence alignment. *Briefings in Bioinformatics*. Vol. 5, pp. 150 -163.

Kuster, E.; Willians, S.T. (1964). Selection of media for isolation of streptomycetes. *Nature*. Vol.202, pp.928-929.

Lee, J. C. et al. (1996). Torreyanic acid: a selectively cytotoxic quinone dimer from the endophytic fungus *Pestalotiopsis microspora*. *Journal of Organic Chemistry*. Vol. 61. pp. 3232-3233.

Lima, M.R.F.; Luna, J.S.; Santos, A.F.; et al. (2006) Anti-bacterial activity of some Brazilian medicinal plants. *Journal of Ethnoph.* Vol. 105, pp. 137-147.

Liu, L. (2011) Bioactive metabolites from the plant endophyte *Pestalotiopsis fici*. *Mycology* Vol. 2, Iss. 1.

Lorenzi, H. (2002) *Árvores Brasileiras – manual de identificação e cultivo de plantas arbóreas nativas do Brasil*. 4ªed. Ed. Instituto Plantarum. Vol. 1, pp. 24,

Marinho, A. M. R.; Rodrigues-Filho, E.; Moitinho, M. L. R. & Santos, L. S. (2005). Biologically active polyketides produced by *Penicillium janthinellum* isolated as an endophytic fungus from fruits of *Melia azedarach*. *J. Braz. Chem. Soc.* Vol.16, pp. 280-283.

Maruna, M.; Sturdikova, M.; Liptaj, T. et al. (2010) Isolation, structure elucidation and biological activity of angucycline antibiotics from an epiphytic yew streptomycete. *Journal of Basic Microbiol.* Vol. 50, pp.1-8.

Melo, F.M.P.; Moraes, L.A.B. et al., (2009). Antifungal compound produced by the cassava endophyte *Bacillus pumilus* MAIIIM4A, *Scientia Agricola*. Vol. 66, no. 5, pp. 583-592.

Mytinger, L., & Williamson, G. B. (1987). The invasion of *Schinus* into saline communities of Everglades National Park. *Fla. Sci.* Vol. 50, pp. 7-12.

Momesso, L.S. et al. (2008). Chaetoglobosinas produzidas por Chaetomium globosum, fungo endofítico associado a *Viguiera robusta* Gardn. (Asteraceae). *Quím. Nova*. Vol.31, n.7, pp. 1680-1685.

Monciardini P, Sosio M, Cavaletti L et al. (2002) New PCR primers for the selective amplification of 16S rDNA from diferent groups of actinomycetes. *FEMS Microbiol Ecol* Vol.42, pp.419-429.

Ordóñez, V.P.; Veja, E;M.; Melagón, A.O. (2006) Phytochemical study of native plant species used in traditional medicine in Loja Province. *Lyonia*. Vol.10, pp. 6-71.

Oliveira, C.M.; Silva, G.H.; Regasini, L.O.; Zanardi, L.M.; Evangelista, A.H.; Young, M.C.; Bolzani, V.S.; Araujo, A.R.; (2009). Bioactive metabolites produced by *Penicillium* sp. 1 and sp. 2, two endophytes associated with *Alibertia macrophylla* (Rubiaceae). Z *Naturforsch* C. Vol. 64, pp. 824-830.

Oliveira, M. N.; et al. (2011).Novel anthraquinone derivatives produced by *Pestalotiopsis guepinii*, an endophytic of the medicinal plant *Virola michelii* (Myristicaceae). *J. Braz. Chem. Soc.* Vol.22, n.5, pp. 993-996. ISSN 0103-5053.

Pastre, R.; et al. (2007). Diversidade de policetídeos produzidos por espécies de *Penicillium* isoladas de *Melia azedarach* e *murraya paniculata*. *Quím. Nova*. Vol.30, n.8, pp. 1867-1871.

Peixoto Neto, P.A.S.; Azevedo, J.L.; Caetano, L.C. (2004). Microrganismos endofíticos em plantas: status atual e perspectivas. *Boletín Latinoamecano y del Caribe de Plantas Medicinales y Aromáticas*. Santiago. Vol. 3, pp. 69-72.

Petrini, O. (1991). Fungal endophytes of tree leaves. In: ANDREWS, J. H.; HIRANO, S. S. (Eds.). *Microbial Ecology of Leaves*. New York: Springer-Verlag, pp. 179-197.

Pontecorvo, G., et al. (1953). The genetics of *Aspergillus nidulans*. *Advan. Genet.* Vol.5, pp. 141-238.

Queires LCS, Rodrigues LEA (1998). Quantificação das substâncias fenólicas totais em órgãos da Aroeira *Schinus terebenthifolius* (Raddi). Braz Arch Biol Technol. Vol. 41, pp. 247-253.

Queires, L.C. et al. (2006). Polyphenols purified from the Brazilian aroeira plant (*Schinus terebinthifolius, Raddi*) induce apoptotic and autophagic cell death of DU145 cells. Anticancer Research, Vol.26, n°1A, pp. 379-387.

RIBAS, M.O. *et al.* (2006). Efeito da *Schinus terebenthifolius* Raddi sobre o processo de reparo tecidual das lesões ulceradas induzidas na mucosa bucal do rato. *Rev. Odonto Cienc.* - Fac. Odonto/PUCRS. Vol.21, n° 53, pp. 245-252.

Raeder, U.; Broda, P. (1985). Rapid preparation of DNA from filamentous fungi. *Letters in Applied Microbiology*, Oxford. Vol.1, pp. 17-20.

Ramos, H. P.; Braun, G. H; Pupo, M. T. & Said, S. (2010). Antimicrobial activity from endophytic fungi *Arthrinium* state of *Apiospora montagnei* Sacc. and *Papulaspora immersa*. *Braz. Arch. Biol. Technol.*Vol.53, n.3, pp. 629-632.

Rocha, R.; et al. (2009). Selection of endophytic fungi from comfrey (*Symphytum officinale* L.) for in vitro biological control of the phytopathogen *Sclerotinia sclerotiorum* (Lib.). *Braz. J. Microbiol.* Vol.40, n.1 pp. 73-78.

Rodrigues, I.M.C.; Souza Filho, A.P.S.; Ferreira, F.A. (2009). Estudo fitoquímico de *Senna alata* por duas metodologias. *Planta Daninha.* Vol. 27, pp. 507-513.

Rodrigues-Heerklotz, K. F., Drandarov, K., Heerklotz, J., Hesse, M. and Werner. C. (2001). Guignardic acid, a novel type of secondary metabolite produced by endophytic fungus *Guignardia* sp.: isolation, structure elucidation and asymmetric synthesis. *Helv. Chim. Acta*, Vol.84, pp.3766-3771.

Rosa, L. H. et al. (2010). Leishmanicidal, trypanocidal, and cytotoxic activities of endophytic fungi associated with bioactive plants in Brazil. *Braz. J. Microbiol.* Vol. 41, pp. 420-430.

SEMA -SECRETARIA DO ESTADO DO MEIO AMBIENTE. (1995). *Lista vermelha de plantas ameaçadas de extinção no Paraná.* Curitiba, SEMA. p. 130.

Schmourlo, G., Mendonça-Filho, R.R., Alviano, C.S., Costa, S.S. (2005). Screening of antifungal agents using ethanol precipitation and bioautography of medicinal and food plants. *Journal of Ethnoph.* Vol.96, pp.563-568.

Silva, G.S.; Furtado, N.A.J.C.; Pupo, M.T.; et al. (2004). Antibacterial activity from *Penicillium corylophilum* Dierckx. *Microbiol Research.* Vol.159, pp. 317-322.

Silva, G. H. et al. (2010). Citocalasinas produzidas por *Xylaria* sp., um fungo endofítico de Piper aduncum (piperaceae). *Quím. Nova.* Vol.33, n.10, pp. 2038-2041.

Siqueira, V. Conti, R., de Araújo, J., Souza-Motta, C. (2011). Endophytic fungi from the medicinal plant *Lippia sidoides* Cham. and their antimicrobial activity. *Symbiosis.* Vol. 53, n. 2, pp. 89-95.

Silva, G. H.; Teles, H. L.; Trevisan, H. C. et al., (2005). New bioactive metabolites produced by *Phomopsis cassiae*, an endophytic fungus in *Cassia spectabilis*. *Journal of the Brazilian Chemical Society.* Vol. 16, no. 6 B, pp. 1463-1466.

Soares, D.G.S. *et al.* (2007). Atividade Antibacteriana *in vitro* da Tintura de Aroeira (*Schinus terebinthifolius*) na Descontaminação de Escovas Dentais Contaminadas pelo *S. mutans*. *Pesq. Bras. Odontoped. Clin. Integr.* Vol. 7, n3, pp. 253-257.

Swofford, D. L., (1998). *PAUP: phylogenetic analysis using parsimony* (and other methods). Version 4.00. Sinauer Associates, Sunderland, MA.

Stierle, A.; Strobel, G.; Stierle, D.; (1993).Taxol and taxane production by *Taxomyces andreanea*, an endophytic fungus of Pacific yew. *Science.* Vol. 260, pp. 214-216.

Strobel, G. A. (2002). Rainforest endophytes and bioactive products .*Critical Review Biotechnologic.*Vol. 22, pp. 315-333.

Strobel, G. A.; Daisy, B. H. (2003). Biosprospecting for Microbial Endophytes and Their Natural Products. *Microbiology and Molecular Biology Reviews.* Vol. 67, pp 491-502.

Strobel, G. A.; Long, D. M. (1998). Endophytic microbes embody pharmaceutical potential. *ASM News.* Vol. 64, pp. 263-268.

Suay, I.; Arenal, F.; Asensio, F. J. et al. (2000). Screening of basidiomycetes for antimicrobial activities. *Anton van Leeuw.* Vol. 78, pp.129 139.

Teles, H. L.; Silva, G. H.; Castro-Gamboa, I.; Bolzani, V. S.; Pereira, J. O.; Costa-Neto, C. M.; Haddad, R., Eberlin, M. N., Young, M. C. M., Araújo, A. R. (2006). Benzopyrans from *Curvularia* sp., an endophytic fungus associated with *Ocotea corymbosa* (Lauraceae). *Phytochemistry*. Vol. 66, pp. 2363-2367.

White, T.J., Bruns, T.D., Lee, S. and Taylor, J.W. (1990). Amplification and direct sequencing of fungal ribosomal RNA genes for phylogenetics. In: *PCR Protocols: A Guide to Methods and Applications* (eds. M.A. Innis, D.H. Gelfand, J.S. Sninsky and T.J. White). Academic Press, New York: 315-322.

11

The Natural Antimicrobial Chromogranins/Secretogranins-Derived Peptides – Production, Lytic Activity and Processing by Bacterial Proteases

Ménonvè Atindehou*, Rizwan Aslam*, Jean-François Chich, Youssef Haïkel, Francis Schneider and Marie-Hélène Metz-Boutigue
Biomatériaux et Ingénierie Tissulaire, University of Strasbourg, Strasbourg France

1. Introduction

1.1 Multidrug antibiotic resistance and innate immunity

Multidrug-resistant organisms, such as methicillin-resistant *Staphylococcus aureus* (MRSA) and Vancomycin-resistant enterococci (VRE) have important infection control implications in all healthcare stings. Multidrug antibiotic resistance is a worldwide crucial health problem and the production of new potent antibiotics, acting alone or in combination is urgent. In addition, a major factor in the emergence of antibiotic resistant organisms is the overuse of antibiotics in the hospital or the community. To overcome this abuse, numerous efforts are undertaken to reduce antibiotics prescription and/or promote synergistic effects by others molecules.

Indeed, stimulating organism defense is a promising way to struggle against pathogens. The innate immune system is, since 2 billion years, the primary defense in most living organisms and antimicrobial peptides (AMPs) are fundamental components of the innate immune defense of multicellular organisms, either animal or vegetal (Bulet et al., 2004; Aerts et al. 2008; Manners, 2007).

1.2 The antimicrobial peptides

The antimicrobial peptides (AMPs) have been well conserved throughout the evolution and they ensure the organism's defense against a large number of pathogens. They serve as endogenous antibiotics that are able to rapidly kill bacteria, fungi and viruses. Interestingly, they are not toxic for the host cells. Taking into consideration the diversity of the living beings, it is presumed that a large number of specific antibiotic peptides have been developed during evolution, allowing a protection of each organism in various conditions and the last years it has clearly appeared that many of these peptides, in addition to their direct antimicrobial activity, also have a wide range of functions in modulating both innate and adaptive immunity. Most of these are small molecules (less than 40 aminoacids) but some can be proteins. To date more than 1414 antibacterial, antifungal and 107 antiviral peptides have been

* These authors contributed equally

identified, (antimicrobial peptides database http://aps.unmc.edu/AP/main.php), including peptides from several tissues and cell types from invertebrates, plants and mammals (Wang Z. & Wang G. 2004). Among them are found cytokines and chemokines, several neuropeptides and fragments derived from proteins exhibiting antimicrobial activity. They carry an average of 40-50 percent hydrophobic residues in such a structure that the folded peptide adopts an amphipathic profile. These properties are important for their microbial killing mechanism: the cationic character of AMPs induces an electrostatic attraction to the negatively-charged phospholipids of microbial membranes and their hydrophobicity aids the integration into the microbial cell membrane, leading to membrane disruption. Furthermore, the amphipathic structure also allows the peptides to be soluble both in aqueous environments and in lipid membranes (Yeaman & Yount 2003).

In mammals, the most well studied AMPs are human defensins and cathelicidins (Zanetti, 2004; Yang et al., 2002). Furthermore, some large proteins such as lysozyme, caseins, hemoglobin, lactalbumin, secretory phospholipase A2 and lactoferrin display antimicrobial activity against numerous microorganisms. Several of them, such as lysozyme and phospholipase A2 are ubiquitous and secreted by a large number of cells (*i.e.* epithelial cells, leukocytes and Paneth cells in the small intestine) (Keshav, 2006).

Because a large number of AMPs were identified in gut and skin, in the first part of this chapter we report a review of the well-studied AMPs expressed in these tissues and in the second part we present recent data relative to the new active CGs-derived peptides in relation with pathogens involved with intestine diseases, skin infections and sepsis.

1.3 Gut and antimicrobial peptides

Gastrointestinal mucosa is a large host-environmental interface, showing a remarkable organization (Figure 1) and operating several functions including the digestive absorptive processes and the nutrients peristaltism, but also a physical and immunological protection of the body against microbes and a reconnaissance between commensal and pathogenic microorganisms.

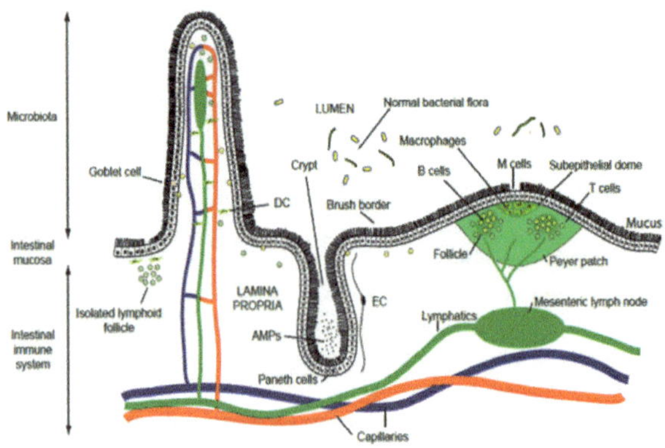

Fig. 1. Schematic representation of the gut epithelium. The different cellular actors involved in innate and/or adaptative immunity are represented. (DC: dendritic cells ; EC: enterochromaffin cells.)(According to Metz-Boutigue, M.H. et al., Curr Pharm Des.2010;16(9):1024-39).

Lamina propria is a conjunctive tissue composed of fibroblasts, immune cells and collagen. It also contains capillaries and lymphatic vessels. Epithelial cells, or enterocytes, are disposed on a single layer separating the *lumen* from the *lamina propria*. These cells are tightly bound by tight junctions forming an impermeable barrier to commensal flora and to pathogens. Brush-border *microvilli* are present on the apical surface of absorptive enterocytes, representing a large absorbing surface and allowing of microorganisms to the gut. In contrast, microfold cells are not present in *microvilli* (Figure 1); these cells express cathepsin E (a proteolytic enzyme) and Toll-like receptors able to secrete proinflammatory cytokines and chemokines. The main function of microfold cells is the transport of antigens from the lumen to the subepithelial lymphoid tissue and thus to the adaptive immune system.

Several anatomical structures are present along the gastrointestinal tractus. Peyer's patches are lymphoid structures containing B and T cells, macrophages and dendritic cells (Figure 1). Lieberkühn crypts are found in the small intestine and they constitute the basis of the intestinal *villi* (Figure 1). They contain multipotent stem cells and cells, involved in gastrointestinal immunity. Two other cellular types are also present in intestine: i) goblet cells synthesize and secrete large quantities of mucin, ii) enterochromaffin cells that originate from neural crest synthesize serotonin (5-HT) and numerous neuropeptides (Figure 1).

In addition to humoral and cellular immunity, non-immunological defense mechanisms represent an important line of intestinal defenses. Some of these protective factors have been amply documented: pancreatic and gastric juices, intestinal motility and intestinal flora (Sarker, 1992).

Mucosal epithelial cells and Paneth cells produce a variety of AMPs (defensins, cathelicidins, cryptdin related peptides, bactericidal/permeability increasing protein (BPI), chemokine CCL20 and bacteriolytic enzymes such as lysozyme and group IIA phospholipase A2 (Müller et al., 2005). In addition to their direct role in killing pathogenic microorganisms, AMPs are involved in attraction of leukocytes, alarming the adaptive immune system and neutralizing the proinflammatory bacterial molecules (Müller et al., 2005).

Lysozyme

Lysozyme is synthesized and secreted by Paneth cells, macrophages, neutrophils and epithelial cells (Mason & Taylor, 1975; Satoh et al., 1988). Its role and selectivity towards microbes are the same as in skin.

Lactoferrin

Lactoferrin (LF) exhibits a wide spectrum of antimicrobial and immunotropic properties (Artym et al., 2005). In contrast to caseins, LF is particularly resistant to proteolytic degradation in alimentary tract. LF is absorbed from the intestine by means of specific receptors located on brush border cells. Orally administered LF stimulates both local and systemic immune responses. It suppresses the growth of pathogenic bacteria, while promoting the multiplication of non-pathogenic *Lactobacillus sp.* and *Bifidobacterium sp.* (Artym et al., 2005).

Studies on mice showed LF to be protective against bacteremia and endotoxemia. LF inhibits the activity of proinflammatory cytokines, nitric oxide and reactive forms of oxygen. Furthermore, LF promotes the differentiation of T and B cells from their immature precursors and increases the activity of NK and LAK (lymphokine activated killer) cells (Artym et al., 2005).

Phospholipase A2

The hydrophobic layer of phosphatidylcholine (PC) overlies and protects the surface of the gastrointestinal (GI) tract, contributing to barrier integrity. In addition, phospholipase A2 is synthesized by Paneth cells and this enzyme hydrolyses bacterial membrane phospholipids to generate both free fatty acids and lysophospholipids. An important prerequisite for the action of phospholipase A2 is the successful binding to the phospholipids surface. *In vitro* studies utilizing recombinant enzymes and artificial phospholipids substrates have shown that phospholipases act on anionic phospholipids (phosphatidylglycerol, phosphatidylserine and phosphatidylethanolamine), but are inactive with phosphatidylcholine due to the lack of high affinity binding (Wu et al., 2010). During critical illness such as sepsis, gut barrier integrity may be compromised, which could be related to degradation of PC. Pretreatment with an orally active sPLA(2) inhibitor blocks the LPS-induced increase in GI permeability, and may suggest a new approach to reinforce the GI mucosal barrier and prevent complications from endotoxin in trauma in other septic conditions (Zayat et al., 2008).

Cathelicidins

Cathelicidin LL-37/hCAP18 is synthesized by neutrophils, where it was first identified (Romeo et al., 1988) and epithelial cells of the colon (Hase et al., 2002). *In vitro*, it has chemotactic properties for monocytes, macrophages and T cells (Koczulla et al., 2003). LL-37 is found in sites of inflammation where it modifies dendritic cells (DCs) differentiation, relying innate and adaptive immunity. *In vitro*, modified DCs had, among others characteristics induced by the peptide, enhanced secretion of Th-1 inducing cytokines and promoted Th1 responses (Davidson et al., 2004). LL-37 acts synergistically with IL-1-beta to increase the production of suppressive cytokines (IL-6 and IL-10) and chemokines MCP-1 and MCP-3 by macrophages (Yu et al., 2007). It acts *via* the transcription factor CREB and the activation of phosphorylation of the kinase Akt. In LPS-stimulated monocytes, LL-37 inhibits the release of TNF-alpha modulating inflammatory response induced by LPS, endotoxins and other agonists of TLRs (Mookherjee et al., 2006).

RNAses

Angiogenin-4 (Ang-4) is a member of the ribonucleases family. This protein is synthesized by Paneth cells and is similar to RNase 7 found in skin. Its secretion is stimulated by exposure to LPS. Ang-4 kills *E. faecalis* and *L. monocytogenes* at concentrations as low as 1 μM, whereas its concentration in crypts can be 1000 times greater (Hooper et al., 2003). Similarly to defensins, it is sensitive to salt concentration and is potentially cytotoxic to eukaryotic cells (Saxena et al., 1992).

C-type lectins

C-type lectins HIP/PAP are synthesized in human by enterocytes and Paneth cells. The same protein exists in mouse and is named RegIII gamma. These lectins bind Gram-positive peptidoglycan and act by direct killing. Several members of this family are found in gastrointestinal tissues (Dieckgraefe et al., 2002).

Defensins

As in skin, defensins have a direct antimicrobial role as well as immunomodulatory function. Alpha-defensins are synthesized by Paneth cell in the gastrointestinal tractus (Porter et al., 2002). Alpha-defensin expression does not require microbe induction since they are synthesized in germ-free conditions (Putsep et al., 2000) and/or prenatally (Mallow et al., 1996). In transfected mouse, it was shown that the alpha-defensin hBD-5 protects efficiently against *Salmonella typhimurium*, demonstrating the direct antimicrobial effect of this peptide. In mouse, alpha-defensins are named cryptdins and several families of peptides related to cryptdins are regrouped under the term CRS (Cryptdin Related Sequences). Interestingly, these CRS can form homo- or heterodimers, thus allowing a combinatorial diversity to struggle against pathogens (Hornef et al., 2004).

Beta-defensins are expressed in enterocytes of the small and large intestines. 28 beta-defensin encoding genes have been identified in human genome, but only 8 were found to be expressed. hBD-1 is constitutively expressed in absence of stimulus or bacterial infection (O'Neil et al., 1999), while some nutrients can stimulate its production in cell lines (Sherman et al., 2006). In mouse, an infection by the *Cryptosporidium* parasite resulted in a down-regulation of mBD-1 (Zaalouk et al., 2004), while *in vitro*, sporozoites are killed by this defensin. Some authors conclude on an unique and important regulation of hBD-1, during small intestine infections (Dann et Eckmann, 2007). hBD-2 is not constitutively expressed, but is induced by an infection or by proinflammatory stimuli (O'Neil et al., 1999). hBD-3 and -4 are inducible and particularly expressed in crypt regions (Fahlgren et al., 2004). Defensins can also act as chemotactic agents for immune cells in a similar way to that described for the skin.

Bactericidal Permeability Increasing protein

Bactericidal/permeability increasing protein (BPI), a constituent of primary neutrophil granules, is a potent natural antibiotic and anti-BPI antibodies are detected during infectious enteritis. In addition, BPI is a target antigen for anti-neutrophil cytoplasmic antoantibodies in inflammatory bowel diseases such as Crohn's disease and ulcerative colitis (Walmsley et al., 1997).

Neuropeptides

Enterochromaffin cells (EC) (Siddique et al., 2009) (Figure 1) are enteroendocrine cells present in the intestine, especially colon (Kuramoto et al., 2007) and containing large amounts of serotonin (5-HT). These cells can sense luminal content before its basolaterally release, and activate afferent neuron endings within *lamina propria*, allowing information exchange between gut and central nervous system (Hansen & Witte et al., 2008). Besides this important role, EC secrete also numerous other products, among which VIP (Zanner et al., 2004), Substance P (Heitz et al., 1976), CgA, CgB and secretogranin II/CgC (Cetin & Grube, 1991) and melatonin (Raikhlin et Kvetnoy, 1976).

Despite the crucial role of these cells, their sparse repartition and their low number did not allowed their extensive study. However, the BON cells were proposed as a model (Kim et al., 2001), that will enhance further research. When EC were stimulated by odors, they released serotonin, showing that these cells can also be stimulated by spices and fragrances (Braun et al., 2007). Moreover, a new method was proposed allowing isolating and purifying EC from biopsies (Modlin et al., 2006).

1.4 Skin and antimicrobial peptides

Mammal skin is an essential defense barrier against external aggressions, such as microbial pathogens, oxidant stress, chemical aggressions, mechanical insults, burns etc. For a long time, skin was considered as a simple physical barrier, but it is in a process of continual regeneration and has its own immunological, histological and nervous responses to environment.

Skin is composed of three layers, from inside to outside (Figure 2): i) *hypodermis* or subcutaneous tissue, ii) *dermis*, or *corium*, with a 3 to 5 mm thickness, iii) *epidermis*, with a thickness varying from 0.06 to 0.8 mm. *Epidermis* can be subdivided itself into four layers : *stratum basale*, *stratum spinosum*, *stratum granulosum* and *stratum corneum* (Figure 2). The deeper layers are composed of keratinocytes, melanocytes, Langerhans cells, Merkel cells and malpighian cells (Figure 2). Epidermis is composed as a gradient of differentiated keratinocytes, synthesizing keratine in *stratum granulosum*, and losing nuclei and organelles.

Skin, and more specifically *stratum corneum*, acts as a barrier in several ways (Elias, 2007). Corneocytes and extracellular matrix represent a physical barrier ("brick wall" model) (Figure 2).

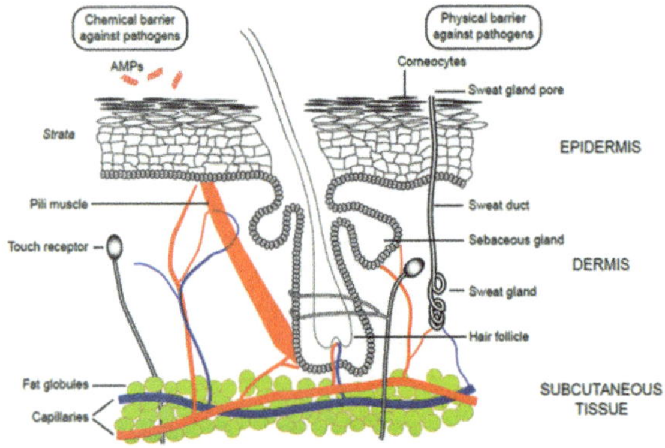

Fig. 2. Schematic representation of the different skin layers, adapted from different sources. A: Epidermis, dermis and subcutaneous tissues are shown with the different structures composing them. (according to Metz-Boutigue, M.H. et al., Curr Pharm Des. 2010;16(9):1024-39).x

The slightly acidic surface (pH~ 5.0), as well as the low hydration level of the skin represents a hostile area for pathogens, such as *Staphylococcus aureus*. Lipids (ceramides, cholesterol, free fatty acids) and their metabolic products present in *stratum corneum* act also as antimicrobial defense. Last, constitutive (and/or inducible) expression of antimicrobial peptides and proteins helps to maintain skin integrity and to prevent pathogen colonization. On the contrary, the surface of healthy skin is ideal for the growth of the normal cutaneous microflora (*Micrococcacea*, i.e. *Staphylococcus epidermidis* and *Corynebacteriacea*) that colonizes skin, competes with pathogens for nutrients and synthesizes antimicrobial compounds. These evolutionary conserved components of the innate immune system can act as direct antimicrobial agents and exert a role as immunomodulatory molecules in normal skin and during skin diseases, such as atopic dermatitis or psoriasis.

Lysozyme

Lysozyme is the first antimicrobial protein found in human skin. It was located in cytoplasm of epidermal cells in granular layers and in malpighian cells present in the *stratum spinosum* layer (Ogawa et al., 1971; Papini et al., 1982). Lysozyme is mainly active against Gram-positive bacteria (*S. aureus*), but is also active against Gram-negative bacteria, acting probably as a control of bacterial growth. Still recently, the contribution of lysozyme to cutaneaous defense was subjected to debate since it was not detected in *stratum corneum* as well as in washing fluid. However, it was recently detected in skin wash of adults, and lysozyme concentration was 5 times higher in newborn skin than in adult (Walker et al., 2008), confirming its status of antimicrobial molecule, as well as giving it an important role in preventing infections in newborn children.

Lactoferricin

Lactoferricin is an antimicrobial peptide originally produced by pepsin digestion of lactoferrin. It is active against Gram-positive, Gram-negative bacteria and also against *Candida albicans* (Bellamy et al., 1993). This molecule was also detected in skin wash of adult and newborn children (Walker et al., 2008). Synthesized by melanocytes, cutaneous lactoferrin is an iron-binding protein with antibacterial properties due to its ability to sequester iron in biological fluids or to destabilize bacterial membranes, limiting microorganism proliferation and adhesion. It has also immunomodulatory properties by up and down regulating immune cells involved in inflammatory processes (Legrand et al., 2005). The protective anti-inflammatory role of lactoferrin is due to its ability to bind free ferric ion acting as an anti-oxidant (Walker et al., 2008). It can bind to LPS and their receptors during an infection as well (Legrand et al., 2005). Expression of virulence factors of *S. aureus* is modulated by transferrin and lactoferrin (Kansal et al., 2005), demonstrating that these iron-binding proteins play an important role in the host pathogen interaction in skin and in mucosal tissue probably by LPS or its receptors binding.

Dermcidin and its derived peptides

Dermcidin, is constituvely and specifically expressed in the eccrine sweat glands within the dermis of human skin, secreted into the sweat and transported *via* sweat to the epidermal surface (Schittek et al., 2001). It is a 47 amino acids peptide produced from hydrolysis of a 9.3 kDa precursor by cathepsin D (Baechle et al., 2006). It possesses antibacterial properties at low concentration against *S. aureus, E. faecalis, E. coli* and *C. albicans*. The *in vivo* importance of DCD in prevention of infections has been demonstrated by its low expression in patients with atopic dermatitis. It was shown that dermcidin induces the production by SepA of *S. aureus*, a proteolytic virulence factor that cleaves and inactivates dermcidin (Lai et al., 2007). In the eccrine sweat, several proteolytically generated DCD fragments (DCD-1, DCD-1L) have been identified. DCD-1L is the most abundant antimicrobial peptide present in sweat, but other peptides derived from dermcidin by proteolysis are also found (Baechle et al., 2006; Rieg et al., 2006). The distribution of these peptides was found to be different according to the individuals. Most of them have 2 to 4 of the major DCD-derived peptides with the constant presence of at least one of the following peptides: DCD-1L (63-110), LEK-45 (66-110) and SSL-29 (63-91). The authors also showed that the distribution of these peptides is dependent on the body sites, which correlates with the presence of eccrine sweat glands and not with apocrine glands. Body parts in contact with pathogens (arms, face etc.) produce high levels of DCD-derived peptides. The molecular analysis of the antimicrobial activity of dermcidin-derived peptides showed that peptides like DCD-1L or SSL-23 do not disrupt bacterial membranes, but kill bacteria by still unknown mechanisms (Steffen et al., 2006).

Recently, by using a proteomic approach, a dermcidin precursor was found in human cervico-vaginal fluid (Shaw et al., 2007), together with haptoglobin, neutrophil defensin, lysozyme and lactoferrin. Dermcidin precursor was also found in human gestational tissue (Lee Motoyama et al., 2007), where it is proposed to play a role in pregnancy by regulating trophoblastic functions.

Cathelicidin, LL-37, hCAP18

Cathelicidin is found in eccrine gland cells, but also released into circulation. The CAP18 precursor is produced in skin by keratinocytes and is processed within neutrophils, keratinocytes and mast cells by inflammation or injury. In circulation, the mature form is LL-37, after processing of CAP18 by neutrophil-derived elastase and proteinase-3, but other proteases can also produce KS-30 and RK-21, two peptides active against pathogenic bacteria. Cathelicidin expression is also regulated at the transcriptional level by bacterial LPS, cutaneous injury and pro-inflammatory mediators (IL-6, retinoic acid). The LL-37 is intensively studied and besides its wide antibacterial spectrum, it is considered as a mediator between innate and adaptive immunity (Kai-Larsen & Agerberth, 2008) and cell differentiation can also regulate its activity.

RNase A superfamily

Eight known functional RNase A ribonucleases genes are encoding small polypeptides of 15 kDa (Dyer & Rosenberg, 2006). Besides their well-documented ribonuclease activity, some of these proteins display unexpected antimicrobial activities unrelated to their primary function. Eosinophil-derived neurotoxin (EDN/RNase 2) and eosinophil cationic peptide (ECP/RNase 3) are proteins secreted by eosinophilic leukocytes and were primarily tested for their toxic role against parasites. *In vitro*, ECP has also an activity against Gram-positive and Gram-negative bacteria (Lehrer et al., 1989).

RNase A7 was identified as a major agent of the innate immune response of the skin acting on Gram-positive and Gram-negative bacteria and also on *C. albicans* (Harder & Schröder, 2002). RNase 7 transcripts were induced in keratinocyte culture by addition of TNF-alpha, interferon-gamma, interleukin-1 beta and in the presence of bacteria (Harder & Schröder, 2002). More recently, RNase 5 was added to the list of antimicrobial molecules present in skin (*stratum corneum*), and the same authors showed that skin proteases are involved in inhibition of RNases 5 and 7 (Abtin et al., 2009).

Psoriasin (S100A7)

Psoriasin belongs to the S100 family of calcium-binding proteins. This family is composed of 21 genes and 11 proteins that have been found to be expressed in human epidermis or in cultured keratinocytes. Langerhans cells and melanocytes (Boni et al., 1997; Broome et al., 2003) express S100B and Meissner's corpuscules (sensorial receptors localized in the upper part of dermis) express S100P (Del Valle et al., 1994). These proteins possess two EF hands (helix-loop-helix calcium binding domains) and they act probably as calcium sensors. Several functions have been proposed for S100 proteins in keratinocytes, the main role being an implication in skin inflammatory processes (Jinquan et al., 1996). Another role could be keratinocytes membrane remodeling, that occurs during differentiation: psoriasin and another member of the S100 family, calgranulin-A (S100A9), have been shown to have their expression correlated with the degree of keratinocyte differentiation, suggesting that they are involved in this process (Martinsson et al., 2005]. A third role could be an involvement in the formation of calcium channels, in conjunction with annexins. Other postulated roles concern S100 proteins as substrate for transglutaminase, resulting in an incorporation of S100 in the cornified envelope; a last role could be a response to exogenous agents that modulate S100 proteins distribution and consequently their function (Eckert et al., 2004). Psoriasin has been found to be overexpressed in psoriasis. It is produced in *stratum corneum* by keratinocytes (Martinsson et al., 2005) and its basal expression is influenced by extracellular calcium level. Its expression in normal adult tissue is low, but high expression levels were detected in fetal skin, as for transferrin, suggesting a protective role in innate immunity. Psoriasin was found to be the main *E. coli*-cidal agent in the skin. It is a chemotactic agent for neutrophils and $CD4^+$ T cells (Jinquan et al., 1996). Moreover, psoriasin mediates the production of several inflammatory cytokines and chemokines from neutrophils *via* MAPK p38 and ERK activation. It also induces reactive oxygen species production and the exocytosis of alpha-defensins from neutrophils (Zheng et al., 2008).

Defensins

To date 4 defensins (hBD-1 to -4) in neutrophils and 2 defensins (hBD-5 and hBD-6) produced by Paneth cells were identified. The first inducible human defensin, hBD-2, was identified in psoriatic lesions as the most abundant AMP. It was found to be expressed in terminally differentiated keratinocytes, in a structure located in *stratum corneum*, lamellar bodies that contain lipid-rich secretory granules. It is probably released with lipid-like content of these lamellar bodies (Oren et al., 2003). hBD-2 is also up-regulated locally by infections (Radek & Gallo, 2007) or wounds (Butmarc et al., 2004). It has preferential bactericidal properties against Gram-negative bacteria (Harder et al., 1997) and like LL-37, its effect is sensitive to the concentration of NaCl. hBD-2 derived from neutrophils, promotes prostaglandins production and histamine release from mast cells, playing a role in allergic response (Bals et al., 1998). hBD-2 has also chemotactic properties for immature dendritic cells and memory T cells; it was described to bind to CCR-6, the receptor for macrophage inflammatory protein 3 alpha. In monocytes, hBD-2 expression is stimulated by several cytokines (Ganz, 2003; Kanda & Watanabe, 2008) and Il-1 seems to be the major inducer of hBD-2 production. Bacteria can also stimulate the expression of hBD-2 by epithelial cells, in a cytokine-independent pathway. *P. aeruginosa* is a powerful inducer of hBD-2 by primary keratinocytes (Schroeder & Harder, 2006).

hBD-1 was considered as a constitutively expressed antimicrobial peptide and in particularly not induced by proinflammatory cytokines. However, its production can be induced by peptidoglycan or LPS exposure (Sorensen et al., 2005). It is expressed in malpighian layer and in *stratum corneum* (Ali et al., 2001) and this expression is induced by increasing concentration of calcium (Harder et al., 2004), condition that provokes keratinocyte differentiation *in vitro* (Lichti et al., 2008).

hBD-3 has its expression induced by EGF that provokes keratinocytes proliferation in skin wounds (Sorensen et al., 2006).

It has chemotactic properties for monocytes (Garcia et al., 2001). While its expression is not induced by infection, hBD-3 displays a broad spectrum of antimicrobial activities against Gram-positive and Gram-negative bacteria, as well as against fungi (Harder et al., 2001). Regarding the adaptive immune system, hBD-2, 3 and 4 stimulate expression of proinflammatory cytokines, IL-10 and MCP-1 (Niyonsaba et al., 2007). They also stimulate the phosphorylation of STAT-1 and STAT-3 that induce keratinocytes migration and proliferation.

Neuropeptides in skin immunity

It was reported that neuropeptides display antimicrobial activities, linking together nervous and immune system (Radek & Gallo, 2007; Sternberg, 2006). Both systems can influence each other: brain and peripheral nervous system directly influence the activity of innate and adaptive immune system. Immune system can relay signals to the nervous system *via* the production of growth factors and cytokines. For example, stress can induce alterations in the immune response (Webster et al. 2002), or can be elicited by infection or injury with release of neuropeptides (Brogden et al., 2005).

Exchange between both systems can occur at systemic, as well as at regional or local levels (Sternberg, 2006). The first, global level gathers sympathetic nervous system, the hypothalamic-pituitary-adrenal axis and circulating AMPs. The second, local level, is composed of nervous endings, neuropeptide-releasing cells and receptors-exhibiting cells.

At the skin level, important structures, such as Merkel cells (Lucarz & Brand, 2007) localized at the basement membrane, separating epidermis from dermis, are neuropeptide-producing cells, cutaneous nervous cells and target cells. Merkel cells have characteristics of both epidermal and neuroendocrine cells. They are connected to nervous system with terminal sensory synapses and dense-core granules contain CGRP (Calcitonin Gene Related Peptide), VIP (VasoIntestinal Peptide), and CgA (Chromogranin A)-derived peptides (Hartschuh et al., 1989a; Hartschuh et al., 1989b).

Alpha-melanocyte-stimulating hormone (alpha-MSH), a 13 amino-acid peptide, is synthesized by keratinocytes, melanocytes, monocytes and astrocytes (Wikberg et al., 2000). This peptide derives from the pro-opiomelanocortin (POMC) after a processing by a proteolytic cascade (Pritchard & White, 2007), producing also five other peptides. Alpha-MSH acts as an AMP by inhibiting *S. aureus* and *C. albicans* growth at picomolar concentration (Cutuli et al., 2000). Interestingly, the tripeptide KPV (alpha-MSH 11-13) exhibited similar antimicrobial properties (Hiltz & Lipton, 1990; Mandrika et al., 2001; Mugridge et al., 1991), without effect on melanocytes (Sawyer et al. 1990). Alpha-MSH acts in two ways; it has a direct antimicrobial effect at very low concentration and reduces inflammatory responses associated with UV induced epithelial injury (Radek & Gallo, 2007).

2. Structural and biological properties of the antimicrobial peptides derived from chromogranins/secretogranins

2.1 Introduction

Chromogranins/secretogranins (CGs/SGs) constitute the granin family of genetically distinct acidic proteins present in secretory vesicles of nervous, endocrine and immune cells (Helle, 2004). The natural processing of bovine CGs is well described in granules of sympathoadrenal medullary chromaffin cells, where the resulting peptides are co-secreted with the catecholamines (Metz-Boutigue et al., 1993). The numerous cleavage sites are consistent with the specificity of prohormone convertases (PC1/3 and PC2) and carboxypeptidase E (CPE), that reside within chromaffin granules (Metz-Boutigue et al., 1993; Seidah & Chretien 1999). Secretogranin II (SgII), the third member of the chromogranin family is also processed to generate several natural fragments (Metz-Boutigue et al., 1993; Anouar et al., 1998; Marksteiner et al., 1993; Yajima et al., 2004). The discovery that pancreastatin, a chromogranin A (CGA)-derived peptide inhibits insulin secretion from pancreatic beta-cells, initiated the concept of prohormone (Eiden, 1987; tatemoto et al., 1986). The release of these CGs-derived peptides from chromaffin cells results from the nicotinic cholinergic stimulation and regulates several neuroendocrine functions (Helle & Serck-Hanssen, 1975).

Numerous cleavage products of the granins have been characterized, among which some display biological activities (Tatemoto et al., 1986; Aardal et al., 1993; Curry et al., 1992; Fasciotto et al., 1993; Lugardon et al., 2001; Mahata et al., 1997; Strub et al., 1996a,b). Neuroendocrine activities are reported from *in vivo* studies, with modulations of homeostatic processes, such as calcium regulation and glucose metabolism (Helle et al., 2007), cardiovascular functions (Brekke et al., 2002; Corti et al., 2004), gastrointestinal motility (Amato et al., 2005; Ghia et al., 2004a), nociception (Ghia et al., 2004b) tissue repair (Gasparri et al., 1997; Ratti et al., 2000), inflammatory responses (Ceconi et al., 2002; Corti et al., 2000) and as host defense agents during infections (Radek et al., 2008). During the past decade, our laboratory has characterized new antimicrobial CGs-derived peptides (Strub et al., 1996a,b; Metz-Boutigue et al., 1998; Lugardon et al., 2000, 2001; Briolat et al., 2005; Helle et al., 2007) (Figure 3).

Peptide	Location	Sequence	Net charge
CGA			
VS-I	1-76	LPVNSPMNKGDTEVMKC*IVEVISDTLSKPSPMPVSKEC*FETLRGDERILSILRHQNLLKELQDLALQGAKERTHQQ	+3
NCA	4-40	NSPMNKGDTEVMKC*IVEVISDTLSKPSPMPVSKEC*FE	-1
CHR	47-66	RILSILRHQNLLKELQDLAL	+1.5
Chrom	173-194	<u>Y</u>PGPQAKEDSEGP**S**QGPASREK	-1
CAT	344-364	RSMRLSFRARGYGFRGPGLQL	+5
CCA	418-427	LEKVAHQLEE	-2
ProChrom	79-431	HS<u>S</u>YEDELSEVLEK.....	-37
CGB			
Chromb	564-626	SAEFPDFYD<u>S</u>EEQM<u>S</u>PQHTAENEEEKAGQGVLTEEEEKELENLAAMDLELQKIAEKFSGTRRG	-12
SEC	614-626	QKIAEKFSGTRRG	+3
CGC			
Rrf	131-138	RKLKHMRF	+4.5
Kvk	430-443	KVLSRLPYGPGRSK	+4

Fig. 3. The antimicrobial bovine CGs-derived peptides according to the sequence of CGA (P05059), CGB (P23389) and CGC ((P20616) For each antimicrobial peptide the sequence, the location and net charge are indicated. *, cysteine residues of the disulfide bridge; phosphorylated residue are underlined and the glycosylated residue is in bold.

They act at micromolar range against bacteria, fungi, yeasts and are non-toxic for mammalian cells. They are recovered in biological fluids involved in defense mechanisms (serum, saliva) and in secretions of stimulated human neutrophils (Briolat et al., 2005; Lugardon et al., 2000).

These new AMPs are integrated in the concept that highlights the key role of the adrenal medulla in the immunity (Sternberg, 2006) as previously reported for adrenaline and neuropeptide Y that regulate immunity systemically once released from the adrenal medulla. Furthermore, the adrenal medulla contains and releases large amounts of IL-6 and TNF-alpha in response to pro-inflammatory stimuli such as LPS, IL-1 alpha and IL-1 beta (Metz-Boutigue et al., 1998). The discovery of the presence of TLRs on the adrenal cortex cells raises the interesting possibility that the adrenal gland might have a direct role in the response to pathogens, activation of innate immune response and clearing of infectious agents (Sternberg, 2006).

2.2 Antimicrobial peptides derived from chromogranin A

Several new antimicrobial peptides isolated from the granules of chromaffin cells of the bovine adrenal medulla correspond to CGA-derived peptides (Figure 3). The corresponding sequences are highly conserved in human. Interestingly, the main cleavage site in position 78-79 of bCGA and the subsequent remove of the two basic residues K77 and K78 by the carboxipeptidase H (Metz-Boutigue et al., 1993) produces two antimicrobial fragments: vasostatin-I (VS-I; bCGA1-76) (Lugardon et al., 2000) and prochromacin (Prochrom; bCGA79-431) (Strub et al.,1996b). For these N- and C-terminal domains with antimicrobial activities several shorter active fragments were identified: for VS-I, bCGA1-40 (N CgA; NCA) (Shooshtarizadeh et al., 2010), bCGA47-66 (chromofungin; CHR) and for ProChrom, bCGA173-194 (Chromacin; Chrom) (Strub et al., 1996b) and bCGA344-364 (Catestatin; CAT) (Shooshtarizadeh et al., 2010). The unique disulfide bridge of bCGA is present in VS-I and NCA sequences. Two post-translational modifications are important for the expression of the antibacterial activity of Chrom: the phosphorylation of Y173 and the O-glycosylation of S186 [130] (Strub et al., 1996a). Furthermore, it is important to point out that a dimerization motif GXXXG similar to that reported for Glycophorin A (Brosig & Langosch, 1998) is present in the Chrom sequence (G184-G188).

Vasostatin-I

Vasostatin-I (VS-I) displays antimicrobial activity against (i) Gram-positive bacteria (*Micrococcus luteus* and *Bacillus megaterium*) with a minimal inhibitory concentration (MIC) in the range 0.1-1 μM; (ii) against filamentous fungi (*Neurospora crassa, Aspergillus fumigatus, Alternaria brassicola, Nectria haematococca, Fusarium culmorum, Fusarium oxysporum*) with a MIC of 0.5-3 μM and (iii) against yeast cells (*Saccharomyces cerevisiae, Candida albicans*) with a MIC of 2 μM (Lugardon et al., 2000). However VS-I is unable to inhibit the growth of *Escherichia coli* SBS363 and *Escherichia coli* D22. VS-I (Figure 3) possesses structural features specific for antimicrobial peptides, such as a global positive charge (+3), an equilibrated number of polar and hydrophobic residues (20:23) and the presence of a helical region CGA40-65 characterized to be a calmodulin-binding sequence (Lugardon et al., 2001; Yoo, 1992). The loss of the antibacterial activity of CGA7-57 suggests that the N- and C-terminal sequences are essential, nevertheless CGA7-57 is less efficient than VS-I against fungi. Besides, the disulfide bridge is essential for the antibacterial, but not the antifungal property. Altogether, these data suggest that antibacterial and antifungal activities of VS-I have different structural requirements (Lugardon et al., 2001). Interestingly, two helix-helix dimerization motifs important for the interaction with membranes such as LXXXXXXL, present in DAT and dopamine transporter sequences (Torres et al., 2003) are present in the bovine and human VS-I sequences (L42-L49; L57-L64).

Surface interaction of rhodamine-labelled bCGA1-40 was demonstrated using confocal microscopy after incubation of the labeled peptide with *Aspergillus fumigatus, Alternaria brassicola* and *Neurospora crassa* (Blois et al., 2006). In addition, the interaction of bCGA1-40 with monolayers of phospholipids and sterols, as models for the interaction with mammalian and fungal membranes was investigated by the surface tension technique (Blois et al., 2006; Maget-Dana et al., 1999). These studies demonstrated that the N-terminal bCGA1-40 fragment interacts with model membrane phospholipids in a manner consistent with an amphiphilic penetration into membranes in a concentration range relevant for biological activity in mammalian tissue (Blois et al., 2006).

Chromofungin

When VS-I was treated with the endoprotease Glu-C from *Staphylococcus aureus*, one of the generated peptide, chromofungin (CHR), is the shortest active VS-I-derived peptide with antimicrobial activities (Figure 3). It is well conserved during evolution and displays antifungal activity at 2-15 μM against filamentous fungi (*Neurospora crassa, Aspergillus fumigatus, Alternaria brassicola, Nectria haematococca, Fusarium culmorum, Fusarium oxysporum*) and yeast cells (*Candida albicans, Candida tropicalis, Candida neoformans*) (Lugardon et al., 2001). Since this peptide was generated after digestion of the material present in chromaffin secretory vesicles by the endoprotease Glu-C from *S. aureus*, it may be hypothesized that it is produced during infections by this class of pathogens.

The 3-D structure of CHR has been determined in water-trifluoroethanol (50:50) by using ^{1}H-NMR spectroscopy. This analysis revealed the amphipathic helical structure of the sequence 53-56, whereas the segment 48-52 confers hydrophobic character (Lugardon et al., 2001).The importance of the amphipathic sequence for antifungal activity was demonstrated by the loss of such activity against *N. crassa* when two proline residues were substituted for L61 and L64, disrupting the helical structure, the amphipathic character and the dimerization motif helix-helix L57-L64 (Lugardon et al., 2001).

Catestatin

Two CGA-derived fragments bCGA333-364 and bCGA343-362 were characterized after the extensive processing of bCGA by prohormone convertases (PC 1/3 or 2) in chromaffin granules (Taylor et al., 2000). More recently, it was shown that cathepsin L colocalizes with CGA in chromaffin granules. *In vitro* it is able to generate after digestion of recombinant hCGA, a catestatin (CAT)-derived fragment hCGA360-373 (Biswas et al., 2009). In addition to the inhibitory effect of CAT on catecholamine release from chromaffin cells (Mahata et al., 1997), we have shown for this peptide and its shorter active sequence bCGA344-358 (cateslytin, CTL), (Figure 3) a potent antimicrobial activity with a MIC in the low-micromolar range against Gram-positive bacteria (*Micrococcus luteus, Bacillus megaterium* at concentration of 0.8 μM), Gram-negative bacteria (*Escherichia coli D22* at concentration of 8 μM), filamentous fungi (*Neurospora crassa, Aspergillus fumigatus, Nectria haematococca* at concentration of 0.2-10 μM) and yeasts (*Candida albicans, Candida tropicalis, Candida glabrata, Candida neoformans* at concentration of 1.2-8 μM). The sequence of CAT (Figure 3) has been highly conserved during evolution (Briolat et al., 2005). The two human variants P370L and

G364S display antibacterial activity against *M. luteus* with a MIC of 2 and 1 μM, respectively, and against *E. coli* with a MIC of 20 and 10 μM, respectively (Briolat et al., 2005). However, the most active peptide corresponds to the bovine sequence. Bovine CTL, a cationic sequence with a global net charge of +5 (R344, R347, R351, R353, R358) and five hydrophobic residues (M346, L348, F360, Y355, F357) (Figure 3), is able to completely kill bacteria at concentration lower than 10 μM even in the presence of NaCl (0-150 mM) (Briolat et al., 2005). The C-terminal sequence bCGA352-358 is inactive, whereas the N-terminal sequences bCGA344-351 and bCGA 348-358 are antibacterial at 20 μM.

C-terminal CGA-derived fragment

CCA, the C-terminal CGA-derived fragment bCGA418-427 (Figure 3), with a remarkable net charge of -2, displays antifungal activity and belongs to the less abundant anionic AMPs family. It is well conserved during evolution and is homologous to the C-terminal sequence of CGB and the antibacterial peptide SEC (secretolytin) [(Strub et al., 1996b). This peptide was generated *in vitro* after digestion, by the protease Glu-C from *S. aureus*, of the material present in chromaffin secretory vesicles. As previously postulated for CHR, CCA could be generated during infections induced by this pathogen.

2.3 Antimicrobial peptides derived from bovine chromogranin B

To date, the natural C-terminal fragment of bovine CGB (CCB; bCGB 564-626), isolated from chromaffin granules of the adrenal medulla, was found to display antibacterial activity against both *M. luteus* and *E. coli*. The complete inhibition of bacterial growth was observed at a concentration around 1.8 μM (Strub et al., 1996b). This large fragment contains the natural short antibacterial peptide secretolytin (SEC, bCGB614-626) with a net positive charge (+3) (Figure 3). We observed the natural formation of a pyrrolidone glutamic acid at the N-terminal end of SEC and both forms displayed antibacterial activity against *M. luteus*, reaching 100% of growth inhibition at 2 μM (Strub et al., 1996ab). A structure-activity analysis suggests that an alpha-helical amphipathic structure common to SEC and cecropins may account for the antibacterial activity (Strub et al., 1996b).

2.4 Antimicrobial peptides derived from bovine secretogranin II

Because bSGII is weakly expressed in the intragranular matrix of chromaffin secretory vesicles (2% of total proteins), the detection of endogenous AMPs by classical methods was unsuccessful. After *in-silico* analysis, two synthetic peptides with cationic amphipathic sequences were prepared: Rrf and Kvk, which correspond to the sequences bSGII131-138 and bSGII430-443 with respective net charges of +4.5 and 4 (Figure 3). Rrf, completely inhibits the bacterial growth of *M. luteus* and *B. megaterium* with a MIC of 5 and 15 μM, respectively, and Kvk displays antifungal properties at 19 μM against *N. crassa* (Shooshtarizadeh et al., 2010).

3. Interaction of antimicrobial chromogranins-derived peptides with bacterial proteases

The AMPs avoidance mechanisms deployed by bacteria include the proteolytic degradation of the active forms by the bacterial proteases. In order to examine the effects of bacterial proteases on the isolated AMPs derived from CGs, we have tested the effects of *Staphylococcus aureus* V8 protease Glu-C and several supernatants from *S aureus, Salmonella enteretica, Klebsiella oxytoca, Shigella sonnei* and *Vibrio cholera.* By using biochemical methods we have analyzed the degradation of the peptide in presence of bacteria.

Interaction of antimicrobial CGs-derived peptides with proteases from diarrheogenic bacteria Bacteria were isolated from patients of the Strasbourg Civil Hospital by the Bacteriology Institute, University of Strasbourg, (EA-4438). The four strains have a clinical interest because apart from inducing diarrhea, they may cause other infections.

Thus, *Klebsiella* was involved in the occurrence of post-antibiotic diarrheas (Gorkiewicz 2009). Many studies show that *Klebsiella oxytoca* is also involved in nosocomial infections for newborns or adults (Biran et al., 2010) *Klebsiella* infections may also be commensal (Tsakris et al., 2011). *Klebsiella oxytoca* has also been associated with hemorrhagic colitis (Hoffmann et al., 2010) and intercurrent colitis in Crohn's disease (Plessier et al. 2002). *Salmonella* destroys infected cells and the infection continues through blood (sepsis) or through lymphatic vessel (typhoid fever). Salmonella cause also gastrointestinal infections. *Shigella sonnei* and *Vibrio cholera* non O1 cause inflammation of the intestinal mucosa by producing the Shiga toxin.

Klebsiella oxytoca, Salmonella enterica, Shigella sonnei, and Vibrio cholera develop phenomena of antibiotic resistance. Thus, *Salmonella* was reported to be resistant for the action of Ciprofloxacine (Medalla et al., 2011) and Ceftriaxone (Su et al., 2011).

Concerning CgA, we have tested bovine, rat and human CAT corresponding to the sequences bCgA344-364, rCgA6344-364 and hCgA352-372, bovine CTL located at bCgA344-358, two short fragments hCgA360-372 and the conserved tetrapeptide LSFR (bCgA348-351). In addition, we have tested a scrambled peptide relative to the sequence of bovine CAT and the procatestatin fragment bCgA332-364.

We have found antimicrobial activities only for the bovine CAT and CTL, showing that CTL is the shorter active fragment and that it corresponds to the active domain of CAT. Procatestatin was inactive in similar experimental conditions. Bovine CAT and CTL were active against *Klebsiella oxytoca, Salmonella enterica* and *Vibrio cholera* at 100 μM and 50 μM respectively and against *Shigella Sonnei* at 50 μM and 25 μM. In addition, CHR and the C-terminal fragment (CgA387-431) were inactive for concentration up to 100 μM. In contrast, CTL is active at 30 μM against the four pathogens.

Three CgB-derived peptides (CgB58-62, CgB279-291, and CgB547-560) and secretoneurin corresponding to SgII189-254 were examined against the four strains in order to analyse their degradation by bacterial proteases. By using HPLC we have compared the profiles of the peptide alone and the peptide with the inoculated medium.

These experiments show that except CTL all the peptides are completely degraded by the bacteria. To illustrate these data, we present on Figure 4, the profiles relative to CAT and CTL in presence of buffer with *Salmonella enterica*. The complete peptide and the processed form are analysed by sequencing and mass spectrometry (MALDI-TOF).

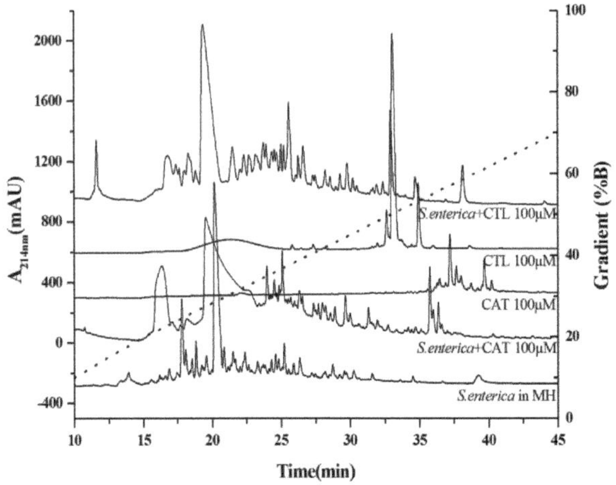

Fig. 4. Analysis by HPLC of the catestatin (CAT) and cateslytin (CTL) degradation by *Salmonella enterica*. The HPLC system is composed by a Dionex chromatogram, Germerong, Germany), using a Nucleosil 300-5 C18 column (4×250 mm, particle size 5 µm, porosity 300 Å; Macherey Nagel, Düren, Germany). The solvent system consisted of 0.1% (v/v) trifluoroacetic acid in water (solvent A) and 0.09% (v/v) trifluoroacetic acid in 70% acetonitrile in milliQ water (solvent B). Elutions were performed at a flow rate of 700 µL min−1 using the gradient indicated on the chromatogram.

3.1 Interaction of antimicrobial Cgs-derived peptides with proteases from *Staphylococcus aureus*

After incubation with *S. aureus* V8 protease Glu-C of the proteic intragranular material of chromaffin cells present in the adrenal medulla, 21 new peptides were isolated by HPLC and analysed by sequencing and mass spectrometry. These peptides were tested against Gram positive bacteria (*Micrococcus luteus* and *S. aureus*), Gram negative bacteria (*Escherichia coli*), fungi (*Neurospora crassa*) and yeast (*Candida albicans*). They are not antibacterial but 5 peptides corresponding to CgA47-60, CgA418-426 and CgB 279-291, CgB 450-464 and CgB470-486 display antifungal activity at the micromolar range against *N. crassa*. Thus, *S. aureus* subverts innate immunity to degrade the antibacterial Cgs/Sgs-derived peptides and produce new antifungal peptides (manuscript in preparation).

Four antimicrobial CgA derived peptides (CHR CgA47-66, bovine CAT CgA344-364, human CgA352-372 and CTL CgA344-358) were incubated in presence of staphylococcal supernatants from S1 (a Methicillin resistant strain) and S2 (a non-resistant strain). CTL, the active domain of CAT, is able to completely kill *S. aureus* at 30 µM, but the two others peptides are inactive. By using a proteomic analysis (HPLC, sequencing and mass spectrometry) we demonstrated that CHR and CTL were not degraded by supernatants, whereas bovine and human CAT are processed to produce several fragments (Figure 5).

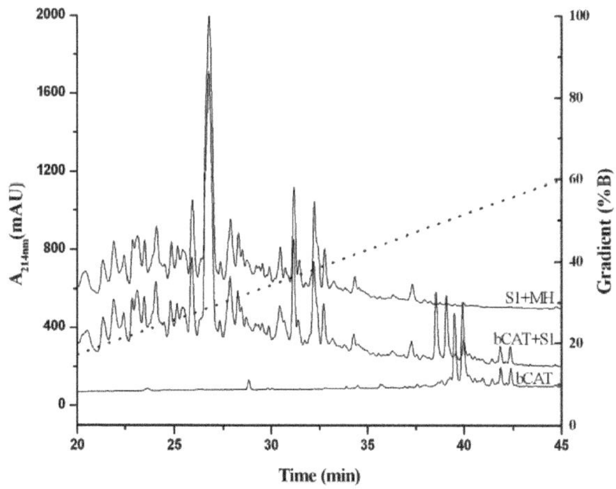

Fig. 5. Analysis by HPLC of the catestatin (CAT) degradation by a methicillin resistant *Staphylococcus aureus* (MRSA). The HPLC system is composed by a Dionex chromatograph, (Germerong, Germany), using a Nucleosil 300-5 C18 column (4×250 mm, particle size 5 µm, porosity 300 Å; Macherey Nagel, Düren, Germany). The solvent system consisted of 0.1% (v/v) trifluoroacetic acid in water (solvent A) and 0.09% (v/v) trifluoroacetic acid in 70% acetonitrile in milliQ water (solvent B). Elutions were performed at a flow rate of 700 µL min−1 using the gradient indicated on the chromatogram.

4. Synergy of the combination of antimicrobial peptides with antibiotics

The emergence of multi-drug resistant bacteria (MDR), with therapeutic failure against *Staphylococcus aureus* (MRSA), *Klebsiella pneumonia, Acinebacter baumannii and Pseudomonas aeruginosa* have paved the way to develop new therapeutic agents by the help of the synergism. In addition the highly toxic effects of antibiotics have shifted the research focus to discover new peptides with broad spectrum of activity and less toxicity. Synergy is the combined activity of two antimicrobial agents that can never be attained by any one of them singly (Serra et al., 1977). Numerous AMPs demonstrate broad spectrum of activity against pathogens, interacting directly with membranes or acting with a specific mode. They represent interesting candidates to synergistically act with antibiotics.

4.1 For *Staphylococcus aureus* MRSA

Most of the patients can prone to serious bacterial infections caused mainly by the multi-resistant microorganisms, *Staphylococcus aureus* coagulase negative spp are one of them. These coagulase negative strains (MRSA) have got approximately 90% of methicillin resistance due to β-lactam resistance (Silva et al., 2011). Story just not stopped here, but still it continues, some of the staphylococcal strains got resistance to the other drugs such as Vancomycin, which was previously widely used against the MRSA infections, and to treat infections of central nervous system, bone infections and sometimes for the pulmonary infections which require a more concentrations to get treated (Dehority, 2010). *S. aureus* have also developed resistance to the Vancomycin due to the use at low level concentrations and recently, *S. aureus* was isolated that had got the *VanA* gene from the *Enterococcus spp* (Sievert et al., 2008) which leads to drug resistance.

In our group, we have examined the synergically effects of three CGA-derived peptides (CAT, CTL and CHR) with Minocyclin, Amoxicillin and Linezolide. To demonstrate that antimicrobial peptides are able to reduce the doses of antibiotics used and to potentiate the activity of antibiotics, antimicrobial tests were carried out by combining the antibiotic peptides at doses below the MIC. The comparison was made with the antibiotic or peptide separately at the same doses.

Minocyclin has a MIC of 2 μg/ml alone against the *S. aureus* ATCC 49775, but when it was combined with CTL at a concentration corresponding to 75% of the MIC, the, concentration of Minocycline was lowered to 0.5 μg/ml. Similar data were obtained by the use of the two others peptides (Figure 6). Thus we demonstrate that amidated bCTL acts synergistically with Minocycline against *S. aureus.* In addition CTL acts synergistically with Voriconazole against *Candida albicans* and *Candida tropicalis.*

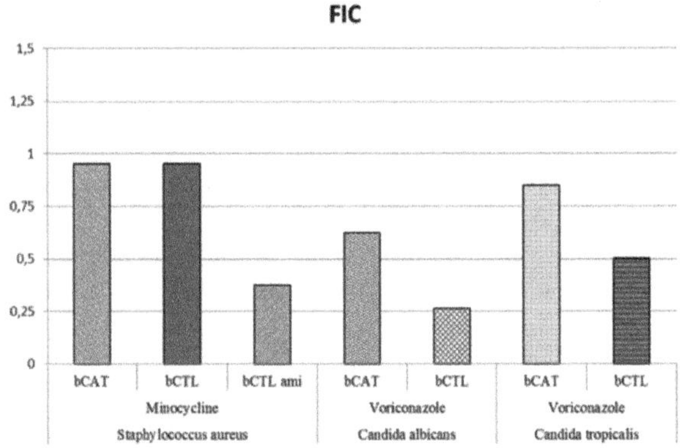

Fig. 6. Fractional inhibitory concentration (FIC) of the chromogranin derived peptides combined with the antimicrobials (Minocycline against the *Staphylococcus aureus* and Voriconazole against *Candida albicans* and *Candida tropicalis*). FIC in range of ≤0.5 gives a synergistic effect, ≤0.5 - <2 is an additive effect but if more than 2 have an antagonistic effect.

4.2 From *Shigella*

Some of the strains of *Shigella* got resistance to antibiotics. A 9-year study of shigellosis in Malaysia, show that 58.4% of the studied strains were resistant to tetracyclin and 53.8% to trimetropin-sulfamethoxasol (Banga Singh et al., 2011). In China, another study establish for *Shigella* the resistance to aztrenam (30,8%), ampicillin (92,3%), piperacilline (61,5%), ceftazidime (30,8%), cefotaxime (30,8%), gentamicine (53,8%) (Zhang et al., 2011). Furthermore, *Vibrio cholera* was also described to develop several resistances against antibiotics (Lamrani et al., 2010).

In conclusion these studies show that CGA-derived AMPs potentiate the effects of antibiotic drugs. One could imagine a mechanism in which the peptide would favor the destabilization of the membrane allowing the antibiotic to rapidly penetrate inside the bacterial cells and thus to reach its site of action.

5. Chromogranin A, a new marker of severity

In clinical practice, CGA has been used as a marker of pheochromocytomas (O'Connor et al., 1984), carcinoid tumors (O'Connor & Deftos, 1986; Syversen et al., 1993), neuroblastomas (Hsiao et al., 1990), neuroendocrine tumors (Berruti et al., 2005), and neurodegenerative diseases (Rangon et al., 2003). Recent data have shown CGA to be a useful prognostic indicator in patients with chronic heart failure (Omland et al., 2003, suggesting that CGA may have some association with cardiovascular diseases. Furthermore, a pilot study has shown CGA to be a predictor of mortality in patients with acute myocardial infarction (Estensen et al., 2006). Characterization of the severity of organ failures and prediction of patient outcome are of major importance for physicians who care for critically ill patients. Multiple organ failure (MOF) remains the main problem in intensive care because of its impact on morbidity, mortality, and resources (Baue et al., 1998). MOF can develop as a consequence of multiple causes, such as infection, systemic inflammatory response syndrome (SIRS), myocardial infarction, septic shock, leading to the activation of various endogenous cascades, cellular dysfunction and death (Baue et al., 1998).

In a recent study we have evaluated whether unselected critically ill patients at ICU (Hautepierre Hospital, Strasbourg, France) admission demonstrate increased plasma CGA concentrations and whether CGA can be of any interest in the care of patients at high risk of death. Patients older than 18 years were recruited consecutively over 3 months during 2007. Exclusion criteria included: duration of stay >24 h and conditions known to increase CGA concentrations independently of acute stress [i.e., a history of documented neuroendocrine tumors (O'Connor & Deftos, 1986) or chronic treatment with proton pump inhibitors before admission (Giusti et al., 2004). Patients who required surgical interventions were also excluded. Of the 120 participants included in the study, 70 patients had a primary diagnosis severe infection, and 50 had a SIRS. Serum CGA concentrations were measured with a commercial sandwich RIA kit (a gift of Cisbio Bioassays, Marcoule, France. In the central 95% of the healthy population, serum CGA concentrations range from 19μg/L to 98μg/L. In neuroendocrine system tumors, the CGA serum concentration varies from the typical range up to 1200 μg/L, depending on the biological and structural characteristics of the tumor, as well as on the extent of tumor spread (Degorce et al., 1999). As a control Procalcitonin (PCT) concentrations were measured on the Kryptor system (Brahms Diagnostic) with the time-resolved amplified cryptate emission methodology in accordance with the manufacturer's recommendations. The Simplified Acute Physiological Score II (SAPS II) and the Logistic Organ Dysfunction System (LODS) score were calculated at admission according to published standards (Levy et al., 2003; Le Gall et al., 1993). Our data show that CGA concentration was positively but weakly correlated with age, PCT concentration, creatinine concentration, SAPS II, and LODS score (P <0.001 for all variables) and was correlated with CRP concentration (Zhang et al., 2008). Thirty-three deaths occurred during the median follow- up time of 23 days. The death rates for CGA and PCT are shown by quartiles in Figure 7. Statistical analysis revealed a significant difference in death rates between CGA quartile 4 and CGA quartiles 1, 2, and 3 (P < 0.001, log-rank test). The death rate for CGA quartile 3 was also significantly different from that of CGA quartile 1 (P= 0.033).

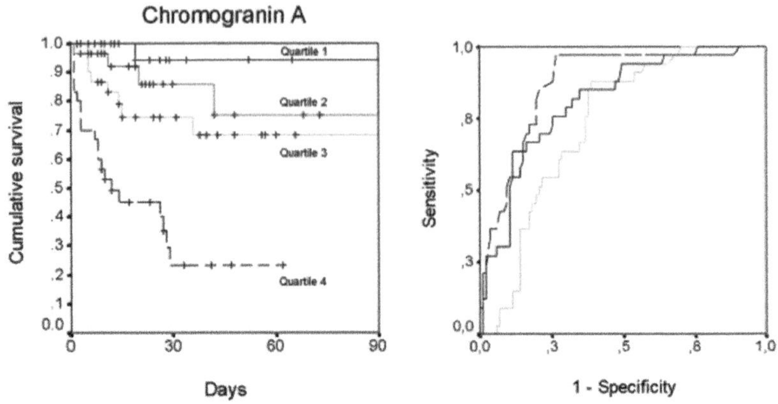

Fig. 7. Kaplan-Meier analysis: cumulative incidence of death by CGA and PCT quartiles. (A), Median (interquartile range) for CGA concentration data: quartile 1, 35 _g/L (30-53 _g/L); quartile 2, 84 _g/L (77-94 _g/L); quartile 3, 174 _g/L (151-197 _g/L); quartile 4, 563 _g/L (355-974 _g/L). Each quartile includes 30 patients.
(B), ROC curve to test the ability of CGA (black line), SAPS II (black dashed line), and PCT (gray dashed line) to predict outcome.

ROC curves for CGA, PCT, and SAPS II are shown in Figure 7. To assess the best positive likelihood ratio, we chose the cutoff value that was associated with the best specificity. For CGA, we chose a cutoff value of 255μg/L, which produced a sensitivity of 0.63 and a specificity of 0.89 (positive likelihood ratio, 5.73; negative likelihood ratio, 0.42; AUC, 0.82). A cutoff value of 65 for SAPS II produced a sensitivity of 0.61 and a specificity of 0.85 (positive likelihood ratio, 4.07; negative likelihood ratio, 0.46; AUC, 0.87). For a PCT cutoff value of 4.82 μg/L, sensitivity and specificity were 0.60 and 0.71, respectively (positive likelihood ratio, 2.07; negative likelihood ratio, 0.56; AUC, 0.73). To conclude, in this clinical study of critically ill nonsurgical patients, we demonstrate that plasma CGA is a strong and independent prognostic in consecutive critically ill nonsurgical patients. The over expression of complete CGA suggests that for these patients the processing machinery to procuce antimicrobial peptides in not correct.

6. Insertion of synthetic antimicrobial chromogranins-derived peptides in biomaterials

The surface of medical devices is a common site of bacterial and fungal adhesion, first step to the constitution of a resistant biofilm leading frequently to chronic infections. In order to prevent such complications, several physical and chemical modifications of the device surface have been proposed. In a previous study, we experimented a new type of topical antifungal coating using the layer-by-layer technique. The nanometric multilayer film obtained by this technique is functionalized by the insertion of a CgA-derived antifungal peptide (CGA 47-66, Chromofungin). We show that the embedded peptide keeps its antifungal activity by interacting with the fungal membrane and penetrating into the cell. *In vitro* studies demonstrated that such an antifungal coating is able to inhibit the growth of yeast *Candida albicans* by 65% and completely stop the proliferation of filamentous fungus *N.crassa*. The cytotoxicity of such a coating was also assessed by growing human gingival fibroblasts at its surface. Finally, the antifungal coating of poly (methylmethacrylate), a widely used material for biomedical devices, is successfully tested in an *in vivo* oral candidiasis rat model (Etienne et al., 2005).

7. Conclusions

CGs family emerges as prohormones able to modulate homeostatic processes in response to excessive stimulations such as microbial infections. The studies concerning the expression of CGs and their antimicrobial peptides in patients with inflammatory diseases and the correlation with the proteolytic processes occurring in these pathologies vs. controls are crucial to understand the involvement of these prohormones and their derived peptides in innate and adaptive immunities. Calcium is a universal secondary messenger involved in many cellular signal transduction pathways, regulating crucial functions such as secretion, cell motility, proliferation and cell death. The calcium-dependent immunomodulatory properties of CHR and CAT are important for the understanding of their involvement in inflammatory mechanisms. In sum, these linear peptides may represent prototypic lead molecules useful for the development of new therapeutic agents and also biomaterials.

8. Acknowledgement

This study was funded by INSERM, the University of Strasbourg (UDS) and INRA (JFC). We are grateful to financial assistance from the Odontology Faculty of the University of Strasbourg (MA, RA). We thank Charlotte Bach for the excellent technical assistance, Bernard Guérold for the preparation of the synthetic peptides, Thomas Lavaux for fruitful discussions, Cisbio Bioassays Research and Development for providing the ELISA kit required for CGA dosages, EA44-38 for the isolation of bacteria and the preparation of bacterial supernatants and Martine Rivet for the preparation of the manuscript.

9. References

Aardal, S., Helle, K.B., Elsayed, S., Reed, R.K. & Serck-Hanssen, G. (1993). Vasostatins, comprising the N-terminal domain of chromogranin A, suppress tension in isolated human blood vessel segments. *Journal of Neuroendocrinology*, Vol. 5, No. 4, (August 1993), pp. 405-412, ISSN: 0953-8194.

Abtin, A., Eckhart, L., Mildner, M., Ghannadan, M., Harder, J., Schroder, J.M. & Tschachler, E. (2009). Degradation by stratum corneum proteases prevents endogenous RNase inhibitor from blocking antimicrobial activities of RNase 5 and RNase 7. *Journal of Investigative Dermatology*, Vol. 129, No. 9, (March 2009), pp. 2193-2201, ISSN: 0022-202X.

Aerts A.M., François, I.E., Cammue, B.P. & Thevissen, K. (2008). The mode of antifungal action of plant, insect and human defensins. *Cellular and Molecular Life Science*, Vol. 65, No. 12, (July 2008), pp. 2069-2079, ISSN: 1420-682X.

Ali, R.S., Falconer, A., Ikram, M., Bissett, C.E., Cerio, R. & Quinn, A.G. (2001). Expression of the peptide antibiotics human beta defensin-1 and human beta defensin-2 in normal human skin. *Journal of Investigative Dermatology*, Vol. 117, No. 1, (July 2001), pp.106-111, ISSN: 0022-202X.

Amato, A., Corti, A., Serio, R. & Mule, F. (2005). Inhibitory influence of chromogranin A N-terminal fragment (vasostatin-1) on the spontaneous contractions of rat proximal colon. *Regulatory Peptides*, Vol. 130, No.1-2, (August 2005), pp. 42-47, ISSN: 0167-0115.

Anouar, Y., Yon, L., Desmoucelles, C., Leprince, J., Breault, L., Gallo-Payet, N. & Vaudry, H. (1998). Identification of a novel secretogranin II-derived peptide in the adult and fetal human adrenal gland. *Endocrinology Research* Vol. 24, No. 3-4, (August-November 1998), pp. 731-736, ISSN: 0743-5800.

Artym, J., Zimecki, M., Kuryszko, J. & Kruzel, M.L. (2005). Lactoferrin accelerates reconstitution of the humoral and cellular immune response during chemotherapy-induced immunosuppression and bone marrow transplant in mice. *Stem Cells Development*, Vol. 14, No.5, (October 2005), pp. 548-555, ISSN: 1547-3287.

Baechle, D., Flad, T., Cansier, A., Steffen, H., Schittek, B., Tolson, J., Herrmann, T., Dihazi, H., Beck, A., Mueller, G.A., Mueller, M., Stevanovic, S., Garbe, C., Mueller, C.A. & Kalbacher H. (2006). Cathepsin D is present in human eccrine sweat and involved in the postsecretory processing of the antimicrobial peptide DCD-1L. *Journal of Biological Chemistry*, Vol. 281, No.9, (March 2006), pp. 5406-5415, ISSN: 0021-9258.

Bals, R., Wang, X., Zasloff, M. & Wilson, J.M. (1998). The peptide antibiotic LL-37/hCAP-18 is expressed in epithelia of the human lung where it has broad antimicrobial activity at the airway surface. *Proceedings of National Academy of Sciences of the United States of America*, Vol. 95, No. 16, (August 1998), pp. 9541-9546, ISSN: 0027-8424.

Banga Singh, K.K., Ojha, S.C., Deris, Z.Z., & Rahman, R.A. (2011). A 9-year study of shigellosis in Northeast Malaysia: Antimicrobial susceptibility and shifting species dominance, *Journal of Public Health*, Vol. 19, No. 3, (June 2011), pp. 231-236, ISSN: 1613-2238.

Baue, A.E., Durham, R. & Faist, E. (1998). Systemic inflammatory response syndrome (SIRS), multiple organ dysfunction syndrome (MODS), multiple organ failure (MOF): are we winning the battle? *Shock*, Vol. 10, No. 2, (August 1998), pp. 79-89, ISSN: 1073-2322.

Bellamy, W., Wakabayashi, H., Takase, M., Kawase, K., Shimamura, S. & Tomita, M. (1993). Killing of Candida albicans by lactoferricin B, a potent antimicrobial peptide derived from the N-terminal region of bovine lactoferrin. *Medical Microbiology and Immunology*, Vol. 182, No .2, (May 1993), pp. 97-105, ISSN: 0300-8584.

Berruti, A., Mosca, A., Tucci, M., Terrone, C., Torta, M., Tarabuzzi, R., Russo, L., Cracco, C., Bollito, E., Scarpa, R.M., Angeli, A. & Dogliotti, L. (2005). Independent prognostic role of circulating chromogranin A in prostate cancer patients with hormone-refractory disease. *Endocrine Related Cancer*, Vol. 12, No. 1, (March 2005), pp.109-117, ISSN: 1351-0088.

Biran, V., Gaudin, A., Mariani-Kurdjian, P., Doit, C., Bingen, E. & Aujard, Y. (2010). Implication of extended-spectrum beta-lactamase enterobacteriaceae in nosocomial infections in neonates. *Archives de Pédiatrie*, Vol. 17, Suppl 4, (September 2010), pp. S150-153, ISSN: 0929-693X.

Biswas, N., Rodriguez-Flores, J.L., Courel, M., Gayen, J., Vaingankar, S.M., Mahata, M., Torpey, J.W., Taupenot, L., O'Connor, D.T. & Mahata, S.K. (2009). Cathepsin L colocalizes with chromogranin A in chromaffin vesicles to generate active peptides. *Endocrinology*, Vol. 150, No. 8, (August 2009), pp. 3547-3557, ISSN: 0013-7227.

Blois, A., Holmsen, H., Martino, G., Corti, A., Metz-Boutigue, M.H. & Helle, K.B. (2006). Interactions of chromogranin A-derived vasostatins and monolayers of phosphatidylserine, phosphatidylcholine and phosphatidylethanolamine. *Regulatory Peptides*, Vol. 134, No. 1, (March 2006), pp. 30-37, ISSN: 0167-0115.

Boni, R., Burg G., Doguoglu, A., Ilg, E.C., Schafer, B.W., Mulle, B. & Heizmann, C.W. (1997). Immunohistochemical localization of the Ca2+ binding S100 proteins in normal human skin and melanocytic lesions. *The British Journal of Dermatology*, Vol. 137, No. 1, (July 1997) pp. 39-43, ISSN: 0007-0963.

Braun, T., Voland, P., Kunz, L., Prinz, C. & Gratzl, M. (2007). Enterochromaffin cells of the human gut: sensors for spices and odorants. *Gastroenterology*, Vol. 132, No. 5), (May 2007), pp. 1890-1901, ISSN: 0016-5085.

Brekke, J.F., Osol, G.J. & Helle KB. (2002). N-terminal chromogranin-derived peptides as dilators of bovine coronary resistance arteries. *Regulatory Peptides*, Vol. 105, No. 2, (May 2002), pp. 93-100, ISSN: 0167-0115.

Briolat, J., Wu, S.D., Mahata, S.K., Gonthier, B., Bagnard, D., Chasserot-Golaz, S., Helle, K.B., Aunis D & Metz-Boutigue MH. (2005). New antimicrobial activity for the catecholamine release-inhibitory peptide from chromogranin A. *Cellular and Molecular Life Science*, Vol. 62, No. 3, (February 2005), pp. 377-385, ISSN: 1420-682X.

Broome, A.M., Ryan, D. & Eckert, R.L. (2003). S100 protein subcellular localization during epidermal differentiation and psoriasis. *The Journal of Histochemistry and Cytochemistry*, Vol. 51, No. 5, (May 2003), pp. 675-685, ISSN: 0022-1554.

Bulet, P., Stocklin, R. & Menin, L. (2004). Anti-microbial peptides: from invertebrates to vertebrates. *Immunological reviews*, Vol. 198, (April 2004), pp. 169-184, ISSN: 0105-2896.

Butmarc, J., Yufit, T., Carson, P. & Falanga, V. (2004). Human beta-defensin-2 expression is increased in chronic wounds. *Wound repair and regeneration*, Vol. 12, No. 4, (July-August 2004), pp. 439-443, ISSN: 1067-1927.

Ceconi, C., Ferrari, R., Bachetti, T., Opasich, C., Volterrani, M., Colombo, B., Parrinello, G; & Corti A. (2002). Chromogranin A in heart failure; a novel neurohumoral factor and a predictor for mortality. *European heart journal*, Vol. 23, No. 12, (June 2002), pp. 967-974, ISSN: 0195-668X.

Cetin, Y. & Grube, D. (1991). Immunoreactivities for chromogranin A and B, and secretogranin II in the guinea pig entero-endocrine system: cellular distributions and intercellular heterogeneities. *Cell and tissue research*, Vol. 264, No. 2, (May 1991), pp. 231-241, ISSN: 0302-766X.

Corti, A., Ferrari, R. & Ceconi, C. (2000). Chromogranin A and tumor necrosis factor-alpha (TNF) in chronic heart failure. *Advances in experimental medicine and biology*, Vol. 482, pp. 351-359, ISSN: 0065-2598.

Corti, A., Mannarino, C., Mazza, R., Angelone, T., Longhi, R. & Tota, B. (2004). Chromogranin A N-terminal fragments vasostatin-1 and the synthetic CGA 7-57 peptide act as cardiostatins on the isolated working frog heart. *General and comparatative endocrinology*, Vol. 136, No. 2, (April 2004), pp. 217-224, ISSN: 0016-6480.

Curry, W.J., Shaw, C., Johnston, C.F., Thim, L. & Buchanan, K.D. (1992). Isolation and primary structure of a novel chromogranin A-derived peptide, WE-14, from a human midgut carcinoid tumour. *FEBS letters*, Vol. 301, No. 3, (April 1992), pp. 319-321, ISSN: 0014-5793.

Cutuli, M., Cristiani, S., Lipton, J.M. & Catania, A. (2000). Antimicrobial effects of alpha-MSH peptides. *Journal of leukocyte biology*, Vol. 67, No. 2, (February 2000), pp. 233-239, ISSN: 0741-5400.

Dann, S.M. & Eckmann, L. (2007). Innate immune defenses in the intestinal tract. *Current opinion in gastroenterology*, Vol. 23, No. 2, (March 2007), pp. 115-120, ISSN: 0267-1379.

Davidson, D.J., Currie, A.J., Reid, G.S., Bowdish, D.M., MacDonald, K.L., Ma, R.C., Hancock, R.E. & Speert, D.P. (2004). The cationic antimicrobial peptide LL-37 modulates dendritic cell differentiation and dendritic cell-induced T cell polarization. *The journal of immunology*, Vol. 172, No. 2, (January 2004), pp. 1146-1156, ISSN: 0022-1767.

Degorce, F., Goumon, Y., Jacquemart, L., Vidaud, C., Bellanger, L., Pons-Anicet, D., Seguin, P., Metz-Boutigue, M.H. & Aunis, D. (1999). A new human chromogranin A (CgA) immunoradiometric assay involving monoclonal antibodies raised against the unprocessed central domain (145-245). *British journal of cancer*, Vol. 79, No.1, (january 1999), pp. 65-71, ISSN: 0007-0920.

Dehority, W. (2010). Use of vancomycin in pediatrics. *The pediatric infectious disease*, Vol. 29, No. 5, (may 2010), pp. 462-463, ISSN: 0891-3668.

Del Valle, M.E., Vazquez, E., Represa, J., Malinovsky, L. & Vega, J.A. (1994). Immunohistochemical localization of calcium-binding proteins in the human cutaneous sensory corpuscles. *Neuroscience letters*, Vol. 168, No. 1-2, (February 1994), pp. 247-250, ISSN: 0304-3940.

Dieckgraefe, B.K., Crimmins, D.L., Landt, V., Houchen, C., Anant, S., Porche-Sorbet, R. & Ladenson, J.H. (2002). Expression of the regenerating gene family in inflammatory bowel disease mucosa: Reg Ialpha upregulation, processing, and antiapoptotic activity. *Journal of investigative medicine*, Vol. 50, No. 6, (November 2002), pp. 421-434, ISSN: 1081-5589.

Dyer, K.D. & Rosenberg, H.F. (2006). The RNase a superfamily: generation of diversity and innate host defense. *Molecular diversity* Vol. 10, No. 4, (November 2006), pp. 585-597, ISSN: 1381-1991.

Eckert, R.L., Broome, A.M., Ruse, M., Robinson, N., Ryan, D. & Lee, K. (2004). S100 proteins in the epidermis. *The journal of investigative dermatology*, Vol. 123, No. 1, (July 2004), pp. 23-33, ISSN: 0022-202X.

Eiden, L.E. (1987). Is chromogranin a prohormone? *Nature*, Vol. 325, No. 6102, (January 1987), pp. 301, ISSN: 0028-0836.

Elias, P.M. (2007). The skin barrier as an innate immune element. *Seminars in immunopathology* Vol. 29, No. 1, (April 2007), pp. 3-14, ISSN: 1863-2297.

Estensen, M.E., Hognestad, A., Syversen, U., Squire, I., Nq, L., Kickshus, Dickstein, K., Omland, T. (2006). Prognostic value of plasma chromogranin A levels in patients with complicated myocardial infarction. *American heart journal,* Vol. 152, No.5, (november 2006), pp. 927.e1-6, ISSN : 0002-8703.

Etienne, O., Gasnier, C., Taddei, C., Voegel, J.C., Aunis, D., Schaaf, P., Metz-Boutigue, M.H., Bolcato-Bellemin, A.L. & Egles, C. (2005). Antifungal coating by biofunctionalized polyelectrolyte multilayered films. Biomaterials, Vol. 26, No. 33, (November 2005), pp. 6704-6412, ISSN: 0142-9612.

Fahlgren, A., Hammarstrom, S., Danielsson, A. & Hammarstrom, M.L. (2004). beta-Defensin-3 and -4 in intestinal epithelial cells display increased mRNA expression in ulcerative colitis. *Clinical and experimental immunology,* Vol. 137, No. 2, (August 2004), pp. 379-385, ISSN: 0009-9104.

Fasciotto, B.H., Trauss, C.A., Greeley, G.H. & Cohn, D.V. (1993). Parastatin (porcine chromogranin A347-419), a novel chromogranin A-derived peptide, inhibits parathyroid cell secretion. *Endocrinology,* Vol. 133, No. 2, (August 1993), pp. 461-466, ISSN: 0013-7227.

Forrester, J.S., Diamond, G., Chatterjee, K. & Swan, H.J. (1976). Medical therapy of acute myocardial infarction by application of hemodynamic subsets (second of two parts). *The New England journal of medicine,* Vol. 295. No. 25, (December 1976), pp 1404-1413, ISSN: 0028-4793.

Ganz, T. (2003). Defensins: antimicrobial peptides of innate immunity. *Nature Review Immunology,* Vol. 3, No. 9, (September 2003), pp. 710-720, ISSN: 1474-1733.

Garcia, J.R., Jaumann, F., Schulz, S., Krause, A., Rodriguez-Jimenez, J., Forssmann, U., Adermann, K., Kluver, E., Vogelmeier, C., Becker, D., Hedrich, R., Forssmann, W.G, & Bals, R. (2001). Identification of a novel, multifunctional beta-defensin (human beta-defensin 3) with specific antimicrobial activity. Its interaction with plasma membranes of Xenopus oocytes and the induction of macrophage chemoattraction. *Cell and tissue research,* Vol. 306, No. 2, (November 2001), pp. 257-264, ISSN: 0302-766X.

Gasparri, A., Sidoli, A., Sanchez, L.P., Longhi, R., Siccardi, A.G., Marchisio, P.C. & Corti, A. (1997). Chromogranin A fragments modulate cell adhesion. Identification and characterization of a pro-adhesive domain. *The journal of biological chemistry,* Vol. 272, No. 33, (August 1997), pp. 20835-20843, ISSN: 0021-9258.

Ghia, J.E., Crenner, F., Metz-Boutigue, M.H., Aunis, D., Angel, F. (2004b). The effect of a chromogranin A-derived peptide (CgA4-16) in the writhing nociceptive response induced by acetic acid in rats. *Life Science,* Vol. 75, No.15, (August 2004), pp. 1787-1799, ISSN: 0024-3205.

Ghia, J.E., Crenner, F., Rohr, S., Meyer, C., Metz-Boutigue, M.H., Aunis, D. & Angel F. (2004a). A role for chromogranin A (4-16), a vasostatin-derived peptide, on human colonic motility. An in vitro study. *Regulatory Peptides,* Vol. 121, No. 1-3, (September 2004) pp. 31-39, ISSN: 0167-0115.

Giusti, M., Sidoti, M., Augeri, C., Rabitti, C. & Minuto, F. (2004). Effect of short-term treatment with low dosages of the proton-pump inhibitor omeprazole on serum chromogranin A levels in man. *European journal of endocrinology,* Vol. 150, No. 3, (March 2004), pp: 299-303, ISSN: 0804-4643.

Gorkiewicz, G. (2009). Nosocomial and antibiotic-associated diarrhoea caused by organisms other than Clostridium difficile. *International journal of antimicrobial agents,* Vol. 33, Suppl 1, (March 2009), pp. S37 41, ISSN: 0924 8579.

Hansen, M.B. & Witte, A.B. (2008). The role of serotonin in intestinal luminal sensing and secretion. *Acta physiologica* Vol. 193, No. 4, (August 2008), pp. 311-323, ISSN: 1748-1708.

Harder, J., Bartels, J., Christophers, E. & Schroder, J.M. (1997). A peptide antibiotic from human skin. *Nature,* Vol. 387, No. 6636, (June 1997), pp. 861 ISSN: 0028-0836.

Harder, J., Bartels, J., Christophers, E. & Schroder, J.M. (2001). Isolation and characterization of human beta -defensin-3, a novel human inducible peptide antibiotic. *The journal of biological chemistry,* Vol. 276, No. 8, (February 2001), pp. 5707-5713, ISSN: 0021-9258.

Harder, J. & Schroder, J.M. (2002). RNase 7, a novel innate immune defense antimicrobial protein of healthy human skin. *The journal of biological chemistry,*Vol. 277, No. 48, (November 2002), pp. 46779-46784, ISSN: 0021-9258.

Harder, J., Meyer-Hoffert, U., Wehkamp, K., Schwichtenberg, L. & Schroder, J.M. (2004). Differential gene induction of human beta-defensins (hBD-1, -2, -3, and -4) in keratinocytes is inhibited by retinoic acid. *The journal of investigative dermatology,* Vol. 123, No. 3, (September 2004), pp. 522-529, ISSN: 0022-202X.

Hartschuh, W., Weihe, E. & Yanaihara, N. (1989a). Immunohistochemical analysis of chromogranin A and multiple peptides in the mammalian Merkel cell: further evidence for its paraneuronal function? *Archives of histology and cytology,* Vol. 52, Suppl., pp. 423-431, ISSN: 0914-9465.

Hartschuh,W., Weihe, E. & Egner, U. (1989b). Chromogranin A in the mammalian Merkel cell: cellular and subcellular distribution.*The journal of investigative dermatology,* Vol. 93, No. 5, (November 1989), pp. 641-648, ISSN: 0022-202X.

Hase, K., Eckmann, L., Leopard, J.D., Varki, N. & Kagnoff, M.F. (2002). Cell differentiation is a key determinant of cathelicidin LL-37/human cationic antimicrobial protein 18 expression by human colon epithelium. *Infection and Immunity,* Vol. 70, No. 2, (February 2002), pp. 953-963, ISSN: 0019-9567.

Heitz, P., Polak, J.M., Timson, D.M. & Pearse, A.G. (1976). Enterochromaffin cells as the endocrine source of gastrointestinal substance P. *Histochemistry,* Vol. 49, No. 4, (November 1976), pp. 343-347, ISSN: 0301-5564.

Helle, K.B. & Serck-Hanssen, G. (1975). The adrenal medulla: a model for studies of hormonal and neuronal storage and release mechanisms. *Molecular and Cellular Biochemistry,* Vol. 6, No. 2, (February 1975), pp. 127-146, ISSN: 0300-8177.

Helle, K.B. (2004). The granin family of uniquely acidic proteins of the diffuse neuroendocrine system: comparative and functional aspects. *Biological review of the Cambridge Philosophical Society,* Vol. 79, No. 4, (November 2004), pp. 769-794, ISSN: 1464-7931.

Helle, K.B., Corti, A., Metz-Boutigue, M.H., & Tota, B. (2007). The endocrine role for chromogranin A: a prohormone for peptides with regulatory properties. *Cellular and molecular life science,* Vol. 64, No. 22, (November 2007), pp. 2863-2886, ISSN 1420-682X.

Hiltz, M.E. & Lipton, J.M. (1990). Alpha-MSH peptides inhibit acute inflammation and contact sensitivity. *Peptides,* Vol. 11, No. 5, (September-October 1990), pp. 979-982, ISSN: 0196-9781.

Hoffmann, K.M., Deutschmann, A., Weitzer, C., Joainig, M., Zechner, E., Hogenauer, C. & Hauer, A.C. (2010). Antibiotic-associated hemorrhagic colitis caused by cytotoxin-producing Klebsiella oxytoca. *Pediatrics,* Vol. 125, No. 4, (April 2010), pp. e960-963, ISSN: 0031-4005.

Hooper, L.V., Stappenbeck, T.S., Hong, C.V. & Gordon, J.I. (2003). Angiogenins: a new class of microbicidal proteins involved in innate immunity. *Nature immunology,* Vol. 4, No. 3, (March 2003), pp. 269-273, ISSN: 1529-2908.

Hornef, M.W., Putsep, K., Karlsson, J., Refai, E. & Andersson, M. (2004). Increased diversity of antimicrobial peptides by covalent dimer formation. *Nature immunology* Vol. 5, No. 8, (August 2004), pp. 836-843, ISSN: 1529-2908.

Jinquan, T., Vorum, H., Larsen, C.G., Madsen, P., Rasmussen, H.H., Gesser, B., Etzerodt, M., Honore, B., Celis, J.E. & Thestrup-Pedersen, K. (1996). Psoriasin: a novel chemotactic protein. *The journal of investigative dermatology,* Vol. 107, No. 1, (July 1996), pp. 5-10, ISSN: 0022-202X.

Kai-Larsen, Y. & Agerberth, B. (2008). The role of the multifunctional peptide LL-37 in host defense. *Frontiers in bioscience,* Vol. 1, No. 13, (May 2008), pp. 3760-3767, ISSN: 1093-4715.

Kanda, N. & Watanabe, S. (2008). IL-12, IL-23, and IL-27 enhance human beta-defensin-2 production in human keratinocytes. *European journal of immunology,* Vol. 38, No.5, (May 2008), pp. 1287-1296, ISSN: 0014-2980.

Kansal, R.G., Aziz, R.K. & Kotb, M. (2005). Modulation of expression of superantigens by human transferrin and lactoferrin: a novel mechanism in host-Streptococcus interactions. *The Journal of infectious diseases,* Vol. 191, No.12, (June 2005), pp. 2121-2129, ISSN: 0022-1899.

Keshav, S. (2006). Paneth cells: leukocyte-like mediators of innate immunity in the intestine. *Journal of leukocyte biology,* Vol. 80, No. 3, (September 2006), pp. 500-508, ISSN: 0741-5400.

Kim, M., Cooke, H.J., Javed, N.H., Carey, H.V., Christofi, F. & Raybould, H.E. (2001). D-glucose releases 5-hydroxytryptamine from human BON cells as a model of enterochromaffin cells. *Gastroenterology,* Vol. 121, No.6, (Dec 2001), pp.1400-1406, ISSN 0016-5085

Koczulla, R., von Degenfeld, G., Kupatt, C., Krotz, F., Zahler, S., Gloe, T., Issbrucker, K., Unterberger, P., Zaiou, M., Lebherz, C., Karl, A., Raake, P., Pfosser, A., Boekstegers, P., Welsch, U., Hiemstra, P.S., Vogelmeier, C., Gallo, R.L., Clauss, M. & Bals, R. (2003). An angiogenic role for the human peptide antibiotic LL-37/hCAP-18. *The Journal of clinical investigation,* Vol. 111, No.11, (June 2003), pp.1665-1672, ISSN: 0021-9738.

Kuramoto, H., Kadowaki, M., Sakamoto, H., Yuasa, K., Todo, A. & Shirai, R. (2007). Distinct morphology of serotonin-containing enterochromaffin (EC) cells in the rat distal colon. *Archives of histology and cytology,* Vol. 70, No.4, (November 2007), pp. 235-241, ISSN: 0914-9465.

Lai, Y., Villaruz, A.E., Li ,M., Cha, D.J., Sturdevant, D.E., & Otto, M. (2007). The human anionic antimicrobial peptide dermcidin induces proteolytic defence mechanisms in staphylococci. *Molecular microbiology,* Vol. 63, No.2, (January 2007), pp. 497-506, ISSN: 0950-382X.

Lamrani Alaoui, H., Oufdou, K., & Mezrioui, N.E. (2010). Determination of several potential virulence factors in non-o1 Vibrio cholerae, Pseudomonas aeruginosa, faecal coliforms and streptococci isolated from Marrakesh groundwater. *Water science and technology*, Vol. 61, No.7, pp. 1895-1905, ISSN: 0273-1223.

Lee Motoyama J.P., Kim-Motoyama, H., Kim, P., Nakagama, H., Miyagawa, K. & Suzuki, K. (2007). Identification of dermcidin in human gestational tissue and characterization of its proteolytic activity. *Biochemical and biophysical research communications*, Vol. 357, No.4, (June 2007), pp. 828-833, ISSN: 0006-291X.

Le Gall, J.R., Lemeshow, S. & Saulnier, F. (1993). A new simplified acute physiology score (SAPS II) based on a european/north american multicenter study. *The journal of the American medical association*. Vol. 27, No.17, (may 1994), pp.1321, ISSN: 0098-7484.

Legrand, D., Elass, E., Carpentier, M. & Mazurier, J. (2005). Lactoferrin: a modulator of immune and inflammatory responses. *Cellular and molecular life science*, Vol. 62, No.22, (November 2005), pp. 2549-2559, ISSN: 1420-682X.

Lehrer, R.I., Szklarek, D., Barton, A., Ganz, T., Hamann, K.J. & Gleich, G.J. (1989). Antibacterial properties of eosinophil major basic protein and eosinophil cationic protein. *Journal of immunology*, Vol. 142, No.2, (June 1989), pp. 4428-4434, ISSN: 0022-1767.

Levy, M.M., Fink, M.P., Marshall, J.C., Abraham, E., Angus, D. Cook, D., Cohen, J., Opal, S.M., Vincent, J.L. & Ramsay, G. (2003). International sepsis definitions conference. *Intensive care*, Vol. 29, No.4, (april 2003), pp.530-538, ISSN: 0342-4642.

Lichti, U., Anders, J. & Yuspa, S.H. (2008). Isolation and short-term culture of primary keratinocytes, hair follicle populations and dermal cells from newborn mice and keratinocytes from adult mice for in vitro analysis and for grafting to immunodeficient mice. *Nature Protocols*, Vol. 3, No.5, (April 2008), pp. 799-810, ISSN: 1750-2799.

Lucarz, A. & Brand, G. (2007). Current considerations about Merkel cells. *European journal of cell biology*, Vol. 86, No.5, (May 2007), pp. 243-251, ISSN: 0171-9335.

Lugardon, K., Raffner, R., Goumon, Y., Cort, A., Delmas, A., Bulet, P., Aunis, D. & Metz-Boutigue, M.H. (2000). Antibacterial and antifungal activities of vasostatin-1, the N-terminal fragment of chromogranin A. *Journal of biological chemistry*, Vol. 275, No. 15, (April 2000), pp. 10745-10753, ISSN: 0021-9258.

Lugardon, K., Chasserot-Golaz, S., Kieffer, A.E., Maget-Dana, R., Nullans, G., Kieffer, B., Aunis, D. & Metz-Boutigue M.H. (2001). Structural and biological characterization of chromofungin, the antifungal chromogranin A-(47-66)-derived peptide. *Journal of biological chemistry*, Vol. 276, No.38, (September 2001), pp. 35875-35882, ISSN: 0021-9258.

Maget-Dana, R. (1999). The monolayer technique: a potent tool for studying the interfacial properties of antimicrobial and membrane-lytic peptides and their interactions with lipid membranes. *Biochemica and biophysica acta*, Vol. 1462, No. 1-2, (December 1999), pp. 109-140, ISSN: 0006-3002.

Maget-Dana, R., Metz-Boutigue, M.H. & Helle, K.B. (2002). The N-terminal domain of chromogranin A (CgA1-40) interacts with monolayers of membrane lipids of fungal and mammalian compositions. *Annals of New York Academy of Sciences*, Vol. 971, (October 2002), pp. 352-354, ISSN: 0077-8923.

Mahata, S.K., O'Connor, D.T., Mahata, M., Yoo, S.H., Taupenot, L., Wu, H., Gill, B.M. & Parmer, R.J. (1997). Novel autocrine feedback control of catecholamine release. A discrete chromogranin a fragment is a noncompetitive nicotinic cholinergic antagonist. *Journal of clinical investigation*, Vol. 100, No. 6, (September 1996), pp. 1623-1633, ISSN: 0021-9738.

Mallow, E.B., Harris, A., Salzman, N., Russell, J.P., DeBerardinis, R.J., Ruchelli, E. & Bevins, C.L. (1996). Human enteric defensins. Gene structure and developmental expression. *The Journal of biological chemistry*, Vol. 271, No.8, (February 1996), pp. 4038-4045, ISSN: 0021-9258.

Mandrika, I., Muceniece, R. & Wikberg, J.E. (2001). Effects of melanocortin peptides on lipopolysaccharide/interferon-gamma-induced NF-kappaB DNA binding and nitric oxide production in macrophage-like RAW 264.7 cells: evidence for dual mechanisms of action. *Biochemical pharmacology*, Vol. 61, No.5, (March 2001), pp. 613-621, ISSN: 0006-2952.

Manners, J.M. (2007). Hidden weapons of microbial destruction in plant genomes. *Genome biology*, Vol. 8, No.9, pp. 225, ISSN: 1465-6906.

Marksteiner, J., Kirchmair, R., Mahata, S.K., Mahata, M., Fischer-Colbrie, R., Hogue-Angeletti, R., Saria, A. & Winkler H. (1993). Distribution of secretoneurin, a peptide derived from secretogranin II, in rat brain: an immunocytochemical and radioimmunological study. *The European journal of neuroscience*, Vol. 54, No. 4, (June 1993), pp. 923-944, ISSN: 0306-4522.

Martinsson, H., Yhr, M. & Enerback, C. (2005). Expression patterns of S100A7 (psoriasin) and S100A9 (calgranulin-B) in keratinocyte differentiation. *Experimental dermatology*, Vol. 14, No. 3, (March 2005), pp. 161-168, ISSN: 0906-6705.

Mason, D.Y. & Taylor, C.R. (1975). The distribution of muramidase (lysozyme) in human tissues. *Journal of clinical pathology*, Vol. 28, No.2, (February 1975), pp. 124-132, ISSN: 0021-9746.

Medalla, F., Sjölund-Karlsson, M., Shin, S., Harvey, E., Joyce, K., Theobald, L., Nygren, B.N., Pecic, G., Gay, K., Austin, J., Stuart, A., Blanton, E., Mintz, E. D., Whichard, J. M. & Barzilay, E. J. (2011). Ciprofloxacin-resistant Salmonella enterica Serotype Typhi, United States, 1999-2008. *Emerging Infectious Diseases*, Vol. 17, No. 6, (June 2011), pp. 1095-1098, ISSN: 1080-6040.

Metz-Boutigue, M.H., Garcia-Sablone, P., Hogue-Angeletti, R. & Aunis D. (1993). Intracellular and extracellular processing of chromogranin A. Determination of cleavage sites. *European journal of biochemistry*, Vol. 217, No. 1, (October 1993), pp. 247-257, ISSN: 0014-2956.

Metz-Boutigue, M.H., Goumon, Y., Lugardon, K., Strub, J.M. & Aunis, D. (1998). Antibacterial peptides are present in chromaffin cell secretory granules. *Cellular and molecular neurobiology*, Vol. 18, No. 2, (April 1998), pp. 249-266, ISSN: 0272-4340.

Modlin, I.M., Kidd, M., Pfragner, R., Eick, G.N. & Champaneria, M.C. (2006). The functional characterization of normal and neoplastic human enterochromaffin cells. *Journal of clinical endocrinology and metabolism*, Vol. 91, No.6, (June 2006), pp. 2340-2348, ISSN: 0021-972X.

Mookherjee, N., Brown, K.L., Bowdish, D.M., Doria, S., Falsafi, R., Hokamp, K., Roche, F.M., Mu, R., Doho, G.H., Pistolic, J., Powers, J.P., Bryan, J., Brinkman, F.S. & Hancock, R.E. (2006). Modulation of the TLR-mediated inflammatory response by the human defense peptide LL-37. *Journal of immunology*, Vol. 176, No. 4, (February 2006), pp. 2455-2464, ISSN: 0022-1767.

Mugridge, K.G., Perretti, M., Ghiara, P. & Parente, L. (1991). Alpha-melanocyte-stimulating hormone reduces interleukin-1 beta effects on rat stomach preparations possibly through interference with a type I receptor. *European journal of pharmacology*, Vol. 197, No. 2-3, (May 1991), pp. 151-155, ISSN: 0014-2999.

Müller, C.A., Autenrieth, I.B. & Peschel, A. (2005). Innate defenses of the intestinal epithelial barrier. *Cellular and molecular life sciences*, Vol. 62, No. 12, (June 2005), pp. 1297-1307, ISSN: 1420-682X.

Niyonsaba, F., Ushio, H., Nakano, N., Ng, W., Sayama, K., Hashimoto, K., Nagaoka, I., Okumura, K. & Ogawa, H. (2007). Antimicrobial peptides human beta-defensins stimulate epidermal keratinocyte migration, proliferation and production of proinflammatory cytokines and chemokines. *Journal of investigative dermatology*, Vol. 127, No. 3, (March 2007), pp. 594-604, ISSN: 0022-202X.

Ogawa, H., Miyazaki, H. & Kimura, M. (1971). Isolation and characterization of human skin lysozyme. *Journal of investigative dermatology*, Vol. 57, No. 2, (August 1971), pp. 111-116, ISSN: 0022-202X.

Omland, T., Dickstein, K. & Syversen, U. (2003). Association between plasma chromogranin A concentration and long-term mortality after myocardial infarction. *The American journal of medicine*, Vol. 114, No. 1, (January 2003), pp. 25-30, ISSN: 0002-9343.

O'Neil, D.A., Porter, E.M., Elewaut, D., Anderson, G.M., Eckmann, L., Ganz, T. & Kagnoff, M.F. (1999). Expression and regulation of human beta-defensins hBD-1 and hBD-2 in intestinal epithelium. *Journal of immunology*, Vol. 163, No. 12, (December 1999), pp. 6718-6724, ISSN: 0022-1767.

Oren, A., Ganz, T., Liu, L. & Meerloo, T. (2003). In human epidermis, beta-defensin 2 is packaged in lamellar bodies. *Experimental and molecular pathology*, Vol. 74, No.2, (April 2003), pp. 180-182, ISSN: 0014-4800.

Papini, M., Simonetti, S., Franceschini, S., Scaringi, L. & Binazzi, M. (1982). Lysozyme distribution in healthy human skin. *Archives of dermatological research*, Vol. 272, No. 1-2, pp. 167-170, ISSN: 0340-3696.

Plessier, A., Cosnes, J., Gendre, J.P. & Beaugerie, L. (2002). Intercurrent Klebsiella oxytoca colitis in a patient with Crohn's disease. *Gastroenterologie clinique et biologique*, Vol. 26, No. 8-9, (August-September 2002), pp. 799-800, ISSN: 0399-8320.

Porter, E.M., Bevins, C.L., Ghosh, D. & Ganz, T. (2002). The multifaceted Paneth cell. *Cellular and molecular life sciences*, Vol. 59, No. 1, (January 2002), pp. 156-170, ISSN: 1420-682X.

Pritchard, L.E. & White, A. (2007). Neuropeptide processing and its impact on melanocortin pathways. *Endocrinology* Vol. 148, No. 9, (September 2007), pp. 4201-4207, ISSN: 0013-7227.

Putsep, K., Axelsson, L.G., Boman, A., Midtvedt, T., Normark, S., Boman, H.G. & Andersson, M. (2000). Germ-free and colonized mice generate the same products from enteric prodefensins. *Journal of biological chemistry*, Vol. 275, No. 51, (December 2000), pp. 40478-40482, ISSN: 0021-9258.

Radek, K.A. & Gallo, R. (2007). Antimicrobial peptides: natural effectors of the innate immune system. *Seminars in Immunopathology*, Vol. 29, No. 1, (April 2007), pp. 27-43, ISSN: 1863-2297.

Radek, K.A., Lopez-Garcia, B., Hupe, M., Niesman, I.R., Elias, P.M., Taupenot, L, Mahata, S.K., O'Connor, D.T. & Gallo, R.L. (2008). The neuroendocrine peptide catestatin is a cutaneous antimicrobial and induced in the skin after injury. *The Journal of Investigative Dermatology*, Vol. 128, No. 6, (June 2008) pp. 1525-1534, ISSN: 0022-202X.

Raikhlin, N.T. & Kvetnoy, I.M. (1976). Melatonin and enterochromaffin cells. *Acta Histochemica*, Vol. 55, No. 1, pp. 19-24, ISSN: 0065-1281.

Rangon, C.M., Haik, S., Faucheux, B.A., Metz-Boutigue, M.H., Fierville, F., Fuchs, J.P, Hauw, J.J. & Aunis, D. (2003). Different chromogranin immunoreactivity between prion and a-beta amyloid plaque. *Neuroreport*, Vol. 14, No. 5, (April 2003), pp.755-758, ISSN: 0959-4965.

Ratti, S., Curnis, F., Longhi, R., Colombo, B., Gasparri, A., Magni, F., Manera, E., Metz-Boutigue, M.H. & Corti A. (2000). Structure-activity relationships of chromogranin A in cell adhesion. Identification of an adhesion site for fibroblasts and smooth muscle cells. *The Journal of biological chemistry*, Vol. 275, No. 38, (September 2000), pp. 29257-29263, ISSN: 0021-9258.

Rieg, S., Seeber, S., Steffen, H., Humeny, A., Kalbacher, H., Stevanovic, S., Kimura, A., Garbe, C., Schittek, B. (2006). Generation of multiple stable dermcidin-derived antimicrobial peptides in sweat of different body sites. *The Journal of investigative Dermatology*, Vol. 126, No. 2, (February 2006), pp. 354-365, ISSN: 0022-202X.

Romeo, D., Skerlavaj, B., Bolognesi, M. & Gennaro, R. (1988). Structure and bactericidal activity of an antibiotic dodecapeptide purified from bovine neutrophils. *The Journal of biological chemistry*, Vol. 263, No. 20, (July 1988), pp. 9573-9575, ISSN: 0021-9258.

Sarker, S.A. & Gyr, K. (1992). Non-immunological defence mechanisms of the gut. *Gut*, Vol. 33, No. 7, (July 1992), pp. 987-993, ISSN: 0017-5749.

Satoh, Y., Ishikawa, K., Tanaka, H., Oomori, Y. & Ono, K. (1988). Immunohistochemical observations of lysozyme in the Paneth cells of specific-pathogen-free and germ-free mice. *Acta Histochemical*, Vol. 83, No. 2, pp. 185-188, ISSN: 0065-1281.

Sawyer, T.K., Staples, D.J., Castrucci, A.M., Hadley, M.E., al-Obeidi, F.A., Cody, W.L. & Hruby, V.J. (1990). Alpha-melanocyte stimulating hormone message and inhibitory sequences: comparative structure-activity studies on melanocytes. *Peptides*, Vol. 11, No. 2, (March 1990), pp. 351-357, ISSN: 0196-9781.

Saxena, S.K., Rybak, S.M., Davey, R.T., Jr., Youle, R.J. & Ackerman, E.J. (1992). Angiogenin is a cytotoxic, tRNA-specific ribonuclease in the RNase A superfamily. *The Journal of biological chemistry*, Vol. 267, No. 30, (October 1992), pp. 21982-21986, ISSN: 0021-9258.

Schittek, B., Hipfel, R., Sauer, B., Bauer, J., Kalbacher, H., Stevanovic, S., Schirle, M., Schroeder, K., Blin, N., Meier, F., Rassner, G. & Garbe, C. (2001). Dermcidin: a novel human antibiotic peptide secreted by sweat glands. *Nature immunology*, Vol. 2, No. 12, (December 2001), pp. 1133-1137, ISSN: 1529-2908.

Schroder, J.M. & Harder, J. (2006). Antimicrobial skin peptides and proteins. *Cellular and molecular life sciences*, Vol. 63, No. 4, (February 2006), pp. 469-486, ISSN: 1420-682X.

Seidah, N.G. & Chretien, M. (1999). Proprotein and prohormone convertases: a family of subtilases generating diverse bioactive polypeptides. *Brain research*, Vol. 848, No. 1-2, (November 1999), pp. 45-62, ISSN: 0006-8993.

Serra, P., Brandimarte, C., Martino, P., Carlone, S., & Giunchi, G. (1977). Synergistic treatment of enterococcal endocarditis: in vitro and in vivo studies. *Archives of internal medicine*, Vol. 137, No. 11, (November 1977), pp. 1562-1567, ISSN: 0003-9926.

Shaw, J.L., Smith, C.R. & Diamandis, E.P. (2007). Proteomic analysis of human cervico-vaginal fluid. *Journal of proteome research*, Vol. 6, No. 7, (July 2007), pp. 2859-2865, ISSN: 1535-3893.

Sherman, H., Chapnik, N. & Froy, O. (2006). Albumin and amino acids upregulate the expression of human beta-defensin 1. *Molecular immunology*, Vol. 43, No. 10, (April 2006), pp.1617-1623, ISSN: 0161-5890.

Shooshtarizadeh, P., Zhang, D., Chich, J.F., Gasnier, C., Schneider, F., Haïkel, Y., Aunis, D. & Metz-Boutigue, M.H. (2010). The antimicrobial peptides derived from chromogranin/secretogranin family, new actors of innate immunity. Regulatory peptides, Vol. 165, No. 1, (November 2009), pp. 102-110, ISSN: 0167-0115.

Siddique, Z.L., Drozdov, I., Floch, J., Gustafsson, B.I., Stunes, K., Pfragner, R., Kidd, M. & Modlin, I.M. (2009). KRJ-I and BON cell lines: defining an appropriate enterochromaffin cell neuroendocrine tumor model. *Neuroendocrinology* Vol. 89, No. 4, (March 2009), pp. 458-470, ISSN: 0028-3835.

Sievert, D.M., Rudrik, J.T., Patel, J.B., McDonald, L.C., Wilkins, M.J. & Hageman, J.C. (2008). Vancomycin-resistant Staphylococcus aureus in the United States, 2002-2006. *Clinical infectious diseases*, Vol. 46, No. 5, (March 2008), pp. 668-674, ISSN: 1058-4838.

Silva, L.V., Araújo, M.T., Santos, K.R. & Nunes, A.P. (2011). Evaluation of the synergistic potential of vancomycin combined with other antimicrobial agents against methicillin-resistant Staphylococcus aureus and coagulase-negative Staphylococcus spp strains. *Memorias do Instituto Oswaldo Cruz*, Vol. 106, No. 1, (February 2011), pp. 44-50, ISSN: 0074-0276.

Sorensen, O.E, Thapa, D.R., Rosenthal, A., Liu, L., Roberts, A.A. & Ganz, T. (2005). Differential regulation of beta-defensin expression in human skin by microbial stimuli. *Journal of immunology*, Vol. 174, No. 8, (April 2005), pp. 4870-4879, ISSN: 0022-1767.

Sorensen, O.E., Thapa, D.R., Roupe, K.M., Valore, E.V., Sjobring, U., Roberts, A.A., Schmidtchen, A. & Ganz, T. (2006). Injury-induced innate immune response in human skin mediated by transactivation of the epidermal growth factor receptor. *The Journal of clinical investigation*, Vol. 116, No. 7, (July 2006), pp. 1878-1885, ISSN: 0021-9738.

Steffen, H., Rieg, S., Wiedemann, I., Kalbacher, H., Deeg, M., Sahl, H.G., Peschel, A., Gotz, F., Garbe, C. & Schittek, B. (2006). Naturally processed dermcidin-derived peptides do not permeabilize bacterial membranes and kill microorganisms irrespective of their charge. *Antimicrobial agents and chemotherapy*, Vol. 50, No. 8, (August 2006), pp. 2608-2620, ISSN: 0066-4804.

Sternberg, E.M. (2006). Neural regulation of innate immunity: a coordinated nonspecific host response to pathogens. *Nature review immunology*, Vol. 6, No. 4, (April 2006), pp. 318-328, ISSN: 1474-1733.

Strub, J.M., Goumon, Y., Lugardon, K., Capon, C., Lopez, M., Moniatte, M., Van Dorsselaer, A., Aunis, D. & Metz-Boutigue, MH. (1996a). Antibacterial activity of glycosylated and phosphorylated chromogranin A-derived peptide 173-194 from bovine adrenal medullary chromaffin granules. *The Journal of biological chemistry,* Vol. 271, No. 45, (November 1996), pp. 28533-28540, ISSN: 0021-9258.

Strub, J.M., Hubert, P., Nullans, G., Aunis, D. & Metz-Boutigue, M.H. (1996b). Antibacterial activity of secretolytin, a chromogranin B-derived peptide (614-626), is correlated with peptide structure. *Federation of European Biochemical Society Letters,* Vol. 379, No. 3, (February 1996), pp. 273-278, ISSN: 0014-5793.

Su, L.H., Teng, W.S., Chen, C.L., Lee, H.Y., Li, H.C., Wu, T.L. & Chiu, C.H. (2011). Increasing ceftriaxone resistance in Salmonellae, Taiwan. *Emerging infectious diseases, Vol.* 17, No. 6, (June 2011), pp. 1086-1090, ISSN: 1080-6040.

Syversen, U., Mignon, M., Bonfils, S., Kristensen, A. & Waldum, H.L. (1993). Chromogranin A and pancreastatin-like immunoreactivity in serum of gastrinoma patients. *Acta oncologica,* Vol. 32, No. 2, pp. 161-165, ISSN: 0284-186X.

Tatemoto, K., Efendić, S., Mutt, V., Makk, G., Feistner, G.J. & Barchas, J.D. (1986). Pancreastatin, a novel pancreatic peptide that inhibits insulin secretion. *Nature,* Vol. 324, No. 6096, (December 1986), pp. 476-478, ISSN: 0028-0836.

Taylor, C.V., Taupenot, L., Mahata, S.K., Mahata, M., Wu, H., Yasothornsrikul, S., Toneff, T., Caporale, C., Jiang, Q., Parmer, R.J., Hook, V.Y. & O'Connor, D.T. (2000). Formation of the catecholamine release-inhibitory peptide catestatin from chromogranin A. Determination of proteolytic cleavage sites in hormone storage granules. *The Journal of biological chemistry,* Vol. 275, No. 30, (July 2000), pp. 22905-22915, ISSN: 0021-9258.

Torres, G.E., Carneiro, A., Seamans, K., Fiorentini, C., Sweeney, A., Yao, W.D. & Caron, M.G. (2003). Oligomerization and trafficking of the human dopamine transporter. Mutational analysis identifies critical domains important for the functional expression of the transporter. The *Journal of biological chemistry,* Vol. 278, No. 4, (January 2003), pp. 2731-2739, ISSN: 0021-9258.

Tsakris, A., Poulou, A., Markou, F., Pitiriga, V., Piperaki, E.T., Kristo, I. & Pournaras, S. (2011). Dissemination of clinical isolates of Klebsiella oxytoca harboring CMY-31, VIM-1, and a New OXY-2-type variant in the community. *Antimicrobial agents and chemotherapy,* Vol. 55, No. 7, (July, 2011), pp. 3164-3168, ISSN: 0066-4804.

Walker, V.P., Akinbi, H.T., Meinzen-Derr, J., Narendran, V., Visscher, M. & Hoath, S.B. (2008). Host defense proteins on the surface of neonatal skin: implications for innate immunity. *The Journal of pediatrics,* Vol. 152, No. 6, (July 2008), pp. 777-781, ISSN: 0022-3476.

Walmsley, R.S., Gillen, C.D. & Allan, R.N. (1997). Prognosis and management of Crohn's disease in the over-55 age group. *Postgraduate medical journal,* Vol. 73, No. 858, (April 1997), pp. 225-229, ISSN: 0032-5473.

Wang, Z. & Wang, G. (2004). APD: the Antimicrobial Peptide Database. *Nucleic acids research,* Vol. 32, (January 2004), pp. D590-592, ISSN: 0305-1048.

Webster, J.I., Tonelli, L. & Sternberg, E.M. (2002). Neuroendocrine regulation of immunity. *Annual review of immunology,* Vol. 20, (October 2001), pp. 125-163, ISSN: 0732-0582.

Wikberg, J.E., Muceniece, R., Mandrika, I., Prusis, P., Lindblom, J., Post, C. & Skottner, A. (2000). New aspects on the melanocortins and their receptors. *Pharmacological research,* Vol. 42, No. 5, (November 2000), pp. 393-420, ISSN: 1043-6618.

Yajima, A., Ikeda, M., Miyazaki, K., Maeshima, T., Narita, N. & Narita, M. (2004). Manserin, a novel peptide from secretogranin II in the neuroendocrine system. *Neuroreport.*, Vol. 15, No. 11, (August 2004), pp. 1755-1759, ISSN: 0959-4965.

Yang, D., Biragyn, A., Kwak, L.W. & Oppenheim, J.J. (2002). Mammalian defensins in immunity: more than just microbicidal. *Trends in immunology*, Vol. 23, No. 6, (June 2002), pp. 291-296, ISSN: 1471-4906.

Yeaman, M.R. & Yount, N.Y. (2003). Mechanisms of antimicrobial peptide action and resistance. *Pharmacological reviews*, Vol. 55, No. 1, (March 2003), pp. 27-55, ISSN: 0031-6997.

Yoo, S.H. (1992). Identification of the Ca(2+)-dependent calmodulin-binding region of chromogranin A. *Biochemistry*, Vol. 31, No. 26, (July 1992), pp. 6134-6140, ISSN: 0006-2960.

Yu, .J, Mookherjee, N., Wee, K., Bowdish, D.M., Pistolic, J., Li, Y., Rehaume, L. & Hancock R.E. (2007). Host defense peptide LL-37, in synergy with inflammatory mediator IL-1beta, augments immune responses by multiple pathways. *Journal of immunology*, Vol. 179, No.11, (December 2007), pp. 7684-7691, ISSN: 0022-1767.

Zaalouk, T.K., Bajaj-Elliott, M., George, J.T. & McDonald, V. (2004). Differential regulation of beta-defensin gene expression during Cryptosporidium parvum infection. *Infection and immunity*, Vol. 72, No.5, (May 2004), pp. 2772-2779, ISSN 0019-9567

Zanetti, M. (2004). Cathelicidins, multifunctional peptides of the innate immunity. *Journal of leukocyte biology*, Vol. 75, No. 1, (January 2004), pp. 39-48, ISSN: 0741-5400.

Zanner, R., Gratzl, M. & Prinz, C. (2004). Expression of the endocytic proteins dynamin and amphiphysin in rat gastric enterochromaffin-like cells. *Journal of Cell Science*, Vol. 117, No. pt11, (May 2004), pp. 2369-2376, ISSN: 0021-9533.

Zayat, M., Lichtenberger, L.M. & Dial, E.J. (2008). Pathophysiology of LPS-induced gastrointestinal injury in the rat: role of secretory phospholipase A2. *Shock*, Vol. 30, No. 2, (August 2008), pp. 206-211, ISSN: 1073-2322.

Zhang, D., Lavaux, T., Voegeli, A.C., Lavigne, T., Castelain, V., Meyer, N., Sapin, R., Aunis, D., Metz-Boutigue, M.H. & Schneider, F. (2008). Prognostic value of chromogranin A at admission in critically ill patients: a cohort study in a medical intensive care unit. *Clinical chemistry*, Vol. 54, No. 9, (September 2008), pp. 1497-1503, ISSN: 0009-9147.

Zhang, R., Zhou, H.W., Cai, J.C., Zhang, J., Chen, G.X., Nasu, M. & Xie, X.Y. (2011). Serotypes and extended-spectrum beta-lactamase types of clinical isolates of Shigella spp. from the Zhejiang province of China. *Diagnostic Microbiology and infectious disease*, Vol. 69, No. 1, (January 2011), pp. 98-104, ISSN: 0732-8893.

Zheng, Y., Niyonsaba, F., Ushio, H., Ikeda, S., Nagaoka, I., Okumura, K. & Ogawa, H. (2008). Microbicidal protein psoriasin is a multifunctional modulator of neutrophil activation. *Immunology*, Vol. 124, No. 3, (July 2008), pp. 357-367, ISSN: 0019-2805.

12

Quinolones: Synthesis and Antibacterial Activity

Pintilie Lucia
National Institute for Chemical-Pharmaceutical Research and Development, Bucharest Romania

1. Introduction

After the concept of selective toxicity in chemotherapy was introduced at the beginning of the 20th century, (Ehrlich, 1913), classes of substances with antibacterial properties, produced by microorganisms or created through synthesis were obtained. After the discovery of penicillin, the first antibiotic introduced in clinical use in man in 1940s, a large number of different types of antibiotics were produced. Antibiotics such as beta-lactams, macrolides, aminoglycozides and tetracyclines were discovered and introduced during an extremely short period. These were obtained either by isolation from fungi or by chemically modification of the naturally isolated substrates. These dominated the antimicrobial industry, while synthetically obtained substances only played a minor role. (Chu & Fernandes, 1991)

In 1962, G. Y. Lesher and his collaborators introduced the first quinolone derivative, nalidixic acid (1-ethyl-1,4-dihydro-7-methyl-4-oxo-1,8-naphthyridine-3-carboxilyc acid), (1, Lesher et al. 1962) which had moderate activity against gram-negative organisms and was used for treating urinary tract infections. In the following years, a large gamma of derivatives from common elements were synthesized, which could be grouped by: cinoline (cinoxacin), pyrido-pyrimidine (pipemidic acid; piromidic acid), naphthyridine (nalidixic acid) and quinolones (oxolinic acid, miloxacin , tioxacin, etc.). These derivatives, with differentiated structures, have 2 common pharmacological properties, which allowed them to be classified as first generation biologically active derivatives with quinolone structure. The two common characteristics for first generation quinolones are:

- a narrow antibacterial spectrum, designed especially for enterobacteriaceae;
- a pharmacokinetic which allows for rapid elimination and reduced tissue absorption, only allowing them to be used as urinary antiseptics.

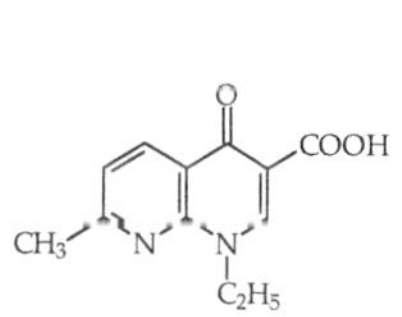

Nalidixic Acid

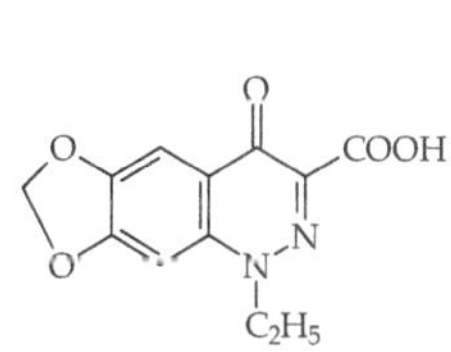

Cinoxacine

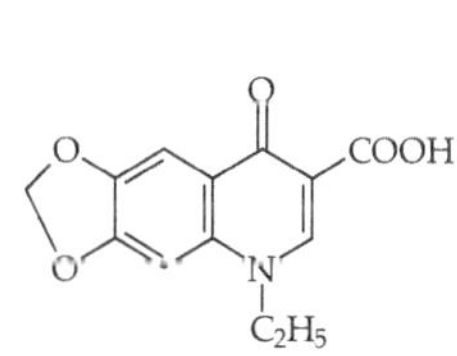

Oxolinic Acid

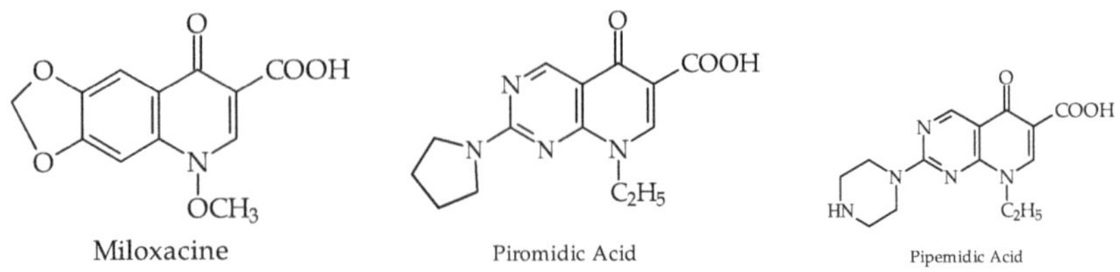

Fig. 1. First-generation quinolones.

The success of first generation quinolones spurred the research in this area, which led to the obtainment through synthesis, after 1980, of a new series of compounds with stronger antibacterial properties and a broader spectrum of antibacterial activity which included gram positive and gram negative organisms, and which where defined by their ability to be applied on all localized infections. Koga and his collaborators introduced Norfloxacin into clinical use in 1980, the first quinolone with a fluorine atom substituted at the C-6 position and a piperazine C-7. Norfloxacin (Koga et al. 1980) was the first quinolone with increased antimicrobial activity, acting on a large spectrum of gram positive and gram negative microorganisms, including Pseudomonas aeruginosa.

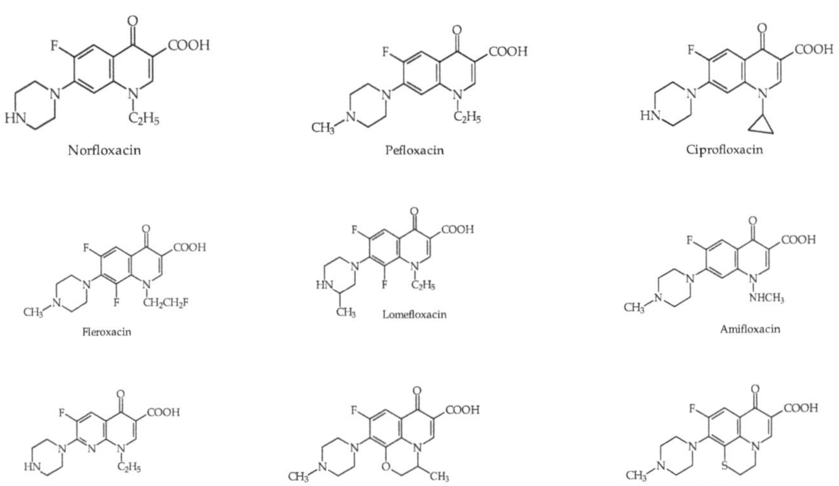

Fig. 2. Second-generation quinolones.

Research in the field of derivatives with a quinolone structure have lead to new compounds obtained recently, which have been classified as third and fourth generation systemic quinolones, largely effective against Staphilococcus aureus. Their large antibacterial spectrum includes anaerobes, Chlamydia and Mycoplasma. (Brighty & Gootz, 2000)

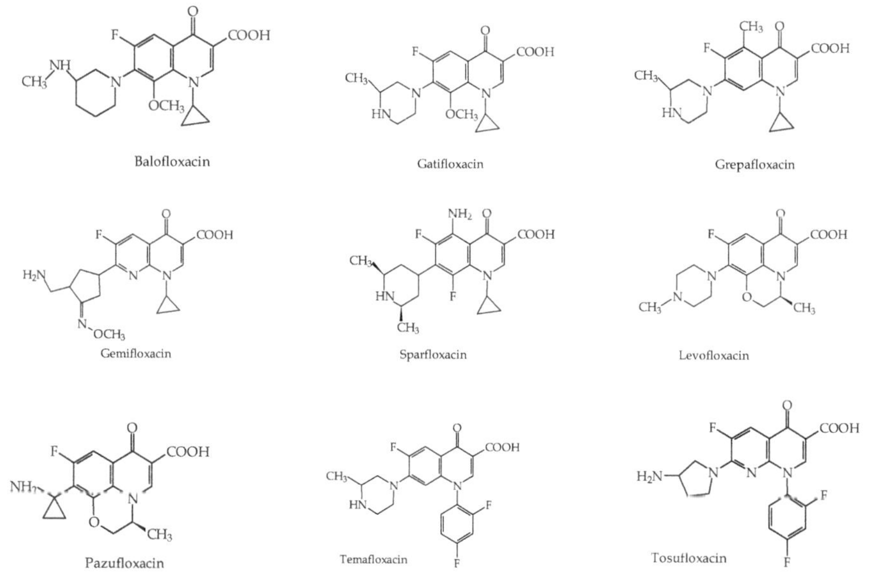

Fig. 3. Third- generation quinolones.

The four generations have the following common aspects: an identical mechanism of action by inhibition the A subunit of DNA-gyrasa, an exclusively chromosomal bacteria resistance and some similar bacteria effects: photo toxicity, neurotoxicity, cartilage toxicity.

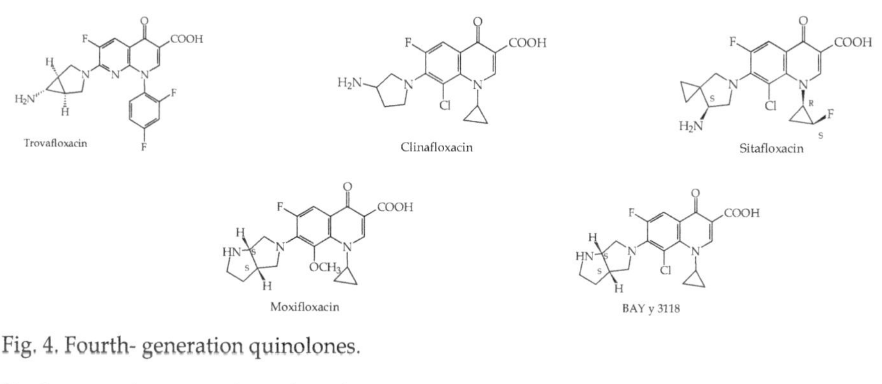

Fig. 4. Fourth- generation quinolones.

Until now a large number of antibacterial substances belonging to the above mentioned class have been used in medicine. Quinolones are used when treating infections of the urinary tract, the respiratory tract, intestinal infections, ear/nose/throat infections, STD's, soft tissue and skin infections, meningitis caused by gram negative and Staphilococci bacteria, liver and bile infections, septicemia and endocarditis, prophylaxis and surgical infections and on patients with immune deficiencies.

The mechanism of action of quinolone antibacterial agents involves the inhibition of DNA gyrase (a bacterial topoisomerase II) resulting in a rapid bactericidal effect.

The antibacterial activity of quinolones (measured in terms of MIC), however, is the result of the combination of bacterial cell penetration and DNA gyrase inhibitory activity. The antibacterial activity of quinolones depends not only on the bicyclic heteroaromatic system combining the 1,4-dihydro-4-pyridine-3-carboxylic acid moiety and an aromatic ring, but also on the nature of the peripheral substituents and their spatial relationships. These substituents exert their influence on bacterial activity by providing additional affinity for bacterial enzimes, enhancing cell penetration or altering the pharmacokinetics.

The research for an ideal quinolone continues worldwide. Such a quinolone must be biologically active on a large spectrum of gram positive and gram negative bacteria, aerobes and anaerobes and mycobacteria, must have as few side effects as possible, excellent solubility in water and oral bioavailability.

In figure 5, the most common synthesized chemical variations obtained during the research for new quinolones with antibacterial activity, are visible.

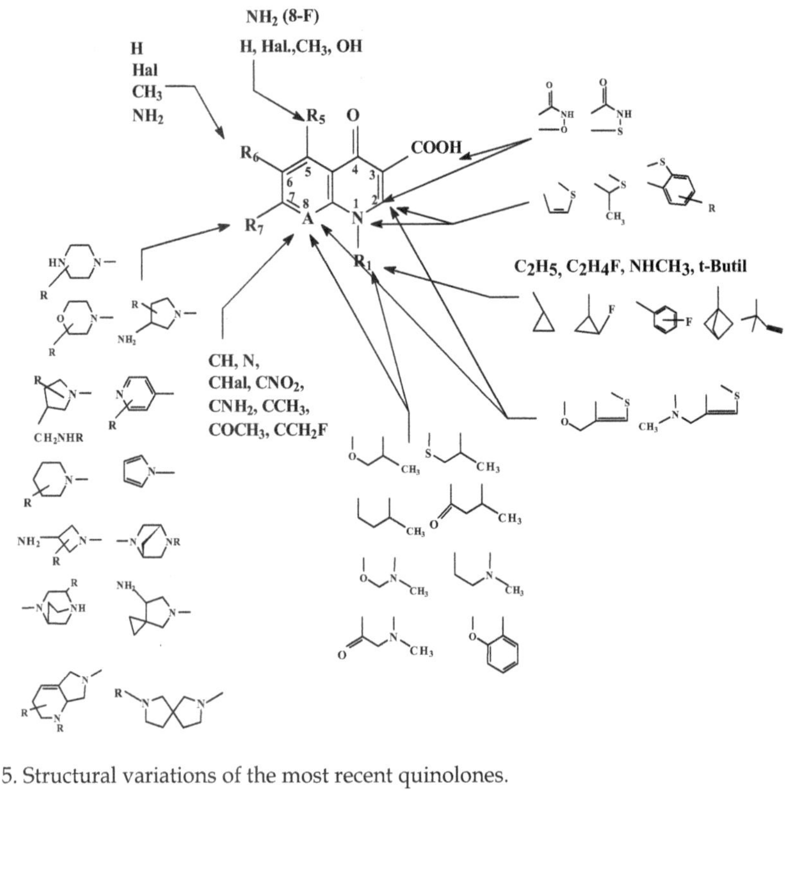

Fig. 5. Structural variations of the most recent quinolones.

2. Quinolones: Structural features and method of synthesis

2.1 Structural features

Quinolone derivatives are an important class of antibacterial agents with wide action. Basic structure of these compounds (Figure 6) is a bicyclic structure, which contains a ring of type *A* 4-piridinona combined with aromatic or heteroaromatic ring *B*. The ring type *A* 4-piridinona is a ring with absolute necessity: an unsaturation in position 2-3, a free acid function in position 3 and a substituent at nitrogen in position 1.

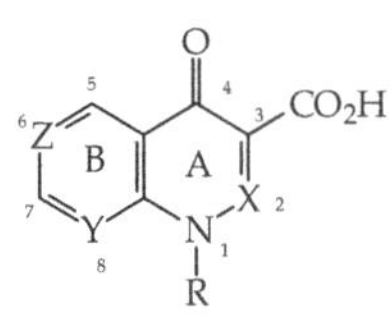

Fig. 6. Basic structure of quinolones.

2.1.1 Bicyclic quinolones

Position 1

The studies on quinolones indicated that in order for the compound to have antibacterial activity, the N-1 position requires a substituent. Many quinolones contain in N-position : ethyl (norfloxacin, pefloxacin, lomefloxacin) , fluoroethyl (fleroxacin), vinyl, clloroethyl, trifluoroethyl, aminoethyl,, cyclopropyl (ciprofloxacin), *t*-butyl, bicyclopentyl,*p*-fluorophenyl,2,4-difluorophenyl (Scott 1997)

Position 2

Quinolones contain at C-2 hydrogen (R_2=H). The replacement at hydrogen has generally proven to be disadvantageous. However, some compounds containing a suitable C-1, C-2 ringhave recently been shown to possess biological activity. (Figure7 -Segawa 1992) (Figure 8 - Scott 1997)

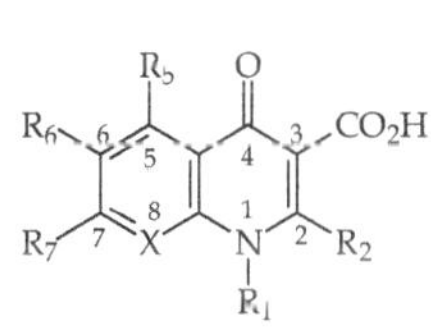

Fig. 7. Basic structure of bicyclic quinolones.

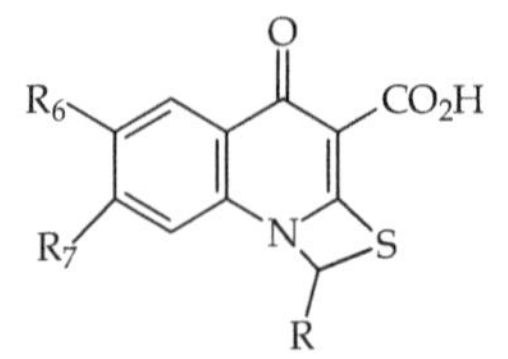

R = H, methyl, ethyl, substituted phenyl

R_6= F, Cl

R_7= heterocycle

Fig. 8. 7-Substituted-6-halo-4-oxo-4H-[1,3]-thiazeto[3,2]quinolin-3-carboxilyc acid.

Position 3

The C-3 carboxylic acid moiety is most commonly encountered. (Chu &Fernandes1991) . In the late of 1980s, a modification was described that eliminated the need for C-3 carboxylic acid. A fused izothiazolone ring was identified as serving as a carboxylic acid mimic,The compound A-62824 (Figure 9) have been found with biological activity.

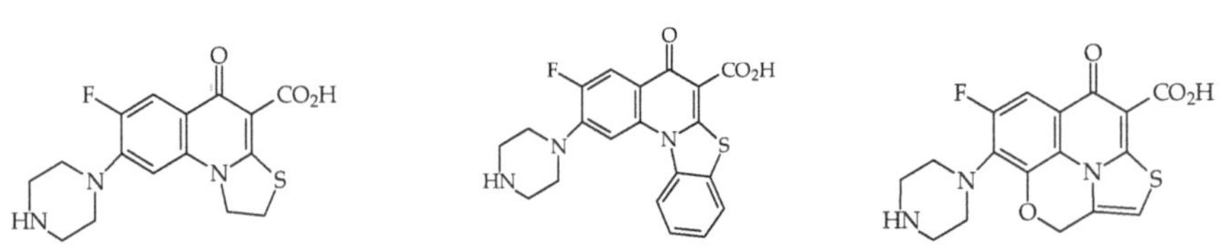

Fig. 9. Quinolones with sulfur substituent at C-2.

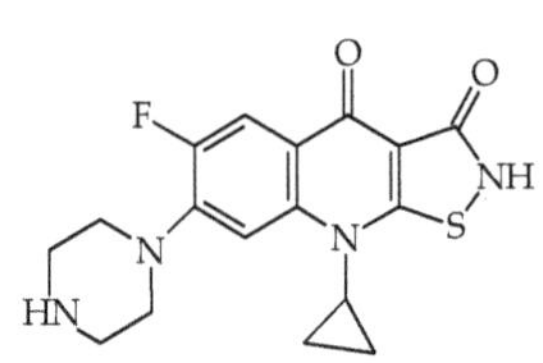

Fig. 10. A-62824.

Position 4

The C-4 oxo group of the quinolones nucleus is generally considered to be essential for antibacterial activity.

Position 5

The choice of the C-5 substituent appears to be dictated by the the steric regulations and the nature of the N-1 and C-8 substituent (Chu &Fernandes1991). (R_5 = methyl, halogen, amino when X = CF).

Position 6

The nature of the C-6 substituent have a great impact on the DNA-gyrase inhibitory activity and cell penetration. (Domagala et al. 1986). The R_6 can be H, Cl, F, NO_2, NH_2, CN, CH_3SCH_3, $COCH_3$) (Koga et al. 1980)

Position 7

The choice of the C-7 substituent is a key issue which continues to guide the design of new antibacterial quinolones. The R_7 can be substituted/unsubstituted piperazines, aminopyrrolidines, aminoalkylpyrrolidines, (Figure 5) (Chu & Fernandes 1991) (Scott 1997).

Position 8

The most common variations at the C-8 position is hydrogen atom (X= CH) or a nitrogen atom(a naphthyridine) (X=N). However, compact, liophilic group (X = CF,C-CF_3,, CCl, C-OCH_3) increase the antibacterial activity. (Chu & Fernandes 1991) (Scott 1997).

2.2 Method of synthesis

Gould-Jacobs method

The quinolones are of synthetic origin. (Chu & Fernandes, 1991). The most common synthetic methodology to prepare quinolone derivatives is Gould-Jacobs method (Figure 11). This method is used mainly for synthesis of compounds with N-1 alkyl substituents, and consists in the condensation of anilines (II) with diethyl ethoxymethylenemalonate (EMME) and cyclization of the obtained anilinomethylenemalonate. Termal cyclization can be carried out in dowterm (Koga, et al.1980), clorsulfonic acid, oleum acid or a mixture of clorosulfonic acid and oleum acid (Saukaita & Gupton, 1996). The key intermediary obtained (IV or X) will undergo a alkylation (Koga et al. 1980), cycloalkylation with bromo-cyclopropane (Kazimierozaack & Pyznar, 1987), (Sanjose&Ulpiano 1986), or with 1-bromo-1-ethoxy-cyclopropane, arylation with *para*-nitro-clorofenil or 2,4-dinitro-clorofenil (Raddl & Zikan, 1989) in order to insert the substituent in position 1 of the quinolone nucleus. The ethyl esther (V) undergoes a hydrolysis reaction, and the quinoline-3-carboxylic acid (VI), following regiospecific substitution of the 7-chloro group leads to the final compounds (VIII). Figure 11 illustrates also, methods for synthesis of 1-cyclopropyl-quinolones starting to anilines of formula II.Anilines (II) is reacted with 1-bromo-1-ethoxy-cyclopropane (Ramos & Garcia 1994)(Scriewer et al. 1988) or a cyclopropyl-metalic compound (McGuirk 1989). Alternatively, N-ethyl substituted anilines of formula XV may be formed by reductive amination with an appropiate aldehyde and a suitable reducing agent: diborane, palladium on carbon with hydrogen, sodium borohydride or sodium cyanoborohidride (McGuirk 1989) (Ramos 1994). N-isopropyl substituted quinolones may be form by alkylation with isopropylbromide (Pintilie et al. Sept. 2009), (Pintilie et al, oct.2009),(Pintilie et al. 2010), of compounds IV. (Figure 11).

The modified Gould-Jacobs method will also be used, where the diethyl ethoxymethylenemalonate reacts with monosubstituted N aniline (XVII) (Figure 12). The aniline (XVII) is obtained by reductive amination of ketones and aldehydes with sodium borohydride-acetic acid (Itoh & Kato 1984) or triacetoxyborohydride. (Pintilie et al.2009). (Pintilie et al. 2010).

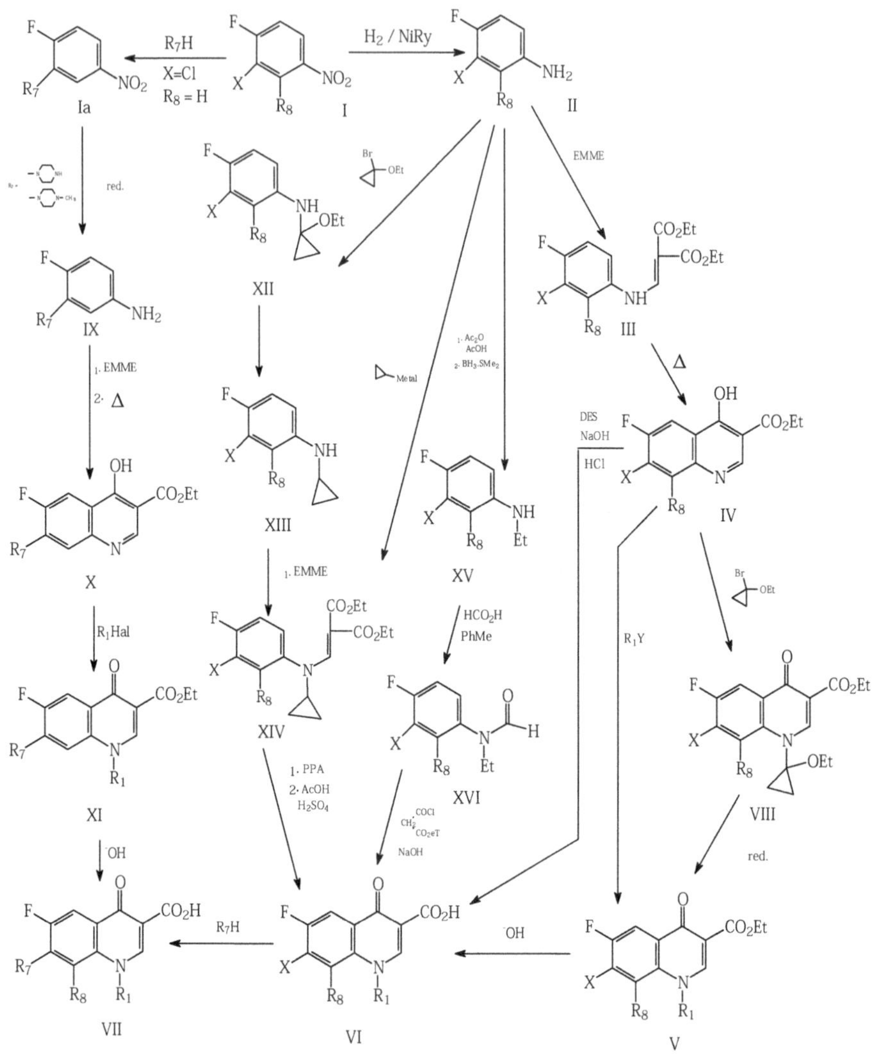

Fig. 11. Gould-Jacobs method.

Method requiers the reaction of isatoic anhydride with sodium ethyl formyl acetate

Another synthesis method requiers the reaction of isatoic anhydride with sodio ethyl formyl acetate (Figure 13). 2,4,5-trihalobenzoic acid (XX) is reacted with an appropiate amine, and then is treated with the compound :R_2R_3CO ($R_2 = R_3 =$ Cl, CCl_3O or $R_2= C_{1\text{-}10}$alkyl and $R_3 =$ Cl) to produce benzoxazindione (XXII). The benzoxazindione (XXII) is then condensed with compound ($HOCH{=}CHCO_2Et$) to provide key compound (V).

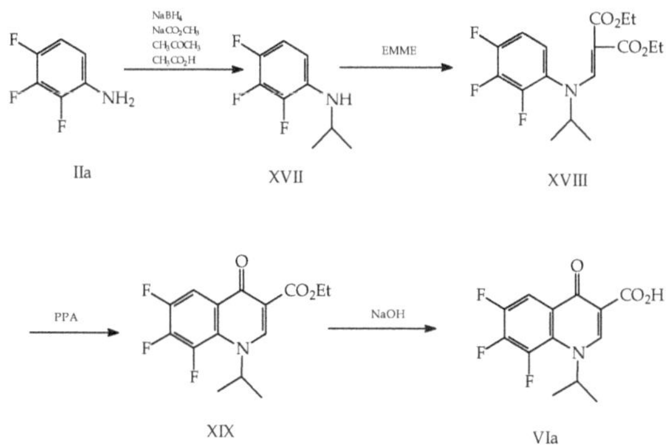

Fig. 12. The modified Gould-Jacobs method.

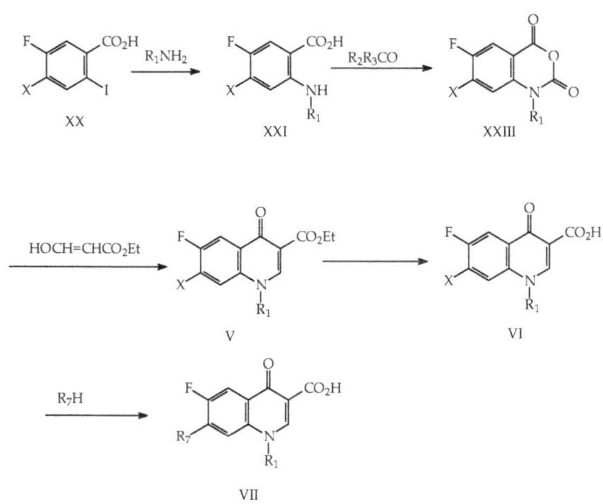

Fig. 13. Method requiers the reaction of isatoic anhydride with sodium ethyl formyl acetate

Intramolecular nucleophilic displacement cyclization route to quinolones (a)

An efficient and regiospecific synthesis via an intramolecular nucleophilic displacement cyclization reaction was reported. (Chu,1985) (Figure 14).

Key compund (III) can be obtained by:

- reaction of benzoic acid chloride (I) with ethyl malonic acid; the compound (II) give the compund (III).(Petersen & Grohe 1984a), (Petersen & Grohe 1984b),
- acetophenone (Ia) is condensed with diethyl carbonate in the presence of sodium hydride(Chu et al. 1985)

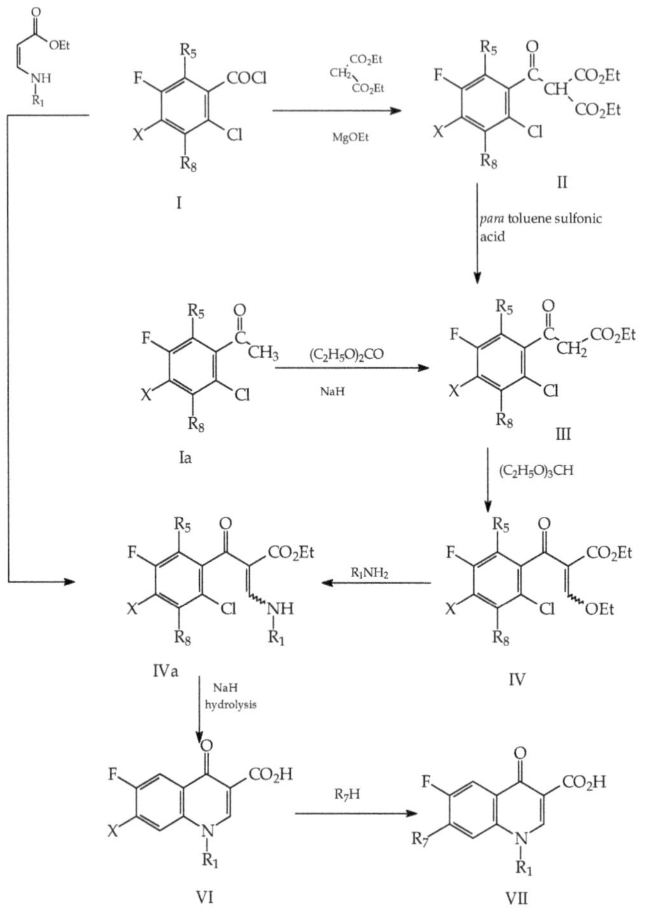

Fig. 14. Intramolecular nucleophilic displacement cyclization route to quinolones (a).

Intermediates (III) reacts with acetic anhydride in the presence trietilortoformiate to produce 3-ethoxy-2-benzoyl-ethyl acrylate (IV). Compound (IV) is further reacted with an appropriate amine in dichloromethane at room temperature to provide 3-anilino-2-benzoyl-ethyl acrylate (IVa).

Compound (IVa) can be also obtained directly from benzoic acid chloride (I). (Chu & Fernandes 1991).

Treatment with a base induces cyclization to produce the quinolone (V).

Intramolecular nucleophilic displacement cyclization route to quinolones (b)

A synthesis method similar to that described above is shown in Figure 15. This method involves intramolecular cyclization of the compound (VIII).(Egawa et al. 1987).

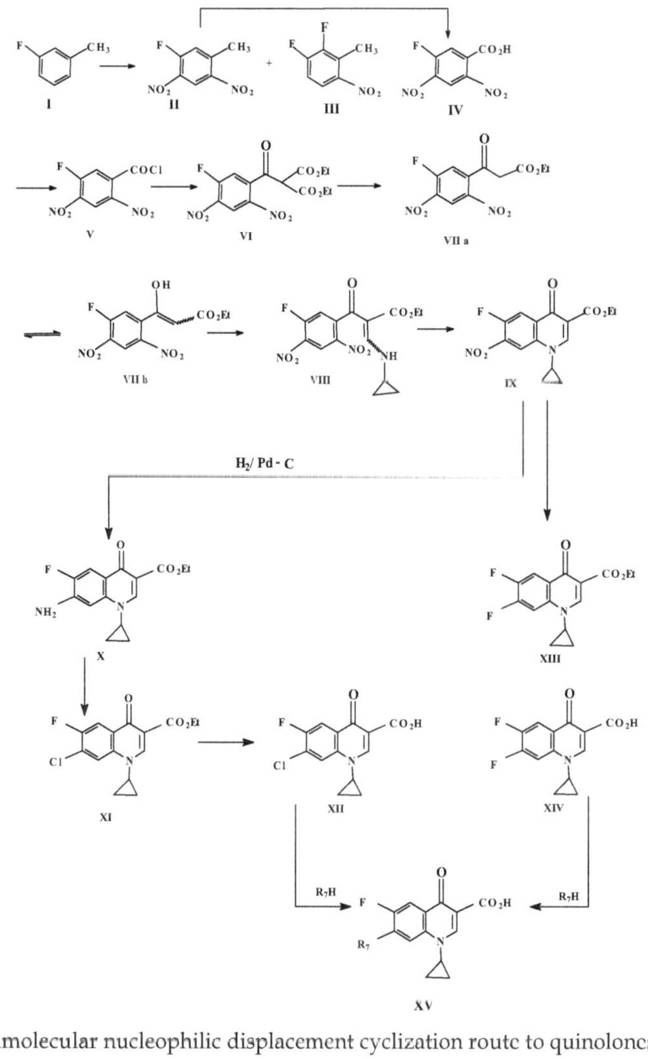

Fig. 15. Intramolecular nucleophilic displacement cyclization route to quinolones (b).

2.3 Structure of the new compounds

This paper presents experimental data regarding the synthesis of several quinolones with general formula: (Figure 16)

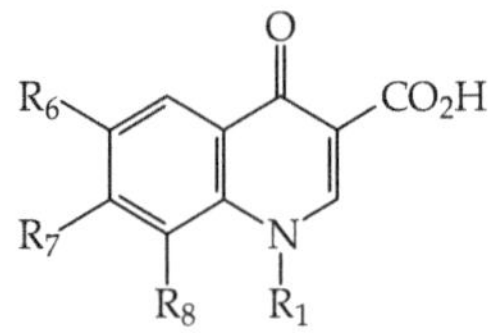

Fig. 16. The structure of the new compounds.

R_1 = ethyl, isopropyl, 2-buthyl, 2-penthyl, benzyl, alyl, *p*-nitro-phenyl, *p*-amino-phenyl;
R_6 = hydrogen, fluor, chlor, methyl;
R_7 = 3-methyl-piperazinyl, 4-methyl-piperazinyl, piperidinyl, 3-methyl-piperidinyl, 4-methyl-piperidinyl, pirolidinyl, morpholinyl, homopiperazinyl;
R_8 = hydrogen,chlor, methyl. methoxy, nitro

2.4 Synthesis pathway

The synthesis of the novel quinolones followed a Gould-Jacobs cyclization process (Figure 17). An appropriate unsubstituted aniline (1) is reacted with diethylethoxy methylene malonate (EMME) to produce the resultant anilinomethylenemalonate (2). A subsequent thermal process induces Gould-Jacobs cyclization to afford the corresponding 4-hidroxy-quinoline-3-carboxylate ester (3). (R_6 = fluoro, chloro, methyl, hydrogen) (Pintilie et al. 2009a) (Pintilie et al. 2009b),(Pintilie et al. 2010).

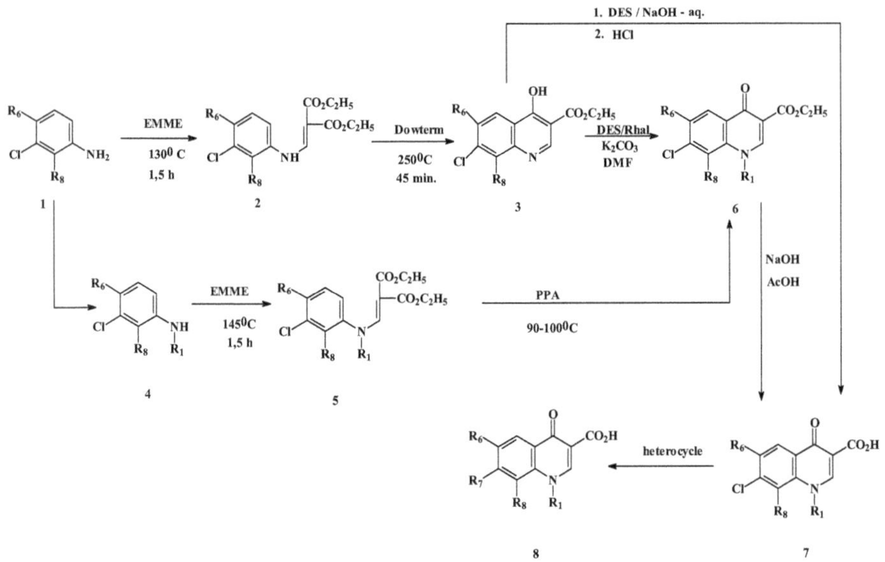

Fig. 17. Synthesis of the new quinolones.

The following operation is the alkylation of the 4-hidroxy-quinoline-3-carboxylate ester (3). which is usually accomplished by reaction with a suitable alkyl halide, dialkyl sulphates, aril halide to produce the qinolone 3-carboxylate ester (6). (R_1 = ethyl, alyl, benzyl, *p*-nitrophenyl) (Pintilie et al. 2003a) (Pintilie et al. 2003b),(Pintilie et al. 2003c)(Pintilie & Nita 2011).

A modified approach resorts to the use of a monosubstitued aniline (4) as a starting material which avoids subsequent N-1-amine alkylation (R_1 = isopropyl, 2-butyl, 2-pentyl). (Pintilie et al. 2009a) (Pintilie et al. 2009b),(Pintilie et al. 2010). A strong acid (such as polyphosphoric acid) is often needed to induce cyclization directly resulting in the formation of N-isopropyl-4-oxo-quinolone-3-carboxylate ester (6) (R_1 = isopropyl, 2-butyl, 2-pentyl). In either case, the final manipulation is acid or basic hydrolysis to cleave the ester generating the biologically active free carboxylic acid (7). The biologically active free carboxylic acid (7) was also obtained from the corresponding 4-hidroxy-quinoline-3-carboxylate ester (3) by alkylation with dialkyl sulphates in presence of alkali, for example the reaction it can conveniently be carried out in aqueous 40 % sodium hydroxide solution. The displacement of 7-chloro group with a heterocycle yielded compounds (8).

The synthesis of new 1-aryl quinoline-3-carboxilyc acids is according Figure 18. compound (3) (R_6=F,Cl,CH_3) is direct N-arylation. Treatment of (3) with potasium carbonate in DMSO and *p*-fluoro-nitrobenzene yielded 9). The esters were hydrolized to the appropiate acids (10) by refluxing with a mixture of hydrochloric and acetic acids. Upon treatment with a heterocycle yielded compounds (11). The 1-(*p*-amino-phenyl)-quinoline-3-carboxylic acids (12) can be prepared by a common reduction of nitro group using sodium dithionite.

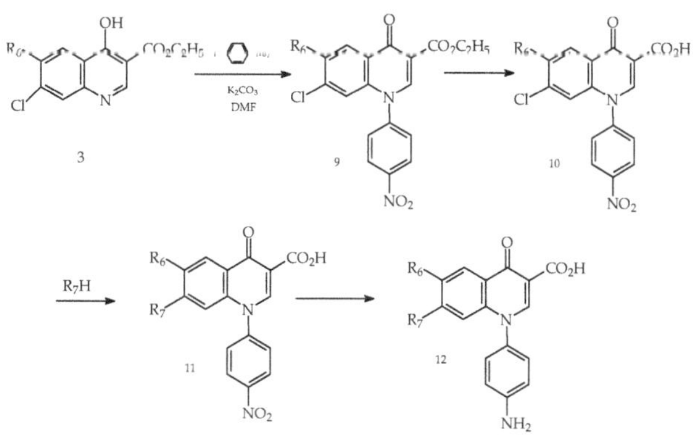

Fig. 18. Sinthesys of 1-aryl-quinolones.

The sinthesys of the new 8-substituted quinoline-3-carboxylic acids is according Figure 19. 8-Chloro-quinoline-3-carboxylic acids (13) was synthesized from 8-unsubstituted qinoline-3-carboxilyc acids by chlorination with sulfuryl chloride. 8-Methoxy-quinoline-3-carboxilyc acids (14) was prepared allowing compound (13) to act with alkali metalic alcholate.

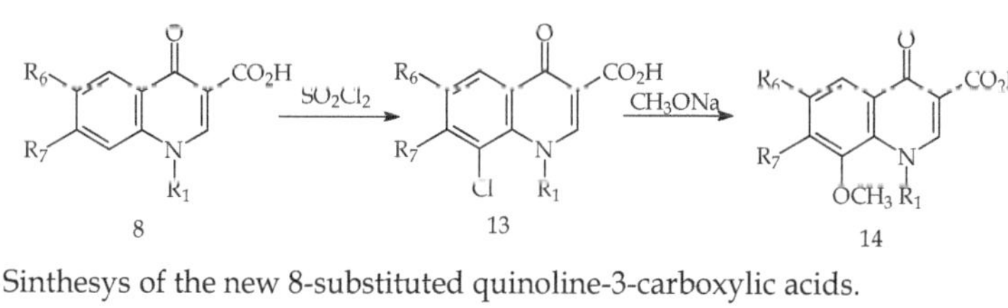

Fig. 19. Sinthesys of the new 8-substituted quinoline-3-carboxylic acids.

2.5 New compounds: Structure and antimicrobial activity

2.5.1 Structure of the new compunds

A series of new 4-oxo-1,4-dihydro-quinoline-3-carboxylic acids was synthesized. (Figure 20) (Table 1).

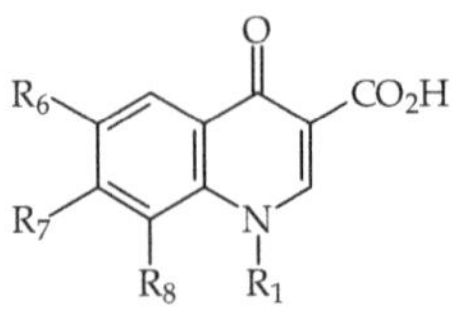

Fig. 20. Structure of the new compounds.

Quinolones	R_1	R_6	R_7	R_8	m.p. (^{0}C)	Reference
Q 83 $C_{18}H_{21}FN_2O_3$	ethyl	F	4-methyl-piperidin-1-yl	H	235-237	Pintilie et al. (2003b)
Q 85 $C_{18}H_{20}ClFN_2O_3$	ethyl	F	4-methyl-piperidin-1-yl	Cl	201-202,5	Pintilie et al. (2003b)
PQ 1 $C_{19}H_{23}FN_2O_4$	ethyl	F	4-methyl-piperidin-1-yl	OCH_3	170	Pintilie et al. (2003b)
PQ 12 $C_{19}H_{23}FN_2O_3$	*iIso*-propyl	F	4-methyl-piperidin-1-yl	H	253	Pintilie et al. (2003b)
PQ 11 $C_{23}H_{23}FN_2O_3$	benzyl	F	4-methyl-piperidin-1-yl	H	240-242	Pintilie et al. (2003b)
PQ 4 $C_{19}H_{21}FN_2O_3$	alyl	F	4-methyl-piperidin-1-yl	H	168-170	Pintilie et al. (2003b)
FPQ 24 $C_{18}H_{21}FN_2O_3$	ethyl	F	3-methyl-piperidin-1-yl	H	189,4	Pintilie et al. (2009b)
6ClPQ 24 $C_{18}H_{21}ClN_2O_3$	ethyl	Cl	3-methyl-piperidin-1-yl	H	216,4-218,4	Pintilie et al. (2009b)
PQ 24 $C_{19}H_{23}FN_2O_3$	*iIso*-propyl	F	3-methyl-piperidin-1-yl	H	209,1-211,7	Pintilie et al. (2009b)
PQ 22 $C_{18}H_{21}FN_3O_3$	*iIso*-propyl	F	3-methyl-piperazin-1-yl	H	215-218	Pintilie et al. (2009b)
PQ 23 $C_{17}H_{19}FN_2O_4$	*iIso*-propyl	F	morpholin-1-yl	H	266-268	Pintilie et al. (2009b)
FPQ 25 $C_{16}H_{17}FN_2O_4$	ethyl	F	morpholin-1-yl	H	257,4-258,7	Pintilie et al. (2009b)
6ClPQ 25 $C_{16}H_{17}ClN_2O_4$	ethyl	Cl	morpholin-1-yl	H	267,1-269,2	Pintilie et al. (2009b)
6ClPQ 27 $C_{17}H_{20}FN_3O_3$	ethyl	Cl	3-methyl-piperazin-1-yl	H	170,5-171,4	Pintilie et al. (2009b)

Quinolones	R_1	R_6	R_7	R_8	m.p. (^0C)	Reference
FPQ 28 $C_{16}H_{16}ClFN_2O_4$	ethyl	F	morpholin-1-yl	Cl	244,6-244	Pintilie et al. (2009b)
6MeQ 83 $C_{19}H_{24}N_2O_3$	ethyl	CH_3	4-methyl-piperidin-1-yl	H	240-242	Pintilie et al. (2003a)
6MePQ 12 $C_{20}H_{26}N_2O_3$	*iIso*-propyl	CH_3	4-methyl-piperidin-1-yl	H	234-235	Pintilie et al. (2003a)
6MePQ 11 $C_{24}H_{26}N_2O_3$	benzyl	CH_3	4-methyl-piperidin-1-yl	H	218-220	Pintilie et al. (2003a)
6MePQ 4 $C_{20}H_{24}N_2O_3$	alyl	CH_3	4-methyl-piperidin-1-yl	H	244-246	Pintilie et al. (2003a)
HQ 83 $C_{18}H_{22}FN_2O_3$	ethyl	H	4-methyl-piperidin-1-yl	H	240-242	Pintilie et al. (2003c)
HPQ 12 $C_{19}H_{24}N_2O_3$	*iIso*-propyl	H	4-methyl-piperidin-1-yl	H	234-235	Pintilie et al. (2003c)
HPQ 11 $C_{23}H_{24}N_2O_3$	benzyl	H	4-methyl-piperidin-1-yl	H	218-220	Pintilie et al. (2003c)
HPQ 4 $C_{19}H_{22}N_2O_3$	alyl	H	4-methyl-piperidin-1-yl	H	244-246	Pintilie et al. (2003c)
HPQ 21 $C_{18}H_{23}N_3O_3$	*iIso*-propyl	H	4-methyl-piperazin-1-yl	H	239-240	Pintilie et al. (2009a)
HPQ 24 $C_{18}H_{22}N_2O_3$	ethyl	H	3-methyl-piperidin-1-yl	H	190,1-192,1	Pintilie et al. (2009a)
HPQ 25 $C_{16}H_{18}N_2O_4$	ethyl	H	morpholin-1-yl	H	267,3-269	Pintilie et al. (2009a)
HPQ 27 $C_{17}H_{21}N_3O_3$	ethyl	H	3-methyl-piperazin-1-yl	H	191,3-192,6	Pintilie et al. (2009a)
HPQ 31 $C_{19}H_{24}N_2O_3$	2-butyl	H	4-methyl-piperidin-1-yl	H	181,4-183	Pintilie et al. (2009a)
HPQ 51 $C_{19}H_{24}N_2O_3$	2-pentyl	H	4-methyl-piperidin-1-yl	H	138,5-140,5	Pintilie et al. (2009a)
PQ 3 $C_{22}H_{20}FN_3O_5$	*p*-nitro-phenyl	F	4-methyl-piperidin-1-yl	H	204-206	Pintilie& Nita (2011)
PQ 7 $C_{21}H_{19}FN_4O_5$	*p*-nitro-phenyl	F	Homopiperazin-1-yl	H	128-130	Pintilie& Nita (2011)
6ClPQ 3 $C_{22}H_{20}ClN_3O_5$	*p*-nitro-phenyl	Cl	4-methyl-piperidin-1-yl	H	202-205	Pintilie& Nita (2011)
6McPQ 3 $C_{23}H_{23}N_3O_5$	*p*-nitro-phenyl	CH_3	4-methyl-piperidin-1-yl	H	222-224	Pintilie& Nita (2011)
APQ 3 $C_{22}H_{22}FN_3O_3$	*p*-amino-phenyl	F	4-methyl-piperidin-1-yl	H	284-285,5	Pintilie& Nita (2011)
A6MePQ 3 $C_{23}H_{22}N_3O_3$	*p*-amino-phenyl	CH_3	4-methyl-piperidin-1-yl	H	250-253	Pintilie& Nita (2011)

Table 1. 4-Oxo- 1,4-dihydro-quinoline-3-carboxylic acids synthesized in this paper.

2.5.2 Antibacterial activity of the new compunds

The new compounds were evaluated for "in vitro" activity by determining minimum inhibitory concentration against of bacteria *Escherichia. Coli, Staphylococcus. Aureus and Pseudomonas .aeruginosa,* by agar dilution method (Buiuc 1998) (NCCLS 2003). (Table 2).

Quinolone	Minimum inhibitory concentration µg/ml			Referances
	E. coli	S. aureus	P. aeruginosa	
Q 83	3,12 (a)	1,56 (c)	6,25 (e)	Pintilie et al. (2003b)
Q 85	3,12 (a)	0,39 (c)	6,25 (e)	Pintilie et al. (2003b)
PQ 1	3,12 (a)	0,78 (c)	3,12 (e)	Pintilie et al. (2003b)
PQ 4	12,5 (a)	1,56 (c)	6,25 (e)	Pintilie et al. (2003b)
FPQ 24	2,00 (a)	0,50 (b)	32,00 (d)	Pintilie et al. (2009b)
6ClPQ 24	8,00 (a)	2,00 (b)	>128 (d)	Pintilie et al. (2009b)
PQ 24	8,00 (a)	2,00 (b)	64,00 (d)	Pintilie et al. (2009b)
PQ 22	0,50 (a)	4,00 (b)	8,00 (d)	Pintilie et al. (2009b)
6ClPQ 25	4,00 (a)	2,00 (b)	128 (d)	Pintilie et al. (2009b)
FPQ 25	0,125 (a)	0,06 (b)	8,00 (d)	Pintilie et al. (2009b)
FPQ 28	0,125 (a)	0,06 (b)	8,00 (d)	Pintilie et al. (2009b)
HPQ 21	8,00 (a)	64,00 (b)	>128 (d)	Pintilie et al. (2009a)
HPQ 25	8,00 (a)	64,00 (b)	>128 (d)	Pintilie et al. (2009a)
HPQ 27	>128 (a)	32,00 (b)	>128 (d)	Pintilie et al. (2009a)
PQ 3	12,50 (a)	25,00 (c)	12,50 (e)	Pintilie& Nita (2011)
APQ 3	12,50 (a)	0,78 (c)	12,50 (e)	Pintilie& Nita (2011)
PQ 7	12,50 (a)	3,12 (c)	12,50 (e)	Pintilie& Nita (2011)

a. Escherichia. coli ATCC 25922, b. Staphylococcus. aureus ATCC29213, c. Staphylococcus. aureus ATCC29223, d. Pseudomonas .aeruginosa ATCC27813,e. Pseudomonas .aeruginosa ATCC27853

Table 2. "In vitro" antibacterial activity of the new quinolones.

3. Conclusion

In conclusion, were synthesized new quinolones and was investigated their antibacterial activity. The results indicate that substituent combinations in the quinolone ring, might produce powerful antibacterial agents such as compound: FPQ-28 (1-ethyl-6-fluoro-7-morpholinyl-8-chloro-1,4-dihydro-4-oxo-quinoline-3-carboxylic acid), (Figure 21) in concordance with the QSARs studies (Tarko et al. 2008), showed excellent „in vitro" activity against *E. Coli* ATCC 25922 (MIC 0,125 µg/mL) and *S.aureus ATCC29213* (MIC 0,06 µg/mL).

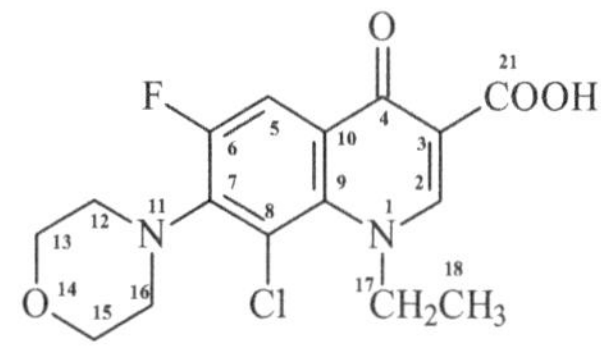

FPQ - 28

Fig. 21. 1-Ethyl-6-fluoro-7-morpholinyl-8-chloro-1,4-dihydro-4-oxo-quinoline-3-carboxylic acid -FPQ 28

^{1}H-NMR(dmso-d6, δ ppm, *J* Hz): 8.97(s, 1H, H-2); 8.07(d, 1H, H-5, 11.8); 4.89(q, 2H, H-17, 7.2); 3.82(m, 4H, sist. A_2B_2, H-13-15); 3.37(m, 4H, sist. A_2B_2, H-12-16); 1.46(t, 3H, H-18, 7.2).
^{13}C-NMR(dmso-d6, δ ppm, *J* Hz): 175.56(C-4); 166.12(C-21); 154.95(d, $J(^{13}C-^{19}F)$=254.8, C-6);158.37(Cq); 153.04(C-2); 125.94(Cq); 124.76(Cq); 116.86(Cq); 111.57(d, $J(^{13}C-^{19}F)$=23.5, C-5); 98.35(C-3); 67.23(C-13-15); 53.64(C-12-16); 51.58(C-17); 16.14(C-18).
FT-IR(solid in ATR, ν cm^{-1}): 3056; 2957; 2895; 2849; 1717; 1615; 1558; 1532; 1492; 1435; 1376; 1300; 1253; 1207; 1102; 1033; 980; 920; 890; 846; 803; 740; 651; 528; 464.

4. References

Brighty, K & Gootz, T. (2000) Chemistry and Mechanism of action of the quinolone antibacterial, In: *The Quinolones Third Edition*, Vincent Andriole, pp. 33-97, Academic Press, ISBN 978-0-12-059517-4

Chu, D.T.W., Fernandes P., Claiborne, A.K., Pihuleac, E., Norden, C.W., Maleczka, J.R.E. & Pernet, A.G. (1985). Synthesis and structure-activity relationships of novel arylfluoroquinolone antibacterial agents. *Journal of Medicinal Chemistry*, Vol. 28, No.12, (dec. 1985), pp. 1558-1564, ISSN-0022-2623

Chu, D.T.W. & Fernandes, P. (1991). Recent developments in the field of quinolone antibacterial agents, In : *Advances in drug research Vol. 21*, Bernard Testa, pp. 39-144, Academic Press, ISBN 0-12-013321-0, London ; San Diego ; New York

Domagala, J.M., Heifetz, C.L., Mich, T.F. & Nichols, J.B., (1986) 1-Ethyl-7-[3-[(ethylamino)methyl]-1-pyrrolidinyl]-6,8-difluoro-1,4-dihydro-4-oxo-3-quinoline carboxylic acid. New quinolone antibacterial with potent gram-positive activity. *Journal of Medicinal Chemistry*, Vol. 29, No. 4, (apr. 1986), pp. 445-448, ISSN-0022-2623

Buiuc, D. (1998) Determinarea sensibilității la medicamente antimicrobiene: tehnici cantitative, în "Microbiologie clinică", vol. I, 1998, pp. 438-442. Editura Didactică şi Pedagogică, Bucureşti.

Egawa, H., Kataoka, M., Shibamori K., Miyamoto, J.N. & Matsumoto, J. (1987) A new synthetic route to 7-halo-1-cyclopropyl-6-fluoro-1,4-dihydro-4-oxoquinoline-3-carboxylic acid, an intermediate for the synthesis of quinolone antibacterial agents. *Journal of Heterocyclic Chemistry*, Vol.24, (1987), pp 181-185, ISSN -0022-152X

Itoh, Y & Kato, H. (1984) Ger. Offen *Patent* DE 34 33 924 , 1984.

Kazimierozaack, J. & Pyznar, B. (1987). PL *Patent* 154 525, 1987.

Koga, H., Itoh, A. & Murayama, S.,(1980) Structure-activity relationships of antibacterial 6,7- and 7,8-disubstituted 1-alkyl-1,4-dihydro-4-oxoquinoline-3-carboxylic acids. *Journal of Medicinal Chemistry*, Vol. 23, No.12, (dec. 1980), pp. 1358-1363, ISSN-0022-2623

Lesher, G. Y., Foelich, E. J., Garnett, M. D., Bayley, J. H. & Brundage, P. R., (1962). 1,8 Naphtyridine derivatives, a new class of chemotherapeutic agents. *Journal of Medicinal Chemistry,* Vol. 5, No. 5, (sept. 1962), pp. 259-279, ISSN-0022-2623

McGuirk, P.R. (1989), EP *Patent,* EP 0348 099, 1989.

Petersen, U. & Grohe, K. (1984a). Ger. Offen *Patent* DE 32 485 05, 1984.

Petersen, U. & Grohe, K. (1984b). Ger. Offen *Patent* DE 32 485 06, 1984.

Pintilie, L., Oniscu, Draghici, C., Caproiu, M.T., Alexandru, N., Damian, E., Dobrovolschi, D. & Diaconu, L. (2003a). 6Methyl-quinolones with biological activity. *Romanian Biotechnological Letters,* Vol. 8, No. 2, (april. 2003), pp 1163-1168. ISSN 1224-5984

Pintilie, L., Oniscu,Voiculescu Gh., Draghici, C., Caproiu, M.T., Alexandru, N., Paraschiv, I., Damian, E., Dobrovolschi, D. & Diaconu, L. (2003b). Synthesis and antibacterial activity of some novel fluoroquinolones. *Romanian Biotechnological Letters,* Vol. 8, No. 2, (april. 2003), pp 1197-1204. ISSN 1224-5984

Pintilie, L., Oniscu,Voiculescu Gh., Draghici, C., Caproiu, M.T., Alexandru, N. & Damian, E., (may 2003). Synthesis of some novel desfluoroquinolones. *Romanian Biotechnological Letters,* Vol. 8, No. 3 (may.2003), pp. 1303-1309. ISSN 1224-5984

Pintilie, L., Negut, C., Oniscu, C., Caproiu, M.T., & Nechifor, M. (2009a). Synthesis and antibacterial activity of some novel desfluoroquinolones. *Revista de chimie,* Vol. 60, No.9, (sept.2009)pp. 871-975, ISSN 0034-7752

Pintilie, L., Negut, C., Oniscu, C., Caproiu, M.T., Nechifor, M, Iancu, L., Ghiciuc, C. & Ursu R. (2009b). Synthesis and antibacterial activity of some novel quinolones. *Romanian Biotechnological Letters,* Vol. 14, No. 5, (oct. 2009), pp. 4756-4767, ISSN 1224-5984

Pintilie, L., Nita, S. & C., Caproiu. (2010). Synthesis of new 7-chloro-8-substituted-1,4-dihydro-4-oxo-quinolin-3-carboxylic acids. *Revista de chimie,* Vol. 61, No.8, (aug.2010) pp. 745-749, ISSN 0034-7752

Pintilie, L. & Nita S.,(2011). RO *Patent application* RO A/00554. 15.06.2011

Radl, S. & Zikan, V. (1989). Synthesis of some 1-aryl-1,4-dihydro-4-oxo-quinoline-3-carboxylic acids and their antibacterial activity. *Collect. Czech.Chem.Commun.,* Vol.54, No. 8, (1989), pp 2181-2189, ISSN – 0010-0765

Ramos, G. A. (1994) ES *Patent* ES 2 049 631, 1994.

Ramos, G. A. & Garcia, N. J. (1994) ES *Patent* ES 2 046 091, 1994.

Saukaita, J.C. & Gupton, F.B. (1996). U.S. *Patent* 5 430 150 (1996)

Sanjose, M.I. & Ulpiano M. (1986). ES *Patent* ES 548 375, 1986

Scott, L.D. (1997), Quinolone antibacterial, In: *Antibacterial Chemotherapeutic Agents,* pp 298-345, Blackie Academic&Professional, London , ISBN 10 0751402893

Scriewer, M., Petersen, U & Grohe, K. (1988). Ger. Offen Patent DE 3808 118, 1988.

Segawa, J., Kitano, M., Kazuno,K., Matsuoka,M., Shirahase, I., Ozaki, M., Matsuda, M., Tomii,Y. & Kise, M. (1992). Studies on pyridonecarboxylic acids. 1. Synthesis and antibacterial evaluation of 7-substituted-6-halo-4-oxo-4H-[1,3]thiazeto[3,2-a]quinoline-3-carboxylic acids. . *Journal of Medicinal Chemistry,* Vol. 35, No.25, (dec. 1992), pp. 4727-4738, ISSN-0022-2623

Tarko, L., Pintilie, L., Negut, C., Oniscu, C. & Caproiu, M.T. (2008).QSARs on bactericidal activity of 3-carboxy-4-quinolones. *Revista de Chimie,* Vol. 59, No. 2 (febr. 2008), pp.185-194, ISSN 0034-7752

*** National Committee on Clinical Laboratory Standards (NCCLS) (2003) *Antimicrobial Susceptibility Standards* (ATS), ed. 2003, for M7 (CMI) şi M100

13

Superbugs: Current Trends and Emerging Therapies

Amy L. Stockert and Tarek M. Mahfouz
The Raabe College of Pharmacy, Ohio Northern University
USA

1. Introduction

1.1 An era before antibiotic treatments

Modern pharmaceutical advancements have placed us in an era where fatalities due to common communicable diseases such as pneumonia or plague are rare. It is difficult to imagine a time when antibiotics were not used as the "fix all" for common illnesses, and even used in cases where antibiotic treatment is not indicated. Although we generally take current treatments for granted, it is important to point out that historically speaking, available treatments for bacterial illnesses were not developed until nearly one-third of the way through the 20th century. It is the accidental discovery of penicillin in 1928 by Alexander Fleming that is considered perhaps one of the largest medical advancements of modern medicine (Bellis, n.d). Prior to the discovery and subsequent development of penicillin, epidemics and pandemics were more frequent, more prominent, and carried larger death tolls.

Early records identify epidemics of plague in Egypt as early as 1650BC, although it is not clear whether it was plague or influenza (Austin, 2003; Daileader, 2007; Wade, 2010). The first major plague outbreak, which is now considered the beginning of the first plague pandemic, began in the Byzantine Empire around 541. The "Black Death" which affected Europe and Asia from 1338 to 1351 claiming 100,000,000 lives marks the beginning of the second plague pandemic and carries the largest death toll to date. The "Black Death" plague re-occurred in several smaller outbreaks including the 1665 "Great Plague of London" as well as outbreaks in France, Spain, and Vienna. The third plague pandemic began in 1873 in China and eventually spread to India, South Africa, North America, South America, and Australia. The death toll in Hong Kong and India from this pandemic breached 12,500,000 before 1957 (Williams, 1997).

Plague Pandemic	Death Toll	Location
1st Pandemic (Byzantine Plague) c541-c639	~25,000,000	Southern Europe
2nd Pandemic 1338-1665 (Black Death, 1338-1351)	>100,000,000*	N. Europe, Asia
3rd Pandemic 1873-1957	>12,500,000	Europe, N. Asia, India, China

Table 1. Comparison of death toll and location for historical plague pandemics (Austin, 2003; Daileader, 2007; Wade, 2010; Williams, 1997). *Death toll from black death period only.

As mortality trends are examined prior to the development of penicillin, it is easy to observe the effect that penicillin had on survival rates. Although we see a substantial number of fatalities, predominately in India, related to the third pandemic of plague, it is important to observe not only the difference in population at the time, but also length of time that continued outbreaks occurred. For example, it is roughly estimated that 75-200 million people were lost during the 14th century outbreaks, with a large geographical range including Northern European climates (England and France) in addition to Southern European regions such as Italy and Southern Spain. Recent studies suggest that this represented approximately 20% of the population in Northern European regions, and a striking 75-80% of the population in Europe's Southern countries (Daileader, 2007). The most recent plague pandemic started roughly in 1873 in China and spread throughout India, the Americas, South Africa and Australia claiming more than 12.5 million (in China and India alone) before the late 1950s. This particular pandemic encompassed a larger geographical region, albeit during a time of more expedited travel. Although the death toll associated with this plague pandemic is large, the plague of the 14th century claimed at least six times more individuals during a time when there were fewer people. Hong Kong experienced a prolonged and repeated outbreak for a few years which claimed approximately 90% of their population (an estimated 8600 total losses) (Pryor, 1975). Despite these isolated large death rates, the actual count of lives lost throughout the eight decades included in this most recent pandemic is extremely low when compared to those from the Black Death.

One might assume that the discovery and subsequent mass production of penicillin is related to this decrease in fatalities. Although the development of penicillin as well as other antibiotics or alternative treatments likely played a substantial role in ultimately stopping the pandemic, it is most definitely not that simple. Generally speaking, the following major differences existed this time around as compared to the first and second pandemics: 1) Penicillin was mass produced and readily available near the end of the third pandemic. 2) Increased travel opportunity and trade lines contributed to the increase in affected regions. 3) Scientific studies have suggested that this plague was not as contagious. 4) There were considerably larger populations during this pandemic. 5) Population density in the regions with highest fatality were high. 6) This pandemic (approximately 84 years $^{+}/_{-}$ 2 years) was shorter than the first (approximately 98 years $^{+}/_{-}$ 40 years) and second (approximately 327 years). 7) The population in general had a better understanding of the spread of disease. 8) Scientists and medical personnel had adopted better practices. 9) Drastic measures were taken to stop spreading. These differences are indeed relative, but do not necessarily suggest that "penicillin stopped the plague." In fact, these differences suggest that development of a drug that the organism thought to be responsible for each plague, *Yersinia pestis,* is susceptible to, was not the "cure all end all" for the disease. Nor will current antibiotics be the cure all for current and emerging diseases. Some of these differences suggest that without penicillin, the third pandemic could have been worse, or longer, or more deadly. For example, few people died despite the fact that more people were likely exposed and the pandemic ended sooner than the others. Figure 1 shows a graph of total reported infectious diseases of bacterial nature in the United States beginning in 1944 with the first available Morbidity and Mortality Weekly Report Summary (MMWR, 1994-2011).

In contrast however, some of these differences suggest that increased knowledge aided in the control of infection. Consider when comparing these pandemics, the trends within each pandemic. For example, during the second pandemic, there was little understanding about how to control infection; consequently we see a prolonged pandemic. During the third pandemic, we assume greater knowledge about infection control, we see shorter pandemics. After adding another variable, these seemingly related correlations lose strength. Consider also during the third pandemic, that the largest number of fatalities occurred during the first half of the pandemic, a time which perhaps surprisingly does not correlate to the availability of penicillin. The conclusion that should be drawn from these correlations is that the plague from the third pandemic likely differed enough that even without penicillin or increased knowledge of infection, the determents of the "Black Death" would not have been repeated. One then has to decide if the fact that our "miracle" drug may not have saved us should bring comfort as we face the emergence of other new "plagues" with no drugs to combat them, or whether the fact that the development of penicillin, if not solely responsible for stopping the plague, suggests that the development of new drugs may also not solve the "superbug" attack. As decision is considered, contemplate the following: It is most likely that genetic differences between the plague of the third pandemic and that of the second is responsible for the difference in outcomes, a difference in this case that likely spared much of the world's population; it is also these differences in genetics that are converting our bugs into "superbugs", perhaps this time not in our favor.

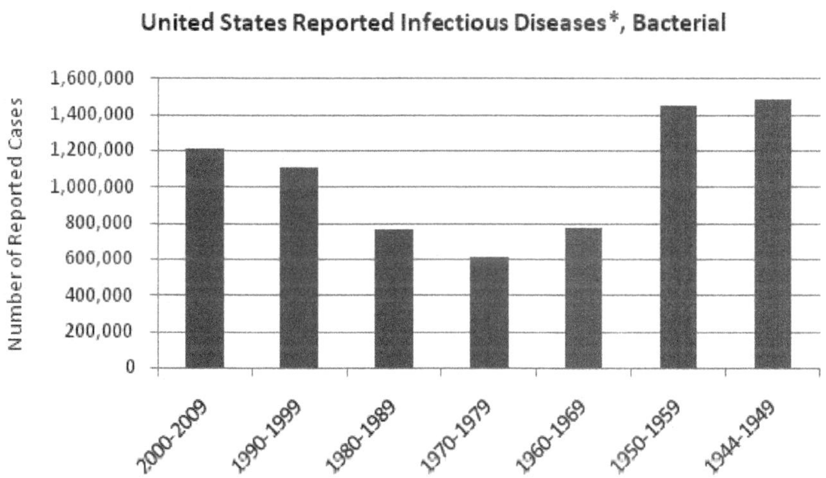

Fig. 1. Reported Bacterial Based Infectious Disease in the United States 1944-2009, population corrected. Data were compiled by the authors using The Center for Disease Control Morbidity and Mortality Weekly Reports 1944-2000. *Included diseases Cholera, *E. coli* O157:H7, *Meningococcal* disease, Pertussis, Plague, Salmonellosis, *Streptococcal* disease (invasive, Group A), *Streptococcus pneumoniae* (drug resistant, invasive disease), Syphilis, Tuberculosis, Typhoid fever.

1.2 Emergence of the "superbug"

The term "superbug" is readily used in the media and to some extent well understood by the public. The media has provided the public with a perceived understanding of the term, but unfortunately has not provided the same understanding of the implications of such "superbugs". Many of the references which are readily viewable on the internet are magazine articles that provide only bits of information with questionable accuracy. In general, the public thinks of a "superbug" as a uniquely contagious, potentially fatal infection that is not treatable with current medicines. Although the most important consideration is really the "superbug's" resistance to current antibiotics, the most prevalent issues to the public seem to be the endless number of dangerous nouns that can be preceded with the term "super." The concern over the development of the next pandemic of a "super-contagious" or "super-fatal" infection fuels the fear of the public. Although today's "superbugs" are certainly contagious, they are not necessarily any more contagious than today's "non-superbugs." Likewise, they are not necessarily more inherently fatal than "non-superbugs." Chances of fatality are higher because of the difficulty in treating and killing the bacteria.

Another public misconception comes from the perceived rarity of these "superbugs." Even with the media announcing that hospital bugs have moved out of the hospital and into the community, in general it seems that the public still views their presence as rare and is shocked and frightened by reports of infections near their community. People in general find it disheartening to know that *MRSA* (methicillin resistant *Staphylococcus aureus*) is commonly found in many gyms for example. Studies demonstrate that the presence of "superbugs" such as *MRSA* is growing, so are the numbers of cases of infections growing as well? If it is everywhere, why don't we all have it? The key here is the same thing that leads to a difference in plague outcomes between the second and third pandemics: genetic differences. In lay terms, some bugs (note the intentional absence of "super") are more infectious than others, some people are more likely to get an infection than others, some infections are easier to treat than others, and some bugs are more susceptible to antibiotics than others. Considering all these differences, the only reliable way to define a "superbug" is scientifically, based on evidence.

Ironically, the scientific definition of "superbug" doesn't have to differ much from the media definition, so long as the implications of the "superbugs" are understood clearly. Based on science, the term "superbug" refers to a bacterial organism which either is inherently or has developed resistance to at least one current antibiotic that would have typically been used to treat said bacteria. For example, the most well known type of hospital infection is staph, which when used to describe a post-operative infection is usually *Staphylococcus aureus*. Typical *Staphylococcus aureus* infections are treated with the penicillin class of antibiotics, such as nafcillin, oxacillin, dicloxacillin and methicillin. The more these infections were treated with these antibiotics, the better *Staphylococcus aureus* became at resisting the treatment. *MRSA*, stands for methicillin resistant *Staphylococcus aureus* and is perhaps the most well known "superbug."

It is important to differentiate that technically viruses cannot be considered "superbugs". The term "bug" is reserved for bacterial organisms, however, it is very common to find the phrase "superbug" applied to both bacteria and viruses in the media, and occasionally even in the scientific arena. The fact that these terms have both been included stems from the fact that both have the ability to mutate and both are infectious. Many viral infections develop accompanying bacterial infections as well, further complicating the differentiation. Comparison of infection trends makes it difficult to strictly separate the two as well because many viral related illnesses result in death from the subsequent development of bacterial infections. Many bacteria develop virulent strains, a term which is used to describe the degree of infectious nature, not indicating that the bacteria are a virus.

1.3 Current and emerging threats

The list of current "superbugs" is undefined. New strains of bacteria showing drug resistance are rapidly being identified. In 2006, the Antimicrobial Availability Task Force (AATF) of the Infectious Disease Society of America generated a list of drug resistant pathogens that was published in *Clinical Infectious Disease* (Talbot et al., 2006). Six pathogens were identified as "high-priority" for concern including: *Acinetobacter baumannii, Aspergillus* species, extended spectrum β-lactamase (ESBL)-producing Entrerbacteriaceae, vancomycin-resistant *Enterococcus faecium*, *Pseudomonas aeruginosa*, and methicillin-resistant *Staphylococcus aureus* (*MRSA*). The AATF selected this list of bacterial and fungal pathogens based on the following characteristics: current clinical and/or public health concern in the United States (based on high infection incidence and substantial morbidity), infection with high attributable mortality rates, unique virulence or resistance factors rendering current therapeutics ineffective, and a lack of substantial or novel drug candidates (primarily those that had few candidates in the phase 2 or 3 trials).

The gram negative bacterium *Acinetobacter baumannii* was included on the list because despite its historical lack of virulence, an increased number of severe infections have been identified. These infections have been identified as both hospital-acquired as well as community-acquired. A survey of infection in US intensive care units has indicated an increase of hospital acquired *Acinetobacter* pneumonia from 1.4% in 1975 to 6.9% in 2003. From 1975 to 2003 significant but smaller increases in bloodstream infection, surgical site infection, and urinary tract infection were also observed (Gaynes & Edwards, 2005). Increased incidence of *Acinetobacter* infections with drug-resistance have also been observed in military personnel with war-related injuries and survivors of the 2004 tsunami.

The inclusion of *Aspergillus* species on the list due to the increasing nature of invasive infections observed in immunocomprimised individuals (Maschmeyer & Ruhnke, 2004). Infections from *Aspergillus* fungi have a 50-60% mortality rate (Boucher et al., 2004). Additionally, several current treatments for *Aspergillus* infections require improvement both in the realm of efficacy as well as patient tolerace and safety. The top three drugs of choice for treatment of aspergillosis only have an approximate success rate of 40% (Walsh et al., 1999, 2002, 2004 as cited in Talbot et al., 2006). These include amphotericin B deoxycholate, which is highly toxic unless administered in lipid formulation; caspsofungin, which only has FDA approval for second-line defense which is based on a study with a relatively small number of individuals; and voriconazole, which has documented common drug-drug interactions (Johnson & Perfect, 2003; Boucher et al., 2004).

Escherichia coli and *Klebsiella* species strains producing the extended spectrum β-lactamase (ESBL) were selected for the list due to common infection in the urinary, biliary or gastrointestinal tracts. There is also a common occurrence in trauma injury and surgical sites as well as a high incidence of hospital acquired pneumonia and postoperative meningitis (Decré et al., 2004; Kang et al., 2004; Meyer et al., 1993; Paterson et al., 2004a, 2004b; Quale et al., 2002; Weiner et al., 1999 as cited in Talbot et al., 2006). A 2001 survey for US intensive care units identified 11.2% and 16.2% occurrence of ESBL production in *E. coil* and *Klebsiella* species, respectively (Biedenbach et al., 2004; Streit et al., 2004). The most alarming observation is the large increase in the percentage of resistant pathogens relative to total reported cases. During a 2 year period, 56 out of 57 samples collected of *Klebsiella oxytoca* exhibited multi-drug resistance (Decré et al., 2004 as cited in Talbot et al., 2006). A survey of 91 ESBL-producing *Klebsiella* species indicated resistance to gentamicin in 84% of the samples. Resistance to tri-methoprim-sulamethoxazole (70%), piperacillin-tazobactam (60%), and ciprofloxacin (51%) was also observed (Schwaoer et al., 2005).

Limited treatment options and increased infections have led to the high-risk classification of vancomycin-resistant *Enterococcus faecium.* Recently high rates of resistance to glycopeptides treatment have been observed in the United States compounded with an increased incidence of *Enterococcus faecium* blood infection in patients, particularly infections related to catheter use (Murray, 2000; Wisplinghoff et al., 2004). High-risk patients, such as those that have received a liver transplant or have cancer, face a disturbingly high rate of infection near 70% (National Nosocomial Infections Surveillance [NNIS] System Report, 2004; Streit et al., 2004; Wisplinghoff et al., 2004).

The severity of infections caused by *Pseudomonas aeruginosa* warrant the inclusion of this gram negative bacterium. Immunocompromised patients face potential fatal invasive infections (Maschmeyer & Braveny, 2000). *Pseudomonas aeruginosa* threatens a wide range of ages and includes lower respiratory and urinary tract infections. Infections occurring in patients with cystic fibrosis, often result in severe inflammation causing fatal damage to the lung tissue (Rajan & Saiman, 2002). Incidence of intensive care unit acquired pneumonia caused by *Pseudomonas aeruginosa* are increasing to approximately two times the rates observed in 1975. Similarly the infection rates of the urinary tract and surgical sites have doubled (NNIS System Report, 2004). Like other members of the "superbug" list, the rate at which *Pseudomonas aeruginosa* has developed drug resistance is distressing. From 1997 to 2001 resistance to fluoroquinolones increased 37%, resistance to imipenem increased 32%, resistance to ceftazidime increased 22%, resistance to multiple-drugs increased 4% (NNIS System Report, 2003; Obritsch et al., 2004).

The last pathogen included on the 2006 "superbug" list is perhaps the most well known, methicillin-resistant *Staphylococcus aureus* (*MRSA*). It is currently estimated that approximately 4 out of 1000 patients discharged from the hospital have a *MRSA* infection (Kuehnert et al., 2005). *MRSA* infections are more prominent in surgical or dialysis patients as well as premature infants. Hospital acquired *MRSA* infections were among the first identified and resulted in higher mortality rates. Recently, concern has risen over the number of cases occurring in the community, particularly in a crowed population. Currently vancomycin is the primary therapeutic used to combat *MRSA* infections, but strains showing vancomycin resistance are emerging (Fridkin et al., 2003). Hospitalizations due to *MRSA* infections, regardless of the cause of infection, have increased from 127,000 in 1999 to

280,000 in 2005 (Kallen et al., 2010; Klein et al., 2007; Klevens et al., 2007). Table 2 below summarizes the 2006 list of "superbug" threats as well as the reason for inclusion on the threat list.

Pathogen	Reason for list inclusion
Acinetobacter baumannii	Multi-drug resistant, hospital- and community-acquired, increasing incidence
***Aspergillus* species**	Current drugs with low efficacy and/or side effects including drug-drug interactions, high mortality rate, increased invasive infections
ESBL-producing Entrerbacteriaceae	Increasing incidence, rapidly increasing drug-resistance, multi-drug resistance
vancomycin-resistant *Enterococcus faecium*	Increasing incidence of blood infections, high infection rates, increasing infection rates across patient care areas
Pseudomonas aeruginosa	Severity of infections, high mortality rate in high risk patients, increasing incidence, increasing resistance, multi-drug resistance
methicillin-resistant *Staphylococcus aureus* (MRSA)	Increasing resistance, hospital- and community-acquired, increasing incidence, rapid resistance development to current therapeutics

Table 2. Summary of AATF List of Drug Resistant Pathogens requiring concern, 2006.

Although not included on the 2006 AATF list, several additional organisms should be considered due to the emergence of similar characteristics. One such organism that should be added to a list of concern is *Clostridium difficle.* This organism has been identified as number one identifiable cause of diarrhea in HIV infected patients (Sanchez et al., 2005). Estimates suggest that drug-resistant and virulent form *Clostridium difficle* played a role in nearly 300,000 hospitalizations in 2005, a two-fold increase from 2000 before the virulent strain was prevalent. This study also suggested the fatality rate increased from 1.2% to 2.2% from 2000 to 2004 (Zilberberg et al., 2008). Infection with *Clostridium difficle* results in production of two toxins, A and B. New evidence suggests that toxin B provides the virulent nature of *Clostridium difficle* (Lyras et al., 2009). Another organism which has rising concern over the development of multi-drug resistance is *Neisseria gonorrhoeae,* the bacteria that causes gonorrhea. As early as the 1970s, the United States has seen strains of *Neisseria gonorrhoeae,* resistant to penicillin and tetracycline. Many of the more recent strains have developed resistance to fluoroquinolines. Just reported in 2011, a multi-drug resistant strain known as H041 was identified in Japan (Ohnishi et al., 2011). Food-bourne diseases are also beginning to demonstrate resistance. Salmonella strains that are resistant to ciprofloxacin have recently emerged. An estimated 3.3 million cases of salmonella poisoning were reported in North American and Europe between 1999 and 2008, although these cases include both resistant and non-resistant strains (Le Hello et al., 2011; McConnell, 1999). Other diseases of particular concern that were included on the Notifiable Disease List in 2009 produced by the Center for Disease Control (CDC) include: *Streptococcal* species, *Streptococcus pneumoniae,* vancomycin-resistant *Staphylococcus aureus* (*VRSA*), *Mycobacterium tuberculosis, Neisseria meningitidis, Bordetella pertussis, Vibrio cholera*

(Christensen et al., 2009; Lynch et al., 2009; Morbidity and Mortality Weekly Report [MMWR], 2009; Phares et al., 2008; Robinson et al., 2001; Tanaka et al., 2003). Although in some of these cases antibiotic resistance is already observed, they are included primarily because of the availability of case reports with these diseases. Figure 2 represents a comparison of total reported cases of Streptococcal disease, invasive, group A to those that were drug resistant in the United States from 2002 to 2007. The percentage of cases that showed drug resistance are shown for each year. These data do not suggest a large increase in the number of reported cases but a trend of increasing resistance. Also, infections caused by these bacteria exhibit characteristics and trends similar to those bacterium that have been placed on the AATF list.

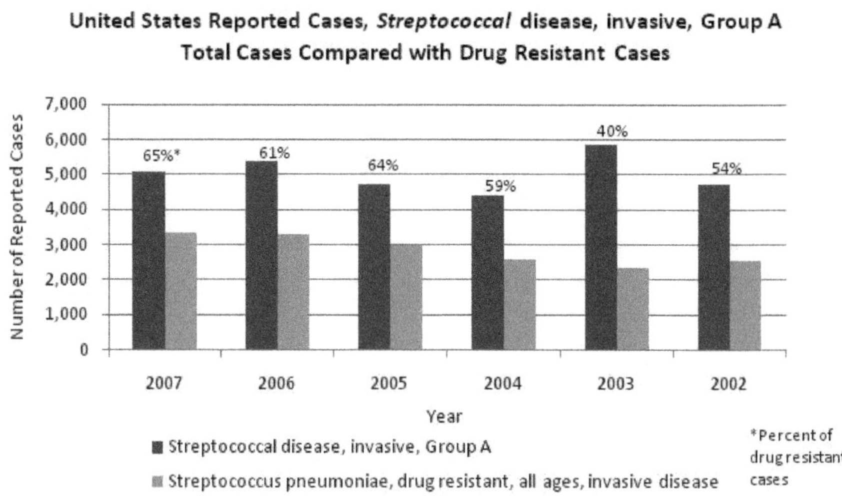

Fig. 2. The total number of *Streptococcal* disease (invasive, group A) cases reported in the United States between 2002 and 2007 compared to the number of cases that demonstrated drug-resistance (shown as a percentage each year.) Data were compiled by the authors from the Center for Disease Control Morbidity and Mortality Weekly Reports, 2002-2007.

2. How did bugs become "super?"

2.1 Antibiotic misuse

Perhaps the most commonly known cause of the development of antibiotic resistance is the so-called misuse of antibiotics. This phrase refers not only to the patient's adherence to antibiotic prescription instructions, but also to the doctors that prescribe antibiotics unnecessarily. Many times problems with over prescription of antibiotics comes from the patients demand. Perhaps doctors are concerned with patient satisfaction or wish to decrease the likelihood of a follow up visit for a viral illness which could result in a bacterial infection. It is possible that the patients have developed an expectation to leave the doctor's office with prescription in hand. Regardless of the reason, antibiotics administered for unnecessary purposes, including non-bacterial infections and prophylaxis, encourage the development and the spread of antibiotic resistance. Considering one study that estimated over 90% of all infections are viral, yet over half the US patients are taking antibiotics for these viral infections (*Science Daily*, 2005).

A study published in *Science* in 2010 utilized a genomic approach to examine single nucleotide polymorphisms using a high resolution second generation DNA sequencing platform. Researchers examined two samples: one was a global collection ranging from 1982 to 2003 and the second was a collection from Thailand over a seven month period. Sample one represents a random population while the second samples are limited to a single transmission. The data suggests specific European samples from the global collection relate to those collected from the Thailand hospital. The complete set of data allowed phylogenic analysis and an estimation of time since the evolution of the resistance. The researchers observed that 28.9% of the homoplasies identified had direct links to current therapeutics, providing strong evidence that the misuse of antibiotics in today's medical practice is a major contributor to the development of resistance. Furthermore, this study has allowed an estimate of one single nucleotide polymorphism every six weeks, an essentially unimaginable rate in evolutionary time (Harris et al., 2010).

The second part of this concern is patient adherence. This usually stems from the fact that antibiotic treatment, assuming it is a non-resistant bug, usually improves clinical symptoms within 1 to 3 days. Patients have difficulty continuing to take the prescription when their symptoms have been alleviated. They also have a tendency to "save" the rest of the prescription in case they need it again in the future. The contribution of this action to antibiotic resistance is simple: initial treatment kills most of the bacteria, particularly those susceptible to the antibiotic; those with some minor susceptibility to the antibiotic survive and thrive as the dosing is waned. Essentially this is an acceleration of "survival of the fittest." Bacteria that have been able to survive, reproduce and pass along whatever genetic variance they carry which provides resistance.

Recent reports have warned the overuse of antibiotics as prophylaxis in the food industry, although there is some controversy over the actual contribution to food animal antibiotic administration to the growing problem of global "superbug" problems (Singer et al., 2003). It is proposed that unnecessary use of antibiotics in food animals will contribute to resistance in the same ways as over prescribing and lack of adherence in the human population.

2.2 Common household "superbug" advancement

Although antibiotic misuse is perhaps the most publicized cause of "superbug" development, several similar mechanisms advance the resistant strains as well. Antibacterial soap is one example in which a large sample of weaker bugs is being killed, allowing the tough survivors to expand their gene pool. Many antibacterial products contain the ingredient triclosan, which functions by inhibiting essential fatty acid synthesis. Surviving bacteria develop a resistance to triclosan and are therefore not affected by future triclosan based cleansing. Laboratory experiments demonstrate that *E. coli* variants which developed resistance to triclosan did so via a mutation in the *fab1* gene. *Fab1* encodes the enzyme enoyl reductase, an enzyme essential for fatty acid metabolism, a mechanism untouched by most of today's antibiotics (Levy, 2000). Further experiments suggest two hours (4-8 hours for resistant strains) are required to kill 90% of susceptible *E. coli* when treated with soap containing 150 μg/ml triclosan (Levy, 2000).

The thought of "superbug" advancement in your home can be disturbing, but understanding where bacteria and fungi are found, where they live, and what strains they are can help educate the public about cleanliness in the home. It is important to point out here that my mentioning cleanliness in a review on "superbugs," one might imagine that evidence suggests we need to use more antibacterial cleaners and clean more, however, this is not necessarily the case. Most likely what is required is a solid education about the spread of the organisms, most importantly how to wash your hands. In reality, what is really required is not a better cleaner or more cleaning, but longer cleaning. A recent article in *Popular Mechanics* examined places in your home where microorganisms are likely thriving and identified the top five: refrigerator (particularly the vegetable drawer), dishwasher, air around the trash can and the trash can itself, washing machine, and the shower head. Presented results indicated that 23.4% of the bacteria found in the refrigerator was *Klebsiella pneumoniae;* the potentially infectious bacteria *Pseudomonas aeruginosa* were found in the washing machine; bacteria samples collected from the trash and the air around the trash contained *Staphylococcus aureus,* approximately 33% of which were methicillin resistant; *Exophiala* fungi capable of infecting humans was found in the dishwasher; and *Mycobacterium avium,* a bacteria that is usually benign but can infect immunocompromized individuals, was found in the shower head (Grunbaum, web, 2011). The important point to take from both of these "household" examples is that any cleansing treatment (hands, body, and refrigerator) must be approached with sufficient cleanser and sufficient time to ensure that maximal bacteria or fungus has been extinguished.

2.3 Resistant gene transfer

Misuse of antibiotics and antibacterial products have forded bacteria the opportunity to evolve resistance via one or more mechanisms of DNA alteration. Generally speaking, the result of these DNA alterations is either a modification that allows the bacteria to modify the drug chemically, rapidly remove the drug from the cell or prevent drug entry into the cell, or prevents binding of the drug by modifying the drug's target site. Likewise, certain bacteria are inherently resistant to some antibiotics. For example, gram negative bacteria are resistant to a number of antibiotics that are typically effective for gram positive bacteria, such as vancomycin. This resistance comes from the outer cell membrane layer that surrounds gram negative bacteria but not gram positive bacteria (Ibezim, 2005). The most pressing concern, however, is the rate of spread of so called acquired resistance. Acquired resistance refers to the presence of DNA encoding resistance, either through mutations or so called horizontal gene transfer (which is the exchange of resistance genes among different bacterial species). Mutations are thought to occur about one in every 10^8 to 10^9 bacteria (Todar, 2009). Once bacteria develop a mutation that allows it to survive in the presence of antibiotics, this trait is passed on via a process known as vertical gene transfer through the replication of DNA and growth of new cells. Of these two processes, it is horizontal gene transfer that contributes most considerably to the mass wave of resistant bacteria.

Bacteria are equipped with a variety of mechanisms capable of gene exchange including conjugation, transduction, and transformation which are all methods of horizontal gene transfer. Likewise, bacteria can undergo gene exchange by sequence specific mechanisms such as transposition. Conjugation refers the interaction between two bacterial cells through a sex pillus, which allows polymerase mediated duplication of plasmid DNA to be transferred or exchanged. Oftentimes, these plasmid molecules contain a gene which encodes resistance. The second method, transduction, also involves incorporation of new DNA. Transduction involves transfer of genetic material via a bacteriophage, which injects DNA with potential resistance genes included into a host cell. Infection stimulates the production of new phage molecules with both phage DNA and host cell DNA, which upon infection into another host cell will result in incorporation of the original host cell DNA (presumably containing a resistance gene) into the chromosome of the newly infected cell. Fragmented pieces of DNA from donor cells, which may confer resistance, are taken up by new cells via the process of transformation (Tortora, 2003).

Likewise, bacteria can undergo gene exchange by sequence specific mechanisms such as transposition. Transposition occurs when a resistance gene is flanked with genes encoding enzymes known as transpoase. These enzymes, together with sequences of DNA known as insertion sequences, when expressed, facilitate the transfer and insertion of the resistance gene into host DNA. This mechanism is referred to as horizontal gene transfer because the gene sequence along with DNA encoding machinery for further transposition activity are incorporated in a cross-over like process between two strands of DNA (Tortora, 2003).

Thus far, a variety of genes have been identified that confer resistance when expressed. One of the most widely publicized was the New Dehli Metallo-β-lactamase (NDM-1) (Kumarasamy et al., 2010). The NDM-1 gene encodes an enzyme known as carapenemase, which is a β-lactamase that acts specifically on carbanpenem antibiotics, a class which until recently reserved for infections demonstrating resistance to other antibiotics. Likewise the β-lactamase activity affords organisms carrying this gene resistance to all β-lactam antibiotics, including cephalosporins, many glycopeptides, monobactams, and penicillins (Walsh, 2008). The gene is capable of horizontal gene transfer and has been observed in select strains of *E. coli* and *Klebsiella pneumoniae* (Yong et al., 2009).

3. Current, emerging, and needed therapies

3.1 Current therapies

Many of the existing therapies for bacterial infections function via similar mechanisms of action. In general antibiotics inhibit one of three cellular mechanisms including: protein synthesis (aminoglycosides, macrolides, tetracyclines, and others including streptomycin, chloramphenicol, linezolid, quinupristin/dalfopristin); cell wall synthesis (carbapenems, cephalosporins, glycopeptides, and penicillins); or topoisomerase activity (quinolones) (Lexi Comp, Inc., 2011). There are a few select antibiotics that have a unique mechanism of action including: daptomycin, which binds to the cell membrane and causes rapid depolarization thus inhibiting synthesis of nucleic acids and proteins; trimethoprin sulfamethoxazole, which interferes substantially with bacterial folic acid synthesis; and metronidazole, which results in breakdown of DNA helical structure (Lexi-Comp, Inc., 2011). Table 3 summarizes selected current antibiotics used for bacterial disease and infection, specifically those currently indicated for infections caused by organisms that have been added to the "superbug" list.

Generic	Common Uses
Aminoglycosides	
Gentamicin	Infections due to gram- organisms & gram+ *Staphylococcus*
Kanamycin	Infections caused by *E. coli, E. aerogenes, K. pneumoniae, Acinetobacter* spp
Carbapenems	
Imipenem/ Cilastatin	Infections of LRT, UT, bone, skin; infections due to gram+ bacteria (*S. aureus, Streptococcus* spp), resistant gram- bacilli (including EBSL-producing *E. coli, Klebsiella* spp, *Enterobacter* spp, *P. aeruginosa*)
Meropenem	Meningitis caused by *S. pneumoniae, N. meningitidis*; skin infections
Cephalosporins	
Cefotaxime	Infections of RT, skin, bone, UT due to gram(- bacilli (not *Pseudomonas*), gram+ cocci (not enterococcus), many penicillin-resistant pneumococci.
Cefepime	UTIs due to *E. coli, K. pneumoniae*; infections of skin due to methicillin-susceptible staphylococci; pneumonia due to *S. pneumoniae, K. pneumoniae, Enterobacter* spp; *Enterobacter* spp
Glycopeptides	
Vancomycin	Infections caused by staphylococcal spp, streptococcal spp, *C. difficile*
Lipopeptide	
Daptomycin	Infections due to gram+ organisms; endocarditis caused by MSSA or *MRSA*
Macrolides	
Azithromycin	Infections of U/LRT, skin; CAP, infections due to *S. aureus, S. pneumoniae*
Clarithromycin	Infections due to *S. pneumoniae, S. aureus, S. pyogenes,*
Penicillins	
Ampicillin	Infections due to non-β-lactamase-producing organisms, streptococci, pneumococci, meningococci, some *Salmonella, Enterobacter, Klebsiella*
Penicillin G	Sepsis, pneumonia, endocarditis, meningitis; infections due to gram+ organisms (generally not *S. aureus*), some gram- organisms
Quinolones	
Ciprofloxacin	Infections of the UT, LRT, skin, bone infections; gonorrhea; HAP
Levofloxacin	CAP, MDRSP, HAP, UTI, skin infections
Moxifloxacin	CAP, MDRSP, bronchitis, skin infections, intra-abdominal infections
Sulfonamides	
Trimethoprim-Sulfamethoxazole	UTIs due to *E. coli, Klebsiella* & *Enterobacter* spp, bronchitis due to S. *pneumoniae*
Tetracyclines	
Doxycycline	Infections caused by *Chlamydia, Mycoplasma, N. gonorrhoeae, Clostridium, B. anthracis*, uncommon gram- & + organisms; syphilis; CAP
Others	
Chloramphenicol	Infections due to organisms resistant to other antibiotics caused by *N. meningitidis, Salmonella*; vancomycin-resistant enterococci
Linezolid	HAP caused by *S. aureus* (including *MRSA*) or *S. pneumoniae* (including multidrug-resistant strains), skin infections, CAP caused by gram+ organisms, Vancomycin-resistant *E. faecium* (VRE) infections

Table 3. Selected antibiotic therapeutics and selected common uses. Data were compiled with Lexi-Comp Online in August 2011. Spp=species; CAP=community acquired pneumonia; MDRSP = multidrug-resistant *S. pneumoniae;* U/LRT = upper/lower respiratory tract; UTI = urinary tract infection; HAP = hospital acquired pneumoniae (Lexi-Comp, Inc., 2011).

In regards to the specific organisms which have documented resistant strains, the following drugs demonstrate efficacy: The imipenem/cilastatin combination has been effective against resistant gram negative bacilli such as the ESBL-producing *E.coli* and *Klebsilla* species and the *Enterobacter* species and *Psendomonas aeruginosa.* Ceftoaxime has demonstrated efficacy against some penicillin-resistant pneumococci. Treatment of *MRSA* and *MSSA* has been successful with daptomycin. The primary quinolones used for drug resistant *S. pneumoniae* are levofloxacin and moxifloxacin. Chloramphenicol, although quite toxic, has demonstrated activity against many vancomycin-resistant enterococci. Perhaps the most notable is linezolid, which is a newer antibiotic designed to inhibit bacterial protein synthesis, albeit by binding the bacterial 23S ribosomal RNA of the 50S subunit and preventing formation of the 70S subunit. This antibiotic has been effective against vancomycin-resistant *Enterococcus faecium* (VRE), nosocomial pneumonia caused by both methicillin susceptible and methicillin resistant forms of *Staphylococcus aureus* as well as *Streptococcus pneumoniae* including those that are multidrug resistant. Also of worthy attention is the relatively few side effects documented for patients treated with linezolid (Lexi-Comp, Inc., 2011). Table 4 summarizes selected infections as well as recommended and alternative treatment combinations.

Pathogen	Recommended Adult Drug Therapy	Alternative Drug Therapy
Pseudomonas Aeruginosa	Ceftazidime plus Aminoglycosides or Penicillins, Extended-Spectrum plus Aminoglycosides or Cefepime plus Aminoglycosides	Imipenem and Cilastatin or Meropenem plus Aminoglycosides or Ciprofloxacinplus Penicillins, extended Spectrum or Aztreonam
Aspergillus Species	Voriconazole	Amphotericin B (Lipid Complex), Echinocandins, Itraconazole, Posaconazole
Sallmonella Species	Cephalosporins, 3rd Generation	Ampicillin, Sulfamethoxazole and Trimethoprim, Chloramphenicol, Ciprofloxacin
Enterococcus Species	Penicillin G plus (Gentamicin or Streptomycin) or Ampicillin plus (Gentamicin or Streptomycin); Vancomycin-resistant Enterococcus: Linezolid, Quinupristin and Dalfopristin, Doxycycline, Choramphenicol	Vancomycin plus Gentamicin or Penicillin G Plus Streptomycin or Ampicillin plus Streptomycin
Staphylococcus aureus, Methicillin-Resistant	Vancomycin	Daptomycin, Doxycycline, linezolid, Quinupristin and Dalfopristin, Sulfamethoxazole and Trimethoprim
Clostridium difficle	Metronidazole	vancomycin
Neisseria gonorrhoeae	Cefixime, Ceftriaxone	Monotherapy: Cefotaxime, Spectinomycin
Bordetella pertussis	Erythromycin	Azithromycin, Clarithromycin, Tetracycline, Sulfamethoxazole and Trimethoprim, Chloramphenicol

Table 4. Summary of selected infectious organisms and the recommended and alternative treatments (Lexi-Comp, Inc., 2011).

3.2 Emerging therapies

In the recent years there have been a few significant developments of new antibiotics. Ceftaroline, often referred to as a 5th generation cephalosporin, has shown activity against multidrug resistant gram positive bacteria (Bazan et al., 2009; Steed & Ryback, 2010).

Ceftaroline fosamil is a prodrug form which is rapidly converted to the active form after administered (Bazan et al., 2009). Like other cephalosporins, it binds to penicillin binding proteins (PBP), but differs from other β-lactams in that it has a high affinity for PBP2a, which is unique to *MRSA* (Steed & Ryback, 2010). Ceftaroline has been successfully used for the treatment of skin and skin structure infections caused by methicillin resistant *S. aureus, S. pyogenes, S. agalactiae, E. coli, K. oxytoca,* and *K. pneumoniae* (Bazan et al., 2009; Product insert, 2010; Saravolatz et al., 2010a, 2011b; Snydman et al., 2010; Steed & Ryback, 2010). The most common side effects reported were diarrhea, nausea, constipation, vomiting, increased transaminases, hyperkalemia, rash, and phlebitis (Hester et al., 2011).

Another recent addition to approved antibiotics is telavancin. Telavancin is a lipoglycopeptide derivative of vancomycin that inhibits bacterial cell wall synthesis (Saravolatz et al., 2009). When compared to vancomycin, talavancin has demonstrated effectiveness in treatment of skin and skin structure infections caused by methicillin resistant *S. aureus, S. pyogenes, S. agalactiae, S. pneumoniae,* and vancomycin resist*ant E. faecalis* (Stryjewski et al., 2006a, 2006b, 2008c). The drug has also been explored for use in hospital acquired pneumonia (Rubinstein et al., 2011). The most common side effects reported included: nausea, vomiting, foamy urine, and disturbance in taste (Medical Letter, 2010).

A recent carapenem, doripenem, has demonstrated a broad spectrum of antimicrobial activity against gram positive and negative bacteria including *P. aeruginosa* (included some cabapenems resistant strains) (Jones et al., 2004; Lister, 2007; Mushtaq et al., 2004). Doripenem is indicated for complicated intra-abdominal and urinary tract infections due to enterococci, anaerobes, and *P. aeruginosa* as well as hospital acquired pneumonia resulting from *Klebsiella, Enterobacter, Acinetobacter,* and *Serratia* species or in some cases *S. aureus* (Medical Letter, 2007; Solomkin et al., 2003). Aside from allergic reactions, the most commonly reported side effects included: headache, nausea, diarrhea, rash, and phlebitis (Horiuchi et al., 2006).

Retapamulin is a recently approaved topical antibiotic effective for treatment of impetigo due to *S. pyogenes* and methicillin-susceptible *S. aureus* (Rittenhouse et al., 2006). Activity against *MRSA* has been observed *in vitro* (Rittenhouse et al., 2006). This antibiotic is derived from fermentation of fungi and represents the first in a class of antibiotics known as pleuromutilins. Drugs from this class interfere with bacterial protein synthesis by acting on the 50S subunit of the ribosome (Yan et al., 2006). Reported side effects are minimal and included only site irritation (Parish et al., 2008; Parish et al., 2006).

Lastly, consideration of some not yet approved but promising antibiotics is warranted. In early 2011, results of a phase 3 clinical trial for a new antibiotic called fidaxomicin were published (Louie et al., 2011). Fidaxomicin starts a new class of antibiotics referred to as macrocycles. The drug offers a narrow range of activity as it is designed specifically for *C. difficile* (Louie et al., 2011). The clinical studies reported that fidaxomicin treated patients had fewer recurrent episodes of *C. difficle* infection than patients taking vancomycin (Louie et al., 2011). Another potential antibiotic worth considering is referred to as kibdelomycin, which was selected based on screening against multiple engineered strains of S. aureus. Although the structure identified was unique, it was found to function as a type II topoisomerase inhibitor and has demonstrated activity primarily against gram positive bacteria. Although it functions as a topoisomerase inhibitor, it is unique in the fact that it specifically inhibits the ATPase activity of bacterial type II topoisomerases (Phillips et al., 2011). Another promising publication in *Nature* suggests that a new inhibitor (GSK299423) has demonstrated broad spectrum activity by inhibiting DNA gyrase. The promising detail about this inhibitor is that crystal structures have indicated that the inhibitor binds to a non-catalytic site on the DNA gyrase, as compared to the binding site for most fluoroquinolones, thus representing a new class of antibiotics and making this a prime target for further development (Bax et al., 2010).

3.3 Therapeutic concerns and the need for continued antibiotic development

The concern over the current antibiotics available is that the majority function via one or two general mechanisms. Currently the carbapenems are "last line" therapy for many resistant bacteria; the emergence of the NDM-1 gene demonstrates not only an organism's ability to withstand treatment from the majority of available antibiotics, but also demonstrates the threat of effective transposition based spreading from the gene. Many "newer" antibiotics function via some slight variation of previous mechanisms, for example inhibiting protein synthesis by binding one of the ribosomal subunits at a different location or a with a different affinity. Bacteria are likely to rapidly develop resistance mechanisms for antibiotics that function so similarly. Currently there are very few approved antibiotics with novel mechanisms and the "drug development pipeline" does not include a substantial number of new designs.

The emergence of the multidrug resistance element NDM-1 suggests the urgency for the development of drastically novel function antibiotics. The over publicized, and perhaps mis-publicized, evolution of "superbugs" has forced both public and government attention to the uncertain nature of our microbial defense. The necessity of government support through funding is essential in order to develop drugs that are positioned to enter the "pipeline." Considering the time required for drug development, the risk of global spread of resistance is alarming.

4. Conclusion

4.1 Prevention of antibiotic resistance

Data clearly demonstrate a rise in the number of resistant organisms as well as in increase in the number of multidrug resistant bacteria. Based on the relative mutation rate and gene transfer rates, there is indeed a global concern over a future inability to treat bacterial infection effectively and without toxic side effects. Today's medical treatments and surgical capabilities have advanced modern medicine just as the discovery and development of penicillin marked a turning point in therapeutics. Emerging resistant mechanisms and organisms place the world on a path not only similar to an era before penicillin, but also to an era where medical surgical procedures become impossible to the risk of infection. New multidrug resistance elements, in particular, NDM-1, is concerning because of its potential to travel between species and produce "superbugs" at rates well beyond the limit of natural selection. History has demonstrated that organisms have been able to develop resistant mechanisms rapidly once introduced to new antibiotics, and in particular once introduced to a new class of antibiotics. Continued responsible use of antibiotics is currently the best way to attempt to slow down the development of resistant strains. Careful attention should be paid to when antibiotics are prescribed, but even more importantly which antibiotics are prescribed. It is extremely important to reserve new antibiotics for strains that have demonstrated resistance to other drugs. Infatuation with "hot" new drugs has the potential to accelerate the selection of resistant organisms and render the new drugs ineffective as well. Consideration for patient compliance is also important; ensuring that the full course of antibiotic is taken will produce maximal eradication of the bacteria, leaving no remaining cells to pass on their "secret" of survival.

4.2 Spread the research and spread the word

Financial cutbacks by large drug companies and governmental funding cuts have slowed the potential for development of novel antibiotics. Although the high risk - high payoff drug development programs are waning, smaller research groups and companies are in a position to collaborate and share promising results thereby forming a network of antibiotic development team members. In recent years, the pressure to "develop and sell" outweighed the pressure to "develop and share". Perhaps with the economic setbacks, the "develop and share" model will accelerate design of new drugs. The importance of sharing knowledge with colleagues is evident, but the necessity of correctly explaining our current state to the general public should be equally considered. A clear understanding of the investment, both time and financial, required to bring a drug to market needs to be highlighted so that everyone has the motivation to slow the spread of resistance and give the drug development industry an opportunity to excel.

5. References

The Choice of Antibacterial Drugs. (2001). *Medical Letter on Drugs and Therapeutics*, Vol. 43, No. 1111-2, pp. (69-78) ISBN 0025-732X

Vibativ (Telavancin) for Skin and Skin Structure Infections. (2009). *Journal of Drugs in Dermatology*, Vol. 8, No. 12, pp. (1151-1151) ISBN 1545-9616

Telavancin (Vibativ) for Gram-Positive Skin Infections. (2010). *Medical Letter on Drugs and Therapeutics*, Vol. 52, No. 1329, pp. (1-2) ISBN 0025-732X

Apostol, M., et al. (2009). Trends in Perinatal Group B Streptococcal Disease-United States, 2000-2006 (Reprinted from MMWR, Vol 58, Pg 109-112, 2009). *Jama-Journal of the American Medical Association*, Vol. 301, No. 12, pp. (1218-1220) ISBN 0098-7484

Appelbaum, P.C., et al. (2009). *Activity of Telavancin against Staphylococci and Enterococci Determined by MIC and Resistance Selection Studies.* Antimicrobial Agents and Chemotherapy, Vol. 53, No. 10, pp. (4217-4224) ISBN 0066-4804

Austin, A.S. (2003). *A pest in the land: new world epidemics in a global perspective.* University of New Mexico Press, ISBN 0826328717 Retrieved from: <http://openlibrary.org/books/OL8167121M/A_Pest_in_the_Land>

Balasubramamian, J. et al. (2011) Bad Bugs No Drugs - A Review on NDM-1. *International Journal of Pharma and Bio Sciences,* Vol. 2, No. 1, pp. (B-62- B67), ISSN 0975-6299, Retrieved from: <www.ijpbs.net>

Bax, B.D., et al. (2010). Type IIA Topoisomerase Inhibition by a New Class of Antibacterial Agents. *Nature,* Vol. 466, No. 7309, pp. (935-U951) ISBN 0028-0836

Bazan, J.A., et al. (2009). Newer β-Lactam Antibiotics: Doripenem, Ceftobiprole, Ceftaroline, and Cefepime. *Infectious Disease Clinics of North America,* Vol. 23, No. 4, pp. (983-+) ISBN 0891-5520

Bellis, M. (n.d.) History of Penicillin, In: *About.Com Inventors,* August 12, 2011, Available from: < http://inventors.about.com/od/pstartinventions/a/Penicillin.htm>

Biedenbach, D.J., et al. (2004). Occurrence and Antimicrobial Resistance Pattern Comparisons among Bloodstream Infection Isolates from the Sentry Antimicrobial Surveillance Program (1997-2002). *Diagnostic Microbiology and Infectious Disease,* Vol. 50, No. 1, pp. (59-69) ISBN 0732-8893

Boucher, H.W., et al. (2004). Newer Systemic Antifungal Agents - Pharmacokinetics, Safety and Efficacy. *Drugs,* Vol. 64, No. 18, pp. (1997-2020) ISBN 0012-6667

Cardo, D., et al. (2004). National Nosocomial Infections Surveillance (NNIS) System Report, Data Summary from January 1992 through June 2004, Issued October 2004. *American Journal of Infection Control,* Vol. 32, No. 8, pp. (470-485) ISBN 0196-6553

Chinedum, I.E. (2005). Microbial Resistance to Antibiotics. *African Journal of Biotechnology,* Vol. 4, No. 13, pp. (1606-1611) ISBN 1684-5315

Christensen, K.L.Y., et al. (2009). Infectious Disease Hospitalizations in the United States. *Clinical Infectious Diseases,* Vol. 49, No. 7, (Oct), pp. (1025-1035) ISBN 1058-4838

Daileader, P. (2007). *The Late Middle Ages.* The Teaching Co., Chantilly, VA

Decre, D., et al. (2004). Outbreak of Multi-Resistant *K. oxytoca* Involving Strains with Extended-Spectrum β-Lactamases and Strains with Extended-Spectrum Activity of the Chromosomal β-Lactamase. *Journal of Antimicrobial Chemotherapy,* Vol. 54, No. 5, (Nov), pp. (881-888) ISBN 0305-7453

Fridkin, S.K., et al. (2003). Epidemiological and Microbiological Characterization of Infections Caused by *S. aureus* with Reduced Susceptibility to Vancomycin, U.S, 1997-2001. *Clinical Infectious Diseases,* Vol. 36, No. 4, pp. (429-439) ISBN 1058-4838

Gaynes, R., et al. (2005). Overview of Nosocomial Infections Caused by Gram-Negative Bacilli. *Clinical Infectious Diseases,* Vol. 41, No. 6, pp. (848-854) ISBN 1058-4838

Grunbaum, M. 5 Places in Your Home that are Breeding Superbugs. *Popular Mechanics,* Retrieved from < http://www.popularmechanics.com/science/health/5-places-in-your-home-that-are-breeding-superbugs>

Hays, J.N. (2005). *Epidemics and pandemics: their impacts on human history.* ABC-CLIO, Inc. ISBN 9781851096589. Retrieved from: <http://0- ebooks.ohiolink.edu.polar.onu.edu/xtf-ebc/view?docId=tei/abc/DISWHE/DISWHE.xml&query=&brand =default>

Hecker, J.F.C. (1835). *The epidemics of the middle ages.* Sherwood, Gilbert and Piper. Retrieved from: <http://books.google.com/books?id=lDynaxN2Q-cC>

Horiuchi, M., et al. (2006). Absence of Convulsive Liability of Doripenem, a New Carbapenem Antibiotic, in Comparison with β-Lactam Antibiotics. *Toxicology,* Vol. 222, No. 1-2, (May 1), pp. (114-124) ISBN 0300-483X

Johnson, M.D. & Perfect, J.R. (2003). Caspofungin: First Approved Agent in a New Class of Antifungals. *Expert Opinion on Pharmacotherapy*, Vol. 4, No. 5, (May), pp. (807-823) ISBN 1465-6566

Jones, R.N., et al. (2004). Activities of Doripenem (S-4661) against Drug-Resistant Clinical Pathogens. *Antimicrobial Agents and Chemotherapy*, Vol. 48, No. 8, (Aug), pp. (3136-3140) ISBN 0066-4804

Kallen, A.J., et al. (2010). Health Care-Associated Invasive *MRSA* Infections, 2005-2008. *Journal of the American Medical Association*, Vol. 304, No. 6, (Aug 11), pp. (641-648) ISBN 0098-7484

Kang, C.I., et al. (2004). Bloodstream Infections Due to Extended-Spectrum β-Lactamase-Producing *E. coli* and *K. pneumoniae*: Risk Factors for Mortality and Treatment Outcome, with Special Emphasis on Antimicrobial Therapy. *Antimicrobial Agents and Chemotherapy*, Vol. 48, No. 12, pp. (4574-4581) ISBN 0066-4804

Klevens, R.M., et al. (2007). Invasive Methicillin-Resistant *S. aureus* Infections in the U.S. *Journal of the American Medical Association*, Vol. 298, No. 15, (Oct 17), pp. (1763-1771) ISBN 0098-7484

Kuehnert, M.J., et al. (2005). Methicillin-Resistant – *S. aureus* Hospitalizations, U.S. *Emerging Infectious Diseases*, Vol. 11, No. 6, (Jun), pp. (868-872) ISBN 1080-6040

Lexi-Comp, Inc. (2011). August 22, 2011, Available from: <http://online.lexi.com/crlsq/servlet/crlonline>

Lister, P.D. (2007). Carbapenems in the USA: Focus on Doripenem. *Expert Review of Anti-Infective Therapy*, Vol. 5, No. 5, (Oct), pp. (793-809) ISBN 1478-7210

Louie, T.J., et al. (2011). Fidaxomicin versus Vancomycin for *C. difficile* Infection. *New England Journal of Medicine*, Vol. 364, No. 5, pp. (422-431) ISBN 1533-4406

Lynch, M.F., et al. (2009). Typhoid Fever in the U.S., 1999-2006. *Journal of the American Medical Association*, Vol. 302, No. 8, pp. (859-865) ISBN 0098-7484

Maschmeyer, G. & Braveny, I. (2000). Review of the Incidence and Prognosis of *P. aeruginosa* Infections in Cancer Patients in the 1990s. *European Journal of Clinical Microbiology & Infectious Diseases*, Vol. 19, No. 12, pp. (915-925) ISBN 0934-9723

Maschmeyer, G. & Ruhnke, M. (2004). Update on Antifungal Treatment of Invasive Candida and *Aspergillus* Infections. *Mycoses*, Vol. 47, No. 7, pp. (263-276) ISBN 0933-7407

McConnell, H. (1999). Antibiotics and Superbugs. *Futurist*, Vol. 33, No. 2, (Feb), pp. (9-9) ISBN 0016-3317

Meyer, K.S., et al. (1993). Nosocomial Outbreak of *Klebsiella* Infection Resistant to Late-Generation Cephalosporins. *Annals of Internal Medicine*, Vol. 119, No. 5, (Sep 1), pp. (353-358) ISBN 0003-4819

Murray, B.E. (2000). Drug Therapy: Vancomycin-Resistant Enterococcal Infections. *New England Journal of Medicine*, Vol. 342, No. 10, (Mar 9), pp. (710-721) ISBN 0028-4793

Mushtaq, S., et al. (2004). Doripenem versus *P. aeruginosa* in Vitro: Activity against Characterized Isolates, Mutants, and Transconjugants and Resistance Selection Potential. *Antimicrobial Agents and Chemotherapy*, Vol. 48, No. 8, (Aug), pp. (3086-3092) ISBN 0066-4804

Obritsch, M.D., et al. (2004). National Surveillance of Antimicrobial Resistance in *P. aeruginosa* Isolates Obtained from Intensive Care Unit Patients from 1993 to 2002. *Antimicrobial Agents and Chemotherapy*, Vol. 48, No. 12, pp.(4606-4610) ISBN 0066-4804

Ohnishi, M., et al. (2011). Is *N. gonorrhoeae* Initiating a Future Era of Untreatable Gonorrhea?: Detailed Characterization of the First Strain with High-Level Resistance to Ceftriaxone. *Antimicrobial Agents and Chemotherapy*, Vol. 55, No. 7, (Jul), pp. (3538-3545) ISBN 0066-4804

Parish, L.C., et al. (2006). Topical Retapamulin Ointment (1%, Wt/Wt) Twice Daily for 5 Days versus Oral Cephalexin Twice Daily for 10 Days in the Treatment of Secondarily Infected Dermatitis: Results of a Randomized Controlled Trial. *Journal of the American Academy of Dermatology*, Vol. 55, No. 6, (Dec), pp. (1003-1013) ISBN 0190-9622

Parish, L.C. & Parish, J.L. (2008). Retapamulin: A New Topical Antibiotic for the Treatment of Uncomplicated Skin Infections. *Drugs of Today*, Vol. 44, No. 2, (Feb), pp. (91-102) ISBN 1699-3993

Paterson, D.L., et al. (2004). Antibiotic Therapy for *K. pneumoniae* Bacteremia: Implications of Production of Extended-Spectrum β-Lactamases. *Clinical Infectious Diseases*, Vol. 39, No. 1, (Jul 1), pp. (31-37) ISBN 1058-4838

Phares, C.R., et al. (2008). Epidemiology of Invasive Group B Streptococcal Disease in the United States, 1999-2005. *Journal of the American Medical Association*, Vol. 299, No. 17, (May 7), pp. (2056-2065) ISBN 0098-7484

Phillips, J.W., et al. (2011). Discovery of Kibdelomycin, a Potent New Class of Bacterial Type II Topoisomerase Inhibitor by Chemical-Genetic Profiling in *S. aureus*. *Chemistry & Biology*, Vol. 18, No. 8, (Aug 26), pp. (955-965) ISBN 1879-1301

Product Information for *Tefarlo*. (2010). Forest. St. Louis, MO 63042.

Pryor, E.G. (1975). The Great Plague of Hong Kong. *Journal of the Hong Kong Branch of the Royal Asiatic Society* Vol. 15, pp. (61-70), ISSN 1991-7295

Quale, J.M., et al. (2002). Molecular Epidemiology of a Citywide Outbreak of Extended-Spectrum β-Lactamase-Producing *K. pneumoniae* Infection. *Clinical Infectious Diseases*, Vol. 35, No. 7, (Oct 1), pp. (834-841) ISBN 1058-4838

Rittenhouse, S., et al. (2006). Selection of Retapamulin, a Novel Pleuromutilin for Topical Use. *Antimicrobial Agents and Chemotherapy*, Vol. 50, No. 11, (Nov), pp. (3882-3885) ISBN 0066-4804

Robinson, K.A., et al. (2001). Epidemiology of Invasive *S. pneumoniae* Infections in the U.S., 1995-1998 - Opportunities for Prevention in the Conjugate Vaccine Era. *Journal of the American Medical Association*, Vol. 285, No. 13, pp. (1729-1735) ISBN 0098-7484

Rosen, W. (2007). *Justinian's flea: plague, empire, and the birth of Europe*. Penguin. ISBN 9780670038558. Retrieved from: <http://books.google.com/books?id=2oA2Lbiv4xAC>

Rubinstein, E., et al. (2011). Telavancin versus Vancomycin for Hospital acquired Pneumonia Due to Gram-Positive Pathogens. *Clinical Infectious Diseases*, Vol. 52, No. 1, (Jan 1), pp. (31-40) ISBN 1058-4838

Sanchez, T.H., et al. (2005). Bacterial Diarrhea in Persons with HIV Infection, United States, 1992-2002. *Clinical Infectious Diseases*, Vol. 41, No. 11, (Dec 1), pp. (1621-1627) ISBN 1058-4838

Saravolatz, L., et al. (2010). In Vitro Activity of Ceftaroline against Community-Associated Methicillin-Resistant, Vancomycin-Intermediate, Vancomycin-Resistant, and Daptomycin-Nonsusceptible *S. aureus* Isolates. *Antimicrobial Agents and Chemotherapy*, Vol. 54, No. 7, (Jul), pp. (3027-3030) ISBN 0066-4804

Saravolatz, L.D., et al. (2009). Telavancin: A Novel Lipoglycopeptide. *Clinical Infectious Diseases*, Vol. 49, No. 12, (Dec 15), pp. (1908-1914) ISBN 1058-4838

Saravolatz, L.D., et al. (2011). Ceftaroline: A Novel Cephalosporin with Activity against Methicillin-Resistant *S. aureus*. *Clinical Infectious Diseases*, Vol. 52, No. 9, (May 1), pp. (1156-1163) ISBN 1058-4838

Schwaoer, M.J., et al. (2005). High Levels of Antimicrobial Coresistance among Extended-Spectrum-β-Lactamase-Producing Enterobacteriaceae. *Antimicrobial Agents and Chemotherapy*, Vol. 49, No. 5, (May), pp. (2137-2139) ISBN 0066-4804

Snydman, D.R., et al. (2011). In Vitro Activity of Ceftaroline against a Broad Spectrum of Recent Clinical Anaerobic Isolates. *Antimicrobial Agents and Chemotherapy*, Vol. 55, No. 1, (Jan), pp. (421-425) ISBN 0066-4804

Solomkin, J.S., et al. (2003). Guidelines for the Selection of Anti-Infective Agents for Complicated Intra-Abdominal Infections. *Clinical Infectious Diseases*, Vol. 37, No. 8, (Oct 15), pp. (997-1005) ISBN 1058-4838

Solomon, S., et al. (2003). National Nosocomial Infections Surveillance (NNIS) System Report, Data Summary from January 1992 through June 2003, Issued August 2003. *American Journal of Infection Control*, Vol. 31, No. 8, (Dec), pp. (481-498) ISBN 0196-6553

Steed, M.E. & Rybak, M.J. (2010). Ceftaroline: A New Cephalosporin with Activity against Resistant Gram-Positive Pathogens. *Pharmacotherapy*, Vol. 30, No. 4, (Apr), pp. (375-389) ISBN 0277-0008

Streit, J.M., et al. (2004). Assessment of Pathogen Occurrences and Resistance Profiles among Infected Patients in the Intensive Care Unit: Report from the Sentry Antimicrobial Surveillance Program (North America, 2001). *International Journal of Antimicrobial Agents*, Vol. 24, No. 2, (Aug), pp. (111-118) ISBN 0924-8579

Stryjewski, M.E., et al. (2006). Telavancin versus Standard Therapy for Treatment of Complicated Skin and Skin Structure Infections Caused by Gram-Positive Bacteria: Fast 2 Study. *Antimicrobial Agents and Chemotherapy*, Vol. 50, No. 3, (Mar), pp. (862-867) ISBN 0066-4804

Stryjewski, M.E., et al. (2008). Telavancin vs. Vancomycin for the Treatment of Complicated Skin and Skin-Structure Infections Caused by Gram-Positive Organisms. *Clinical Infectious Diseases*, Vol. 46, No. 11, pp. (1683-1693) ISBN 1058-4838

Stryjewski, M.E., et al. (2005). Telavancin vs. Standard Therapy for Treatment of Complicated Skin and Soft-Tissue Infections Due to Gram-Positive Bacteria. *Clinical Infectious Diseases*, Vol. 40, No. 11, (Jun 1), pp. (1601-1607) ISBN 1058-4838

Study Explores Antibiotic Misuse. (2005). *Science Daily*, August 27, 2011, Available from: < http://www.sciencedaily.com /releases/2005/01/050111162856.htm>

Summary of Notifiable Diseases, United States, 2009 (2011) *MMWR: Morbidity and Mortality Weekly Report*, Vol. 58, No. 53, (May 2011), pp. (996-998), Retrieved from: <http://www.cdc.gov/mmwr>

Summary of Notifiable Diseases, United States, 2008 (2010) *MMWR: Morbidity and Mortality Weekly Report*, Vol. 57, No. 54, (June 2010), pp. (1-94), Retrieved from: <http://www.cdc.gov/mmwr>

Summary of Notifiable Diseases, United States, 2007 (2009) *MMWR: Morbidity and Mortality Weekly Report*, Vol. 56, No. 53, (July 2009), pp. (1-94), Retrieved from: <http://www.cdc.gov/mmwr>

Summary of Notifiable Diseases, United States, 2006 (2008) *MMWR: Morbidity and Mortality Weekly Report*, Vol. 55, No. 53, (March 2008), pp. (1-94), Retrieved from: <http://www.cdc.gov/mmwr>

Summary of Notifiable Diseases, United States, 2005 (2007) *MMWR: Morbidity and Mortality Weekly Report*, Vol. 54, No. 53, (March 2007), pp. (2-92), Retrieved from: <http://www.cdc.gov/mmwr>

Summary of Notifiable Diseases, United States, 2004 (2006) *MMWR: Morbidity and Mortality Weekly Report*, Vol. 53, No. 53, (June 2006), pp. (1-79), Retrieved from: <http://www.cdc.gov/mmwr>

Summary of Notifiable Diseases, United States, 2003 (2005) *MMWR: Morbidity and Mortality Weekly Report*, Vol. 52, No. 54, (April 2005), pp. (1-85), Retrieved from: <http://www.cdc.gov/mmwr>

Summary of Notifiable Diseases, United States, 2002 (2004) *MMWR: Morbidity and Mortality Weekly Report*, Vol. 51, No. 53, (April 2004), pp. (1-84), Retrieved from: <http://www.cdc.gov/mmwr>

Summary of Notifiable Diseases, United States, 2001 (2003) *MMWR: Morbidity and Mortality Weekly Report*, Vol. 50, No. 53, (May 2003), pp. (1-108), Retrieved from: <http://www.cdc.gov/mmwr>

Summary of Notifiable Diseases, United States, 2000 (2002) *MMWR: Morbidity and Mortality Weekly Report*, Vol. 49, No. 53, (June 2002), pp. (1-102), Retrieved from: <http://www.cdc.gov/mmwr>

Summary of Notifiable Diseases, United States, 1999 (2001) *MMWR: Morbidity and Mortality Weekly Report*, Vol. 48, No. 53, (April 2001), pp. (1-104), Retrieved from: <http://www.cdc.gov/mmwr>

Summary of Notifiable Diseases, United States, 1998 (1999) *MMWR: Morbidity and Mortality Weekly Report*, Vol. 47, No. 53, (December 1999), pp. (1-93), Retrieved from: <http://www.cdc.gov/mmwr>

Summary of Notifiable Diseases, United States, 1997 (1998) *MMWR: Morbidity and Mortality Weekly Report*, Vol. 46, No. 54, (November 1998), pp. (1-87), Retrieved from: <http://www.cdc.gov/mmwr>

Summary of Notifiable Diseases, United States, 1996 (1997) *MMWR: Morbidity and Mortality Weekly Report*, Vol. 45, No. 53, (October 1997), pp. (1-87), Retrieved from: <http://www.cdc.gov/mmwr>

Summary of Notifiable Diseases, United States, 1995 (1996) *MMWR: Morbidity and Mortality Weekly Report*, Vol. 44, No. 53, (October 1996), pp. (1-87), Retrieved from: <http://www.cdc.gov/mmwr>

Summary of Notifiable Diseases, United States, 1994 (1995) *MMWR: Morbidity and Mortality Weekly Report*, Vol. 43, No. 53, (October 1995), pp. (1-74), Retrieved from: <http://www.cdc.gov/mmwr>

Summary of Notifiable Diseases, United States, 1993 (1994) *MMWR: Morbidity and Mortality Weekly Report*, Vol. 42, No. 53, (October 1994), pp. (1-73), Retrieved from: <http://www.cdc.gov/mmwr>

Talbot, G.H., et al. (2006). Bad Bugs Need Drugs: An Update on the Development Pipeline from the Antimicrobial Availability Task Force of the Infectious Diseases Society of America (Vol 42, Pg 657, 2006). *Clinical Infectious Diseases*, Vol. 42, No. 7, (Apr 1), pp. (1065-1065) ISBN 1058-4838

Tanaka, M., et al. (2003). Trends in Pertussis among Infants in the U.S., 1980-1999. *Journal of the American Medical Association*, Vol. 290, No. 22, pp. (2968-2975) ISBN 0098-7484

Todar, K. (2009). *The Microbial World*, University of Wisconsin, Madison, Retrieved from: <http://textbookofbacteriology.net/themicrobialworld/bactresanti.html>

Tortora, G.J. (Ed.) (2003). *Microbiology: an introduction*, Benjamin Cummings, IBSN 0805376143, Menlo Park, Ca.

Wade, N. (2010). Europe's Plagues Came from China, Study Finds, In: *The New York Times*, August 18, 2011, Available From: <http://www.nytimes.com/2010/11/01 /health/01plague.html>

Walsh, T.J., et al. (1999). Liposomal Amphotericin B for Empirical Therapy in Patients with Persistent Fever and Neutropenia. *New England Journal of Medicine*, Vol. 340, No. 10, (Mar 11), pp. (764-771) ISBN 0028-4793

Walsh, T.J., et al. (2002). Voriconazole Compared with Liposomal Amphotericin B for Empirical Antifungal Therapy in Patients with Neutropenia and Persistent Fever. *New England Journal of Medicine*, Vol. 346, No. 4, pp. (225-234) ISBN 0028-4793

Walsh, T.J., et al. (2004). Caspofungin vs. Liposomal Amphotericin B for Empirical Antifungal Therapy in Patients with Persistent Fever and Neutropenia. *New England Journal of Medicine*, Vol. 351, No. 14, pp. (1391-1402) ISBN 0028-4793

Walsh, T.R. (2008). Clinically Significant Carbapenemases: An Update. *Current Opinion in Infectious Diseases*, Vol. 21, No. 4, (Aug), pp. (367-371) ISBN 0951-7375

Walsh, T.R., et al. (2010). Emergence of a New Antibiotic Resistance Mechanism in India, Pakistan, and the UK: A Molecular, Biological, and Epidemiological Study. *Lancet Infectious Diseases*, Vol. 10, No. 9, (Sep), pp. (597-602) ISBN 1473-3099

Wiener, J., et al. (1999). Multiple Antibiotic-Resistant *Klebsiella* and *E. Coli* in Nursing Homes. *Journal of the American Medical Association*, Vol. 281, No. 6, (Feb 10), pp. (517-523) ISBN 0098-7484

Williams, B. (1997). *Infectious Diseases in History: a guide to causes and effects*. In: urbanrim.org. uk August 12, 2011, Available from: <http://urbanrim.org.uk/diseases.htm# Plague>

Wisplinghoff, H., et al. (2004). Nosocomial Bloodstream Infections in US Hospitals: Analysis of 24,179 Cases from a Prospective Nationwide Surveillance Study. *Clinical Infectious Diseases*, Vol. 39, No. 7, (Oct 1), pp. (1093-1093) ISBN 1058-4838

Yan, K., et al. (2006). Biochemical Characterization of the Interactions of the Novel Pleuromutilin Derivative Retapamulin with Bacterial Ribosomes. *Antimicrobial Agents and Chemotherapy*, Vol. 50, No. 11, (Nov), pp. (3875-3881) ISBN 0066-4804

Zilberberg, M.D., et al. (2008). Increase in *C. difficile*-Related Hospitalizations among Infants in the US, 2000-2005. *Pediatric Infectious Disease Journal*, Vol. 27, No. 12, (Dec), pp. (1111-1113) ISBN 0891-3668

14

Antibacterial Agents in Dental Treatments

Saeed Rahimi[1], Amin Salem Milani[1], Negin Ghasemi[2,*] and Shahriar Shahi[1]
[1]Dental and Periodontal Research Center,
Faculty of Dentistry, Tabriz University of Medical Sciences,Tabriz,
[2]Department of Endodontics,
Faculty of Dentistry, Tabriz University of Medical Sciences,Tabriz,
Iran

1. Introduction

Because progressive increase in serious transmissible diseases over the last few decades, every health care specialty that involves contact with mucosa, blood or blood contamination, like dentistry, should regulate regarding sterilization and disinfection. Dental patients and dental health-care workers may be exposed to a variety of microorganisms via blood or oral or respiratory secretions. These microorganisms may include cytomegalovirus, *hepatitis B virus (HBV), hepatitis C virus (HCV), herpes simplex virus types 1* and 2, *human immunodeficiency virus (HIV), Mycobacterium tuberculosis, staphylococci, streptococci,* and other viruses and bacteria; specifically, those that infect the upper respiratory tract (Blently, 1994). Infections may be transmitted in the dental operatory through several routes, including direct contact with blood, oral fluids or other secretions; indirect contact with contaminated instruments, operatory equipment or environmental surfaces or contact with airborne contaminants present in either droplet spatter or aerosols of oral and respiratory fluids. Infection via any of these routes requires that all three of the following conditions be present (commonly referred to as "the chain of infection": a susceptible host; a pathogen with sufficient infectivity, numbers to cause infection and a portal through which the pathogen may enter the host) (Burkhart, 1970). Effective infection-control strategies are intended to break one or more of these "links" in the chain, thereby preventing infection. A set of infection-control strategies common to all health-care delivery settings should reduce the risk of transmission of infectious diseases caused by blood-borne pathogens such as *HBV* and *HIV*. Because all infected patients cannot be identified by medical history, physical examination, or laboratory tests, it is recommended that blood and body fluid precautions be used consistently for all patients. In dentistry, beside personal protections like eyewear, gloves and gowns, pretreatment mouth rinse, rubber dam and high velocity air evacuation are the other considerations regarding infection control (Hackney, 1989). Suitable sterilization and disinfection of instruments are inseparable parts of infection control puzzle. So, discussion about the techniques and agents used in sterilization and disinfection is very important, nowadays. In this chapter we mention the antibacterial agents used in sterilization and disinfection in dentistry.

* Corresponding Author

2. Antibacterial agents used in sterilization and disinfection

There are several methods and materials for disinfection. In this chapter, we will discuss the most common antibacterial agents that are used in sterilization and disinfection in dentistry. Disinfectants are substances that are applied to non-living objects to destroy microorganisms that are living on the objects. There are several criteria for Classification of chemical disinfectants that mentioned below (Favero&Bond, 1991):

1. Based on consistency
   a. Liquid (E.g., Alcohols, Phenols)
   b. Gaseous (Formaldehyde vapor, Ethylene oxide)
2. Based on spectrum of activity

Regarding spectrum activity disinfectants have three levels (Table 1).

	Vegetative cells	Mycobacteria	Spores	fungi	viruses	example
High level	+	+	+	+	+	Ethylene Oxide, Glutaraldehyde, Formaldehyde
Intermediate level	+	+	-	+	+	Phenolics, halogens
Low level	+	-	-	+	+/-	Alcohols, quaternary ammonium compounds

Table 1. levels of disinfectants spectrum activity

3. Based on mechanism of action
   a. Action on membrane (E.g., Alcohol, detergent)
   b. Denaturation of cellular proteins (E.g., Alcohol, Phenol)
   c. Oxidation of essential sulphydryl groups of enzymes (E.g., H_2O_2, Halogens)
   d. Alkylation of amino-, carboxyl- and hydroxyl group (E.g., Ethylene Oxide, Formaldehyde)
   e. Damage to nucleic acids (Ethylene Oxide, Formaldehyde)

An ideal disinfectant should have following properties (Crawford, 1983):

1. Should have wide spectrum of activity
2. Should be able to destroy microbes within practical period of time
3. Should be active in the presence of organic matter
4. Should make effective contact and be wettable
5. Should be active in any pH
6. Should be stable
7. Should have long shelf life
8. Should be speedy
9. Should have high penetrating power
10. Should be non-toxic, non-allergenic, non-irritative or non-corrosive
11. Should not have bad odor
12. Should not leave non-volatile residue or stain
13. Efficacy should not be lost on reasonable dilution
14. Should not be expensive and must be available easily

It should be mentioned that the efficacy of disinfectant depends on contact time, temperature, type and concentration of the active ingredient, the presence of organic matter, the type and quantum of microbial load.

2.1 Alcohols

The action mechanisms of this subgroup of disinfectant are coagulation of protein, dehydration of cells and disruption of membranes (Moorer, 2003). Alcohols, usually ethanol or isopropanol, are sometimes used as a disinfectant, but more often as an antiseptic. A 70% aqueous solution is more effective at killing microbes than absolute alcohols. Because water facilitates diffusion through the cell membrane; 100% alcohol typically denatures only external membrane proteins. A mixture of 70% ethanol or isopropanol diluted in water is effective against a wide spectrum of bacteria, though higher concentrations are often needed to disinfect wet surfaces (Brent, 2009). Additionally, high-concentration mixtures (such as 80% ethanol + 5% isopropanol) are required to effectively inactivate lipid-enveloped viruses (such as *HIV, hepatitis B, and hepatitis* C). 70% ethyl alcohol is used as antiseptic on skin. Isopropyl alcohol is preferred to ethanol. It can also be used to disinfect surfaces. It is used to disinfect clinical thermometers. Methyl alcohol kills fungal spores, hence is useful in disinfecting inoculation hoods (Engelenburg, 2002). Alcohols have some disadvantages. They can be a fire hazard. Also, they have limited residual activity due to evaporation, which results in brief contact times unless the surface is submerged, and have a limited activity in the presence of organic material. They are skin irritants and inflammable (Lodgsdon, 1994).

2.2 Aldehydes

The other subgroup of disinfectants is aldehydes that act through alkylation of amino, carboxyl-or hydroxyl group, and probably damage nucleic acids. They have a wide microbiocidal activity and are sporocidal and fungicidal (Crawford, 1983). The most popular of this subgroup are formaldehyde and gluteraldehyde. 40% formaldehyde (formalin) is used for surface disinfection. 10% formalin with 0.5% tetraborate sterilizes clean metal instruments. 2% gluteraldehyde is used to sterilize thermometers, cystoscopes, bronchoscopes, centrifuges, anasethetic equipments etc. An exposure of at least 3 hours at alkaline pH is required for action by gluteraldehyde. 2% formaldehyde at 40°C for 20 minutes is used to disinfect wool and 0.25% at 60°C for six hours to disinfect animal hair and bristles (Favero&Bond, 1991). Disadvantages of these agents are: Vapors are irritating and must be neutralized by ammonia, have poor penetration, leave non-volatile residue, activity is reduced in the presence of protein. Some bacteria have developed resistance to glutaraldehyde, and it has been found that glutaraldehyde can cause asthma and other health hazards; hence ortho-phthalaldehyde is replacing glutaraldehyde (Crawford, 1983).

2.3 Halogens

Halogens for example Chlorine compounds (chlorine, bleach, hypochlorite) and iodine compounds (tincture iodine,iodophores) are oxidizing agents and cause damage by oxidation of essential sulfydryl groups of enzymes. Chlorine reacts with water to form hypochlorous acid, which is microbicidal. Applications of this group are: Tincture of iodine (2% iodine in 70% alcohol) is an antiseptic (Crawford, 1983). Iodine can be combined with neutralcarrier polymers such as polyvinylpyrrolidone to prepare iodophores such as povidone-iodine. Iodophores permit slow release and reduce the irritation of the antiseptic. For hand washing iodophores are diluted in 50% alcohol. 10% Povidone Iodine is used undiluted in pre and postoperative skin disinfection. 0.5% sodium hypochlorite is used in serology and virology. Used at a dilution of 1:10 in decontamination of spillage of infectious material. Mercuric chloride is used as a disinfectant. This group has some disadvantages like: They are rapidly inactivated in the presence of organic matter. Iodine is corrosive and staining. Bleach solution is corrosive and will corrode stainless steel surfaces (Sattar, 1998).

2.4 Hydrogen peroxide

It acts on the microorganisms through its release of nascent oxygen. Hydrogen peroxide produces hydroxyl-free radical that damages proteins and DNA. Hydrogen peroxide is used in hospitals to disinfect surfaces and it is used in solution alone or in combination with other chemicals as a high level disinfectant (Favero&Bond, 1991). It is used at 6% concentration to decontaminate the instruments, equipments such as ventilators. 3%Hydrogen Peroxide Solution is used for skin disinfection. Strong solutions are sporicidal (Sattar, 1998). 1.5-2 % Hydrogen peroxide is used as mouthwashes (Hasturk et al., 2004). It is sometimes mixed with colloidal silver. It is often preferred because it causes far fewer allergic reactions than alternative disinfectants. Decomposition in light, breaking down by catalase and reduction of activity by organic matter is their disadvantages (Favero&Bond, 1991).

2.5 Ethylene oxide

It is an alkylating agent. It acts by alkylating sulfydryl, amino, carboxyl and hydroxyl-groups. It is a highly effective chemisterilant, capable of killing spores rapidly. It is the best method for sterilization of complex instruments, delicate materials, and heat labile articles such as bedding, textiles, rubber, plastics, syringes, disposable petri dishes, heart-lung machine, respiratory and dental equipments (Crawford, 1983). Porous and plastic materials absorb the gas and require aeration for 2 hours, before it is safe to contact skin and tissues. It has a sweet odor, readily polymerizes and is flammable. Since it is highly flammable, it is usually combines with CO2 (10% CO2+ 90% EO) or dichlorodifluoromethane. It requires presence of humidity. But, it is highly toxic, irritating to eyes and skin, highly flammable, mutagenic and carcinogenic.

2.6 Phenol

Phenolic materials for example 5% phenol, 1-5% Cresol, 5% Lysol (a saponified cresol), hexachlorophene or chlorhexidine act by disruption of membranes, precipitation of proteins and inactivation of enzymes. They act as disinfectants at high concentration and as antiseptics at low concentrations (Weber et al., 1999).They are bactericidal, fungicidal, mycobactericidal but are inactive against spores and most viruses. They are not readily inactivated by organic matter. Chlorhexidine can be used in an isopropanol solution for skin disinfection, or as an aqueous solution for wound irrigation. It is often used as an antiseptic hand wash. 20% Chlorhexidine gluconate solution is used for pre-operative hand and skin preparation and for general skin disinfection (Favero&Bond, 1991). 0.12 -0.2 % Chlorhexidine are used as mouthwash. It is also used as root canal irrigant which will be discussed later in this chapter. Chlorhexidine gluconate is also mixed with quaternary ammonium compounds such as cetrimide to get stronger and broader antimicrobial effects (eg. Savlon). Chloroxylenols are less irritative and can be used for topical purposes and are more effective against gram positive bacteria than gram negative bacteria. Hexachlorophene is chlorinated diphenyl and is much less irritative. It has marked effect over gram positive bacteria but poor effect over gram negative bacteria, *mycobacteria,* fungi and viruses. Triclosan is organic phenyl ether with good activity against gram positive bacteria and is effective to some extent against many gram negative bacteria including Pseudomonas. It also has fair activity on fungi and viruses. But it is toxic, corrosive and skin irritant. Chlorhexidine is inactivated by anionic soaps. Chloroxylenol is inactivated by hard water (Crawford, 1983).

2.7 Quaternary ammonium compounds

They are one of the surface active agents and have the property of concentrating at interfaces between lipid containing membranes of bacterial cell and surrounding aqueous medium (Weber et al., 1999). The mechanism of their action is disruption of membrane resulting in leakage of cell constituents. Surface active agents are soaps or detergents. Detergents can be anionic or cationic. Anionics contain negatively charged long chain hydrocarbon .These include soaps and bile salts. If the fat-soluble part is made to have a positive charge by combining with a quaternary nitrogen atom, it is called cationic detergents. Cationic detergents are known as quaternary ammonium compounds (or quat). Typically, quats do not exhibit efficacy against difficult to kill non-enveloped viruses such as norovirus, rotavirus, or polio virus. Newer low-alcohol formulations are highly effective broad-spectrum disinfectants with quick contact times (3–5 minutes) against bacteria, enveloped viruses, pathogenic fungi, and *mycobacteria*. However, the addition of alcohol or solvents to quat-based disinfectant formulas results in the products' drying much more quickly on the applied surface, which could lead to ineffective or incomplete disinfection. Quats are biocides that also kill algae and are used as an additive in large-scale industrial water systems to minimize undesired biological growth. Cetrimide and benzalkonium chloride act as cationic detergents. They are active against vegetative cells, *mycobacteria* and enveloped viruses. They are widely used as disinfectants at dilution of 1-2% for domestic use and in hospitals. This subgroup of disinfectants has several disadvantages as follow: Their activity is reduced by hard water, anionic detergents and organic matter. Pseudomonas can metabolize cetrimide, using them as a carbon, nitrogen and energy source (Favero&Bond, 1991).

3. Antibacterial agents used in dental treatments

Microorganisms are the main cause of pulpal and priapical diaeases. The primary endodontic treatment goal is root canal disinfection and prevention of re-infection of root canal system (Basmadjı-Charles et al., 2002; Shahı et al., 2007; Zand et al.,2010). Besides of aseptic principles like rubber dam placement and correct mechanical instrumentation, root canal irrigants are the important aspect to eradication of microbes from root canals. To increase efficacy of mechanical preparation and bacterial removal, instrumentation must be supplemented with active irrigating solutions. Irrigation is defined as washing out a body cavity or wound with water or medical fluid. The objective of irrigation is both mechanical and biologic. The biologic function is related to their antimicrobial effect and mechanical one is due to flushing out effect (Cheung&Stock, 1993). The ideal irrigant should be germicide and fungicide, nonirritating to tissues, stable in solution, have prolonged antimicrobial effect, not interfere with tissue repair, relatively inexpensive, and non-toxic (Tay et al., 2006). There are several irrigants used in endodontic. In this chapter, we discuss about the properties of routine irrigants used in endodontic field.

3.1 Sodium hypochlorite

Hypochlorite solutions were first used as bleaching agents. Based on the controlled laboratory studies by Koch and Pasteur, hypochlorite then gained wide acceptance as a disinfectant by the end of the 19th century. In World War I, the chemist Henry Drysdale Dakin and the surgeon Alexis Carrel extended the use of a buffered 0.5% sodium hypochlorite solution to the irrigation of infected wounds, based on Dakin meticulous studies on the efficacy of different solutions on infected necrotic tissue (Dakin, 1915). Besides their wide-spectrum, nonspecific killing efficacy on all microbes, hypochlorite preparations are sporocidal, virucidal , and show far greater tissue dissolving effect on necrotic than on vital tissues (Austin & Taylor, 1918) . These features prompted the use of aqueous sodium hypochlorite in endodontics as the main irrigant as early as 1920 (Grossman, 1943). In the endodontic field, NaOCl possesses a broad spectrum antimicrobial activity against microorganisms and biofilms difficult to eradicate from root canals such as Enterococcus, Actinomyces and Candida organisms. Furthermore, sodium hypochlorite solutions are cheap, easily available, and demonstrate good shelf life (Heling et al., 2001; Mahmudpour et al., 2007). Other chlorine-releasing compounds have been advocated in endodontics, such as chloramine-T and sodium dichloroisocyanurate. These, however, never gained wide acceptance in endodontics, and appear to be less effective than hypochlorite at comparable concentration (Dychdala, 1991).There has been controversy over the most suitable concentration of hypochlorite solutions to be used in endodontics. As Dakin original 0.5% sodium hypochlorite solution was designed to treat open wounds, it was surmised that in the confined area of a root canal system, higher concentrations should be used, as they would be more efficient than Dakin solution (Grossman, 1917). The antibacterial effectiveness and tissue-dissolution capacity of aqueous hypochlorite is a function of its concentration, but so is its toxicity (Spyngbergl et al., 1973). However, severe irritations have been reported when 5.25% concentrated solutions were inadvertently forced into the periapical tissues during irrigation or leaked through the rubber dam (Hismann& Hahn, 2000). Furthermore, a 5.25% solution significantly decreases the elastic modulus and flexural strength of human dentin compared to physiologic saline, while a 0.5% solution does not (Sima et al., 2001). This is most likely because of the proteolytic action of concentrated hypochlorite on the collagen matrix of dentin. The reduction of intracanal microbiota, on the other hand, is not any greater when 5% sodium hypochlorite is used as an irrigant as compared to 0.5% (Bystrm&Sundqvist, 1985). From in vitro observations, it would appear that a 1% NaOCl solution should suffice to dissolve the entire pulp tissue in the course of an endodontic treatment session (Sirtes et al., 2005). Hence, based on the currently available evidence, there is no rationale for using hypochlorite solutions at concentrations over 1% wt/vol. This concentration of NaOCl is also used for disinfection of Gutta-percha cones. Reactive chlorine in aqueous solution at body temperature can, in essence, take two forms: hypochlorite (OCL) in pH above 7.6 or hypochlorous acid (HOCl) in pH below 7.6. Both forms are extremely reactive oxidizing agents. Pure hypochlorite solutions as they are used in endodontics have a pH of 12 , and thus the entire available chlorine is in the form of OCl^-. However, at identical levels of available chlorine, hypochlorous acid is more bactericidal than hypochlorite (Zehnder et al., 2002). One way to increase the efficacy of hypochlorite solutions could thus be to lower the pH. It has also been surmised that such solutions would be less toxic to vital tissues than non-buffered counterparts (Kamburis et al., 2003). However, buffering hypochlorite with bicarbonate renders the solution unstable with a decrease in shelf life to less than 1 week. Depending on the amount of the bicarbonate in the mixture and therefore the pH value, the antimicrobial efficacy of a fresh bicarbonate-buffered solution is only slightly higher or not elevated at all compared to that of a non-buffered counterpart (Costigan, 1936). Another approach to improve the effectiveness of hypochlorite irrigants in the root canal system could be to increase the temperature of low-concentration NaOCl solutions. This improves their immediate tissue-dissolution capacity (Abou-Rass &Oglesby, 1981). Furthermore, heated hypochlorite solutions remove organic debris from dentin shavings more efficiently than unheated counterparts (Cunningham&Balekjian, 1980).

3.2 Chlorhexidine

Chlorhexidine is a strong base and is most stable in the form of its salts. The original salts were chlorhexidine acetate and hydrochloride, both of which are relatively poorly soluble in water (Foulkes, 1973). Hence, they have been replaced by chlorhexidine digluconate. It has a cationic molecular component that attaches to negatively charged cell membrane area and causes cell lysis. Chlorhexidine is a potent antiseptic, which is used as a mouth rinse and endodontic irrigant. The later application is based on its substantivity and long-lasting antimicrobial effect which arise from binding to hydroxyapatite. Aqueous solutions of 0.1 to 0.2% concentrations are recommended for that purpose, while 2% is the concentration of root canal irrigating solutions usually found in the endodontic literature (Zamany et al., 2003). It is commonly held that chlorhexidine would be less caustic than sodium hypochlorite (Spngberg et al., 1973). A 2% chlorhexidine solution is irritating to the skin (Foulkes, 1973). As with sodium hypochlorite, heating chlorhexidine of lesser concentration could increase its local efficacy in the root canal system while keeping the systemic toxicity low (Evanov et al., 2004). Despite its usefulness as a final irrigant, chlorhexidine cannot be advocated as the main irrigant in standard endodontic cases, because: (a) chlorhexidine is unable to dissolve necrotic tissue remnants (Naenni et al., 2004), and (b) chlorhexidine is less effective on Gram-negative than on Gram-positive bacteria (Hennessey,1973). In a randomized clinical trial on the reduction of intracanal microbiota by either 2.5% NaOCl or 0.2% chlorhexidine irrigation, it was found that hypochlorite was significantly more efficient than chlorhexidine in obtaining negative cultures (Ringel, 1982). Most important CHX disadvantage is its inability of to dissolve necrotic tissue remnants and chemically clean the canal system.

3.3 Iodine potassium iodine

Iodine potassium iodine is a traditional root canal disinfectant with wide-spectrum antimicrobial activity. It is used in concentrations ranging from 2% to 5%).The oxidizing agent of this substance, iodine, reacts with free sulfhydryl groups of bacterial enzymes cleaving the disulfide bonds. It was manifested that calcium hydroxide-resistant microorganisms could be eradicated with combination of IKI and CHX (Baker et al., 2004). It shows relatively low toxicity in experiments using tissue cultures. An obvious disadvantage of iodine is a possible allergic reaction in some patients (Siren et al., 2004).

3.4 MTAD (Mixture of Tetracyclin, Acid, Detergent)

Biopure MTAD was recently introduced in the market as an antibacterial root canal cleanser .MTAD is a mixture of 3% tetracycline isomer (doxycycline), and 4.25% acid (citric acid), and 0.5% detergent (Tween 80). This biocompatible intracanal irrigant is commercially available as a two-part mix (Torabinejad et al., 2005). One of the characteristic of this solution is a high binding affinity of the doxycycline to dentin (Beltz et al., 2003).In this irrigant, doxycycline hyclate is used instead of its free base, doxycycline monohydrate, to increase the water solubility of this broad-spectrum antibiotic. MTAD has been reported to be effective in removing the smear layer due to citric acid action (Torabinejad et al., 2003), eliminating microbes that are resistant to conventional endodontic irrigants and medications (Shabahang& Torabinejad, 2003) and providing sustained antimicrobial activity. With every new product we are always concerned about the cytotoxicity to the underlying tissue. MTAD was compared with commonly used irrigants and medications The results showed MTAD to be less cytotoxic than eugenol, 3 percent H2O2, $Ca(OH)_2$ paste, 5.25 percent NaOCl, Peridex, and EDTA. It is more cytotoxic than NaOCl at 2.63 percent, 1.31 percent, and 0.66 percent concentrations (Zaung et al., 2003).

3.5 Calcium hydroxide

Residual bacteria in the root canal have been held responsible for failures (Sjugren et al., 1990). It is generally believed that the number of remaining bacteria can be controlled by placing an interappointment medication within the prepared canal (Chong&Pitt Ford, 1992; Rahimi et al.,2010). Calcium hydroxide,$Ca(OH)_2$ is the most common interappointment medication used which requires disinfection period of 7 days (Sjugren et al., 1991). However, some microbes such as *Enterococcus faecalis* (George et al., 2005) and *Candida albicans* (Waltimo et al., 1999) are resistant to it. Therefore, alternative intracanal medications have been sought to improve the eradication of bacteria before obturation. Chlorhexidine gluconate is effective against strains resistant to calcium hydroxide (Delany et al., 1989). Recent studies have suggested that CHX could be used in combination with calcium hydroxide to improve antimicrobial efficacy against calcium hydroxide-resistant microbes (Almyroudi et al., 2002). The high pH of calcium hydroxide formulations (pH=12.5) alters the biologic properties of bacterial lipopolysaccharides in the cell walls of gram-negative species and inactivates membrane transport mechanisms, resulting in bacterial cell toxicity (Siqueira & Lopes, 1999). However, as stated above, *E. faecalis* has been reported to be resistant to this effect as a result of its ability to penetrate the dentinal tubules and adapt to changing environment (George et al., 2005).

3.6 Laser irradiation and photodynamic therapy

Novel approaches to disinfecting root canals have been proposed recently that include the use of high-power lasers (Walsh, 2003) as well as photodynamic therapy (PDT) (Hamblin& Hasan, 2004). High-power lasers function by dose-dependent heat generation, but, in addition to killing bacteria, they have the potential to cause collateral damage such as char dentine, ankylosis roots, cementum melting, and root resorption and periradicular necrosis if incorrect laser parameters are used . Since the introduction of the laser in endodontics in 1971, several lasers were used to eliminating bacteria from root canals. The erbium, chromium: yttrium-scandium-gallium-garnet (Er,Cr:YSGG) laser has highest absorption in water and high affinity to hydroxyapatite, which makes it suitable for use in root canal therapy(Yamazaki et al., 2001; Yavari et al.,2010). Lasers have the ability to clean and effectively disinfect root canals; including eliminating highly resistant species such as *Enterococcus faecalis* (Le Goff et al., 1999). PDT (photodynamic therapy) is a new antimicrobial strategy that involves the combination of a nontoxic photosensitizer and a light source (Demidova&Hamblin., 2004). The excited photosensitizer reacts with molecular oxygen to produce highly reactive oxygen species, which induce injury and death of microorganisms (Wainwright, 1998). It has been established that PS, which possess a pronounced cationic charge, can rapidly bind and penetrate bacterial cells, and, therefore, these compounds show a high degree of selectivity for killing microorganisms compared with host mammalian cells (Maisch et al., 2005). PDT has been studied as a promising approach to eradicate oral pathogenic bacteria (Wilson, 2004) that cause diseases such as periodontitis, peri-implantitis and caries (Walsh, 2003). When PDT followed conventional endodontic therapy, there was significantly more killing and less bacterial growth than was seen after endodontic therapy alone (Garcez et al., 2007).

4. References

Abou-Rass, M. & Oglesby, SW. (1981). The effects of temperature, concentration, and tissue type on the solvent ability of sodium hypochlorite. *J Endod*,Vol.7, pp.376-377,ISSN1887-3554.

Almyroudi, A.; Mackenzie, D. McHugh, S. & Saunders, WP. (2002). .The effectiveness of various disinfectants used as endodontic intracanal medications: an in vitro study. *J Endod*,Vol.28,pp.163-167,ISSN1878-3554.

Austin, JH. & Taylor, HD. (2002). Behavior of hypochlorite and of chloramine-T solutions in contact with necrotic and normal tissue in vivo. *J Exp Med*,No. 27,pp.627-633,ISSN0022-1007.

Baker, N.; Liewehr, F. Buxton, T. & Joyce, A. (2004). Antibacterial efficacy of calcium hydroxide, iodine potassium iodine, betadine and betadine scrub with and without surfactant against E.faecalis in vitro. *Oral Surg Oral Med Oral Pathol*,No.98,pp.359,ISSN1528395X.

Basmadjian-charles, Cl.; Farge, P. & Lebrun, T. (2002). Factors influencing the long-term result of endodontic trearment.*Int Dent J*,Vol.52,pp.81-90,ISSN1309-100X.

Beltz, RE.; Torabinejad, M. & Pouresmail, M. (2003). Quantitative analysis of solubilizing action of MTAD, sodium hypochlorite, and EDTA on bovine pulp and dentin . *J Endod*,Vol.29,pp.334-337,ISSN1878-3554.

Bently, Cd. (1994). Evaluation spatter and aerosol contamination during dental procedure. *J Am Dent Assoc*,Vol.125, pp.579-584,ISSN0002-8177.

Brent, J. (2009). Fomepizole for ethylene glycol and methanol poisoning. *N. Engl. J. Med*,VOL.21,pp.2216-23,ISSN 0028-4793.

Burkhart, NW. & Crawford, JJ. (1997). Critical steps after cleaning: removing debris after sonication. J Am Dent Assoc,Vol.128,pp.456-463,ISSN0002-8177.

Bystrom, A. & Sundqvist, G. (1985) The antibacterial action of sodium hypochlorite and EDTA in 60 cases of endodontic therapy. *Int Endod J, Vol.*18,pp.35-40,ISSN1365-2591.

Cheung, Gs. & stock, CJ. (1993). In vitro cleaning ability of root canal irrigants with and without endosonics. *Int Endod J*,Vol.26,pp.334,ISSN1365-2491.

Chong, BS. & Pitt Ford, TR. (1992). The role of intracanal medication in root canal treatment . *Int Endod J*,Vol.25,pp.97-106,ISSN1365-2491.

Costigan, SM. (1993). Effectiveness of hot hypochlorites of low alkalinity in destroying Mycobacterium tuberculosis. *J Bacteriol*,Vol.32,pp.57-63,ISSN1098-5530.

Crawford, JJ. (1983). Sterilization,disinfection and asepsis in dentistry.In block ss, editor:disinfection,sterilization and preservation. Philadelphia, lea & febiger.

Cunningham, WT. & Balekjian, AY. (1980). Effect of temperature on collagen-dissolving ability of sodium hypochlorite endodontic irrigant . *Oral Surg Oral Med Oral Pathol*, VOL.49,pp.175-177,ISSN1528395X.

Dakin, HD. (1915). On the use of certain antiseptic substances in treatment of infected wounds . *BMJ*,No.2,pp.318-320,ISSN0959-8138.

Delany, GM.; Patterson, SS. Miller, CH. & Newton, CW. (1982). The effect of chlorhexidine gluconate irrigation on the root canal flora of freshly extracted necrotic teeth. *Oral Surg Oral Med Oral Pathol Oral Radiol Endod*,Vol.5,pp.518-523,ISSN1528395X.

Demidova, TN. & Hamblin, MR. (2004). Photodynamic therapy targeted to pathogens. *Int J Immunopathol Pharmacol*,Vol.17,pp.245–254.

Dychdala, GR. (1991). Chlorine and chlorine compounds . In: Block SS editors. Disinfection, sterilization and preservation . Philadelphia: Lea & Febiger.

Engelenburg, FA.; Terpstra, FG. Schuitemaker, H. & Moorer, WR. (2002). The virucidal spectrum of a high concentration alcohol mixture". *The Journal of Hospital Infection*,Vol.51,pp.121–5.

Evanov, C.; Liewehr, F. Buxton, TB. & Joyce, AP. (2004). Antibacterial efficacy of calcium hydroxide and chlorhexidine gluconate irrigants at 37 degrees C and 46 degrees C. *J Endod*,Vol.30,pp.653-657,ISSN1878-3554.

Favero, Ms. & Bond, Ww. (1991). Chemical disinfection in medical materials. In block ss, editor:disinfection,sterilization and preservation. Philadelphia, lea & febiger.

Foulkes, DM. (1973). Some toxicological observations on chlorhexidine . *J Periodontal Res Suppl*,Vol.12,pp.55-60,ISSN1600-0765.

Garcez, AS.; Ribeiro, MS. Tegos, GP. Nuñez, SC. Jorge, AOC. & Hamblin, MR. (2007). Antimicrobial photodynamic therapy combined with conventional endodontic treatment to eliminate root canal biofilm infection. *Lasers Surg Med*,Vol.39,pp.59–66.

George, S.; Kishen, A. & Song, KP. (2005). The role of environmental changes on monospecies biofilm formation on root canal wall by *Enterococcus faecalis*. *J Endod*,Vol.31,pp.867-872,ISSN1878-3554.

Grossman, LI. (1943). Irrigation of root canals. *J Am Dent Assoc*,Vol.30,pp.1915-1917,ISSN0002-8177.

Hackney, RW. (1989). Using a biological indicator to detect potential sources of cross-contamination in the dental operatory. *J Am Dent Assoc*,Vol.129, pp.828-833,ISSN0002-8177.

Halsmann, M. & Hahn, W. (2000). Complications during root canal irrigation , a literature review and case reports . *Int Endod J*,Vol.33,pp.186-193,ISSN1365-2591.

Hamblin, MR. & Hasan,T. (2004). Photodynamic therapy: a new antimicrobial approach to infectious disease?. *Photochem Photobiol Sci*,Vol.3,pp.436–450.

Hasturk, H.; Nunn, M. Warbington, M. & Vandyke, TE. (2004). Efficacy of a fluoridated hydrogen peroxide-based mouthrinse for the treatment of gingivitis: a randomized clinical trial. *J Periodontol*,Vol.75,pp.57-65,ISSN1943-3670.

Heling, I.; Rotstein, I. Dinur, T. Szwec-Levine, Y. & Steinberg, D. (2001). Bactericidal and cytotoxic effects of sodium hypochlorite and sodium dichloroisocyanurate solutions in vitro. *J Endod*,Vol.27,pp.278-280,ISSN1878-3554.

Hennessey, TS. (1973). Some antibacterial properties of chlorhexidine . *J Periodontal Res Suppl*,Vol.12,pp.61-67,ISSN1600-0765.

Kamburis, JJ.; Barker, TH. Barfield, RD. & Eleazer, PD. (2003). Removal of organic debris from bovine dentin shavings . *J Endod*,Vol 29,pp.559-561,ISSN1878-3554.

Le Goff, A.; Morazin-Dautel, A. & Guigand, M. (1999). An evaluation of co2 laser for endodontic disinfection.*J Endod*,Vol.25,pp.105-8,ISSN1878-3554.

Lodgsdon, J.E. (1994). "Ethanol". In Kroschwitz J.I. *Encyclopedia of Chemical Technology*. 9 (4th ed). New York: John Wiley & Sons. p. 820. ISBN0-471-52677-0.

Mahmoudpour, A.; Rahimi, S. Mahmood, S. Soroush MH. Shahi, Sh.&Asl-Aminabadi, N.(2007). Isolation and identification of *Enterococcus faecalis* from necrotic root canals using multiplex PCR. *Journal of Oral Science*, Vol. 49,PP.221-227

Maisch, T.; Bosl, C. Szeimies, RM. Lehn, N. & Abels, C. (2005). Photodynamic effects of novel XF porphyrin derivatives on prokaryotic and eukaryotic cells. *Antimicrob Agents Chemother*,Vol.49,pp.1542–1552.

Moorer, WR. (2003). Antiviral activity of alcohol for surface disinfection. *International Journal of Dental Hygiene*,Vol. 1,pp. 138–42.

Naenni, N.; Thoma, K. & Zehnder, M. (2004). Soft tissue dissolution capacity of currently used and potential endodontic irrigants . *J Endod*,Vol.30,pp.785-,ISSN1878-3554.

Rahimi, S.; Shahi, Sh.Kimyai, S.Khayyam, S.&Abdolrahimi, M.(2010). Effect of calcium hydroxide dressing on microleakage of composite restorations in endodontically treated teeth subsequent to bleaching. *Med Oral Patol Oral Cir Bucal*, Vol.15,pp.413-416.

Ringel, AM.; Patterson, SS. Newton, CW. Miller ,CH. & Mulhern, JM. (1982). In vivo evaluation of chlorhexidine gluconate solution and sodium hypochlorite solution as root canal irrigants . *J Endod*,Vol.8,pp.200-204,ISSN1878-3554.

Shahi, Sh.; Rahimi, S. Yavari, HR. Shakouie, S. Nezafati, S.&Abdolrahimi, M.(2007). Sealing Ability of White and Gray Mineral Trioxide Aggregate Mixed with Distilled Water and 0.12% Chlorhexidine Gluconate When Used as Root-end Filling Materials.*JEndod*,Vol.33,pp.1429-1432, ISSN1878-3554.

Sattar, A. (1998). "A product based on accelerated hydrogen peroxide: Evidence for broad-spectrum activity". *Canadian Journal of Infection Control*,pp.123–130.

Shabahang, S.; Torabinejad, M. (2003). Effect of MTAD on Enterococcus faecalis-contaminated root canals of extracted human teeth. *J Endod*,Vol.29,pp.576-579, ISSN1878-3554.

Siqueira, JF. & Lopes HP. (1999). Mechanisms of antimicrobial activity of calcium hydroxide: critical review. *Int Endod J*,Vol.2,pp.361-369.ISSN 1365-2491.

Sim, TP.; Knowles, JC. Shelton, J. & Gulabivala, K. (2001). Effect of sodium hypochlorite on mechanical properties of dentine and tooth surface strain. *Int Endod J*,Vol.34,pp.120-132,ISSN1365-2591.

Siren, E.;Haapasalo, M. Waltimo, TM. & Qrstavik, D. (2004).In vitro antibacterial effect of calcium hidroxide combind with chlorohexidine or iodide potassium iodine on enterococcus faecalis *Eur J Oral Sci*,Vol.112 ,pp.326-30.ISSN1880-4926.

Sirtes, G.; Waltimo, T. Schaetzle, M. & Zehnder, M. (2005). The effects of temperature on sodium hypochlorite short-term stability, pulp dissolution capacity, and antimicrobial efficacy. *J Endod*,Vol.31,pp.669-671,ISSN1878-3554.

Sjugren, U.; Hogglund, B. Sundqvist, G.& Wing, K. (1990). Factors affecting the long-term results of endodontic treatment. *J Endod*,Vol.16,pp.498-504,ISSN1878-3554.

Sjugren, U.; Figdor, D. Spongberg, L. & Sunquist G. (1991). The antimicrobial effect of calcium hydroxide as a short-term intracranial dressing. *Int Endod,Vol.*24,pp.119-125,ISSN1365-2491

Spyngberg, L.; Engstrm, B.& Langeland, K. (1973). Biologic effects of dental materials. 3. Toxicity and antimicrobial effect of endodontic antiseptics in vitro . *Oral Surg Oral Med Oral Pathol*,Vol.36,pp.856-871,ISSN1528395X.

Tay, Fr.; Pashley, DH. & Loushine, RJ. (2006). Ultrastructure of smear layer-covered intraradicular dentin after irrigation with biopure MTAD. *J Endod*,Vol.32,pp.218-225, ISSN1878-3554.

Torabinejad , M.; Khademi, AA. & Babagoli, J. (2003).A new solution for the removal of the smear layer . *J Endod*,Vol.29,pp.170-175, ISSN1878-3554

Torabinejad, M.; Shabahang, S. & Bahjri K. (2005). Effect of MTAD on postoperative discomfort: a randomized clinical trial. *J Endod*,Vol.31,pp.171-176,ISSN1878-3554.

Wainwright,M. (1998). Photodynamic antimicrobial chemotherapy (PACT). *J Antimicrob Chemother*,Vol.42,pp.13–28.

Walsh, LJ. (2003). The current status of laser applications in dentistry. *Aust Dent J*,Vol.48,pp.146–155,ISSN0045-0421.

Waltimo, T.; rstavik, D. Siren, E. & Haapasalo, M. (1992). In vitro susceptibility of Candida albicans to four disinfectants and their combinations. *Int Endod J*,Vol.32,pp.421-429,ISSN1365-2491.

Weber, DJ.; Barbee, SL. Sobsey, MD. & Rutala WA. (1999). "The effect of blood on the antiviral activity of sodium hypochlorite, a phenolic, and a quaternary ammonium compound". *Infection Control and Hospital Epidemiology*,Vol. 20,pp.821-7.

Wilson, M. (2004). Lethal photosensitisation of oral bacteria and its potential application in the photodynamic therapy of oral infections. *Photochem Photobiol Sci*,Vol.3,pp.412–418.

Yavari, HR.;Rahimi, S. Shahi, Sh. Lotfi, M. Barhaghi, M.&Fatemi, A.(2010). Effect of Er, Cr: YSGG Laser Irradiation on Enterococcus faecalis in Infected Root Canals. *Photomedicine and Laser Surgery*,Vol 23,pp.1-6.

Yamazaki, R.; Goya, C. & Yu, DG. (2001). Effect of Erbium, Chromium:YSGG laser irradiation on root canal walls. *J Endod*,Vol.27,pp. 93-99,ISSN1878-3554.

Zamany, A.; Safavi, K. & Spongberg, LS. (2003). The effect of chlorhexidine as an endodontic disinfectant . *Oral Surg Oral Med Oral Pathol Oral Radiol Endod*,Vol.96,pp.578-581,ISSN1528395X.

Zand, V.;Lotfi, M. Rahimi, S. Mokhtari, H.& Kazemi, A.(2010). A Comparative Scanning Electron Microscopic Investigation of the Smear Layer after the Use of Sodium Hypochlorite Gel and Solution Forms as Root Canal Irrigants.*J Endod*,Vol.36,pp.1234-1237, ISSN1878-3554.

Zehnder, M.; Kosicki, D. Luder, H. Sener, B. & Waltimo, T. (2002). Tissue-dissolving capacity and antibacterial effect of buffered and unbuffered hypochlorite solutions. *Oral Surg Oral Med Oral Pathol Oral Radiol Endod*,Vol.94,pp.756-762,ISSN1528395X.

15

From Synthesis to Antibacterial Activity of Some New Palladium(II) and Platinum(IV) Complexes

Ivana D. Radojević[1], Verica V. Glođović[2], Gordana P. Radić[2], Jelena M. Vujić[3], Olgica D. Stefanović[1], Ljiljana R. Čomić[1] and Srećko R. Trifunović[2]

[1]Department of Biology and Ecology, Faculty of Science, University of Kragujevac, Kragujevac,
[2]Department of Chemistry, Faculty of Science, University of Kragujevac, Kragujevac,
[3]Faculty of Agronomy, University of Kragujevac, Čačak,
Republic of Serbia

1. Introduction

Simultaneously with the rapid development of a wide range of antibacterial agents since the 1940s, bacteria have proved extremely adept at developing resistance to each new employed agent. The rapidly increasing incidence of bacterial resistance to antimicrobial agents has become a serious problem worldwide. Resistance mechanisms have been identified and described for all known antibiotics currently available for clinical use (Fluit et al., 2000).

The synthesis and evaluation of the biological activity of the new metal-based compounds is the field of growing interest. Numerous complexes based on palladium(II) and platina(IV)-ion have been synthesized and their different biological activities have been documented (Agarwal, 2007; Mishra et al., 2007a; Mishra & Kaushik, 2007). The impact of different palladium and platinum complexes on the growth and metabolism of various groups of microorganisms has been studied. Garoufis et al. (2009) reviewed numerous scientific papers on anti-viral, antibacterial and antifungal activity of palladium(II) complexes with different types of ligands (sulfur and nitrogen donor ligands, Schiff base ligands and drugs as ligands). There are other papers in the literature showing different intensity of palladium(II) and platina(IV) complexes activity on various species of bacteria and fungi (Kovala-Demertzi et al., 2001; Brudzinska et al., 2004; Coombs et al., 2005; Guerra et al., 2005; Ali et al., 2006; Manav et al., 2006; Aghatabay et al., 2007; Kizilcikli et al., 2007; Mishra et al., 2007b; Biyala et al., 2008; Al-Hazmi et al., 2008; Vieira et al., 2009).

The aim of this paper is to describe synthesis of some new palladium(II) and platinum(IV) complexes and in vitro research of their antibacterial activities. The second objective is to evaluate the impact these compounds have on probiotic bacteria. Probiotics are used as supplements and they play significant role in protecting and maintaining the balance of intestinal microflora in antibiotic therapy.

2. Experimental

2.1 Chemistry

The palladium(II) and platinum(IV) complexes were obtained by direct reaction of the corresponding starting compounds (K_2PdCl_4 and K_2PtCl_6) and newly synthesized tetradentate or bidentate ligands. The next compounds were synthesized:

- *O,O'*-dipropyl-(*S,S*)-ethylenediamine-*N,N'*-di-2-propanoate (**L1**)
- dichlorido-(*O,O'*-dipropyl-(*S,S*)-ethylenediamine-*N,N'*-di-2-propanoate)-palladium(II) (**C1**)
- *O,O'*-dibutyl-(*S,S*)-ethylenediamine-*N,N'*-di-2-propanoate (**L2**)
- dichlorido-(*O,O'*-dibutyl-(*S,S*)-ethylenediamine-*N,N'*-di-2-propanoate)-palladium(II) (**C2**)
- *O,O'*-dipentyl-(*S,S*)-ethylenediamine-*N,N'*-di-2-propanoate (**L3**)
- dichlorido-(*O,O'*-dipentyl-(*S,S*)-ethylenediamine-*N,N'*-di-2-propanoate)-palladium(II) (**C3**)
- *O,O'*-ethyl-(*S,S*)-ethylenediamine-*N,N'*-di-2-(3-methyl)-butanoate (**L4**)
- chorido((*S,S*)-ethylenediamine-*N*-(*O*-ethyl-2-(3-methyl)-butanoate)-*N'*-2-(3-methyl)-butanoato)-palladium(II) (**C4**)
- tetrachlorido(*O,O'*-diethyl-(*S,S*)-ethylenediamine-*N,N'*-di-2-(3-methyl)butanoate)-platinum(IV) (**C4a**)
- *O,O'*-dipropyl-(*S,S*)-ethylenediamine-*N,N'*-di-2-(3-methyl)-butanoate (**L5**)
- chorido((*S,S*)-ethylenediamine-*N*-(*O*-propyl-2-(3-methyl)-butanoate)-*N'*-2-(3-methyl)-butanoato)-palladium(II) (**C5**)
- *O,O'*-dibutyl-(*S,S*)-ethylenediamine-*N,N'*-di-2-(3-methyl)-butanoate (**L6**)
- chorido((*S,S*)-ethylenediamine-*N*-(*O*-butyl-2-(3-methyl)-butanoate)-*N'*-2-(3-methyl)-butanoato)-palladium(II) (**C6**)
- *O,O'*-dipentyl-(*S,S*)-ethylenediamine-*N,N'*-di-2-(3-methyl)-butanoate(**L7**)
- chorido((*S,S*)-ethylenediamine-*N*-(*O*-pentyl-2-(3-methyl)-butanoate)-*N'*-2-(3-methyl)-butanoato)-palladium(II) (**C7**)
- *O,O'*-diethyl-(*S,S*)-ethylenediamine-*N,N'*-di-2-(4-methyl)-pentanoate (**L8**)
- dichlorido(*O,O'*-diethyl-(*S,S*)-ethylenediamine-*N,N'*-di-2-(4-methyl)-pentanoate)-palladium(II) (**C8**)
- *O,O'*-dipropyl-(*S,S*)-ethylenediamine-*N,N'*-di-2-(4-methyl)-pentanoate (**L9**)
- dichlorido(*O,O'*-dipropyl-(*S,S*)-ethylenediamine-*N,N'*-di-2-(4-methyl)-pentanoate)-palladium(II) (**C9**)
- *O,O'*-dibutyl-(*S,S*)-ethylenediamine-*N,N'*-di-2-(4-methyl)-pentanoate (**L10**)
- dichlorido(*O,O'*-dibutyl-(*S,S*)-ethylenediamine-*N,N'*-di-2-(4-methyl)-pentanoate)-palladium(II) (**C10**)
- *O,O'*-dipentyl-(*S,S*)-ethylenediamine-*N,N'*-di-2-(4-methyl)-pentanoate(**L11**) - dichlorido(*O,O'*-dipentyl-(*S,S*)-ethylenediamine-*N,N'*-di-2-(4-methyl)-pentanoate)-palladium(II) (**C11**)
- S-benzyl-thiosalicylic acid (**L12**)
- *bis*-(S-benzyl-thiosalicylate)-palladium(II) (**C12**)
- S-methyl-thiosalicylic acid (**L13**)

- *bis*-(S-methyl-thiosalicylate)-palladium(II) (**C13**)
- S-ethyl-thiosalicylic acid (**L14**)
- *bis*-(S-ethyl-2-thiosalicylate)-palladium(II) complex (**C14**)
- S-propyl-thiosalicylic acid (**L15**)
- *bis*-(S-propyl-2-thiosalicylate)-palladium(II) (**C15**)
- S-buthyl-thiosalicylic acid (**L16**)
- *bis*-(S-butyl-2-thiosalicylate)-palladium(II) (**C16**)
- *meso*-1,2-diphenyl-ethylenediamine-*N,N*'-di-3-propanoic acid (**L17**)
- dichlorido-(*meso*-1,2-diphenyl-ethylenediamine-*N,N*'-di-3-propanoate)-palladium(II) (**L17a**)
- *s-cis*-dichlorido-(*meso*-1,2-diphenyl-ethylenediamine-*N,N*'-di-3-propanoate)-platinum(IV) (**L17b**)
- *O,O*'-diethyl-(*S,S*)-ethylenediamine-*N,N*'-di-2-propanoate (**L18**)
- tetrachlorido(*O,O*'-diethyl-(*S,S*)-ethylenediamine-*N,N*'-di-2-propanoate)-platinum(IV)(**C18**)
- *O,O*'-diethyl-ethylenediamine-*N,N*'-di-*S,S*-(2,2'-benzyl)acetate (**L19**)
- tetrachorido(*O,O*'-diethyl-ethylenediamine-*N,N*'-di-*S,S*-(2,2'-benzyl)acetate)-platinum(IV) (**C19**)
- *O,O*'-dipropyl-ethylenediamine-*N,N*'-di-*S,S*-(2,2'-benzyl)acetate (**L20**)
- tetrachorido(*O,O*'-dipropyl-ethylenediamine-*N,N*'-di-*S,S*-(2,2'-benzyl)acetate)-platinum(IV) (**C20**)
- *O,O*'-dibutyl-ethylenediamine-*N,N*'-di-*S,S*-(2,2'-benzyl)acetate (**L21**)
- tetrachorido(*O,O*'-dibutyl-ethylenediamine-*N,N*'-di-*S,S*-(2,2'-benzyl)acetate)-platinum(IV) (**C21**)

2.1.1 The synthesis of the ligands - L1, L2, L3 and corresponding palladium(II) complexes – C1, C2, C3

In 50 mL of dry alcohol (1-propanol, 1-butanol or 1-pentanol), saturated with gas HCl, 1.53 g (7.5 mmol) of H_2-*S,S*-eddp was added and the mixture was refluxed for 12 h. The mixture was filtered and left in the refrigerator over night. The obtained white powder was filtered and air-dried.

Complexes were obtained by mixing $K_2[PdCl_4]$ (0.200 g, 0.613 mmol) and equimolar amount of the dpr-*S,S*-eddp·2HCl·3H_2O (**L1**) (0.2546 g, 0.613 mmol), dbu-*S,S*-eddp·2HCl·3H_2O (**L2**) (0.2718 g, 0.613 mmol) or dpe-*S,S*-eddp·2HCl·2H_2O (**L3**) (0.2780 g, 0.613 mmol) esters. During 2 h of stirring 10 cm^3 of water solution of LiOH (0.0294 g, 1.226 mmol) was added in small portions to the reaction mixture. Within this period, pale yellow precipitates of the complexes **C1-C3** were obtained, filtered off, washed with cold water, ethanol and ether and air dried (Vasić et al., 2010) (Fig. 1.).

2.1.2 The synthesis of the ligands - L4, L5, L6, L7 and corresponding palladium(II) complexes – C4, C5, C6, C7

In 50 mL of dry alcohol (ethanol, 1-propanol, 1-butanol or 1-pentanol), saturated with gas HCl, 2.50 g (7.5 mmol) of (H_2-(*S,S*)-eddv) was added and the mixture was refluxed for 12 h. The mixture was filtered off and the filtrate was left for a few days in a refrigerator at 4°C. The esters were recrystallized from hot alcohol used for each reaction.

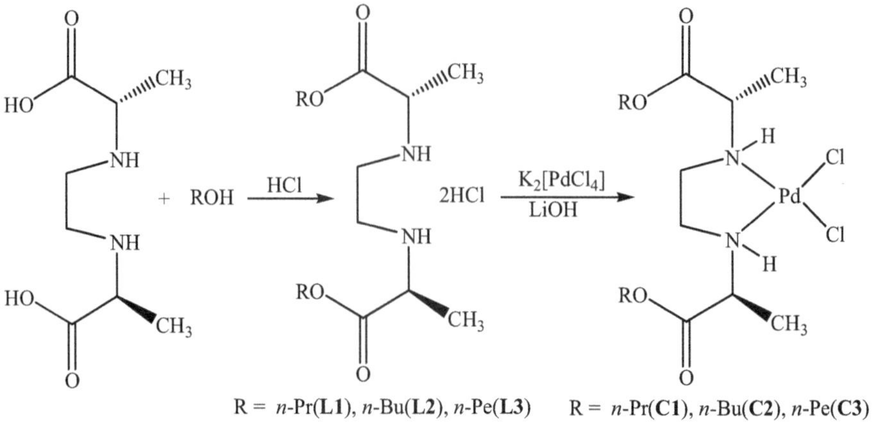

Fig. 1. The preparation of some alkyl esters of H_2-*S,S*-eddp and corresponding palladium(II) complexes

Complexes were obtained by mixing $K_2[PdCl_4]$ (0.200 g, 0.613 mmol) and equimolar amount of the **L4** (0.241 g, 0.613 mmol), **L5** (0.256 g, 0.613 mmol), **L6** (0.273 g, 0.613 mmol) or **L7** (0.290 g, 0.613 mmol) esters. During 2 h of stirring 10 cm^3 of water solution of LiOH (0.0294 g, 1.226 mmol) was added in small portions to the reaction mixture. Within this period, pale yellow precipitates of the complexes **C4-C7** were obtained, filtered off, washed with cold water, ethanol and ether and air dried (Fig.2.). The crystal structure of C4 was confirmed by X-ray analysis (Radić et al., 2010b; 2011a).

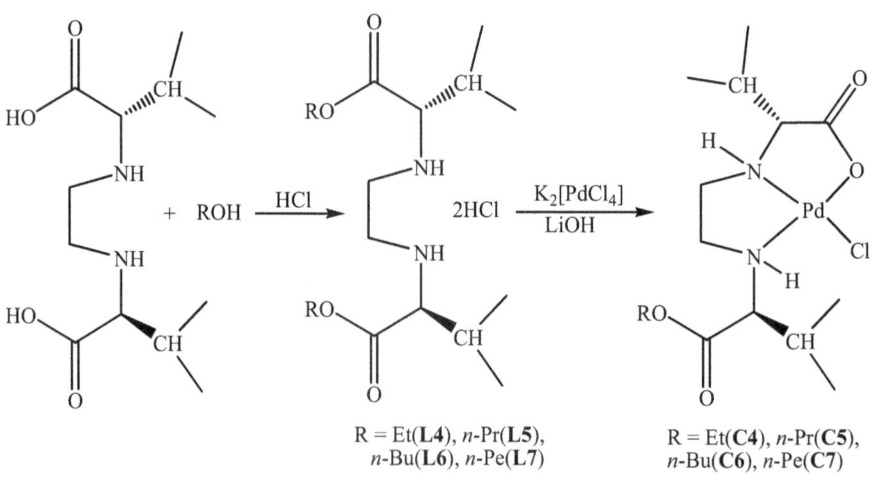

Fig. 2. The preparation of some alkyl esters of H_2-*S,S*-eddv and corresponding palladium(II) complexes

2.1.3 The synthesis of the ligands - L8, L9, L10, L11 and corresponding palladium(II) complexes – C8, C9, C10 and C11

Thionyl choride (4 cm^3, 55 mmol) was introduced into a flask containing 50 cm^3 of corresponding ice cooled alcohol (ethyl, *n*-propyl, n-butyl or *n*-pentyl; anhydrous conditions) for 1 h. After addition of 2 g (5.54 mmol) [(*S,S*)-H_4eddl]Cl_2 the reaction mixture was refluxed for 16 h, filtered off and the filtrate was left for a few days in a refrigerator at 4°C. The esters were recrystallized from the hot alcohol used for each reaction.

Complexes were obtained by mixing $K_2[PdCl_4]$ (0.2 g, 0.61 mmol) and equimolar amount of the **L8**·H_2O (0.267 g, 0.61 mmol), **L9**·H_2O (0.277 g, 0.61 mmol), **L10**·H_2O (0.301 g, 0.61 mmol) or **L11**·H_2O (0.318 g, 0.61 mmol) esters. During 2 h of stirring 10 cm^3 of water solution of LiOH (0.0293 g, 1.22 mmol) was added in small portions to the reaction mixture. Within this period, pale yellow precipitates of the complexes **C8-C11** were obtained, filtered off, washed with cold water, ethanol and ether and air dried (Vujić et al., 2010) (Fig.3.). The crystal structure of **C11** was confirmed by X-ray analysis (Vujić, et al., 2011).

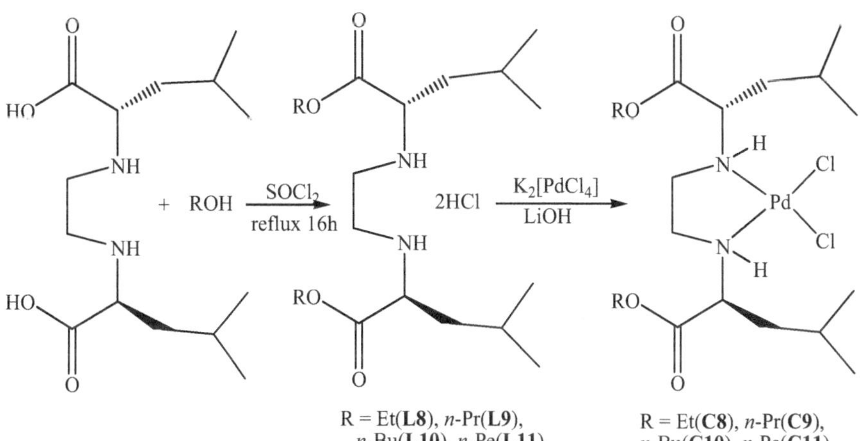

Fig. 3. The preparation of some alkyl esters of H_2-*S,S*-eddl and corresponding palladium(II) complexes

2.1.4 The synthesis of the ligands - L12, L13, L14, L15, L16 and corresponding palladium(II) complexes – C12, C13, C14, C15, C16

The thioacid ligands (**L12**)-(**L16**) were prepared by alkylation of thiosalicylic acid by means of corresponding alkyl halogenides in alkaline water-ethanol solution.

Thiosalicylic acid (1 mmol) was added to a 100 cm^3 round bottom flask containing 50 cm^3 of 30% solution of ethanol in water and stirred. A solution of NaOH (2 mmol in 5 cm^3 of water) was added to acid suspension. The solution became clear. The corresponding alkyl halogenide (2 mmol) was dissolved in 5 cm^3 of ethanol and transferred to the stirred solution. The resulting mixture was kept overnight at 60°C. The reaction mixture was transferred into a beaker and ethanol was evaporated off on a water bath. Diluted hydrochloric acid (2 mol/dm^3) was added to the resulting water solution and S-alkyl thiosalicylic acid was precipitated as a white powder. The liberated acid was filtered off and washed with plenty of distilled water. The product was dried under vacuum overnight.

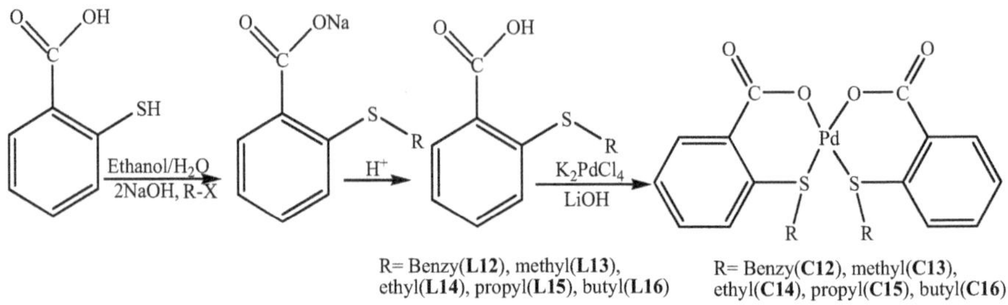

Fig. 4. The preparation of alkyl eters of 2-thiosalicylic acid and corresponding palladium(II) complexes

$K_2[PdCl_4]$ (0.100 g, 0.3065 mmol) was dissolved in 10 cm^3 of water on a steam bath and (S-benzyl)-2-thiosalicylic acid (0.1497 g, 0.613 mmol), (S-methyl)-2-thiosalicylic acid (0.103 g, 0.613 mmol), (S-ethyl)-2-thiosalicylic acid (0.1117 g, 0.613 mmol), (S-propyl)-2-thiosalicylic acid (0.1203 g, 0.613 mmol) or (S-butyl)-2-thiosalicylic acid, (0.1289 g, 0.613 mmol) was added into the solution. The resulting mixture was stirred for 2h and during this time an aqueous solution of LiOH (0.0256 g, 0.613 mmol in 10 cm^3 of water) was introduced. The complexes (**C12- C16**) as a yellow precipitate were filtered, washed with water and air-dried (Radić et al., 2011) (Fig.4.). The crystal structure of **C12** was confirmed by X-ray analysis (Dimitrijević et al., 2011).

2.1.5 The synthesis of the ligand L17 and corresponding palladium(II) complex C17 and corresponding platinum(IV) complex C17a

Benzaldehyde (30 g) was refluxed with ammonium acetate (60 g) for 3 hours. The reaction mixture was cooled and the product was filtered and washed with ethanol. Recrystallization from 1-butanol gave *N*-benzoyl-*N*'-benzylidene-*meso*-1,2-diphenyl-ethylendiamine. Hydrolysis of that compound with 70% sulphuric acid under reflux for 1h gave *meso*-1,2- -diphenyl-ethylenediamine as the basic product of hydrolysis.

3-Chloro-propanoic acid (4.34 g, 0.04 mol) was dissolved in 5 cm^3 of water on ice bath and carefully neutralized with cold water solution of 5 cm^3 NaOH (1.6 g, 0.04 mol). 1,2- Diphenyl--ethylenediamine (4.24 g, 0.02 mol) was added to this solution. The mixture was being stirred for 4 hours at 90°C, and during this period 5 cm^3 NaOH water solution (1.6 g, 0.04 mol) was introduced. After that, 5.6 cm^3 6 mol/dm^3 HCl was added and resulting solution was evaporated to the volume of 7 cm^3; 6 cm^3 *conc.* HCl, 6 cm^3 of ethanol and 6 cm^3 of ether were added to the mixture. The white precipitate of H_2-1,2-dpheddp·2HCl·1.5H_2O (**L17**) was separated by filtration and refined with solution water : ethanol = 1 : 2. The crystal structure of **L17** was confirmed by X-ray analysis (Radić et al., 2010a).

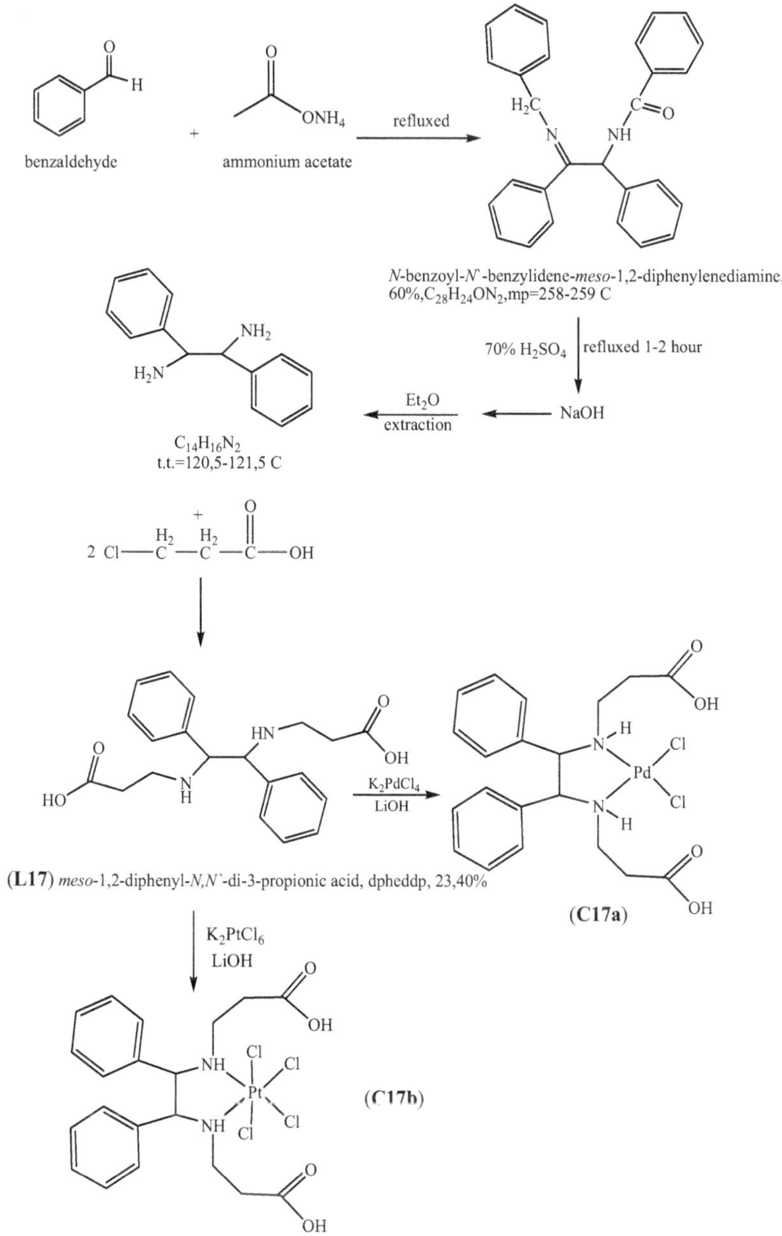

Fig. 5. Reaction pathways in synthesis of *meso*-1,2-diphenyl-ethylenediamine-*N,N'*-di-3- -propionic acid and corresponding palladium(II) and platinum(IV) complexes.

Potassium-hexachloridoplatinate(IV) (0.2 g, 0.411 mmol) was dissolved in 10 cm^3 of water on a steam bath and 1,2-diphenyl-ethylenediamine-*N,N'*-di-3-propanoic acid (0.1876 g, 0.411 mmol) was added. The reaction mixture was heated for 12 hours and during this period 10 cm^3 of LiOH water solution (0.0394 g, 1.65 mmol) was added in small portions and the solution was filtered and evaporated to small volume. The orange precipitate of *s-cis*-[$PtCl_2$(1,2-dpheddp)] **C17b**) was separated by filtration, washed with cold water and air-dried (Fig. 5).

2.1.6 The synthesis of the ligands L4, L18 and corresponding platinum(IV) complexes C4a, C18

$K_2[PtCl_6]$ (0.100 g, 0.205 mmol) and det-(*S,S*)-eddv (0.080 g, 0.205 mmol) were dissolved in 25 cm^3 of water. The reaction mixture was heated on a steam bath for 3 h during which water solution of LiOH·H_2O (0.017 g, 0.41 mmol in 10 cm^3 of water) was introduced. The complex, [$PtCl_4$(det-(*S,S*)-eddv)] (**C4a**), as a yellow precipitate was separated by filtration, washed with water and air-dried (Fig. 6.).

In 50 cm^3 of dry ethanol, saturated with gas HCl, 1.53 g (7.5 mmol) of H_2-*S,S*-eddp was added and the mixture was refluxed for 12 h. The mixture was filtered and left in the refrigerator over night. The obtained white powder of *O,O'*-diethyl-(*S,S*)--ethylenediamine-*N,N'*-di-2-propanoate dihydrochloride, det-*S,S*-eddp·2HCl (**L18**) was filtered and air dried.

$K_2[PtCl_6]$ (0.100 g, 0.205 mmol) and det-(*S,S*)-eddp (0.068 g, 0.205 mmol) were dissolved in 25 cm^3 of water. The reaction mixture was heated on a steam bath for 3 h during which water solution of LiOH·H_2O (0.017 g, 0.41 mmol in 10 cm^3 of water) was introduced. The complex, [$PtCl_4$(det-(*S,S*)-eddp)] (**C18**), as a yellow precipitate was separated by filtration, washed with water and air-dried (Stanković et al., 2011b) (Fig. 7.). The crystal structure of **C18** was confirmed by X-ray analysis (Stanković et al., 2011b).

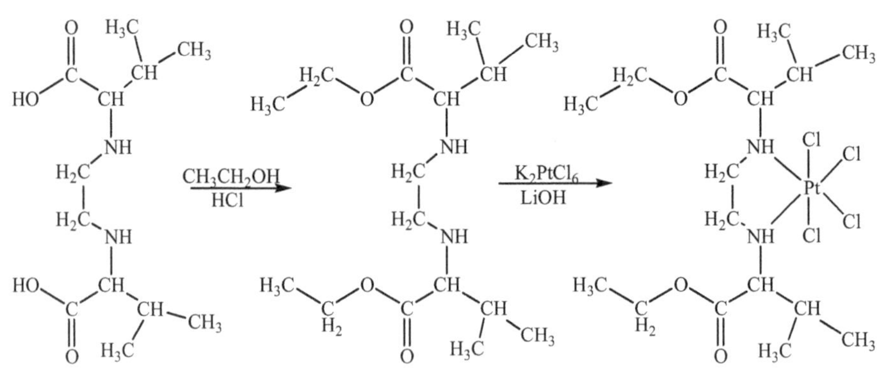

(L4) **(C4a)**

Fig. 6. Synthesis of the ester det-(*S,S*)-eddv·2HCl and platinum(IV) complex

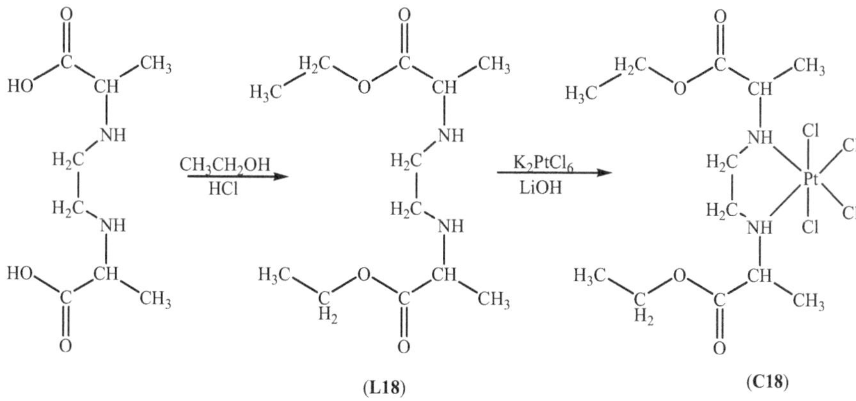

Fig. 7. Synthesis of the ester det-(*S,S*)-eddp·2HCl and platinum(IV) complex

2.1.7 The synthesis of the ligands L19, L20, L21 and corresponding platinum(IV) complexes C19, C20, C21

In 50 cm³ of dry alcohol (ethanol, 1-propanol, 1-butanol) saturated with gaseous HCl, 1.50 g (3.65 mmol) of ethylenediamine-*N,N'*-di-*S,S*-(2,2'-dibenzyl)acetate acid threehydrate (H_2-*S,S*-eddba·3H_2O) was added and the mixture was refluxed for 12 h. The mixture was filtered and left in the refrigerator over night. The obtained white powder was filtered and air-dried.

$K_2[PtCl_6]$ (0.100 g, 0.206 mmol) and 0.206 mmol of R_2-*S,S*-eddba·2HCl (0.100 g of de-*S,S*-eddba·2HCl (**L19**), 0.106 g of dp-*S,S*-eddba·2HCl (**L20**), 0.112 g of db-*S,S*-eddba·2HCl (**L21**)) were dissolved in 15 cm³ of water. The reaction mixture was heated at 40 °C for 12 h and during this period 3.92 cm³ of aqueous 0.105 mol/dm³ LiOH·H_2O (0.412 mmol) were added in small portions The complexes (**C19-C21**) as a yellow-orange precipitates were collected by filtration, washed with water, corresponding alcohol and ether and air-dried (Fig. 8.). The crystal structure of **L20** was confirmed by X-ray analysis (Dimitrijević et al., 2010).

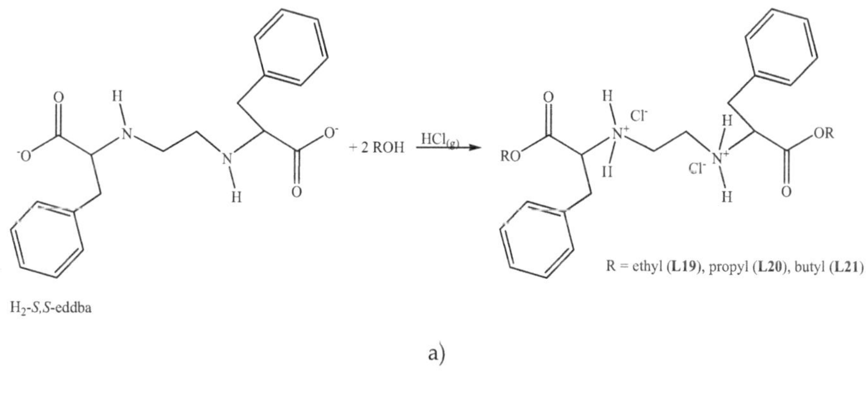

a)

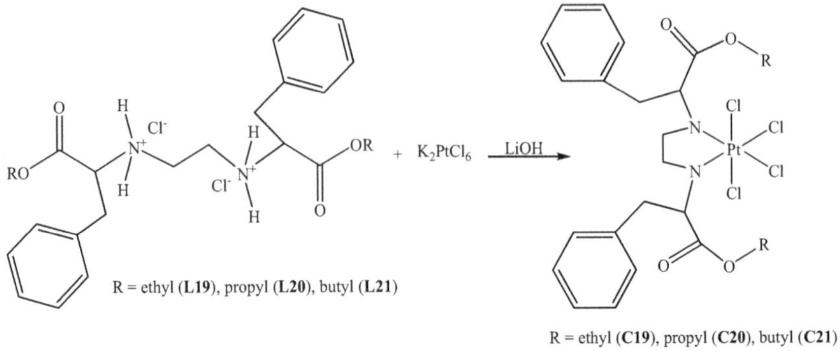

b)

Fig. 8. The synthesis of: a) esters (R_2-*S,S*-eddba·2HCl); b) complexes [$PtCl_4$(R_2-*S,S*-eddba)]

2.2 In vitro antimicrobial assay

2.2.1 Test substances

The tested compounds were dissolved in DMSO and then diluted into nutrient liquid medium to achieve a concentration of 10%. Antibiotic, doxycycline (Galenika A.D., Belgrade), was dissolved in nutrient liquid medium, a Mueller–Hinton broth (Torlak, Beograd).

2.2.2 Test microorganisms

Antimicrobial activity of twenty-one palladium(II) and platinum(IV) complexes and their ligands was tested against 9 species of bacteria: 6 strains of pathogenic bacteria (including 4 standard strains: *Pseudomonas aeruginosa* ATCC 27853, *Enterococcus faecalis* ATCC 29212, *Staphylococcus aureus* ATCC 25923; *Sarcina lutea* ATCC 9341 and 2 clinical isolates: *Escherichia coli* and *Salmonella enterica*) and 3 species of probiotic bacteria (*Bacillus subtilis* IP 5832 PMFKG-P32, *Bifidobacterium animalis subsp. lactis* PMFKG-P33 and *Lactobacillus rhamnosus* PMFKG-P35). All clinical isolates were a generous gift from the Institute of Public Health, Kragujevac. The other microorganisms were provided from a collection held by the Microbiology Laboratory Faculty of Science, University of Kragujevac.

2.2.3 Suspension preparation

Bacterial suspensions were prepared by the direct colony method. The colonies were taken directly from the plate and were suspended in 5 mL of sterile 0.85% saline. The turbidity of initial suspension was adjusted by comparing with 0.5 McFarland's standard (0.5 ml 1.17% w/v $BaCl_2 \times 2H_2O$ + 99.5 ml 1% w/v H_2SO_4) (Andrews, 2005). When adjusted to the turbidity of the 0.5 McFarland's standard, bacteria suspension contains about 10^8 colony forming unites (CFU)/mL. Ten-hold dilutions of initial suspension were additionally prepared into sterile 0.85% saline.

2.2.4 Microdilution method

Antimicrobial activity was tested by determining the minimum inhibitory concentration (MIC) and minimum bactericidal concentration (MBC) by using microdilution plate method with resazurin (Sarker et al., 2007). The 96-well plates were prepared by dispensing 100 μL of nutrient broth into each well. A 100 μL from the stock solution of tested compound (concentration 2000 μg/mL) was added into the first row of the plate. Then, twofold, serial dilutions were performed by using a multichannel pipette. The obtained concentration range was from 1000 μg/mL to 7.81 μg/mL. A 10 μL of diluted bacterial suspension was added to each well to give a final concentration of 5 x 10^5 CFU/mL. Finally, 10 μL resazurin solution was added to each well inoculated with bacteria. Resazurin is an oxidation-reduction indicator used for the evaluation of microbial growth. It is a blue non-fluorescent dye that becomes pink and fluorescent when reduced to resorufin by oxidoreductases within viable cells (Banfi et al., 2003). The inoculated plates were incubated at 37 °C for 24 h. MIC was defined as the lowest concentration of the tested substance that prevented resazurin color change from blue to pink. Doxycycline was used as a positive control. Solvent control test was performed to study an effect of 10% DMSO on the growth of microorganism. It was observed that 10% DMSO did not inhibit the growth of microorganism. Also, in the experiment, the concentration of DMSO was additionally decreased because of the twofold serial dilution assay (the working concentration was 5% and lower). Each test included growth control and sterility control. All tests were performed in duplicate and MICs were constant. Minimum bactericidal concentration was determined by plating 10 μL of samples from wells, where no indicator color change was recorded, on nutrient agar medium. At the end of the incubation period the lowest concentration with no growth (no colony) was defined as minimum bactericidal concentration.

3. Results and discussion

The results of *in vitro* testing of antibacterial activities of the ligands and corresponding palladium(II) and platinum(IV) complex are shown in Table 1-10. For comparison, MIC and MBC values of doxycycline are listed in Table 11. The solvent (10% DMSO) did not inhibit the growth of the tested microorganisms.

The intensity of antimicrobial action varied depending on the species of microorganism and on the type and concentration of tested compounds. The difference between antimicrobial activity of the ligands and corresponding palladium(II) and platinum(IV) complexes is noticed and, in general, the most active were palladium(II) complexes.

The results of antibacterial testing for the ligands (**L1, L2, L3**) and corresponding palladium(II) complexes (**C1, C2, C3**) are shown in Table 1. The results for 3 strains of pathogenic bacteria and 2 species of probiotic bacteria were reported in the paper Vasić et al., (2010). Results for *S. enterica, Staphyl. aureus* ATCC 25923, *S. lutea* ATCC 9341 and *L. rhamnosus* were first presented in this paper. These ligands and complexes, being compared to positive control, showed low to moderate antibacterial activity. MIC and MBC values were in range from <7.81 to >1000 μg/mL, depending on the species of bacteria. Gram-positive bacteria showed higher sensitivity. The most sensitive was *S. lutea* ATCC 9341, where MIC was for **C1** and **C2** <7.81 μg/mL. The best activity at Gram-negative bacteria was shown by **C2** to *P. aeruginosa* ATCC 27853 and *E. coli* (MIC was 31.25 μg/mL). The probiotics showed sensitivity similar to the sensitivity of the other bacteria to the tested compounds. Exception is *B. animalis subsp. lactis* where **L2, C2** and **L3** inhibited its growth at these concentrations: 7.81 μg/mL, 15,63 μg/mL and <7.81 μg/mL.

The results of testing the ligands (**L4, L5, L6, L7**) and their palladium(II) complexes (**C4, C5, C6, C7**) are shown in Table 2 and Table 3. The results of testing for **L4** were reported in the paper by Stanković et al., (2011a; 2011c). The tested ligands, with few exceptions, show very low antimicrobial activity, while palladium(II) complexes show selective and moderate activity. Interestingly, **L6, L7** and **C6, C7** exhibit strong antibacterial activity towards *E. coli*, *Staphyl. aureus* ATCC 25923 and *S. lutea* ATCC 9341, MIC ranged <7.81 μg/mL to 31.25μg/mL. Probiotic bacteria showed high resistance to the effects of tested substances. The most sensitive was *B. subtilis* IP 5832 to **C5** and **C4** (MIC was 7.81μg/mL and 15.63 μg/mL).

The results of testing the ligands (**L8, L9, L10, L11**) and palladium(II) complexes (**C8, C9, C10, C11**) are shown in Table 4 and Table 5. The ligands and complexes, being compared to positive control, with few exceptions, showed low antibacterial activity. MIC and MBC values were in range from <7.8 to >1000 μg/mL, depending on the species of bacteria. **L9, L10** and **L11** showed excellent results to *S. lutea* ATCC 9341 (MIC and MBC <7.81 μg/mL) and **L10** and **L11** to *S. lutea* ATCC 9341, *Staphyl. aureus* ATCC 25923 and *L. rhamnosus* (MIC <7.81 μg/mL). In this case the ligands acted better than corresponding complexes and it is an exception. The complexes have weak antimicrobial activity and some better influence was seen on *B. subtilis* IP 5832 were MIC was in range from 39.06 to 312.5 μg/mL.

The results of testing the ligands (**L12, L13, L14, L15, L16**) and corresponding palladium (II) complexes (**C12, C13, C14, C15, C16**) are shown in Table 6 and Table 7. The results for these testing were accepted for publication in the paper by Radić et al., (2011b). All tested compounds demonstrated selective and moderate antibacterial activity. Tested ligands, with a few exceptions, show very low antimicrobial activity. The activity of corresponding complexes was higher than with the ligands. MICs values for ligands were in range from 250 μg/mL to >1000 μg/mL, and for complexes from 62.5 μg/mL to 1000 μg/mL. The Gram-positive bacteria were more sensitive than the Gram-negative bacteria especially by the activity of the complexes. The best effect was observed in **C16** to *S. lutea* ATCC 9341 were MIC and MBC 62.5 μg/mL. MICs for Gram-negative bacteria were at 500 μg/mL and 1000 μg/mL. The tested complexes (**C13**) and (**C14**) exhibited somewhat stronger antibacterial activity towards *P. aeruginosa* ATCC 27853 (MIC = 250 μg/mL). The probiotics showed sensitivity similar to the sensitivity of the other bacteria (Radić et al., 2011b).

Species	L1		C1		L2		C2		L3		C3	
	MIC	MBC	MIC	MBC	MIC	MBC	MIC	MBC	MIC	MBC	MIC	MBC
Escherichia coli [1]	125	>500	62,5	125	31.3	>500	31,25	> 250	250	>500	125	> 500
Salmonella enterica	>1000	>1000	125	125	nt	nt	250	500	1000	>1000	250	500
Pseud. aeruginosa ATCC 27853 [1]	>500	>500	125	250	>500	>500	31,25	125	250	>500	125	125
Enter. faecalis ATCC 29212 [1]	>500	>500	125	250	125	>500	62,5	250	>500	>500	62,5	250
Staphyl. aureus ATCC 25923	>1000	>1000	62.5	125	nt	nt	62.5	125	250	1000	62.5	125
Sarcina lutea ATCC 9341	1000	1000	<7.8	<7.8	nt	nt	<7.8	15,6	31,25	125	31,25	31,25
Lactobacillus rhamnosus	nt	nt	62.5	500	nt	nt	62.5	250	nt	nt	62.5	125
Bifidobact. animalis subsp. lactis [1]	125	>500	62,5	125	7.81	>500	15,6	125	<7.81	< 31.25	125	> 500
Bacillus subtilis IP 5832 [1]	125	>500	62,5	125	62.5	>500	15,6	125	62.5	>500	62,5	> 500

MIC, minimum inhibitory concentration (μg/mL),
MBC, minimum bactericidal concentration (μg/mL), nt, not tested

Table 1. Antibacterial activity of the ligands (**L1,L2,L3**) and corresponding complexes (**C1, C2, C3**).

[1] Vasić et al., (2010)

Species	L4 [2]		C4		L5		C5	
	MIC	MBC	MIC	MBC	MIC	MBC	MIC	MBC
Escherichia coli	500	1000	125	500	125	1000	125	500
Salmonella enterica	1000	>1000	1000	1000	>1000	>1000	1000	1000
Pseud. aeruginosa ATCC 27853	1000	1000	500	1000	>1000	>1000	500	1000
Enter. faecalis ATCC 29212	500	500	500	1000	>1000	>1000	500	>1000
Staphyl. aureus ATCC 25923	500	500	250	500	250	500	125	500
Sarcina lutea ATCC 9341	31.25	125	250	250	1000	1000	250	250
Lactobacillus rhamnosus	1000	1000	500	1000	nt	nt	500	1000
Bifidobact. animalis subsp. lactis	250	500	125	1000	500	>1000	250	>1000
Bacillus subtilis IP 5832	125	500	15.63	>1000	62.5	>1000	7.81	1000

MIC, minimum inhibitory concentration (μg/mL),
MBC, minimum bactericidal concentration (μg/mL), nt, not tested

Table 2. Antibacterial activity of the ligands (**L4, L5**) and corresponding complexes (**C4, C5**).

Species	L6		C6		L7		C7	
	MIC	MBC	MIC	MBC	MIC	MBC	MIC	MBC
Escherichia coli	15.63	500	31.25	500	15.63	125	<7.81	125
Salmonella enterica	1000	1000	250	500	1000	1000	1000	1000
Pseud. aeruginosa ATCC 27853	>1000	>1000	500	1000	500	>1000	500	1000
Enter. faecalis ATCC 29212	1000	>1000	500	1000	1000	>1000	500	1000
Staphyl. aureus ATCC 25923	31.25	125	125	125	31.25	125	500	500
Sarcina lutea ATCC 9341	31.25	31.25	31.25	31.25	<7.81	<7.81	250	250
Lactobacillus rhamnosus	31.25	250	62.50	125	62.50	250	500	1000
Bifidobact. animalis subsp. lactis	62.50	1000	62.50	1000	62.50	500	125	>1000
Bacillus subtilis IP 5832	250	>1000	500	1000	1000	>1000	500	>1000

MIC, minimum inhibitory concentration (μg/mL),
MBC, minimum bactericidal concentration (μg/mL)

Table 3. Antibacterial activity of the ligands (**L6, L7**) and corresponding complexes (**C6, C7**).

Species	L8		C8		L9		C9	
	MIC	MBC	MIC	MBC	MIC	MBC	MIC	MBC
Escherichia coli	625	>1000	625	>1000	312.5	>1000	>1000	>1000
Salmonella enterica	>1000	>1000	>1000	>1000	>1000	>1000	>1000	>1000
Pseud. aeruginosa ATCC 27853	>1000	>1000	>1000	>1000	>1000	>1000	>1000	>1000
Enter. faecalis ATCC 29212	>1000	>1000	>1000	>1000	>1000	>1000	625	>1000
Staphyl. aureus ATCC 25923	250	500	500	1000	31.25	125	250	500
Sarcina lutea ATCC 9341	250	250	500	500	<7.8	<7.8	250	250
Lactobacillus rhamnosus	1000	1000	500	1000	15.63	125	500	1000
Bifidobact. animalis subsp. lactis	78	>1000	78	>1000	>1000	>1000	>1000	>1000
Bacillus subtilis IP 5832	78.13	>1000	39.06	625	625	>1000	78	>1000

MIC, minimum inhibitory concentration (μg/mL),
MBC, minimum bactericidal concentration (μg/mL)

Table 4. Antibacterial activity of the ligands (**L8, L9**) and corresponding complexes (**C8, C9**).

[2] Stanković et al., (2011a, 2011c)

Species	L10		C10		L11		C11	
	MIC	MBC	MIC	MBC	MIC	MBC	MIC	MBC
Escherichia coli	>1000	>1000	>1000	>1000	625	>1000	312.5	>1000
Salmonella enterica	>1000	>1000	>1000	>1000	>1000	>1000	>1000	>1000
Pseud. aeruginosa ATCC 27853	>1000	>1000	>1000	>1000	>1000	>1000	312.5	>1000
Enter. faecalis ATCC 29212	156.3	>1000	625	>1000	>1000	>1000	156.3	>1000
Staphyl. aureus ATCC 25923	<7.8	125	31.25	125	<7.8	125	500	500
Sarcina lutea ATCC 9341	<7.8	<7.8	31.25	31.25	<7.8	<7.8	250	250
Lactobacillus rhamnosus	<7.8	<7.8	31.25	62.5	<7.8	<7.8	500	1000
Bifidobact. animalis subsp. lactis	>1000	>1000	>1000	>1000	>1000	>1000	625	>1000
Bacillus subtilis IP 5832	>1000	>1000	78	>1000	>1000	>1000	312.5	>1000

MIC, minimum inhibitory concentration (μg/mL),
MBC, minimum bactericidal concentration (μg/mL)

Table 5. Antibacterial activity of the ligands (**L10, L11**) and corresponding complexes (**C10,C11**).

Species	L12		C12		L13		C13		L14		C14	
	MIC	MBC	MIC	MBC	MIC	MBC	MIC	MBC	MIC	MBC	MIC	MBC
Escherichia coli	>1000	>1000	1000	1000	1000	>1000	500	500	1000	>1000	500	500
Salmonella enterica	1000	>1000	1000	1000	1000	>1000	500	500	1000	>1000	500	500
Pseud. aeruginosa ATCC 27853	500	>1000	500	1000	500	>1000	250	500	500	>1000	250	500
Enter. faecalis ATCC 29212	1000	1000	500	500	1000	1000	500	1000	500	1000	250	500
Staphyl. aureus ATCC 25923	500	1000	500	1000	1000	1000	500	1000	1000	1000	500	500
Sarcina lutea ATCC 9341	250	500	250	250	1000	1000	250	250	500	500	250	500
Lactobacillus rhamnosus	>1000	>1000	1000	1000	1000	>1000	500	1000	1000	1000	500	500
Bifidobact. animalis subsp. lactis	500	500	500	1000	500	500	1000	1000	1000	1000	500	500
Bacillus subtilis IP 5832	500	500	500	500	500	500	500	500	1000	>1000	250	500

MIC, minimum inhibitory concentration (μg/mL),
MBC, minimum bactericidal concentration (μg/mL)

Table 6. [3] Antibacterial activity of the ligands (**L12, L13, L14**) and corresponding complexes (**C12, C13, C14**).

Species	L15		C15		L16		C16	
	MIC	MBC	MIC	MBC	MIC	MBC	MIC	MBC
Escherichia coli	1000	>1000	500	500	>1000	>1000	1000	1000
Salmonella enterica	1000	>1000	500	1000	>1000	>1000	1000	1000
Pseud. aeruginosa ATCC 27853	500	>1000	500	1000	500	>1000	500	1000
Enter. faecalis ATCC 29212	500	1000	250	500	1000	1000	500	1000
Staphyl. aureus ATCC 25923	500	1000	500	500	>1000	>1000	500	500
Sarcina lutea ATCC 9341	250	250	500	500	1000	1000	62.5	62.5
Lactobacillus rhamnosus	1000	>1000	500	>1000	>1000	>1000	1000	1000
Bifidobact. animalis subsp. lactis	500	1000	250	500	1000	1000	500	1000
Bacillus subtilis IP 5832	500	500	250	250	1000	>1000	250	500

MIC, minimum inhibitory concentration (μg/mL),
MBC, minimum bactericidal concentration (μg/mL)

Table 7. [4] Antibacterial activity of the ligands (**L15, L16**) and corresponding complexes (**C15,C16**).

---

[3] Radić et al., (2011b)

[4] Radić et al., (2011b)

The results of *in vitro* testing of antibacterial activities of the ligand (**L17**) and corresponding palladium(II) (**C17a**) and platinum(IV) (**C17b**) complexes are shown in Table 8.

Species	L17		C17a		C17b	
	MIC	MBC	MIC	MBC	MIC	MBC
Escherichia coli	>1000	>1000	250	500	>1000	>1000
Salmonella enterica	>1000	>1000	250	500	>1000	>1000
Pseud. aeruginosa ATCC 27853	250	>1000	15.63	500	125	500
Enter. faecalis ATCC 29212	500	>1000	31.25	500	250	500
Staphyl. aureus ATCC 25923	500	>1000	31.25	500	250	500
Sarcina lutea ATCC 9341	500	>1000	62.5	500	125	500
Lactobacillus rhamnosus	125	>1000	62.5	>1000	31.25	>1000
Bifidobact. animalis subsp. lactis	>1000	>1000	31.25	125	250	500
Bacillus subtilis IP 5832	500	>1000	250	500	250	500

MIC, minimum inhibitory concentration (μg/mL),
MBC, minimum microbiocidal concentration (μg/mL)

Table 8. [5]Antibacterial activity of the ligand (**L17**) and corresponding palladium(II) (**C17a**) and platinum(IV) (**C17b**) complexes.

The best activity manifested palladium(II) complex **C17a** with also the best seen result on *P. aeruginosa* ATCC 27853 (MIC 15.63 μg/mL). The same one at Gram-positive bacteria had MIC 31.25 - 62.5 μg/mL. Platinum (IV) complex **C17b** has weaker activity and the best result manifested on *L. rhamnosus* where MIC was 31.25 μg/mL (Radojević et al., 2011).

Species	L4		C4a		L18		C18	
	MIC	MBC	MIC	MBC	MIC	MBC	MIC	MBC
Escherichia coli	500	1000	1000	1000	>1000	>1000	>1000	>1000
Salmonella enterica	1000	>1000	1000	>1000	>1000	>1000	1000	>1000
Pseud. aeruginosa ATCC 27853	1000	1000	1000	>1000	1000	>1000	1000	>1000
Enter. faecalis ATCC 29212	500	500	1000	1000	500	1000	1000	1000
Staphyl. aureus ATCC 25923	500	500	500	1000	500	500	1000	1000
Sarcina lutea ATCC 9341	31.25	125	31.25	62.5	62.5	125	31.25	62.5
Lactobacillus rhamnosus	1000	1000	1000	1000	1000	1000	1000	1000
Bifidobact. animalis subsp. lactis	250	500	500	1000	500	500	1000	>1000
Bacillus subtilis IP 5832	125	500	500	1000	500	500	500	1000

MIC, minimum inhibitory concentration (μg/mL),
MBC, minimum microbiocidal concentration (μg/mL)

Table 9. [6]Antibacterial activity of the ligands (**L4, L18**) and corresponding complexes (**C4a, C18**).

Antibacterial activity of the tested platinum(IV) (**C4a, C18**) complexes and corresponding ligands (**L4, L18**) are shown in Table 9. Results for these testing was reported in the papers Stanković et al., (2011a,c). The ligands and corresponding platinum(IV) complexes demonstrated low antimicrobial activity. There was no difference in activities between the

[5] Radojević et al., (2011)
[6] Stanković et al., (2011a; 2011c)

ligands and corresponding complexes. The ligands and corresponding platinum(IV) complexes showed significant antibacterial activity against *S. lutea* ATTC 9341. MICs values were in range from 31.25 µg/mL to 62.5 µg/mL, and MBCs values were from 62.5 µg/mL to 125 µg/mL. The tested compounds did not affect the growth of Gram-negative bacteria or their activities were very low (MIC ranged from 500 µg/mL to >1000 µg/mL, MBC from 1000 µg/mL to >1000 µg/mL). Also, probiotic bacteria showed high resistance to the effects of tested substances. MICs were from 125 µg/mL to 1000 µg/mL, and MBCs were from 500 µg/mL to >1000 µg/mL (Stanković et al., 2011a,c).

The results of *in vitro* testing of antibacterial activities of the ligands (**L19, L20, L21**) and corresponding platinum(IV) (**C19, C20, C21**) complex are shown in Table 10.

Species	L19		C19		L20		C20		L21		C21	
	MIC	MBC	MIC	MBC	MIC	MBC	MIC	MBC	MIC	MBC	MIC	MBC
Escherichia coli	>1000	>1000	1000	>1000	>1000	>1000	1000	1000	>1000	>1000	1000	1000
Salmonella enterica	>1000	>1000	>1000	>1000	>1000	>1000	1000	1000	>1000	>1000	1000	1000
Pseud. aeruginosa ATCC 27853	>1000	>1000	1000	>1000	>1000	>1000	1000	>1000	>1000	>1000	1000	>1000
Enter. faecalis ATCC 29212	1000	>1000	1000	1000	1000	>1000	250	500	1000	1000	125	500
Staphyl. aureus ATCC 25923	1000	>1000	500	1000	1000	>1000	250	250	1000	>1000	125	250
Sarcina lutea ATCC 9341	1000	>1000	7.81	15.625	1000	>1000	15.625	31.25	1000	>1000	31.25	62.5
Lactobacillus rhamnosus	>1000	>1000	>1000	>1000	>1000	>1000	>1000	>1000	>1000	>1000	>1000	>1000
Bifidobact. animalis subsp. lactis	125	250	1000	1000	<31.25	125	500	500	<31.25	250	125	500
Bacillus subtilis IP 5832	125	250	250	1000	250	250	250	250	250	250	125	250

MIC, minimum inhibitory concentration (µg/mL),
MBC, minimum microbiocidal concentration (µg/mL)

Table 10. Antibacterial activity of the ligands (**L19, L20, L21**) and corresponding complexes (**C19, C20, C21**).

The difference in action between ligands and corresponding complexes can be seen at Gram-positive bacteria. Ligands have significant antimicrobial effect on probiotic bacteria (**L20, L21**), and complexes on Gram-positive bacteria (**C19, C20, C21**). **C21** has better antimicrobial effect than two other complexes. The lowest antimicrobial action of compounds was on Gram-negative bacteria, where tested concentrations of ligands almost didn't have the influence, while corresponding complexes had some better action, but still weak and limited. *L. rhamnosus* also showed similar resistance to the action of tested compounds (none of the tested concentrations had the influence on its growth), while the other probiotic bacteria were more sensitive, especially to the action of ligands, where MIC goes from <31.25 µg/mL to 250 µg/mL. At complexes MIC is in the range from125 µg/mL to 1000 µg/mL.

The gram-positive bacteria were more sensitive than the gram-negative bacteria. The platinum(IV) complexes showed high antibacterial activity against Gram-positive bacteria. MIC values were in range from 7.81 µg/mL to 1000 µg/mL, and MBC values were from 15.63 µg/mL to 1000 µg/mL depending on the species of bacteria. The most sensitive was *S. lutea* ATCC 9341 (MIC values are 7.81 µg/mL, 15.625 µg/mL and 31.25 µg/mL for different complexes.

Species	Doxycycline	
	MIC	MBC
Escherichia coli	7.81	15.625
Salmonella enterica	15.625	31.25
Pseud. aeruginosa ATCC 27853	62.5	125
Enter. faecalis ATCC 29212	7.81	62.5
Staphyl. aureus ATCC 25923	0.224	3.75
Sarcina lutea ATCC 9341	< 0.448	7.81
Lactobacillus rhamnosus	7.81	31.25
Bifidobact. animalis subsp. lactis	31.25	62.5
Bacillus subtilis IP 5832	1.953	15.625

MIC, minimum inhibitory concentration (μg/mL),
MBC, minimum microbiocidal concentration (μg/mL)

Table 11. Antibacterial activity of the positive control - doxycycline

In general, the ligands demonstrated low and selective antimicrobial activity (with few exceptions) and the complexes showed selective and moderate antibacterial activity. MIC values were in range from <7.81μg/mL to >1000 μg/mL and MBC values from 15.625 μg/mL to >1000 μg/mL depending on the species of bacteria. The Gram-positive bacteria were more sensitive than the Gram-negative bacteria. The most sensitive species is *S. lutea* ATCC 9341. Tested probiotics, with a few exceptions, indicate high resistance toward tested compounds. *L. rhamnosus* shows the highest resistance among them. The tested complexes **C1**, **C2**, **C3** and **C17a** exhibit strong activity towards *E. coli*, *P. aeruginosa* ATCC 27853 and *E. faecalis* ATCC 29212. The **L6**, **L7** and **C6**, **C7** exhibit strong antibacterial activity towards *E. coli*. The tested compounds did not affect *S. enterica* or their activities were low. Some activity showed palladium(II) complexes (**C1**, **C2** , **C3**, **C6** and **C17a**). At the ligands the most effective antimicrobial activity show **L6, L7, L9, L10** and **L11** while the most active complexes are **C1, C2, C3, C6** and **C17a.** For eleven ligands (**L1** - **L11**) and corresponding palladium(II) complexes (**C1** - **C11**) antifungal activity is investigated. Palladium(II) complexes showed good antifungal activity opposite to ligands. This study are in keeping with our research to a great extent (Radojević et al., 2010).

4. Conclusion

The intensity of antimicrobial action varied depending on the species of microorganism and on the type of tested compounds. The tested ligands, with few exceptions, show low antimicrobial activity. The difference between antimicrobial activity of the ligands and corresponding palladium(II) and platinum(IV) complexes is noticed and, in general, the most active were palladium(II) complexes. The Gram-positive bacteria were more sensitive than the Gram-negative bacteria. The most sensitive species is *Sarcina lutea* ATCC 9341 and the most resistant is *Salmonella enterica* where the tested compounds did not affect or their activities were low. Tested probiotics, with a few exceptions, also indicate high resistance toward tested compounds.

5. Acknowledgement

The authors are grateful for financial support to the Ministry of Education and Science of Republic of Serbia (projects No. OI172016 and III41010).

6. References

Agarwal, S.K. (2007). Synthesis & Characterization of Some Mixed Ligand Complexes of Pd(II), Rh(III) and Pt(IV) with Carboxylic Hydrazones as Primary and Dithiooxamide as Co-ligand. *Asian Journal of Chemistry*, Vol.19, No.4, pp. 2581-2585, ISSN: 0970-7077

Aghatabay, N. M.; Somer, M.; Senel, M.; Dulger, B. & Gucin, F. (2007). Raman, FT-IR, NMR spectroscopic data and antimicrobial activity of bis[μ_2-(benzimidazol-2-yl)-2-ethanethiolato-*N,S,S*-chloro-palladium(II)] dimer, [(μ_2-$CH_2CH_2NHNCC_6H_4$)$PdCl$]$_2$ C_2H_5OH complex. *European Journal of Medicinal Chemistry*, Vol.42, No.8, (August 2007), pp. 1069-1075, ISSN: 0223-5234

Ali, A.M., Mirza, A.H., Butcher, R.J. & Crouse, K.A. (2006). The preparation, characterization and biological activity of palladium(II) and platinum(II) complexes of tridentate NNS ligands derived from S-methyl- and S-benzyldithiocarbazates and the X-ray crystal structure of the [Pd(mpasme)Cl] complex. *Transition Metal Chemistry*, Vol.31, No.1, (February 2006), pp. 79-87, Print ISSN: 0340-4285, Online ISSN: 1572-901X

Al-Hazmi, G.A., El-Metwally, N.M., El-Gammal, O.A. & El-Asmy, A.A. (2008). Synthesis, spectral characterization and eukaryotic DNA degradation of thiosemicarbazones and their platinum(IV) complexes. *Spectrochimica Acta*, Part A: *Molecular and Biomolecular Spectroscopy*, Vol.69, No.1, (January 2008), pp. 56-61, ISSN: 1386-1425

Andrews, J.M. (2005). BSAC standardized disc susceptibility testing method (version 4). *Journal of Antimicrobial Chemotherapy*, Vol.56, No.1, (July 2005), pp. 60-76, Print ISSN 0305-7453, Online ISSN 1460-2091

Banfi E., Scialino G. & Monti-Bragadin C. (2003). Development of a microdilution method to evaluate Mycobacterium tuberculosis drug susceptibility. *Journal of Antimicrobial Chemotherapy*, Vol.52, No.5, (*November 2003*), pp. 796-800, Print ISSN 0305-7453, Online ISSN 1460-2091

Biyala, M.K., Sharma, K., Swami, M., Fahmi, N. & Vir Singh, R. (2008). Spectral and biocidal studies of palladium(II) and platinum(II) complexes with monobasic bidentate Schiff bases. *Transition Metal Chemistry*, Vol.33, No.3, (April 2008), pp. 377 - 381, Print ISSN: 0340-4285, Online ISSN: 1572-901X

Brudzinska, I., Mikata, Y., Obata, M., Ohtsuki, C. & Yano, S. (2004). Synthesis, structural characterization, and antitumor activity of palladium(II) complexes containing a sugar unit. *Bioorganic & Medicinal Chemistry Letters*, Vol.14, No.10, (17 May), pp. 2533–2536, ISSN: 0960-894X

Coombs, R.R., Ringer, M.K., Blacquiere, J.M., Smith, J.C., Neilsen, J.S., Uh, Y., Gilbert, J.B., Leger, L.J., Zhang, H., Irving A.M., Wheaton, S.L., Vogels, C.M., Westcott, S.A., Decken, A. & Baerlocher, F.J. (2005). Palladium(II) Schiff base complexes derived from sulfanilamides and aminobenzothiazoles. *Transition Metal Chemistry*, Vol.30, No.4, (May 2005), pp. 411-418, Print ISSN: 0340-4285, Online ISSN: 1572-901X

Dimitrijević, D.P., Vujić, J.M., Garcia-Granda, S., Menendez-Taboada, L. & Trifunović S.R. (2010). Synthesis and crystal structure of O,O'-dipropyl-ethylenediamine-N,N'-di-(S,S)-(2,2'-dibenzyl)-acetate dihydrochloride. *Proceedings of XVII Conference of the Serbian Crystallographic Society*, pp. 48, ISBN: 978-86- 6009-004-3, Ivanjica, Serbia, June 3-5, 2010.

Dimitrijević, D.P., Radić G.P., Glođović, V.V., Radojević I.D., Stefanović O.D. , Čomić Lj., Ratković Z.R., Valkonen A., Rissanen, K. & Trifunović, S. R. (2011). Crystal structure of bis-(S-benzyl-thiosalicylate)-palladium(II) complex, [Pd(S-bz-eddp)$_2$]. *Proceedings of XVIII Conference of the Serbian Crystallographic Society*, pp. 44, ISBN: 978-86-7031-194-7, Fruška Gora, Serbia, June 2-4, 2011.

Kizilcikli, I., Kurt, Y.D., Akkurt, B., Genel, A.Y., Birteksöz, S., Ötük, G. & Ülküseven, B. (2007). Antimicrobial Activity of a Series of Thiosemicarbazones and Their ZnII and PdII Complexes. *Folia Microbiologica*, Vol.52, No.1, (January 2007), pp. 15-25, Print ISSN: 0015-5632, Online ISSN: 1874-9356

Kovala-Demertzi, D., Demertzis, M.A., Miller, J.R., Papadopoulou, C., Dodorou, C. & Filousis, G. (2001). Platinum(II) complexes with 2-acetyl pyridine thiosemicarbazone: Synthesis, crystal structure, spectral properties, antimicrobial and antitumour activity, *Journal of Inorganic Biochemistry*, Vol.86, No.2-3, (September 2001), pp. 555-563, ISSN: 0162-0134

Garoufis, A., Hadjikakou, S.K. & Hadjiliadis, N. (2009). Palladium coordination compounds as anti-viral, anti-fungal, anti-microbial and anti-tumor agents. *Coordination Chemistry Reviews*, Vol.253, No.9-10, (May 2009), pp. 1384–1397, ISSN: 0010-8545

Guerra W., de Andrade Azevedo E., de Souza Monteiro A. R., Bucciarelli-Rodriguez M., Chartone-Souza E., Nascimento A. M. A., Fontes A. P. S., Le Moyec L., Pereira-Maia E. C. (2005). Synthesis, characterization, and antibacterial activity of three palladium(II) complexes of tetracyclines. *Journal of Inorganic Biochemistry*, Vol.99, No.12, (December 2005), pp. 2348–2354, ISSN: 0162-0134

Fluit, A.C., Jones, M.E., Schmitz, F.J., Acar, J., Gupta, R., Verhoef, J., & the SENTRY Participants Group. (2000). Antimicrobial susceptibility and frequency of occurrence of clinical blood isolates in Europe from the SENTRY Antimicrobial Surveillance Program, 1997 and 1998. *Clinical Infectious Diseases*, Vol.30, No.3, (March 2000), pp. 454-460, ISSN: 1058-4838

Manav, N., Mishra, A.K. & Kaushik, N. K. (2006). In vitro antitumour and antibacterial studies of some Pt(IV) dithiocarbamate complexes. *Spectrochimica Acta*, Part A: *Molecular and Biomolecular Spectroscopy*. Vol.65, No.1, (September 2006), pp. 32 35, ISSN: 1386-1425

Mishra, A.K. & Kaushik, N.K. (2007). Synthesis, characterization, cytotoxicity, antibacterial and antifungal evaluation of some new platinum (IV) and palladium (II) complexes of thiodiamines. *European Journal of Medicinal Chemistry*, Vol.42, No.10, (October 2007), pp. 1239-1246, ISSN: 0223-5234

Mishra A.K., Mishra, S.B., Manav, N. & Kaushik, N.K. (2007a). Platinum(IV) and palladium(II) thiosemicarbazide and thiodiamine complexes: A spectral and antibacterial study. *Journal of Coordination Chemistry*. Vol.60, No.18, (September 2007) pp. 1923-1932, Print ISSN: 0095-8972, Online ISSN: 1029-0389

Mishra, A.K., Mishra, S.B., Manav, N., Kumar, R., Sharad, R., Chandra, R., Saluja, D. & Kaushik, N.K. (2007b). Platinum (IV) thiohydrazide, thiodiamine and thiohydrazone complexes: A spectral, antibacterial and cytotoxic study. *Spectrochimica Acta* Part A: *Molecular and Biomolecular Spectroscopy*, Vol.66, No.4-5, (April 2007), pp. 1042-1047, ISSN: 1386-1425

Radić, G.P., Glođović, V.V., Garsia-Granda, S., Menéndez-Taboada, L., Ratković, Z.& Trifunović S.R. (2010a). Crystal structure of 1,2-diphenyl-ethylenediamine- N,N'-di-3- propanoic acid dihydrochloride. *Proceedings of XVII Conference of the Serbian Crystallographic Society*, pp. 36, ISBN: 978-86- 6009-004-3, Ivanjica, Serbia, June 3-5, 2010.

Radić, G.P., Glođović, V.V., Heinemann, F.W. & Trifunović, S.R. (2010b). Synthesis and crystal structure of palladium(II) complex with O,O'-diethyl- (S,S)-ethylenediamine-N,N'-di-2-(3-methyl) butanoate. *Proceedings of XVII Conference of the Serbian Crystallographic Society*, pp. 60, ISBN: 978-86-6009-004-3, Ivanjica, Serbia, June 3-5, 2010.

Radić, G.P., Glođović, V.V., Kaluđerović, G.N., Heinemann, F.W. & Trifunović, S. R. (2011a). Palladium(II) complexes with R_2edda derived ligands. Part V. Reaction of O,O'-Diethyl-(S,S)-ethylenediamine-N,N'-di-2-(3-methyl)butanoate with $K_2[PdCl_4]$. *Transition Metal Chemistry*, Vol.36, No.4 , (May 2011), pp. 331–336, ISSN: 0340-4285

Radić, G.P., Glođović, V.V., Radojević, I.D., Stefanović, O.D., Čomić, Lj.R., Ratković, Z.R., Valkonen, A., Rissanen, K. & Trifunović, S.R. (2011b). Synthesis, characterization and antimicrobial activity of palladium(II) complexes with some alkyl derivates of thiosalicylic acids. Crystal structure of *bis*(S-benzyl-thiosalicylate)-palladium(II) complex, $[Pd(S\text{-}bz\text{-}thiosal)_2]$. *Polyhedron*, Accepted, In Press, n.d. ISSN: 0277-5387

Radojević, I., Čomić, Lj., Stefanović, O., Glodjović, V., Vasić, V., Vujić, J. & Trifunović, S. (2010). Antimicrobial activity ligands and their corresponding palladium(II) complexes against Aspergillus species. *Proceedings of ICAR* 2010, *International Conference on Antimicrobial Research*, pp. 475-476, Available from: http://www.formatex.org/icar2010/index.html, Valladolid, Spain, November 3-5, 2010.

Radojević, I., Stefanović, O., Radić, G., Glođović, V., Čomić, Lj. & Trifunović, S. (2011). *In vitro* antimicrobial activity of novel platinum(iv) and palladium(ii) complexes with 1,2-diphenyl-ethylenediamine-n,n'-di-3-propanoic acid. *Proceedings of Preclinical testing of active substances and cancer research, with International Symposium on Anti-Cancer Agents, Cardiotoxicity and Neurotoxicity*, pp. 10-11, ISBN: 978-86-7760-064-8, Kragujevac, Serbia, March 16-18, 2011.

Sarker, S.D., Nahar, L. & Kumarasamy, Y. (2007). Microtitre plate-based antibacterial assay incorporating resazurin as an indicator of cell growth, and its application in the in vitro antibacterial screening of phytochemicals. *Methods,* Vol.42, No.4, (August 2007), pp. 321-324,. ISSN: 1046-2023

Stanković, M., Radić, G., Glođović, V., Radojević, I., Stefanović, O., Čomić, Lj. & Trifunović, S. (2011a). Antimicrobial activity of ethyl esters of (*S,S*)-ethylenediamine-*N,N'*-di-2-propanoic and (*S,S*)- ethylenediamine-*N,N'*-di-2-(3-methyl)-butanoic acids and corresponding platinum(IV) complexes. *Proceedings of Preclinical testing of active substances and cancer research, with International Symposium on Anti-Cancer Agents, Cardiotoxicity and Neurotoxicity,* pp. 9-10, ISBN: 978-86-7760-064-8, Kragujevac, Serbia, March 16-18, 2011.

Stanković, M.Z., Radić, G.P., Glođović, V.V., Klisurić, O.R. & Trifunović, S.R. (2011b). Synthesis and crystal structure of tetrachoride-(O,O'-diethyl-(S,S)-ethylenediamine-N,N'-di-2-propanoato)-platinum(IV). *Proceedings of XVIII Conference of the Serbian Crystallographic Society,* pp. 42, ISBN: 978-86-7031-194-7, Fruška Gora, Serbia, June 2-4, 2011.

Stanković, M.Z., Radić, G.P., Glođović, V.V., Radojević, I.D., Stefanović, O.D., Čomić, L.R., Klisurić, O.R., Djinović, V.M. & Trifunović, S.R., (2011c). Stereospecific ligands and their complexes IX: Synthesis, characterization and antimicrobial activity of ethyl esters of (S,S)-ethylenediamine-N,N'-di-2-propanoic and (S,S)-ethylenediamine-N,N'-di-2-(3-methyl)-butanoic acids and corresponding platinum(IV) complexes: Crystal structure of tetrachloride-(O,O'-diethyl-(S,S)-ethylenediamine-N,N'-di-2-propanoato)-platinum(IV), [PtCl4(det-S,S-eddp)]. *Polyhedron,* In Press, doi: 10.1016/j.poly.2011.05.034, ISSN: 0277-5387

Vasić, G., Glodjović, V., Radojević, I., Stefanović, O., Čomić, Lj. & Trifunović, S. (2010). Stereospecific ligands and their complexes. V. Synthesis, characterization and antimicrobial activity of palladium (II) complexes with some alkyl esters of ethylenediamine-*N,N'*-di-*S,S*-2-propionic acid. *Inorganica Chimica Acta,* Vol.363, No.13, (October 2010), pp. 3606-3610, ISSN: 0020-1693

Vieira, L.M.M., de Almeida, M.V., Lourenço, M.C.S., Bezerra, F.A.F.M. & Fontes, A.P.S. (2009). Synthesis and antitubercular activity of palladium and platinum complexes with fluoroquinolones. *European Journal of Medicinal Chemistry,* Vol.44, No.10, (October 2009), pp. 4107- 4111, ISSN: 0223-5234

Vujić, J.M., Cvijović, M., Kaluđerović, G.N., Milovanović, M., Zmejkovski B.B., Volarević V., Arsenijević N., Sabo, T.J. & Trifunović, S.R. (2010). Palladium(II) complexes with R_2edda derived ligands. Part IV. *O,O'*-dialkyl esters of (*S,S*)-ethylenediamine-*N,N'*-di-2-(4-methyl)-pentanoic acid dihydrochloride and their palladium(II) complexes: Synthesis, characterization and *in vitro* antitumoral activity against chronic lymphocytic leukemia (CLL) cells. *European Journal of Medicinal Chemistry,* Vol.45, No.9, (September 2010), pp. 3601-3606, ISSN: 0223-5234

Vujić, J.M., Garcia-Granda, S., Menendez-Taboada, L. & Trifunović, S.R. (2011). Crystal structure of palladium(II) complex with *O,O'*- dipentil-etilenediamine- *N,N'*-di-(*S,S*)-2(4-methy)-pentanoate ligand. *Proceedings of XVIII Conference of the Serbian Crystallographic Society*, pp. 40, ISBN: 978-86-7031-194-7, Fruška Gora, Serbia, June 2-4, 2011.

16

The Prophylactic Use of Acidifiers as Antibacterial Agents in Swine

V. G. Papatsiros and C. Billinis
School of Veterinary Medicine,
University of Thessaly,
Greece

1. Introduction

In recent decades, acidifiers have emerged as viable alternatives to antibiotics in swine diets, in order to stimulate optimal growth performance and prevent various enteric diseases. Antimicrobials have been used for more than 50 years to enhance growth performance and prevent various pig diseases (Gustafson & Bowen, 1997). There is growing public awareness of the relationship between the feed medication with antimicrobials as growth promoters in livestock diets and the risk of developing cross-resistance of pathogens to antibiotics, threatening animals and human health (Corpet, 1996; Mathew et al. 2007; Hunter et al. 2010). During the last few years, as the use of antibiotics in pig diets has decreased, the use of acidifiers has increased.

Acidifiers can be in organic or inorganic acids or associated salts. As a group of chemicals, organic acids are considered to be any organic carboxylic acid of the general structure R-COOH (including fatty acids and amino acids) (Partanen & Mroz, 1999). Organic acids are widely distributed in plants and animals. They are also produced by microbial fermentation of carbohydrates and other fermentable material, predominantly in the large intestine of pigs. Table 1 shows the common name, chemical name, formula and first pKa- the pH at which the acid is half dissociated - of organic acids that are commonly used as dietary acidifiers in pigs (Partanen & Mroz, 1999).

The activity of most common acids, as well as their beneficial effects is shown in Table 2. Acidifiers have received much attention in pig production due to their beneficial effects on growth performance of pigs (Mahan et al. 1996; Partanen, 2001; Papatsiros et al. 2011). Many acids are available as sodium, potassium or calcium salts and several researchers have proposed their use because of their convenient application and their better effects than those of pure state acids. Table 3 shows a list of the most common salts of acids and their properties. The advantage of salts over free acids is that they are generally odourless and easier to handle in the feed manufacturing process due to their solid and less volatile form. Salts of acids are also less corrosive and may be more soluble in water than free acids (Partanen & Mroz, 1999). Although beneficial effects have been reported from trials using supplements of salts in pig diets (Table 3), other studies have not introduced any positive effects (Biagi et al. 2007; Weber & Kerr, 2008).

Acid	Chemical name	Formula	pKa	Solubility in water	Physical form	Odour / Taste	Production
Formic	Formic Acid	HCOOH	3.75	soluble in all proportions	Liquid (in pure state) Colourles transparent, fuming	Pungent odour Emission of strong odors	**Synthetically:** from methyl formate and formamide, by-product of acetic acid production and by laboratory methods **Naturally:** in many fruits (apples, strawberries and raspberries), honey and nettles
Acetic	Acetic Acid	CH3COOH	4.76	soluble in all proportions	Liquid Colourless, Very volatile	Pungent odour Sour taste	**Synthetically:** by various methods **Naturally:** by bacterial fermentation dietary fibre in the colon
Propionic	2-Propanoic Acid	CH3CH2COOH	4.88	soluble in all proportions	Liquid (in pure state) Oily	Pungent odour Emission of very strong smells	**Synthetically:** from ethyl alcohol and carbon monoxide **Naturally:** by bacteria of genus Propionibacterium, as the end product of their fermentation of dietary fibre in the colon
Butyric	Butanoic Acid	CH3CH2CH2 COOH	4.82	soluble in all proportions	Liquid Oily	Rancind, upleasant odour Acrid taste, with a sweetish after taste (similar to ether)	**Synthetically:** by fermentation of sugar or starch **Naturally:** by bacterial fermentation dietary fibre in the colon
Lactic	2-Hydroxypropanoic Acid	CH3CH(OH) COOH	3.83	very soluble	Liquid (in pure state) colourless or slightly yellow	Rancind, disagreeable odour Sour milk taste	**Synthetically:** from chemicals or organically as a byproduct of corn fermentation. **Naturally:** by bacterial fermentation of carbohydrates such as glucose, sucrose, or lactose by many species (Lactobacillus, Bifidobacterium, Streptococcus) Natural constituent of some feedstuffs
Sorbic	2,4-Hexandienoic Acid	CH3CH:CHCH: CHCOOH	4.76	sparingly soluble	Solid white crystalline powder or granule form	Distinctive odour Midly acrid and sour taste	**Synthetically:** by several different chemical pathways **Naturally:** in certain berries
Fumaric	2-Butenedioic Acid	COOHCH:CH COOH	3.02	sparingly soluble	Solid white crystalline powder	Odourless Tart flavour, fruit-like taste	**Synthetically:** from malic acid **Naturally:** in fumitory (Fumaria officinalis), bolete mushrooms (specifically Boletus fomentarius var. pseudo-igniarius), lichen, and Iceland moss.
Malic	Hydroxybutanedioic Acid	COOHCH2CH (OH)COOH	3.40	soluble in all proportions	Liquid / Solid white crystal or crystalline powder	Odourless Apple taste	**Synthetically:** from maleic anhydride **Naturally:** in apples and in many other fruits (mostly in unripe fruits)
Tartaric	2,3-Dihydroxy-Butanedioic Acid	COOHCH(OH) CH(OH) COOH	2.93	very soluble	Liquid	Strong acid taste	**Synthetically:** by chemical reactions of maleic anhydrid **Naturally:** in many plants (particularly grapes, bananas, tamarinds)
Citric	2-Hydroxy-1,2,3-Propanetricarboxylic Acid	COOHCH2C(OH) (COOH)CH2 COOH	3.13	very soluble	Solid	Odourless Pleasant sour taste	**Synthetically:** by a fermentation process **Naturally:** in a variety of fruits (most notably citrus fruits-lemons, limes) and vegetables
Benzoic acid	Benzenecarboxylic acid	C_6H_5COOH	4.19		Solid colorless crystalline	Highly fragrant odour	**Synthetically:** by partial oxidation of toluene with oxygen **Naturally:** in many plants as an intermediate in the formation of other compounds

Table 1. List of acids and their properties

Inorganic acids added to the pig diets are hydrochloric, sulfuric, and phosphoric acid. Organic and inorganic acids or/and salt form combinations are often used in commercially available acidifiers. The response to mixed acids is generally better than to single acids possibly due to dissociation properties of these acids at various locations in the pig's digestive tract (Hardy 2002; Franco et al. 2005; Partanen et al. 2007; Kasprowicz-Potocka et al. 2009).

Acid	Beneficial effects	
	Antimicrobial activity	**Improvement of growth performance**
Formic	***High antibacterial activity: Coliforms (E. coli - ETEC strains), Salmonella spp.*** Creus et al 2007; Jensen et al. 2001 Knarreborg et al. 2002; Naughton & Jensen 2001 Øverland et al 2007; Tsiloyiannis et al. 2001a	Canibe et al., 2005; Eisemann et al 2007 Jongbloed et al 2000; Mroz, et al 2000 Partanen et al. 2001a,b, 2007 Tsiloyiannis et al. 2001a
Acetic	***Active against bacteria - inhibits the growth of many species of bacteria (E. coli, Salmonella spp) - a lesser extent of yeasts and moulds*** Jensen et al. 2001; Partanen & Mroz 1999	Piva et al. 2002; Roth & Kirchgessner 1988 Valencia 2002
Propionic	***High spectrum of action against fungi and yeasts - Antibacterial activity: Coliforms (E. coli - ETEC strains), Salmonella spp.*** Foegeding & Busta, 1991; Jensen et al. 2001 Knarreborg et al. 2002; Naughton & Jensen 2001 Partanen & Mroz 1999; Tsiloyiannis et al. 2001a	Partanen et al 2007; Tsiloyiannis et al. 2001a
Butyric	***Antibacterial activity: Coliforms (E. coli)*** Knarreborg et al. 2002; Naughton & Jensen 2001	Mroz et al. 2000
Lactic	***High antibacterial activity: Coliforms (E. coli - ETEC strains), Salmonella spp. - Many moulds and yeasts can metabolize it*** Creus et al. 2007; Foegeding & Busta, 1991 Jensen et al. 2001; Knarreborg et al. 2002 Naughton & Jensen 2001; Piva & Grilli 2007 Tsiloyiannis et al. 2001a, b	Jongbloed et al. 2000 Tsiloyiannis et al. 2001a, b
Sorbic	***Antibacterial activity: Coliforms (E. coli - ETEC strains), Salmonella spp. - Active against yeasts, moulds, fungi*** Foegeding & Busta, 1991; Jensen et al. 2001 Øverland et al. 2007; Piva & Grilli 2007	Kirchgessner et al. 1995
Fumaric	***Antibacterial activity: (E. coli - ETEC strains, clostridia)*** Biagi et al. 2003; Knarreborg et al. 2002 Naughton & Jensen 2001; Owusu-Asiedu et al. 2003 Tsiloyiannis et al. 2001a	Giesting *et al.* 1991; Krause et al. 1994 Lawlor et al. 2006; Mroz et al. 2000 Owusu-Asiedu et al. 2003; Risley et al. 1991 Tsiloyiannis et al. 2001a
Malic	***Antibacterial activity: Coliforms (E. coli - ETEC strains) Active against yeasts -*** Partanen & Mroz 1999; Tsiloyiannis et al. 2001a	Kirchgessner et al. 1993; Krause et al. 1994 Tsiloyiannis et al. 2001a
Citric	***Antibacterial activity: Coliforms (E. coli)*** Foegeding & Busta, 1991 Tsiloyiannis et al. 2001a, b	Boling et al. 2000; Krause et al. 1994 Radcliffe et al. 1998; Risley et al 1991 Tsiloyiannis et al. 2001a, b
Benzoic acid	***Antibacterial activity: Coliforms (E. coli)*** Papatsiros et al. 2011; Piva & Grilli 2007	Bühler 2009; Kluge et al. 2006 Maribo et al. 2000

Table 2. Activity of most common acids - Beneficial effects

2. Mechanisms of action

Benefits from the use of dietary acidifiers include positive effects on growth performance and health status (Figure 1). Proposed mechanisms of action include reduction or stabilization of gastric pH, resulting in increased activity of proteolytic enzymes and gastric retention time, and thus led to improvement of protein digestion. Organic acids may influence mucosal morphology or induce alterations in gut microflora through bacteriostatic or bactericidal actions, as well as enhance endogenous enzyme activity, stimulate pancreatic secretions, and they also serve as substrates in intermediary metabolism (Partanen & Mroz, 1999. It is also hypothesized that acidifiers could be related to the reduction of gastric emptying rate, the energy source in intestine, the chelation of minerals, the stimulation of digestive enzymes and the provision of an energy source in the distal gastointestinal tract. Organic acid supplementation can reduce dietary buffering capacity, which is expected to slow down the proliferation and/or colonization of undesirable microbes, e.g. *Escherichia coli*, in the gastro-ileal region, resulting in reduction of scouring (Partanen & Mroz, 1999; Partanen, 2001).

Name	Physical form	Odour	Application possible in	Beneficial effects	
Ca/ K / Na salts				Antimicrobial activity	Improvement of growth performance
Ca salts (eg Ca-formate, Ca-propionate	Solid	Neutral	Feed	Bosi et al. 2005, 2007 Eidelsburger et al. 1992b	Bosi et al. 2006
K salts (eg K-diformate, K-sorbate)	Solid	Neutral	Feed	Canibe et al., 2001 Øverland et al. 2000 Taube et al. 2009	Roth et al. 1996 Mroz et al. 2002 Øverland et al. 2000 Papenbrock et al. 2005 Partanen et al. 2007 Paulicks et al. 2000 Windisch et al 2001
Na salts (eg Na - butyrate, Na- benzoate, Na - formate)	Solid	Rancid / Neutral	Feed	Pallauf & Huter 1993 Kirchgessner & Roth 1990	Piva et al. 2002b Partanen et al. 2007 Mazzoni et al. 2008 Le Gall et al. 2009
Ammonium salts (eg. Amm. formate)	Liquid		Water, feed		Eisemann & Heugte 2007

Table 3. List of most common salts of acids and their properties

The hypothesis that lowering dietary pH with organic acids reduces gastrointestinal pH has been tested in several studies. The low pH of gastric contents is thought to kill many ingested bacteria, while the gastric pH of newly weaned piglets is notably higher than of older pigs. So in newly weaned pigs this protective action may be enhanced by any low pH which is produced by acids in the feed in comparison to the gastric pH (Ravindran & Kornegay, 1993). Moreover, weaned piglets are physiologically immature and may not produce enough hydrochloric acid (HCl) to keep stomach pH at an optimum of approximately 3.5 (Ravindran & Kornegay, 1993). Weaned piglets are physiologically immature and may not produce enough hydrochloric acid (HCl) in order to keep stomach pH at an optimum of approximately 3.5.

The purpose of adding acidifiers in feed, is to lower the pH in the stomach below pH 5, resulting in an increased activity of proteolytic enzymes, improving protein digestibility and inhibiting the proliferation of pathogenic bacteria in the gastointestinal tract (Partanen & Mroz, 1999). At pH=3.5, digestion of proteins and populations of beneficial bacteria (lactobacilli) are maximized and harmful bacteria are inhibited. Organic acids, in a non dissociated form, are lipophilic and can diffuse across bacterial cell membranes to reach the interior of the cell. There, in the relatively high intracellular pH, organic acids dissociate and disrupt the bacterial cell function and this effect may be stronger in some bacteria than in others (Partanen, 2001). A low pH is required for conversion of pepsinogen to pepsin, which is the active form of the most important gastric proteolytic enzymes. Elevated gastric pH may lead to an ineffective gastric proteolysis as a result of limited pepsin activity, and then a greater proportion of protein may enter the small intestine intact, resulting in lower efficiency of digestion and scouring problems (Piva et al. 2002a). In addition, the pH activity profile of pepsin seems to be more active at a low pH. Some results indicate that short-chain fatty acids have a stimulatory effect on both endocrine and exocrine pancreatic secretions in pigs; pancreatic exocrine responses are ranked as: formic acid > lactic acid > acetic acid > butyric acid > propionic acid (Harada et al. 1986).

There are considerable variations in the results of response to acidification due to possible dietary and other factors such as (Mroz, 2005):

- feed palatability,
- type / pKa / dose of supplemented acids,
- type / composition of diets and their acid-base or buffering capacity,
- level of intraluminal production of acids in particular segments of the gastrointestinal tract by inhabiting microflora,
- quantity of fermentable carbohydrate substrates in the diet for bacterial growth,
- colonization and activity resulting in acids production,
- receptors for bacterial colonization on the epithelial villi,
- maternal immunity by vaccinations against pathogens,
- age of pigs,
- hygiene and welfare standards (density/pen, ventilation intensity and area, cleaning frequency etc.)

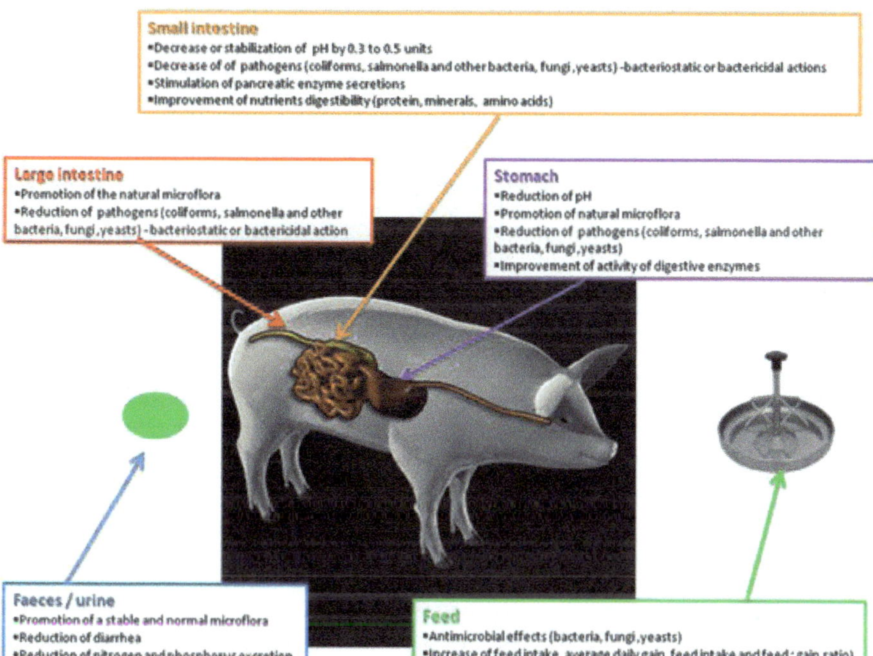

Fig. 1. Mode of action of acidifiers in pig

Dietary buffering capacity varies substantially between different feedstuffs (Bolduan et al. 1988a, 1988b). The acid-buffering capacity is lowest in cereals and cereal by-products, intermediate or high in protein feedstuffs and very high in mineral sources (Jasaitis et al. 1987). Addition of organic acids reduces dietary pH curvili nearly depending on the acid pKa value and buffering capacity (Bolduan et al. 1988a, 1988b) of the diet. The pH-lowering effect of different organic acids is reduced in the following order: tartaric acid>citric-acid>malic acid> fumaric acid>lactic and formic acids>acetic acid> propionic acid. Salts of organic acids have only a small influence on dietary pH, but the addition of protein and mineral sources to the diet weakens the pH-lowering effect of the acid (Roth & Kirchgessner, 1989). It seems reasonable to assume that the buffering capacity of feed can be considerably influenced by the selection of feed ingredients, and it may in part reflect the differences in the effectiveness of acidifiers. In general, organic acids lower dietary buffering capacity, whereas certain salts of organic acids can increase it.

The greatest acidification benefits have been observed in diets formulated from cereals and plant proteins, while the growth-promoting effect in diets containing milk products is small (Giesting et al. 1991). The latter presumably holds true when lactose in milk products is converted to lactic acid by lactobacilli in the stomach, creating the desired reduction in pH and thus reducing the need for diet acidification (Easter, 1988).

2.1 Antimicrobial activity

There are several commercial products with organic acids on the market, all with their own specific chemical and functional properties. As shown in Table 1, the inclusion of organic acids can reduce pH and the feed's buffering capacity, while their antimicrobial effect can prevent the growth of bacteria (especially Gram negative bacterial species, like *Salmonella spp.* and *E. coli*), yeasts and moulds. In the stomach, the pH is decreased, reducing the concentration of all the types of bacteria. In the small intestine, only the organic acids with antibacterial activity are able to inhibit bacteria growth. This is the main reason that the use of these acids has been proposed as a way of preventing or reducing the incidence of diarrhea in young pigs (Jensen et al. 2001; Tsiloyiannis et al. 2001a, 2001b: Piva et al. 2002a; Papatsiros et al. 2011). Thus, the organic acids are divided into two large groups. In the first group are included those with indirect effect on the decrease of the bacterial population by pH reduction and acting mainly on the stomach because the animal organism has the capability of preventing the decline in the acidity in the small intestine by buffering the medium with bicarbonate (fumaric, citric, malic and lactic acids). In the other group, are involved those organic acids (formic, acetic, propionic and sorbic acid), that have the ability to reduce the pH and affect directly Gram- bacteria by interfering in the bacterial cell with complex enzymes. These enzymes destroy the cell membrane and influence the mechanism of DNA duplication which prevents bacterial reproduction (Castro, 2005).

Many studies with dietary acidifiers have shown positive effects in improving growth rate, feed efficiency and acting against bacteria, yeast, fungi, moulds (Table 2), but others have found a negligible and even negative negative response (Radecki et al. 1988; Eidelsburger et al. 1992a; Manzanilla et al. 2004; Štukelj et al. 2010). It is likely that the antimicrobial effects of the organic acid ions, which act by controlling bacterial populations in the upper gastrointestinal tract, are responsible for the beneficial effects of these acids (Roth & Kirchgessner, 1998). Moreover, organic acids can also enhance the effects of antibiotics by improving their absorption (Radecki et al. 1988; Eidelsburger et al. 1992b). In addition, acidifiers can have an initial eradicating effect on bacteria in the feed (Lueck, 1980) and remain there as a first barrier, preventing re-contamination. Even *under good conditions,* all compound feeds have a certain content of germs (bacteria, viruses, fungi and protozoa), which may be proliferate under unfavourable harvest and storage conditions (Schöner, 2001). Preservatives reduce the incidence of germs in the feed and thus the quantity of germs consumed by the animals. The hygienic quality of feed is significantly improved. The addition of organic acid lowers the pH value of the feed and also provides acid-binding capacity.

In fact, organic acids associated with specific antimicrobial activity are short-chain acids (SCFA, C1–C7) and are either simple monocarboxylic acids such as formic, acetic, propionic and butyric acids, or carboxylic acids, bearing a hydroxyl group (usually on the carbon) such as lactic, malic, tartaric, and citric acids. Four organic acids commonly used in feed - formic, acetic, propionic and lactic acid - have a specific ability to penetrate the bacterial cell wall and kill bacteria by interfering with their metabolism. These acids only pass the membrane in non dissociated form. Their primary antimicrobial action (strain-selective growth inhibition or delay) is through pH depression of the diet. However, the ability of organic acids to change from undissociated to dissociated form, depending on the environmental pH, makes them effective antimicrobial agents. When acid is in the undissociated form it can freely diffuse through the semi permeable membrane of micro-organisms into their cell cytoplasm. Once inside the cell, where the pH is maintained near 7, the acid dissociates and suppress cell enzymes (decarboxylases and catalases) and nutrient transport systems (Lueck, 1980). The efficacy of an acid in inhibiting microbes is dependent on its pKa value which is the pH at which 50% of the acid is dissociated. Organic acids with higher pKa values are more effective preservatives and their antimicrobial efficacy is generally improved with increasing chain length and degree of unsaturation (Foegeding & Busta, 1991). In practice this means that the stomach pH has to be lower than 5 for optimal results. Without these specific antimicrobial acids, the pH needs to be very low to destroy bacteria. Some of the above acids' salts, have also shown to have benefits on growth performance. Other acids, such as sorbic and fumaric acid, have some antifungal activity and are short chain-carboxylic acids, containing double bonds. Organic acids are weak acids and are only partly dissociated; most of them, with antimicrobial activity, have a pKa 3 - 5.

In addition, each acid has its own spectrum of antimicrobial activity. Their antimicrobial effects vary from one acid to another, depending on concentration and pH (Chaveerach et al. 2002). For example, lactic acid is more effective in reducing gastric pH and coliforms (Jensen et al. 2001; Tsiloyiannis et al. 2001a; Øverland et al. 2007), whereas other acids, such as formic, propionic have broader antimicrobial activities and they can be effective against bacteria (e.g. coliforms, clostridia, Salmonella), fungi and yeast (Partanen & Mroz, 1999; Bosi et al. 2005; Creus et al. 2007; Øverland et al. 2007). Several reports have shown that the use of organic acids may reduce the coliform burden along the gastrointestinal tract (Bolduan et al. 1988b) and reduce scouring and piglet mortality or control postweaning diarrhea and edema disease in piglets (Tsiloyiannis et al. 2001a, 2001b; Piva et al. 2002a, Papatsiros et al. 2011). The following order of killing potency of coliform bacteria in the gastric digesta at pH 3, 4, and 5, are: propionic<formic<butyric<lactic<fumaric<benzoic were established (Naughton & Jensen, 2001; Knarreborg et al. 2002). Jensen et al. (2001) demonstrated that the potency of these acids against *Salmonella typhiumurium* in gastric digesta at pH4 was in the following order: acetic <formic < propionic < lactic < sorbic < benzoic. Inconsistent results may be due to the variety of diets with different buffering capacities that were used in these experiments. Bacteria are known to develop acid-resistance when exposed to acidic environments for some time (Mroz, 2005).

2.2 Antibacterial activity and growth promoting effects

The beneficial effects of organic acids and their salts on growth performance have been confirmed in several studies. Acidifiers added to pig diets may potentially help improve growth performance (Table 2 & 3) by improving digestive processes through several mechanisms. It is believed that acidifiers can enhance the growth performance by:

a. Improving gut health by promoting the beneficial bacterial growth, while inhibiting growth of pathogenic microbes (through reduction of pH and buffering capacity of diets). A reduced buffering capacity of diets containing organic acids is also expected to slow down the proliferation and/or colonization of undesirable microbes, e.g. *E. coli, clostridia* in the gastro-ileal region (jejunum, cecum) (Partanen & Mroz, 1999; Biagi et al. 2003). In addition organic acids or their salts could not improve the animal growth performance, but they could indirectly increase cecal pH and cecal ammonia concentrations (Biagi et al. 2007).
b. Stimulating - improving pancreatic secretions (Harada et al. 1986), which increase the digestibility, absorption and retention of protein and amino acids (Blank et al 1999, Kemme et al. 1999) and minerals (such as Ca, P, Mg and Zn - particularly Ca and P) (Jongbloed et al. 2000; Valencia, 2002; Omogbenigun et al. 2003) in the diet. Although opposite results have also been reported (Radecki et al. 1988), it is generally considered that dietary organic acids or their salts lower gastric pH, resulting in increased activity of proteolytic enzymes and gastric retention time.
c. Influencing of gut morphology by promoting changes in the digestive function and microbial ecology and fermentation (Piva et al. 2002a; Manzanilla et al. 2004). Some organic acids act positively on microbial growth and ammonia production by pig cecal microflora. Biagi and Piva (2007) noticed that various acids (formic, acetic, propionic, lactic, butyric, sorbic, fumaric, malic, citric, benzoic) can inhibit or enhance cecal bacterial activity and can positively influence pig cecal microflora *in vitro* fermentation reducing ammonia concentrations. It is well known that short-chain fatty acids (acetic, propionic and n-butyric acid) produced by microbial fermentation of carbohydrates stimulate epithelial cell proliferation (Sakata et al. 1995) and the strength of this effect is in the following order: n-butyric>propionic>acetic acid (Sakata, 1987). Increased epithelial cell proliferation has also been observed when short-chain fatty acids are orally given or provided by intravenous or gastrointestinal infusions (Sakata et al. 1995), since dietary organic acids can influence fermentation patterns in the small intestine, and may indirectly influence intestinal morphology. Kirchgessner and Roth (1988) have proposed that organic acids may stimulate intermediary metabolism resulting in improved energy or protein/amino acid utilization.

The use of some organic acids has been found to reduce the formation of biogenic amines (such as cadaverine and putrescin) that are produced particularly in high protein feeds and in feeds, containing added synthetic amino acids. Biogenic amines have unfavourable effects on growth and feed conversion. The growth stimulation effects of formic, acetic and propionic acids are partly caused by their inhibitory effect on biogenic amines (Eckel et al. 1992). However, a clear mode of action has not been fully described yet and the magnitude and consistency of the response may vary, depending on inclusion rate and other dietary factors.

The use of acidifiers appears to be most beneficial in the early period after weaning. Studies demonstrating the improved feed conversion ratio, weight gain and growth-promoting effects of acidifiers indicated that the effect was greater in young pigs than older pigs (Radcliffe et al. 1998; Øverland et al. 2000; Partanen et al. 2007), but there is some evidence that they may be beneficial for improvement of daily gain and feed efficiency in growing-finishing pigs (Øverland et al. 2000; Partanen et al. 2001a; Gauthier 2002; Canibe et al. 2005).

The results of trials including the addition of inorganic acids in pig diets has indicated positive responses on growth performance (Walsh et al. 2007; Stein, 2007), especially during the period after weaning (Mahan et al. 1996, 1999). However, the use of other inorganic acids, such as sulfuric acid, has not shown positive effects on growth performance (Ravindran & Kornegay, 1993). In addition, salts of organic acids, such as formates and diformates can be used to significantly improve growth rate and feed conversion in pigs (Table 3). However, there are also studies with no responses (Biagi et al. 2007) or involving risk factors (Pallauf & Huter, 1993; Øverland et al. 2000). For example, calcium formate decreased feed intake and daily gain (Pallauf & Huter, 1993; Øverland et al. 2000).

3. Risk factors of acidifier use

The use of organic acids in feed appears two main problems:

a. Acidifiers may have a negative effect on diet palatability, when they are added at excessive levels, resulting in lower feed intake or feed refusal (Partanen & Mroz, 1999). Certain acids, e.g. tartaric and formic acids have a strong odour and flavour, and an increasing dietary acid level, which is generally associated with a dramatic decrease in feed intake, as reflected by lower daily gains (Eckel et al. 1992; Kirchgessner et al. 1993). Addition of excessive amounts of formates to the diet may also disturb the acid-base status of pigs leading to metabolic acidosis, which results in decreased feed intake and slower growth (Giesting et al. 1991; Eckel et al. 1992; Eidelsburger et al. 1992e). Organic acids metabolized via the citric-acid cycle, e.g. fumaric and citric-acids, do not seem to cause acidosis, irrespective of their dietary inclusion (Eidelsburger et al. 1992c).
b. Acids at high levels in feed are corrosive to cement and galvanized steel in pig housing, resulting to pose handling and equipment issues to the feed manufacturer. For example, formic acid is the most corrosive for the equipment and it is dangerous to handle, while fumuric acid is easy to handle (Mateos et al. 1999). Salts of organic acids are generally odorless and less corrosive than their acid forms, making them easier to handle in the feed manufacturing process (Jacela et al. 2009).
c. The use of organic acids in their free form, at levels that have been proven to be efficacious, can cause palatability problems (Partanen, 2001), damage the stomachal and duodenal mucosas (Argenzio & Eisemann, 1996), as well as cause bone demineralization (Partanen & Mroz, 1999) and an acidic stress, inducing a resistance mechanism towards organic acids in certain bacteria (Bearson et al. 1997).

In order to minimize these effects, the natural buffering capacity of feeds (related to mineral and protein content) should be evaluated to determine the minimum effective amount of acid to use (Best, 2000). Another strategy to extend the effectiveness of acid supplements and reduce corrosion damage to housing materials is the use of a slow-release form of acids. It consists on the use of organic acids with fatty acids and mono- and diglycerides mixed to form microgranules. A study by Cerchiari (2000) showed that use of these granules, as compared to use of free acids, results in greater feed intake and growth.

4. Conclusion

Due to consumers' concern about the possibility of drug resistance of pathogenic bacteria, there is an urgent need to search for growth promoters other than antibiotics. Dietary acidifiers can actually become the most common and efficacious alternative solution to antibiotics, in order to improve health status and performance of pigs. The use of organic acids in pig production could be part of a general nutritional strategy focusing on a better gastrointestinal health; the goal is better productivity and better meat quality.

5. References

Argenzio, R.A. & Eisemann, J. (1996). Mechanisms of acid injury in porcine gastroesophageal mucosa. *American Journal of Veterinary Research* Vo. 57, No. 4, pp. 564-573, ISSN 0002-9645.

Bearson, S.; Bearson, B. & Foster, J.W. (1997). Acid stress responses in enterobacteria. *FEMS Microbiology Letters*, Vol. 147, No. 2, pp. 173-180, ISSN 1574-6968.

Best, P. (2000). Adding acids to swine diets. *Feed Management*, Vol. 51, No. 5, pp. 19–22, ISSN: 0014-956X.

Biagi, G. & Piva, A. (2007). In vitro effects of some organic acids on swine cecal microflora. *Italian Journal of Animal Science* Vol. 6, No. 4, pp. 361-374, ISSN 1594-4077.

Biagi, G.; Piva, A.; Hill, T.; Schneider, D.K. & Crenshaw, T.D. (2003). Low buffering capacity diets with added organic acids as a substitute for antibiotics in diets for weaned pigs, *Proceedings of the 9th International Symposium on Digestive Physiology in Pigs*, pp. 217-219, (Ball R, ed.) University of Alberta, Department of Agriculture, Food and Nutritional Science, Edmonton, Banff, Alberta, Canada, May 14-17, 2003.

Biagi, G.; Piva, A.; Moschini, M.; Vezzali, E. & Roth, F. (2007). Performance, intestinal microflora, and wall morphology of weanling pigs fed sodium butyrate. *Journal of Animal Science*, Vol. 85, No. 5, pp. 1184-1191, ISSN 0021-8812.

Blank, R.; Mosenthin, R.; Sauer, W.C.; & Huang, S. (1999). Effect of fumaric acid and dietary buffering capacity on ileal and fecal amino acid digestibilities in early weaned pigs. *Journal of Animal Science*, Vol. 77, No. 11, pp. 2974 - 2984, ISSN 0021-8812.

Bolduan, G.; Jung, H.; Schneider, R.; Block, J. & Klenke, B. (1988a). Influence of propionic and formic acids on piglets. *Journal of Animal Physiology and Animal Nutrition*, Vol. 59, No. 2, pp. 72-78, ISSN 1439-0396.

Bolduan, G.; Jung, H.; Schneider, R.; Block, J. & Klenke, B. (1988b) Influence of fumaric acid and propanediol formate on piglets. *Journal of Animal Physiology and Animal Nutrition* 59, No. 1-5, pp. 143 - 149, ISSN 1439-0396.

Boling, S.D.; Webel, D.M.; Mavromichalis, I.; Parsons, C.M. & Baker, D.H. (2000). The effects of citric acid on phytate-phosphorus utilization in young chicks and pigs. *Journal of Animal Science* 78, No. 3, pp. 682-689, ISSN 0021-8812.

Bosi, P.; Mazzoni, M.; Filippi De, S.; Trevisi, P.; Casini, L.; Petrosino, G. & Lalatta-Costerbosa, G. (2006). Nutrient Physiology, Metabolism, and Nutrient-Nutrient Interactions. A Continuous Dietary Supply of Free Calcium Formate Negatively Affects the Parietal Cell Population and Gastric RNA Expression for H1/K1-ATPase in Weaning Pigs. *Journal of Nutrition*, Vol. 136, No. 5, pp. 1229-1235, ISSN 1541-6100.

Bosi, P., Sarli, G., Casini, L., De Filippi, S., Trevisi, P., Mazzoni, M. & Merialdi, G. (2007). The influence of fat protection of calcium formate on growth and intestinal defence in Escherichia coli K88-challenged weanling pigs. *Animal Feed Science and Technology*, Vol. 139, No. 9, pp. 170-185, ISSN ISSN: 0377-8401.

Bosi, P.; Sarli, G.; Casini, L.; De Filippi, S.; Trevisi, P.; Mazzoni, M. & Merialdi, G. (2005). Effect of dietary addition of free or fat-protected calcium formate on growth,intestinal morphology and health of Escherichia coli k88 challenged weaning pigs. Italian Journal of Animal Science, Vol. 4, No. 2, pp. 452-454, ISSN 1594-4077.

Bühler, K.; Buche r B.; Wenk, C. & Broz, J. (2009). Influence of benzoic acid in high fibre diets on nutrient digestibility and VFA production in growing/finishing pigs. *Archives of Animal Nutrition,* Vol. 63, No. 2, pp. 127-136, ISSN 1477-2817.

Canibe, N.; Højberg, O, Højsgaard S. & Jensen B.B. (2005). Feed physical form and formic acid addition to the feed affect the gastrointestinal ecology and growth performance of growing pigs. *Journal of Animal Science, Vol.* 83, No. 6, pp. 1287-1302, ISSN 0021-8812.

Canibe, N.; Steien, S.H.; Overland M. & Jensen, B.B. (2001). Effect of K-diformate in starter diets on acidiy, microflora, and the amount of organic acids in the digestive tract of piglets, and on gastric alterations. *Journal of Animal Science,* Vol. 79, No. 8, pp. 2123 - 2133, ISSN 0021-8812.

Castro, M. (2005). Use of additives on the feeding of monogastric animals. *Cuban Journal of Agricultural Science* 39, p. 439, ISSN 0253-5815.

Cerchiari, E. (2000). Active matrix technology making more of acids. *Pig Progress,* Vol. 16, No. 4, pp. 34-35, ISSN 0031-9775.

Chaveerach, P; Keuzenkamp, D.A; Urlings, H.A.P; Lipman, J.A. & van Knapen, F. (2002). In vitro study on the effect of organic acids on Campylobacter jejuni /coli populations in mixtures of water and feed. *Poultry Science,* Vol. 81, No. 5, pp. 621–628, ISSN 1537-0437.

Corpet, D.E. (1996). Microbiological hazards for humans of antimicrobial growth promoter use in animal production. *Veterinary Medical Review,* Vol. 147, No. 12, pp. 851-862, ISSN 0341-9851.

Creus, E.; Perez, J.F.; Peralta, B.; Baucells, F. & Mateu, E. (2007). Effect of acidified feed on the prevalence of Salmonella in market-age pigs. *Zoonoses and Public Health,* Vol. 54, No. 8, pp. 314-319, ISSN 1863-2378.

Easter, R.A. (1988). *Acidification of diets for pigs.* In Recent Advances in Animal Nutrition, ISBN 0-407-01162-5, pp. 61-71 (Haresign W & Cole DJA, eds). London, Butterworths, UK.

Eckel, B.; Kirchgessner, M, & Roth, F.X. (1992). Influence of formic acid on daily weight gain, feed intake, feed conversion rate and digestibility. *Journal of Animal Physiology and Animal Nutrition,* Vol. 67, No. 2, pp. 93-100, ISSN 1439-0396.

Eidelsburger, U.; Kirchgessner, M. & Roth, F.X. (1992a). Influence of formic acid on daily weight gain, feed intake, feed conversion rate and digestibility. *Journal of Animal Physiology and Animal Nutrition,* Vol. 68, No. 2, pp. 82-92, ISSN 1439-0396.

Eidelsburger, U.; Kirchgessner, M. & Roth, F.X. (1992b). Influence of formic acid, calcium formate and sodium hydrogen carbonate on dry matter content, pH value, concentration of carbonic acids and ammonia in different segments of the gastrointestinal tract. *Journal of Animal Physiology and Animal Nutrition,* Vol. 68, No. 2, pp. 20-32, ISSN 1439-0396.

Eidelsburger, U.; Kirchgessner, M. & Roth, F.X. (1992c). Influence of fumaric acid, hydrochloric acid, sodium formate, tylosin and toyocerin on acid base status. 13. Nutritive value of organic acids in piglet rearing. *Journal of Animal Physiology and Animal Nutrition,* Vol. 68, No. 3, pp. 165- 173, ISSN 1439-0396.

Eidelsburger, U.; Roth FX, & Kirchgessner, M. (1992e). Influence of formic acid, calcium formate and sodium bicarbonate on acid-base status. 9. Effect of organic acids in piglet rearing. *Journal of Animal Physiology and Animal Nutrition, Vol.* 68, pp. 33- 42, ISSN 1439-0396.

Eisemann, J.H. & van Heugten, E. (2007). Response of pig dietary inclusion of formic acid and ammonium formate. *Journal of Animal Science,* Vol. 85, No. 6, pp. 1530-1539, ISSN 0021-8812.

Foegeding, P.M. & Busta F.F. (1991). *Chemical food preservatives.* In: Disinfection, Sterilization and Preservation, ISBN 0812113640, pp. 802- 832 (Block SS, ed). Lea & Febiger, Malvern, Philadelphia, PA.

Franco, L.D.; Fondevila, M.; Lobera, M.B. & Castrillo, C. (2005). Effects of combinations of organic acids in weaned pig diets on microbial species of digestive tract contents and their response on digestibility. *Journal of Animal Physiology and Animal Nutrition,* Vol. 89, No. 3-6, pp. 88–93, ISSN 1439-0396.

Gauthier, R. (2002). *The mode of action of acidifiers and the interest they generate in the growing-finishing phase.* In: Current Developments in Pig Production, French Association of Swine Practitioners, p. 16, Maisons-Alfort, France.

Giesting, D.W.; Ross, M.A. & Easter, R.A. (1991). Evaluation of the effect of fumaric acid and sodium bicarbonate addition on performance of starter pigs fed diets of different types. *Journal of Animal Science,* Vol. 69, No. 6, pp. 2489 – 2496, ISSN 0021-8812.

Gustafson, R.H., Bowen, R.E. (1997). Antibiotic use in animal agriculture. *Journal* of *Applied Microbiology,* Vol. 83, No. 5, pp. 531-541, ISSN: 1365-2672.

Harada, E.; Niiyama, M, & Syuto, B. (1986). Comparison of pancreatic exocrine secretion via endogenous secretin by intestinal infusion of hydrochloric acid and monocarboxylic acid in anesthetized piglets. *Japanese Journal of Physiology,* Vol. 36, No. 5, pp. 843- 856, ISSN 1881-1396.

Hardy, B. (2002). The issue of antibiotic use in the livestock industry. What have we learned? *Animal Biotechnology,* Vol. 13, No. 1, pp. 129–147, ISSN 1049-5398.

Hunter, P.A.; Dawson, S.; French, G.L.; Goossens, H.; Hawkey, P.M.;Kuijper, E.J.; Nathwani D.; Taylor, D.J.; Teale, C.J.; Warren, R.E.; Wilcox, M.H.; Woodford, N.; Wulf, M.W. & Piddock L.J.V. (2010). Antimicrobial-resistant pathogens in animals and man: prescribing, practices and policies. *Journal of Antimicrobial Chemotherapy,* Vol. 65, No. 1, pp. 3-17, ISSN 1460-2091.

Jacela, J.Y.; DeRouchey, J.M.; Tokach, M.D.; Goodband, R.D.; Nelssen, J.L.; Renter, D.G. & Dritz S.S. (2009). Feed additives for swine: Fact sheets – acidifiers and antibiotics. *Journal of Swine Health and Production,* Vol. 17, No. 5, pp. 270–275, ISSN 1066-4963.

Jasaitis, D.K.; Wohlt, J.E. & Evans, J.L. (1987). Influence of feed-ion content on buffering capacity of ruminant feedstuffs in-vitro. *Journal of Dairy Science,* Vol. 70, No. 7, pp. 1391–1403, ISSN 0022-0302.

Jensen BB, Mikkelsen LL, Canibe N, & Høyberg O (2001). *Salmonella in slaughter pigs.* Annual Report 2001 from the Danish Institute of Agricultural Sciences, p.23, Research Centre Foulum, Tjele, Denmark.

Jongbloed, A.W.; Mroz, Z.; van der Weij-Jongbloed, R. & Kemme, P.A. (2000). The effects of microbial phytase, organic acids and their interaction in diets for growing pigs. *Livestock Production Science,* Vol. 67, No. 1/2, pp. 113–122, ISSN 1871-1413.

Kasprowicz-Potocka, M.; Frankiewicz A.; Selwet, M. & Chilomer, K. (2009). Effect of salts and organic acids on metabolite production and microbial parameters of piglets' digestive tract. *Livestock Production Science,* Vol. 126, No. 1-3, pp. 310-313, ISSN 1871-1413.

Kemme, P.A.; Jongbloed, A.W.; Mroz, Z.; Kogut, J. & Beynen, A.C. (1999). Digestibility of nutrients in growing-finishing pigs is affected by Aspergillus niger phytase, phytate and lactic acid levels 1. Apparent ileal digestibility of amino acids. *Livestock Production Science,* Vol. 58, No. 2, pp. 107–117, ISSN 1871-1413.

Kirchgessner, M. & Roth F.X. (1988). Energy value of organic acids in the rearing of piglets and the fattening of pigs. *Übersichten zur Tierernährung,* Vol. 16, pp. 93-108, ISSN 0303-6340.

Kirchgessner, M. & Roth, F.X. (1990). Nutritive effect of calcium formate in combinateion with free acids in the feeding of piglets. *Agribiological Research* 43, No. 1, pp. 53- 64, ISSN 0938-0337.

Kirchgessner, M.; Roth, F.X., & Eidelsburger, U. (1993). Nutritive efficiency of tartaric acid and malic acid in the rearing of piglets. *Journal of Animal Physiology and Animal Nutrition,* Vol. 70, No. 4-5, pp. 216-224, ISSN 1439-0396.

Kirchgessner, M.; Roth, F.X. & Paulicks, B.R. (1995). Nutritive value of sorbic acid in piglet rearing. *Journal of Animal Physiology and Animal Nutrition* 74, No. 4/5, pp. 235 - 242, ISSN 1439-0396.

Kluge, H.; Broz J.; & Eder, K. (2006). Effect of benzoic acid on growth performance, nutrient digestibility, nitrogen balance, gastrointestinal microflora and parameters of microbial metabolism in piglets. *Journal of Animal Physiology and Animal Nutrition,* Vol. 90, No. 7-8, pp. 316-324, ISSN 1439-0396.

Knarreborg, A.; Miquel, N.; Granli, T. & Jensen, B.B. (2002). Establishment and application of an in vitro methodology to study the effects of organic acids on coliform and lactic acid bacteria in the proximal part of the gastrointestinal tract of piglets. *Animal Feed Science and Technology,* Vol. 99, No. 1-4, pp. 131-140, ISSN: 0377-8401.

Krause, D.O.; Harrison, P.C. & Easter, R.A. (1994). Characterization of the nutritional interactions between organic acids and inorganic bases in the pig and chick. *Journal of Animal Science,* Vol. 72, No. 5, pp. 1257-1262, ISSN 0021-8812.

Lawlor, P.G.; Lynch, P.B, & Caffrey, P.J. (2006). Effect of fumaric acid, calcium formate and mineral levels in diets on the intake and growth performance of newly weaned pigs. *Irish Journal of Agricultural and Food Research* 45, No. 1, pp. 61–71, ISSN 0791-6833.

Le Gall, M.; Gallois, M.; Sève, B.; Louveau, I.; Holst, J.J.; Oswald, I.P.; Lallès, J.P. & Guilloteau, P. (2009). Comparative effect of orally administered sodium butyrate before or after weaning on growth and several indices of gastrointestinal biology of piglets. *British Journal of Nutrition,* Vol. 102, No. 9, pp. 1285-1296, ISSN 1475-2662

Lueck, E. (1980). *Antimicrobial Food Additives,* ISBN 354-0100- 563, Springer-Verlag, Berlin.

Mahan, D.C.; Newton, E.A. & Cera, K.R. (1996). Effect of supplemental sodium phosphate or hydrochloric acid in starter diets containing dried whey. *Journal of Animal Science* 74, No. 6, pp. 1217 -1222, ISSN 0021-8812.

Mahan, D.C.; Wiseman, T.D.; Weaver, E. & Russell, L. (1999). Effect of supplemental sodium chloride and hydrochloric acid added to initial diets containing sprayed-dried blood plasma and lactose on resulting performance and nitrogen digestibility of 3-week-old weaned pigs. *Journal of Animal Science* 77, No. 11, pp. 3016-3021, ISSN 0021-8812.

Manzanilla, E.G.; Perez, J.F.; Martin, M.; Kamel, C.; Baucells, F. & Gasa, J. (2004). Effect of plant extracts and formic acid on the intestinal equilibrium of early-weaned pigs. *Journal of Animal Science* 82, No. 11, pp. 3210-3218, ISSN 0021-8812.

Maribo, H.; Jensen, B.B. & Hedemann, M.S. (2000). *Different doses of organic acids to piglets.* Danish Bacon and Meat Council, Report no. 469, Copenhagen, Denmark.

Mateos, G.G.; Salado S, & Gracia, M.I. (1999). *Uso de aditivos como mejorantes de la calidad de las dietas para monogástricos: enzimas y acidificantes.* V Encuentro Regional de Producción de animales Monogástricos. Universidad de Maracay, Venezuela.

Mathew, A.G.; Cissell, R., & Liamthong, S. (2007). Antibiotic Resistance in Bacteria Associated with Food Animals: A United States Perspective of Livestock Production. *Foodborne Pathogens and Disease*, Vol. 4, No. 2, pp. 115-133, ISSN 1535-3141.

Mazzon,i M.; Le Gall, M.; De Filippi, S.; Minieri, L.; Trevisi, P.; Wolinski, J.; Lalatta-Costerbosa, G.; Lallès, J.P.; Guilloteau P. & Bosi P. (2008). Supplemental sodium butyrate stimulates different gastric cells in weaned pigs. *Journal of Nutrition* 138, No. 8, pp.1426-1431, ISSN 1541-6100.

Mroz, Z. (2005). Organic Acids as Potential Alternatives to Antibiotic Growth Promoters for Pigs. *Advances in Pork Production*, Vol. 16, pp. 169 -182, ISSN 1489-1395.

Mroz, Z.; Reese, D.E.; Overland, M.; van Diepen, J.T. & Kogut, J. (2002). The effects of potassium diformate and its molecular constituents on the apparent ileal and fecal digestibility and retention of nutrients in growing-finishing pigs. *Journal of Animal Science*, Vol. 80, No. 3, pp. 681-690, ISSN 0021-8812.

Mroz, Z.; Jongbloed, A.W.;Partanen, K.H.; Vreman, K.; Kemme, P.A. & Kogut, J. (2000). The effects of calcium benzoate in diets with or without organic acids on dietary buffering capacity, apparent digestibility, retention of nutrients, and manure characteristics in swine. *Journal of Animal Science*, Vol. 78, No. 10, pp. 2622-2632, ISSN 0021-8812.

Naughton, P.J. & Jensen, B.B. (2001). A bioreactor system to study survival of Salmonella typhimurium in pig gut content. *Berliner und Münchener Tierärztliche Wochenschrift*, Vol. 114, No. 1, pp. 1-4, *ISSN*: 0005-9366.

Omogbenigun, F.O.; Nyachoti, C.M. & Slominski, B.A. (2003). The effect of supplementing microbial phytase and organic acids to a corn-soybean based diet fed to early-weaned pigs. *Journal of Animal Science*, Vol. 81, No. 7, pp. 1806–1813, ISSN 0021-8812.

Øverland, M.; Granli, T.; Kjos, N.P.; Fjetland, O.; Steien, S.H. & Stokstad, M. (2000). Effect of dietary formates on growth performance, carcass traits, sensory quality, intestinal microflora, and stomach alterations in growing-finishing pigs. *Journal of Animal Science*, Vol. 78, No. 7, pp. 1875–1884, ISSN 0021-8812.

Øverland, M.; Kjos, N.P.; Borg, M. & Sørum, H. (2007). Organic acids in diets for entire male pigs. *Livestock Production Science*, Vol. 109, No. 1-30, pp. 170-173, ISSN 1871-1413.

Owusu-Asiedu, A.; Nyachoti, C.M.; & Marquardt, R.R. (2003). Response of early-weaned pigs to an enterotoxigenic escherichia coli (K88) challenge when fed diets containing spray-dried porcine plasma or pea protein isolate plus egg yolk antibody, zinc oxide, fumaric acid, or antibiotic. *Journal of Animal Science*, Vol. 81, No. 7, pp. 1790-1798, ISSN 0021-8812.

Pallauf, J. & Huter J. (1993). Studies on the influence of calcium formate on growth, digestibility of crude nutrients, nitrogen balance and calcium retention in weaned piglets. *Animal Feed Science and Technology*, Vol. 43, No. 1-2, pp. 65-76, ISSN 1365-2052.

Papatsiros, V.G.; Tassis, P.D.; Tzika, E.D.; Papaioannou, D.S.; Petridou, E.; Alexopoulos, C.; & Kyriakis, S.C. (2011). Effect of benzoic acid and combination of benzoic acid with probiotic containing *Bacillus cereus var. Toyoi* in weaned pig nutrition. *Polish Journal of Veterinary Science*, Vol. 14, No. 1, pp. 117-125, ISSN 1505-1773.

Papenbrock, S.; Stemme, K.; Amtsberg, G.; Verspohl, J. & Kamphues, J. (2005). Investigations on prophylactic effects of coarse feed structure and/or potassium diformate on the microflora in the digestive tract of weaned piglets experimentally infected with Salmonella Derby. *Journal of Animal Physiology and Animal Nutrition*, Vol. 89, No. 3-6, pp. 84-87, ISSN 1439-0396.

Partanen, H.K. & Mroz, Z. (1999). Organic acids for performance enhancement in pig diets. *Nutrition Research Reviews*, Vol. 12, No. 1, pp. 117-145, ISSN 1475-2700.

Partanen, K. (2001). *Organic acids – Their efficacy and modes of action in pigs.* In: Gut Environment of Pigs, Piva, A., Bach Knudsen K.E. and Lindberg, J.E. (Eds), pp. 201-218, ISBN ISBN, 978-1-897676-77-6, Nottingham University Press, Nottingham, UK.

Partanen, K.; Siljander-Rasi, H.; Alaviuhkola, T.; Suomi, K. & Fossi, M. (2001a). Performance of growing-finishing pigs fed medium- or high-fibre diets supplemented with avilamycin, formic acid or formic acid-sorbate blend. *Livestock Production Science,* Vol. 73, No. 2-3, pp. 139-152, ISSN 1871-1413.

Partanen, K.; Jalava, T.; Valaja, J.; Perttila, S.; Siljander-Rasi, H. & Lindeberg, H. (2001b). Effect of dietary carbadox or formic acid and fibre level on ileal and faecal nutrient digestibility and microbial metabolite concentration in ileal digesta of the pig. *Animal Feed Science and Technology,* Vol. 93, No. 3, pp.137-155, ISSN 1365-2052.

Partanen, K., Siljander-Rasi, H., Pentikäinen, J., Pelkonen, S., & Fossi, M. (2007). Effects of weaning age and formic acid-based feed additives on pigs from weaning to slaughter. *Archives of Animal Nutrition,* Vol. 61, No. 5, pp. 336-356, ISSN 1477-2817.

Paulicks, B.R.; Roth, F.X. & Kirchgessner, M. (2000). Effects of potassium diformate (Formi® LHS) in combination with different grains and energy densities in the feed on growth performance of weaned piglets. *Journal of Animal Physiology and Animal Nutrition,* Vol. 84, No. 3–4, pp. 102–111, ISSN 1439-0396.

Piva, A. & Grilli, E. (2007). Role of benzoic, lactic and sorbic acid in vitro swine cecal fermentation. *Veterinary Research Communications,* Vol. 31, No. 1, pp. 401–404, ISSN: 1573-7446.

Piva, A.; Casadei, G. & Biagi, G. (2002a) An organic acid blend can modulate swine intestinal fermentation and reduce microbial proteolysis. *Canadian Journal of Animal Science,* Vol. 82, No. 4, pp. 527-532, ISSN 1918-1825.

Piva, A.; Morlacchini, M.; Casadei, G., Gatta, P.P.; Biagi, G. & Prandini, A. (2002b). Sodium butyrate improves growth performance of weaned piglets during the first period after weaning. *Italian Journal of Animal Science,* Vol. 1, No. 1, pp. 35–41, ISSN 1594-4077.

Radcliffe, J.S.; Zhang, Z. & Kornegay, E.T. (1998). The effects of microbial phytase, citric acid, and their interaction in a corn-soybean meal-based diet for weanling pigs. *Journal of Animal Science,* Vol. 76, No. 7, pp. 1880-1886, ISSN 0021-8812.

Radecki, S.V.; Juhl, M.R. & Miller, E.R. (1988). Fumaric and citric acids as feed additives in starter pig diets: Effect on performance and nutrient balance. *Journal of Animal Science,* Vol. 66, No. 10, pp. 2598-2605, ISSN 0021-8812.

Ravindran, V. & Kornegay E.T. (1993). Acidification of weaner pig diets: A review. *Journal of the Science of Food and Agriculture,* Vol. 62, No. 4, pp. 313–322, ISSN 1097-0010.

Risley, C.R.; Komegay E.T.; Lindemann, M.D. & Weakland, S.M. (1991). Effects of organic acids with and without a microbial culture on performance and gastrointestinal tract measurements of weanling pigs. *Animal Feed Science and Technology,* Vol. 35, No. 3, pp. 259-270, ISSN 1365-2052.

Roth, F.X. & Kirchgessner, M. (1988). Use of acetic acid in pig nutrition. *Landwirtschaftliche Forschung,* Vol. 41, No. 3-4, pp. 253-258, ISSN 0023-8147.

Roth, F.X. & Kirchgessner M. (1989). Significance of dietary pH and buffering capacity in piglet nutrition. 1. pH and buffering capacity in diets supplemented with organic acids. *Landwirtschaftliche Forschung,* Vol. 42, No. 2-3, pp. 157-167, ISSN 0023-8147.

Roth, F.X. & Kirchgessner, M. (1998). Organic acids as feed additives for young pigs—nutritional and gastrointestinal effects. *Journal of Animal Feed Science,* Vol. 7, No. 1, pp. 25–33, ISSN 0377-8401.

Roth, F.X.; Kirchgessner, M. & Paulicks, B.R. (1996). Nutritive use of feed additives based on diformates in the rearing and fattening of pigs and their effects on performance.

Agribiological Research Zeitschrift für Agrarbiologie-Agrikulturchemie-Ökologie, Vol. 49, No. 4, pp. 307–317, ISSN 0938-0337.

Sakata, T. (1987). Stimulatory effect of short-chain fatty acids on epithelial cell proliferation in the rat intestine: a possible explanation for trophic effects of fermentable fibre, gut microbes and luminal trophic factors. *British Journal of Nutrition,* Vol. 58, No. 1, pp. 95-103, ISSN 1475-2662.

Sakata, T.; Adachi, M.; Hashida, M.; Sato, N. & Kojima, T. (1995). Effect of n-butyric acid on epithelial cell proliferation of pig colonic mucosa in short-term culture. *Deutsche Tieraérztliche Wochenschrift,* Vol. 102, No. 4, pp. 163- 164, ISSN 0341-6593.

Schöner, F.J. (2001). Nutritional effects of organic acids. *Cahiers Options Méditerranéennes,* Vol. 54, 55-61, ISSN 0253-1542.

Stein, H. (2007). *Feeding the pig's immune system and alternatives to antibiotics,* Proceedings of London Swine Conference pp. 65–82, ISBN 978-0-9688770-6-7, London, Ontario, Canada.

Štukelj, M.; Valencak, Z.; Krsnik, M. & Svete, A.N. (2010). The effect of the combination of acids and tannin in diet on the performance and selected biochemical, haematological and antioxidant enzyme parameters in grower pigs. *Acta Veterinaria Scandinavica,* Vol. 52, No. 1, p. 19, ISSN 1751-0147.

Taube, V.A.; Neu, M.E.; Hassan, Y., Verspohl, J.; Beyerbach, M. & Kamphues, J. (2009). Effects of dietary additives (potassium diformate/organic acids) as well as influences of grinding intensity (coarse/fine) of diets for weaned piglets experimentally infected with Salmonella Derby or Escherichia coli. *Journal of Animal Physiology and Animal Nutrition,* Vol. 93, No. 3, pp. 350-358, ISSN 1439-0396.

Tsiloyiannis, V.K.; Kyriakis, S.C.; Vlemmas, J. & Sarris, K. (2001a). The effect of organic acids on the control of porcine post-weaning diarrhoea. *Research in Veterinary Science,* Vol. 70, No. 3, pp. 287-293, ISSN 0034-5288.

Tsiloyiannis, V.K.; Kyriakis, S.C.; Vlemmas, J. & Sarris, K. (2001b). The effect of organic acids on the control of post-weaning oedema disease of piglets. *Research in Veterinary Science,* Vol. 70, No. 3, pp. 281-285, ISSN 0034-5288.

Valencia, Z. (2002). Phytase and acetic acid supplementation in the diet of early weaned piglets: effect on performance and apparent nutrient digestibility. *Nutrition Research,* Vol. 22, No. 5, pp. 623-632, ISSN 0271-5317.

Walsh, M.C.; Sholly, D.M.; Hinson, R.B.; Saddoris, K.L.; Sutton, A.L.; Radcliffe, J.S.; Odgaard, R.; Murphy J. & Richert, B.T. (2007). Effects of water and diet acidifi cation with and without antibiotics on weanling pig growth and microbial shedding. *Journal of Animal Science,* Vol. 85, No. 7, pp. 1799–1808, ISSN 0021-8812.

Weber, T.E. & Kerr, B.J. (2008). Effect of sodium butyrate on growth performance and response to lipopolysaccharide in weanling pigs. *Journal of Animal Science,* Vol. 86, No. 2, pp. 442-450, ISSN 0021-8812.

Windisch, W.M.; Gotterbarm, G.G. & Roth, F.X. (2001). Effect of potassium diformate in combination with different amounts and sources of excessive dietary copper on production performance in weaning piglets. *Archiv für Tierernährung,* Vol. 54, No. 2, pp. 87-100, ISSN 0003-942X.

17

Andrographis paniculata (Burm.f) Wall. ex Ness: A Potent Antibacterial Plant

Qamar Uddin Ahmed[1], Othman Abd. Samah[2,*] and Abubakar Sule[2]
[1]*Department of Pharmaceutical Chemistry, Faculty of Pharmacy,*
[2]*Department of Biomedical Science, Faculty of Allied Health Sciences,*
International Islamic University Malaysia, Kuantan, Pahang,
Malaysia

1. Introduction

Antibacterial agents of plant origin have vast therapeutic potential. They are valuable in the treatment of infectious diseases while simultaneously extenuating many of the side effects that are often associated with synthetic antibacterial agents. The beneficial medicinal effects of plant materials typically result from the combinations of secondary metabolites such as alkaloids, steroids, tannins, phenol compounds, flavonoids and resins fatty acids gums which are capable of producing definite physiological action on body (Paul *et al.*, 2006). Nowadays, multiple drug resistance has developed due to indiscriminate use of commercial antimicrobial drugs commonly used in the treatment of infectious disease. In addition to this problem, antibiotics are sometimes associated with adverse side effects on the host including hypersensitivity, immune-suppression and allergic reactions. This situation forced scientists to search for new antimicrobial substances. Giving the alarming incidence of antibiotic resistance in bacteria of medical importance, there is a constant need for new and effective therapeutic agents. Therefore, there is a need to develop alternative antimicrobial drugs for the treatment of infectious diseases from medicinal plants. Biodiversity is a precious source for modern biotechnology. It is a source which potentially holds innovative and sustainable solutions to a broad range of important problems for modern society. Improved cooperation between the natural product chemists and the microbiologists is a productive step to speed up the process of evaluating these potentialities. Moreover, microbiologists and natural product chemists in tropical countries, with the richest flora and fauna placed right at their door step have a very central position. They are essential for building up international scientific cooperation, with the objective of expanding our understanding of biological and biochemical diversity, and based on this bringing forward more biological solutions. The entire process is built on a principle of fairness and equity in sharing of the benefits and respecting the State's sovereign right to its own resources. After figuring out the chemical structures of secondary metabolites, it is considered crucial to know how useful these molecules might be in terms of medicinal properties. During the past 40 years, numerous novel compounds have been isolated from different plants and marine organisms and many of these have been reported to have core biological activities, some of which are of interest from the point of view of potential drug development (Lene, 1996; Gerald, 2001).

In this context, *Andrographis paniculata* (Burm.f.) Wall. ex Nees., could be a potential source to develop new efficacious antibacterial drugs. *A. paniculata* (*Acanthaceae*) (King of Bitters) is an annual herbaceous plant and is widely cultivated and traditionally used in Southern Asia, China and some parts of Europe. *A. paniculata* has been effectively used in traditional Asian medicines for centuries. In traditional medicine, *A. paniculata* is widely used to get rid of a body heat, dispel toxins from the body, prevents common cold, upper respiratory tract infections including sinusitis and fever (Gabrielian *et al.*, 2002) and as an antidote against snakes and insects poisons (Samy *et al.*, 2008). *A. paniculata* has been reported to exhibit various mode of biological activities *in vivo* as well as *in vitro* viz., antiviral (Wiart *et al.*, 2000), anti-inflammatory (Wen *et al.*, 2010), antihuman immunodeficiency virus (HIV) (Calabrese *et al.*, 2000), immunomodulating/immunostimulatory (Iruretagoyena *et al.*, 2005), anticancer activity (Li *et al.*, 2007; Geethangili *et al.*, 2008) and antibacterial activity (Leelarasamee *et al.*, 1990; Singha *et al.*, 2003; Zaidan *et al.*, 2005; Xu *et al.*, 2006; Voravuthikunchai *et al.*, 2006; Mishra *et al.*, 2009; Sahalan *et al.*, 2010; Abubacker and Vasanth, 2010; Kataky and Handique, 2010; Parvataneni and Koduru, 2010; Roy *et al.*, 2010; Sule *et al.*, 2011a, 2011b).

2. Phytochemical investigations of *A. paniculata*

The characteristic secondary metabolites encountered in *A. paniculata* have considerably enhanced its importance in the arena of medicinal plants. It is specifically rated high in therapeutic action in curing liver disorders, common cough and colds in human (Niranjan *et al.*, 2010). *A. paniculata* chiefly contains diterpenes, lactones, and flavonoids. Flavonoids mainly exist in the root, but have also been isolated from the leaves. The aerial parts contain alkanes, ketones, and aldehydes. Although it was initially thought that the bitter substance in the leaves was the lactone andrographolide, later investigations revealed that the leaves contained two bitter principles-andrographolide and a compound named kalmeghin. Four lactones-chuanxinlian A (deoxyandrographolide), B (andrographolide), C (neoandrographolide) and D (14-deoxy-11,12-didehydroandrographolide)-were isolated from the aerial parts in China (Chang and But, 1987). A diterpene glucoside (deoxyandrographolide-19-β-D-glucoside) has been detected in the leaves (Weiming *et al.*, 1982) and six diterpenoids of the ent-labdane type, two diterpene glucosides and four diterpene dimers (bis-andrographolides A, B, C, and D) have been isolated from aerial parts (Matsuda *et al.*, 1994). Two flavonoids identified as 5,7,2′,3′-tetramethoxyflavanone and 5-hydroxy-7,2′,3′-trimethoxyflavone were isolated from the whole plant (Koteswara *et al.*, 2004), while 12 new flavonoids and 14 diterpenoids have been reported from the aerial parts (Chen *et al.*, 2006a, 2006b). Two new flavonoid glycosides and a new diterpenoid (andrographic acid) were recently reported (Li *et al.*, 2007), and two new ent-labdane diterpenoid glycosides were also isolated from the aerial parts of *A. paniculata* (Zhou *et al.*, 2008).

3. Literature review on antibacterial studies of *A. paniculata*

A. paniculata has been extensively used to treat a variety of conditions of infectious origin in traditional systems of medicine. Modern research has investigated it for antimicrobial activity against various pathogenic and non-pathogenic bacteria. For instance, Leelarasamee *et al.* (1990) reported that crude powder suspended in water had no *in vitro* antibacterial activity against *Salmonella, Shigella, Escherichia coli*, and *Staphylococcus aureus*, even at a concentration of

25 mg/mL crude powder. Moreover, administration of a single oral dose of powder, up to 6 g, to healthy volunteers in a randomized crossover manner or daily administration of 0.12-24 g/kg body weight to rats for six months also failed to show any *ex vivo* antibacterial activity. A similar conclusion was also reached by Zaidan *et al.* (2005) who found crude aqueous extract of leaves had no activity against *Escherichia coli* or *Klebsiella pneumoniae* but exhibited significant antimicrobial activity against gram positive *S. aureus*, methicillin-resistant *S. aureus* (MRSA), and gram-negative *Pseudomonas aeruginosa*. However, Singha *et al.* (2003) reported significant antibacterial activity of an aqueous extract and attributed it to the combined effect of andrographolides and arabinogalactan proteins. In contrast, Xu *et al.* (2006) investigated the antimicrobial activity using *A. paniculata* methanolic and aqueous extracts and authentic andrographolide against nine human bacterial pathogens. Their results indicated methanolic extracts of *A. paniculata* to be active against only two of the pathogens, while authentic andrographolide did not show any activity. They concluded that the observed antimicrobial activity was due to other active principle(s) present in the extracts that were used in the investigation. The ethanol extract was also reported to be devoid of significant antibacterial activity against enterohemorrhagic strains of *E. coli* (Voravuthikunchai *et al.*, 2006). In another study, Sahalan *et al.* (2010) reported the antibacterial activity of methanol extract of the leaves of *A. paniculata* against *Staphylococcus aureus, Bacillus subtilis, Streptococcus epidemidis, Escherichia coli, Klebsiella pneumoniae* and *Pseudomonas aeruginosa*. Abubacker and Vasanth (2010) reported the antibacterial value of ethanol leaf extract against pathogenic bacteria *Escherichia coli, Klebsiella peneumoniae, Proteus vulgaris* and *Streptococcus pneumonia*. Bioactive compound andrographolide was isolated from the leaf. The results revealed that the ethanol leaf extract and andrographolide compound are potent in inhibiting these bacteria and this work highlights that the inhibitory effect is on par with standard antibiotics. Kataky and Handique (2010) reported antimicrobial activity of various organic and aqueous extracts of eight-months old micropropagated plantlets of *A. paniculata* against gram negative (*Klebsiella pneumoniae, Escherichia coli, Pseudomonas aeruginosa*), gram positive (*Staphylococcus aureus* and *Bacillus subtilis*) bacteria. Among all tested extracts, chloroform extract showed strong inhibitory activity with all the microbes tested. Out of the five microbial test organisms *Staphylococcus aureus* was the most susceptible. The minimal inhibitory concentration (MIC) of the chloroform extract ranged from 15.625 µg/mL to 31.5 µg/mL. Roy *et al.* (2010) reported the antibacterial potential of chloroform extract of the aerial parts of *A. paniculata* against *E. faecalis* (35 mm), followed by *E. cloacae* (30 mm) *P. aeruginosa* (28 mm) and *E. coli* (25 mm). Least inhibition zone was observed against *S. aureus* (15 mm). Though the inhibition zone observed against *S. typhimurium* was only 18 mm, it is noteworthy when comparing it with that of the control result. Out of the 9 pathogenic strains tested, 7 strains showed inhibition zones comparable with that of the control (amikacin) used. The chloroform extract antimicrobial activity seen against all the tested gram-negative opportunistic and pathogenic bacteria is very encouraging and important considering the role of gram-negative bacteria in noscomial infections leading to increased morbidity and mortality rates. Sule *et al.* (2011a) reported that *A. paniculata* extracts have bactericidal characteristic against most of the Gram positive bacteria and bacteriostatic activity against both Gram negative and Gram positive bacteria.

4. Objective of current study

A. paniculata has already been reported for its significant antibacterial potential by many researchers across the world (Leelarasamee *et al.*, 1990; Singha *et al.*, 2003; Zaidan *et al.*, 2005;

Xu *et al.*, 2006; Voravuthikunchai *et al.*, 2006; Mishra *et al.*, 2009; Sahalan *et al.*, 2010; Abubacker and Vasanth, 2010; Kataky and Handique, 2010; Parvataneni and Koduru, 2010; Roy *et al.*, 2010; Sule *et al.*, 2011a, 2011b). However, no attempt has ever been made to identify and isolate active principles responsible for unleashing its true antibacterial activity. Identification and isolation of active principles from *A. paniculata* might prove promising antibacterial agents through foreseeable future endeavors. Hence, this study was a scrupulous attempt to identify and isolate pure antibacterial compounds from the methanol extract of the whole plant of *A. paniculata* through bioassay guided isolation method.

5. Methods

5.1 Isolation of antibacterial compounds from *A. paniculata*

5.1.1 Collection of plant material and preparation of methanol (MEOH) extract

15 kg fresh whole plant of *A. paniculata* was procured from the botanical garden of Forest Research Institute of Malaysia (FRIM), Kuala Lumpur, Malaysia, during the month of April, 2009. The plant was identified by Dr. Richard Chung Cheng Kong (Ph.D., Taxonomist, FRIM). The voucher specimen (NMPC-Q25) has been deposited in the Herbarium, Faculty of Pharmacy, IIUM, Kuantan, Pahang DM, Malaysia for future references.

The fresh whole plant (15 kg) of *A. paniculata* was cleaned and dried in a protech laboratory air dryer (FDD-720-Malaysia) at 40°C for 7 days and pulverized to powdered form (5.6 kg, 37.33%) using Fritsch Universal Cutting Mill-PULVERISETTE 19-Germany. It was then stored in a desiccators at 2°C until further use. The air dried powder of whole plant (5 kg) of *A. paniculata* was extracted by macerating in double distilled methanol (20.0 L) at room temperature for 24 h, filtered, and evaporated under reduced pressure. The whole process was repeated thrice to ensure maximum yield of methanol soluble compounds from the plant powder. Each time, filtrate was evaporated under reduced pressure (Buchi Rotary Evaporator, R-210) and combined. The dark blackish green residue so obtained was further freeze dried to yield 305 g (6.1%) MeOH extract and was stored at 2°C in labeled sterile bottle until further antibacterial evaluation and isolation of antibacterial compounds.

5.1.2 Source of microorganism and preparation of standard bacterial suspensions

Staphylococcus aureus (IMR S-277), *Streptococcus pyogenes* (IMR S-526), *Micrococcus luteus* (IMR B-7), *Proteus mirabilis* (IMR P-74) and *Pseudomonas aeruginosa* (IMR P-84) were purchased from the Institute for Medical Research (IMR), Kuala Lumpur, Malaysia. The bacterial stock cultures were maintained on nutrient agar slants prior to use. The average number of viable, *S. aureus*, *S. pyogenes*, *M. luteus*, *P. mirabilis* and *P. aeruginosa* organisms per mL of the stock suspensions was determined by means of the surface viable counting technique (Omar, 1974). About 10^7-10^8 CFU/mL was used. Each time, a fresh stock suspension was prepared; the experimental conditions were maintained constant so that suspensions with very close viable counts could be obtained successfully.

5.1.3 *In vitro* antibacterial activity test for MeOH extract and determination of minimum inhibitory concentration (MIC)

The cup-plate agar diffusion method was adopted according to Kokoska *et al.* (2002) to assess the antibacterial activity of the MeOH extract. 0.6 mL of standardized bacterial stock suspensions corresponding to 10^7-10^8 CFU/mL was thoroughly mixed with 60 mL of sterile nutrient agar. 20 mL of the inoculated nutrient agar were distributed into sterile labeled Petri dishes. The agar was left to set at room temperature and in each of these plates, 3 cups 6 mm in diameter were punched using a sterile cork borer allowing at least 30 mm between adjacent wells and the agar discs were removed. Fixed volumes of the plant extract (1000, 500 and 250 μgmL^{-1}) were then introduced into each wells using micro titer-pipette and allowed to diffuse at room temperature for two hours. In separate wells, 30 µg each of gentamicin and vancomycin were added as positive controls whereas 10% DMSO was taken as negative control. The plates were then incubated in the upright position at 37°C for 24 h. Three replicates were carried out for the extract against each of the test organism. After incubation the diameter of the results and growth inhibition zones were measured, averaged and the mean values were recorded.

Micro broth dilution method was used for the determination of MIC values for each plant extract showing antibacterial activity against test pathogens (NCCLS, 2003). Serial dilutions of the extracts were carried out in 10% DMSO (which had no inhibitory activity against test microorganisms) to make 500 μgmL^{-1} final concentration, this was then two fold serially diluted by adding to the broth media in a 96-wells micro titer plates to obtain 250, 125, 62.5, 31.3, 15.6 and 7.81 μgmL^{-1}. Thereafter, 100 µL inoculum (10^8 CFU/mL) was added to each well. Bacterial suspensions were used as negative control, while broth containing standard drug (vancomycin and gentamicin) were used separately as positive controls. The micro titer plates were incubated at 37°C for 24 h. Each extract was assayed in duplicate; one was kept for incubation while the other was kept at 4°C for comparing the turbidity in the wells of micro plate. The MIC values were taken as the lowest concentration of the extracts in the well of the micro titer plate that showed no turbidity after incubation. The turbidity of the wells in the micro titer plate was interpreted as visible growth of microorganisms. Antibacterial index (A_bI) of MeOH whole plant extract of *A. paniculata* was calculated separately as the average value of zone of inhibition against the Gram-positive and Gram-negative bacteria, respectively (Zakaria *et al.*, 2007).

5.1.4 Bioassay guided isolation

To sterilized 8 x 4 cm silica gel 60 F_{254} TLC plates (Merck, Germany), 10 µL of MeOH extract was applied as small spots and the plates were developed in hexane:acetone (2:1) in duplicate (a TLC plate was used as the bioautogram while the other served as a chromatogram for reference in comparison with the bioautograph). The TLC plates were dried in an oven at 25°C for 7 h to activate the plates by absorbing the moisture content from the plates and removing all residual solvents (Veronica *et al.*, 2005).

S. aureus and *P. mirabilis* were used as the indicator microorganisms for the bioautography of antibacterial compounds from the MeOH extract of *A. paniculata*. 200 µL each from broth cultures of *S. aureus* and *P. mirabilis* (adjusted to 10^8 CFU/mL) were mixed with 35 mL molten Mueller-Hinton agar (MHA) at 30°C separately. The suspensions of agar and bacteria were spread aseptically onto the already developed TLC plates in square Petri dishes (8 x 4 cm), allowed for 30 mins to solidify and the plates were incubated at 37°C for 24 h. At the end of incubation time, 0.5% *p*-Iodonitrotetrazolium Violet (INT) was sprayed on the plates for 5 mins. The active antibacterial compounds in the plant extracts formed clear zones of inhibition on the TLC plates against a deep pink back ground of bacterial growth, allowing the chromatographic retention factors (R.f.) observation by viewing under UV light at 254 nm (short wave) and 366 nm (long wave) and comparing with the reference chromatogram (already sprayed with vanillin reagent and heated at 120°C) to note the antibacterial compounds. Vanillin reagent was prepared by dissolving 15 g of vanillin in ethanol (250 mL) and H_2SO_4 (2.5 mL). Vanillin reagent gives different colored spots with different compounds on TLC plate upon heating at 120°C (Rahalison *et al.*, 2007).

5.1.5 Identification and isolation of antibacterial compounds from MeOH extract

100 g MeOH extract was loaded onto column (10 x 50 cm) packed with silica gel 60 particle size 0.063-0.2 mm (70-230 mesh) (Fluka Chemika) as stationery phase, the extracts as the mobile phase and the column was eluted with ten different concentrations of hexane:ethylacetate (9:1-1:9) and finally with ethylacetate:methanol (9:1-1:9) solvent systems (with gradual increase in polarity), 190 fractions were obtained and pooled to give a total of 20 (M_1-M_{20}) similar fractions based on their R.f. values as indicated by TLC plate analysis in chloroform:methanol:ethylacetate ($CHCl_3$:MeOH:EtOAc; 16:0.8:1.2) solvent system. Antibacterial active fractions M_9-M_{13} and M_{16}-M_{18} as indicated by bioautography of the extract afforded two crystallized compounds which were further purified by using preparative column chromatography on silica gel 60 and eluted with hexane:ethylacetate (9:1-1:9) to produce 76 (P_1- P_{76}) fractions. Eluents in test tubes P_1- P_{10}, P_{12}- P_{21}, and P_{22}- P_{35} upon crystallization with absolute ethanol afforded pure antibacterial compound AB-1 (white crystals, 29 mg, R.f. 0.70-$CHCl_3$:MeOH:EtOAc, 16: 0.8: 1.2). Fractions P_{41}- P_{58} upon crystallization with absolute ethanol afforded pure antibacterial compound AB-2 (colourless crystals, 35 mg, R.f. 0.64 ($CHCl_3$:MeOH:EtOAc; 16: 0.8: 1.2), respectively. The purity of both antibacterial compounds were further determined through high performance liquid chromatography (HPLC) and running TLC plates in different binary and ternary solvent systems. Structures of both antibacterial compounds were elucidated through the integration of ^1H- and ^{13}C NMR spectra and comparison of their physical, chemical and spectral data was made with the previous reported data of the same compounds.

3-O-β-D-glucosyl-14-deoxyandrographolides (AB-1): M.P. 242-244°C, UV λ_{max} MeOH nm: 202. IR (cm^{-1}) ν: 3351, 1732, 165, 899. ^1H NMR (600 MHz, in DMSO-*d6*), δ (ppm): 1.25 (o, 1H, C1-CH_2), 1.71 (o, 1H, C1-CH_2), 2.10 (m, 1H, C2-CH_2), 1.98 (m, 1H, C2-CH_2), 3.92 (o, 1H, C3-CH-), 1.3 (m, 1H, C5-CH-), 1.85 (m, 2H, C6-CH_2), 2.4 (m, 2H, C7-CH_2), 3.35 (d, J=8.4 Hz, 1H, C9-CH-), 1.8 (m, 2H, C11-CH_2), 2.6 (m, 1H, C12-CH_2), 2.3 (m, 1H, C12-CH_2), 7.10 (t, 1H, C14-CH-), 4.77 (brs, 2H, C15-CH_2), 4.87 (brs, 1H, C17-CH_2), 4.59 (brs, 1H, C17-CH_2), 1.007 (brs, 3H, C18-CH_3), 4.03 (d, J=9.6 Hz, 1H, C19-CH_2), 3.22 (d, J=9.6, 1H, C19-CH_2), 0.66 (brs, 3H, C20-CH_3), 4.24 (d, J=7.2 Hz, 1H, C1'-CH-), 3.37 (o, 1H, C2'-CH-), 3.39 (o, 1H, C3'-CH-), 3.57 (o, 1H, C4'-CH-), 3.59 (o, 1H, C5'-CH-), 3.84 (dd, J=11.4, 4.8 Hz, 2H, C6'-CH_2), *"o" denotes overlapping signals*; ^{13}C NMR (125.76 MHz, in DMSO*d6*), δ (ppm): 38.19 (C1), 29.72 (C2), 75.04 (C3), 39.56 (C4), 56.44 (C5), 35.97 (C6), 38.44 (C7), 147.30 (C8), 56.18 (C9), 38.89 (C10), 21.72 (C11), 24.46 (C12), 136.02 (C13), 143.84 (C14), 70.11 (C15), 174.33 (C16), 107.08 (C17), 18.93 (C18), 62.61 (C19), 15.41 (C20), 103.10 (C1'), 71.72 (C2'), 72.73 (C3'), 74.03 (C4'), 76.23 (C5'), 70.72 (C6'). From this spectral data and their direct comparison with the previously published spectral data (Zhou *et al.*, 2008) of the same compound, AB-1 was unambiguously identified as 3-*O*-β-D-glucosyl-14-deoxyandrographolide (Fig. 3).

14-deoxyandrographolide (AB-2): M.P. 172-174°C, UV λ_{max} MeOH nm: 223. IR (cm^{-1}) v: 3367, 1736, 1646, 896. ^{1}H NMR (600 MHz, in DMSO-*d6*), δ (ppm): 1.32 (m, 2H, C1-CH_2), 2.04 (brs, 1H, C2-CH_2), 1.99 (o, 1H, C2-CH_2), 3.35 (o, 1H, C3-CH-), 1.46 (o, 1H, C5-CH-), 2.18 (brs, 1H, C6-CH_2), 1.98 (brd, J=6 Hz, 1H, C6-CH_2), 2.45 (t, 2H, C7-CH_2), 3.50 (o, 1H, C9-CH-), 2.43 (dd, J= 4.2, 2.4 Hz, 2H, C11-CH_2), 2.55 (dd, J= 12, 7.2 Hz, 2H, C12-CH_2), 7.10 (brs, 1H, C14-CH-), 4.91 (brs, 2H, C15-CH_2), 4.59 (brs, 1H, C17-CH_2), 4.45 (brs, 1H, C17-CH_2), 1.59 (o, 3H, C18-CH_3), 4.20 (brs, 1H, C19-CH_2), 4.18 (brs, 1H, C19-CH_2), 0.71 (s, 3H, C20-CH_3), *"o" denotes overlapping signals*; ^{13}C NMR (125.76 MHz, in DMSO*d6*), δ (ppm): 38.93 (C1), 37.74 (C2), 80.50 (C3), 64.13 (C4), 55.21 (C5), 28.22 (C6), 37.06 (C7), 148.94 (C8), 55.96 (C9), 42.96 (C10), 24.88 (C11), 23.76 (C12), 146.64 (C13), 127.83 (C14), 66.31 (C15), 172.17 (C16), 108.86 (C17), 22.67 (C18), 74.61 (C19), 15.16 (C20). From this spectral data and their direct comparison with the previously published data (Poonam *et al.*, 2010) of the same compound, AB-2 was unambiguously identified as 14-deoxyandrographolide (Fig. 4).

5.1.6 Minimum inhibitory concentration (MIC) of isolated compounds

The minimum inhibitory concentrations of the isolated compounds AB-1 and AB-2 were determined using the agar dilution method following the standard protocol of the European Committee for Antimicrobial Susceptibility Testing (EUCAST, 2003). The compounds were dissolved in 10% DMSO and 2-fold diluted in MHA to obtain 250, 125, 62.5, 31.3, 15.6 and 7.81 μgmL^{-1}. The mixture of the media and compounds were thoroughly mixed and poured onto pre-labeled sterile Petri dishes on a level surface. Additional Petri dishes containing only the growth media were prepared in the same way so as to serve for comparison of growth of the respective bacteria. The plates were then set at room temperature and dried. The suspensions of the respective bacteria (corresponding to 10^8 CFU/mL) were inoculated onto the series of agar plates. The plates were then incubated at 37°C for 24 h. The experiments were performed in duplicate and MIC values expressed as the lowest concentration of the plant extracts that produced complete suppression of colony of respective bacteria.

5.1.7 Statistical analyses

The experimental results were expressed as mean ± standard deviation (STD) of triplicate experiments. Statistical differences between the antibiotics and inhibition zones formed by the plant extract were detected by analysis of variance (ANOVA) using SPSS 19.0 statistical software (SPSS, Chicago, Illinois, USA) followed by the Tukey test for multiple comparisons between means. P values lower than 0.05 ($p < 0.05$) were considered significantly different whereas P values lower than 0.01 ($p < 0.01$) were considered highly significant.

6. Results

The results of the cup-plate agar diffusion method revealed that MeOH extract of *A. paniculata* whole plant extract do possess antibacterial activity against all 5 bacteria taken into consideration *in vitro* (Table 1). Maximum antibacterial activity was observed against *S. aureus* (19.67 ± 0.76 mm) at 1000 µgmL-1 and the least activity was detected against *P. aeruginosa* (7.00 ± 1.50 mm) at 250 µgmL-1, respectively.

Bacterial strains	Plant Extract	Zones of Inhibition (mm) 1000 μg/ml	500 μg/ml	250 μg/ml	Antibiotics (30 μg)
		Gram Positive Strains			Vancomycin
S. aureus (IMR S-277)	MeOH	19.67 ± 0.76*	18.00 ± 0.50	14.00 ±1.00**	17.00 ± 1.05
M. luteus (IMR B-7)	MeOH	18.50 ± 0.58	15.00 ± 0.89*	13.00 ±0.58**	19.00 ± 0.50
S. pyogenes (IMR S-526)	MeOH	16.00 ± 0.58*	13.00 ± 0.74	10.67 ±1.15**	14.50 ± 1.00
		Gram Negative Strains			Gentamicin
P. mirabilis IMR P-76	MeOH	14.50±0.58**	14.00±0.58**	10.50 ±1.00**	21.33 ± 0.89
P. aeruginosa IMR P-84	MeOH	11.50±0.50**	9.00±1.26**	7.00±1.50**	18.50 ± 0.50

Comparison with antibiotics
**P < 0.01 highly significant
*P < 0.05 significant difference
- No Activity

Table 1. Antibacterial activity of MeOH extract of the whole plant of *A. paniculata*. Numbers indicate the mean diameters of inhibition of triplicate experiments ± standard deviation (SD)

Bioautography of MeOH extract revealed two prominent spots on the bioautogram against *S. aureus* and *P. mirabilis* which were used as an indicator organism and consequently led to the identification and subsequent isolation of two antibacterial compounds viz., an ent-labdane diterpene glycoside (AB-1) and a diterpene lactone (AB-2) as the main active principles. Both compounds were active against *S. aureus* (Fig. 1 & 2) and *P. mirabilis* which were used as indicator organisms in the bioautography technique on TLC plates forming clear zones against pink background of the living microorganisms when compared to the reference chromatogram.

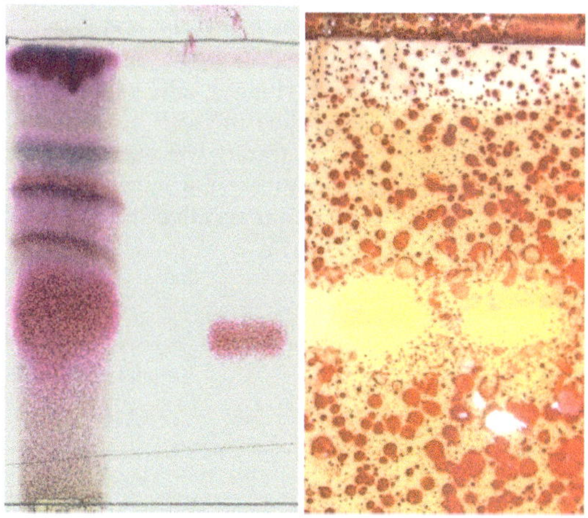

(a) (b)

Fig. 1. Bioautography of AB-1 against *S. aureus*. (a) Referenced chromatogram sprayed with vanillin/H_2SO_4 spray reagent. (b) Bioautogram against *S. aureus*.

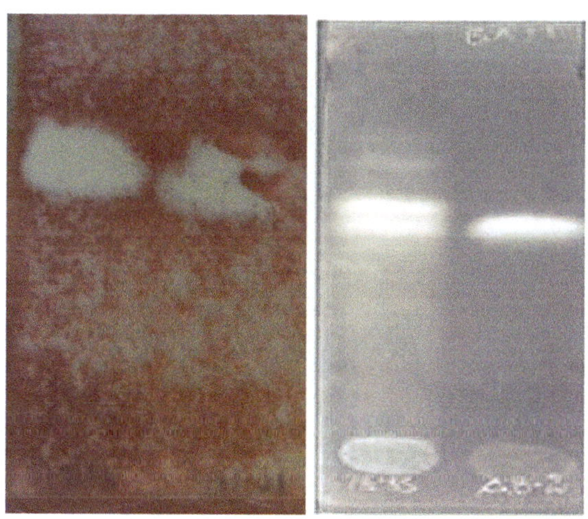

(a) (b)

Fig. 2. Bioautography of AB-2 against *S. aureus*. (a) Bioautogram against *S. aureus*. (b) Referenced chromatogram viewed under UV light.

Minimum inhibitory concentration (MIC) values for MeOH extract and isolated compounds are shown in Table 2. MIC of MeOH extract ranged from 125-250 µgmL^{-1} with the highest MIC value exerted by the extract against *S. pyogenes, P. mirabilis* and *P. aeruginosa* (250 µgmL^{-1}) and the least against *S. aureus* and *M. luteus* (125 µgmL^{-1}). MIC values for both isolated compounds ranged from 15.6-250 µgmL^{-1}. Highest MIC value was exerted by compound AB-1 against *P. aeruginosa* (250 µgmL^{-1}) while the least was exerted by compound AB-2 against *S. aureus* (15.6 µgmL^{-1}), however, no activity was exerted by compound AB-1 against *M. luteus* (Table 2). The MeOH extract's antibacterial index (A_bI) was best against Gram-positive strains tested as compared to the Gram-negative strains with mean inhibition zones of 13.9 mm and 10.4 mm, respectively (Table 3).

	MIC (µg/ml) MeOH Extract	Compounds AB-1	AB-2
Gram Positive			
S. aureus	125	62.5	15.6
M. luteus	125	N/A	125
S. pyogenes	250	125	62.5
Gram Negative			
P. mirabilis	250	125	125
P. aeruginosa	250	250	250

*NA-no activity

Table 2. Minimum inhibitory concentrations (MIC) of the MeOH extract of the whole plant of *A. paniculata* and isolated compounds against bacterial strains

Strains	Activity Index (mm) MeOH Extract
Gram Positive *S. aureus, M. luteus, S. pyogenes*	13.9
Gram Negative *P. mirabilis, P. aeruginosa*	10.4

Table 3. Antibacterial activity indexes (A_bI) of MeOH extract of the whole plant of *A. paniculata*

Compound AB-1 gave positive Legal and Kedde test, suggesting the presence of an α, β-unsaturated lactone in the compound. The ^{1}H- and ^{13}C-NMR spectra of AB-1 revealed signals due to a β-glucopyranosyl group [δ_H 4.24 (d, J=7.2 Hz, 1H)] and δ_C 103.10, 71.72,

72.73, 74.03, 76.23, and 70.72 and the characteristic signals for the double bond containing one hydrogen at carbon 14 in γ-lactone ring were observed at δ 7.10 (t, 1H) in ^{1}HNMR as well as in ^{13}C at δ 143.84, respectively, which corresponds to the 3-*O*-β-D-glucosyl-14-deoxyandrographolide (Zhou *et al.*, 2008) (Fig. 3).

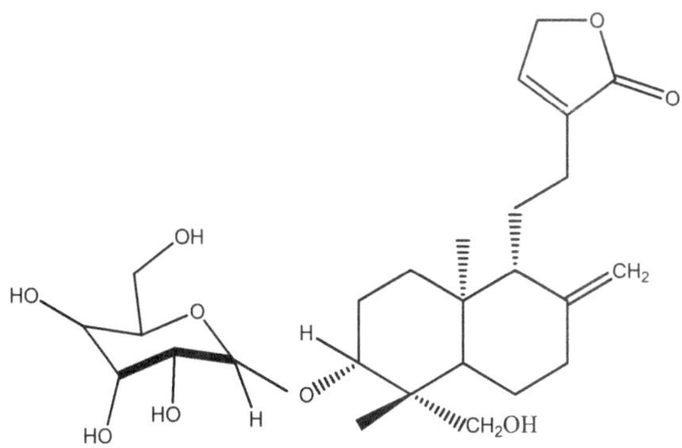

Fig. 3. Structure of AB-1 (3-*O*-β-D-glucosyl-14-deoxyandrographolide) based on ^{1}H- and ^{13}C NMR spectra

AB-2 was also found to be positive for the Legal and Kedde reactions, suggesting the presence of an α, β-unsaturated lactone in the molecule. The characteristic NMR spectral data indicated that compound AB-2 was a labdane-type diterpene with α, β-unsaturated γ-lactone. In the ^{1}H-NMR spectrum of AB-2, two methyl singlets were observed at δ 0.71 and 1.59, respectively. The characteristic exocyclic methylene protons for AB-2 diterpenoids were observed at δ 4.59 (brs, 1H) and 4.45 (brs, 1H) in ^{1}HNMR as well as at δ 108.86 in ^{13}C, respectively. The ^{1}H- and ^{13}C-NMR (in $CDCl_3$) spectra of AB-2 suggested a diterpenoid compound with a structure similar to that of 14-deoxyandrographolide (Poonam *et al.*, 2010) (Fig. 4).

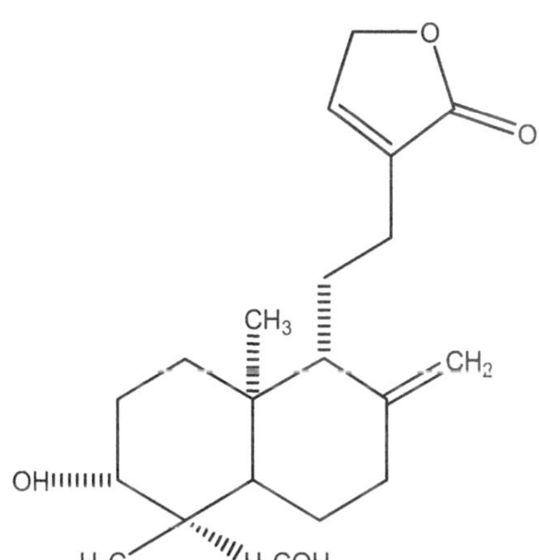

Fig. 4. Structure of AB-2 (14-deoxyandrographolide) based on ^{1}H- and ^{13}C NMR spectra.

7. Discussion

Antibiotics offer the core basis for the effective therapy of chronic bacterial infections. However, the high genetic variability of bacteria enables them to rapidly elude the action of antibiotics by developing antibiotic resistance. As resistance becomes more common, there becomes a greater need for alternative treatments. However, despite a push for new antibiotic therapies, there has been a continued decline in the number of newly approved drugs (Bächi, 2002). According to the World Health Organization (WHO) report on infectious diseases in 2000, overcoming antibiotic resistance is the major issue of the WHO for the next millennium. Hence, the last decade witnessed an increase in the investigations on plants as a source of human disease management (Paul *et al.*, 2006). *A. paniculata* is common throughout Southeast Asia and India and is extensively used by traditional healers for the treatment of a wide variety of ailments (Coon and Ernst, 2004). The antibacterial activity of *A. paniculata* extracts are well known (Leelarasamee *et al.*, 1990; Singha *et al.*, 2003; Zaidan *et al.*, 2005; Xu *et al.*, 2006; Voravuthikunchai *et al.*, 2006; Mishra *et al.*, 2009; Sahalan *et al.*, 2010; Abubacker and Vasanth, 2010; Kataky and Handique, 2010; Parvataneni and Koduru, 2010; Roy *et al.*, 2010; Sule *et al.*, 2011a, 2011b). Whilst many studies have isolated and characterized *A. paniculata* compounds, no study has ever determined the antimicrobial activity of isolated compounds so far. In the present experiment, the MeOH extract of the whole plant of *A. paniculata* showed broad spectrum antibacterial activity. 3-*O*-β-D-glycosyl-14-deoxyandrographolide and 14-deoxyandrographolide were isolated as active principles, which may serve as lead for the development of new pharmaceuticals that might address the unmet therapeutic needs to cure chronic bacterial infections effectively. The obvious fields where the natural product chemist can harvest benefits from a cooperation with the microbiologists are development of bioassay for efficient monitoring of isolation and purification of new compounds; bioassay fingerprinting to help early de-selection of known compounds (hereby supplementing the chemical data and giving additional avenues for tapping into the computerized data bases); activity spectrum to help de-selecting the very toxic compounds; obtaining a sharper focus in the natural product chemistry work on biologically active compounds. Novel and potentially useful may be of more interest than to go exclusively for just novelty (Lene, 1996). Bio-autography provides more information about plant compounds requires a smaller weight of sample and can be used for the bioassay-guided isolation of biological active compounds, simplifying the process of the identification and isolation of the active compounds (Rahalison *et al.*, 2007).

The antibacterial activity measured by the cup-plate agar diffusion method was more prominent on the Gram-positive bacteria (*S. aureus, M. luteus* and *S. pyogenes*) than the Gram-negative bacteria (*P. mirabilis* and *P. aeruginosa*). Gram-positive bacteria were the most susceptible to growth inhibition by MeOH extract of *A. paniculata* whole plant. The greater susceptibility of Gram-positive bacteria has been previously reported for South American (Paz *et al.*, 1995), African (Kudi *et al.*, 1999) and Australian (Palombo and Semple, 2001) plant extracts. Susceptibility differences between Gram-positive and Gram-negative bacteria may be due to cell wall structural differences between these classes of bacteria. Gram-negative bacteria have an outer phospholipid membrane carrying the structural lipopolysaccharide components. This makes the cell wall impermeable to antimicrobial chemical substances. The Gram-positive bacteria tested were more susceptible to the plant extracts because it is well known that all Gram-positive bacteria have an outer peptidoglycan layer which is not an effective permeability barrier. The cell walls of Gram-negative organisms are more complex in lay out than the Gram-positive ones acting as a diffusion barrier and making them less susceptible to the antimicrobial agents than are Gram-positive bacteria (Nikaido, 2003). In the present study, after the first chromatography of the MeOH extract of the whole plant of *A. paniculata* on a silica gel column, the antibacterial activity of the collected fractions were tested against *S. aureus* and *P. mirabilis* using bio-autography on a TLC plate. This revealed that all the fractions except nine were very active against *S. aureus* and *P. mirabilis*. Isolation of these compounds in pure form was achieved by repeated washing of the crystalline matter off the green coloring material with toluene and repeated recrystallization with absolute ethanol and final washing of the crystals with cold methanol. The purity of the sample at every stage of recrystallization was monitored through TLC.

8. Conclusion

The thin layer chromatography bioautography-guided strategy was successfully used to isolate two antibacterial compounds from MeOH extract of *A. paniculata* whole plant for the first time. The 3-*O*-β-D-glycosyl-14-deoxyandrographolide and 14-deoxyandrographolide demonstrated significant antibacterial activities against the selected microbial strains. Quantitative HPLC and TLC analysis confirmed that these isolated compounds are predominate components in whole plant MeOH extract, indicating their significant contribution to the overall antibacterial activity. Further investigation of the activities of these compounds and their potential use in the treatment of bacterial diseases are still sought.

9. References

Abubacker, M.N., S. Vasantha, 2010. Antibacterial activity of ethanolic leaf extract of *Andrographis paniculata* Nees (Acanthaceae) and its bioactive compound andrographolide. *Drug Invention Today* 2: 440-442.

Bächi, B.B., 2002. Resistance mechanisms of Gram-positive bacteria. *J Med Microb.*, 292: 27-35.

Calabrese, C., S.H. Berman, J.G. Babish, M. Xinfang, L. Shinto, M. Dorr, K. Wells, C.A. Wenner, L.J. Standish, 2000. A phase I trial of andrographolide in HIV positive patients and normal volunteers. *Phytotherapy Res.*, 14: 333-338.

Chang, H.M., P.P.H. But, 1987. *Pharmacology and Applications of Chinese Materia Medica.* English translation by Shem Chang-Shing Yeung, Sih Cheng-Yao and Lai-Ling Wang (Chinese Medicinal Material Research Centre, The Chinese University of Hong Kong), Singapore: World Scientific Publishing Co. Pte. Ltd; 2: 918-928.

Chen, L.X., G.X. Qu, F. Qiu, 2006a. Studies on diterpenoids from *Andrographis paniculata. Zhongguo Zhong Yao Za Zhi* 31: 1594-1597.

Chen, L.X., G.X. Qu, F. Qiu, 2006b. Studies on flavonoids of *Andrographis paniculata. Zhongguo Zhong Yao Za Zhi* 31: 391-395.

Coon, J.T., E. Ernst, 2004. *Andrographis paniculata* in the treatment of upper respiratory tract infections: a systematic review of safety and efficacy. *Planta Med.*, 70: 293-298.

European Committee on Antimicrobial Susceptibility Testing (EUCAST), 2003. Discussion document, determination of minimum inhibitory concentrations (MICs) of antibacterial agents by broth dilution. *Clin Microb Infect.*, 9: 1-7.

Gabrielian, E.S., A.K. Shukarian, G.I. Goukasova, G.L. Chandanian, A.G. Panossian, G. Wikman, H. Wagner. 2002. A double blind, placebo-controlled study of *Andrographis paniculata* fixed combination Kan Jang in the treatment of acute upper respiratory tract infections including sinusitis. *Phytomed.*, 9: 589-597.

Geethangili, M., Y.K. Rao, S.H. Fang, Y.M. Tzeng, 2008. Cytotoxic constituents from *Andrographis paniculata* induce cell cycle arrest in Jurkat cells. *Phytotherapy Res.*, 22: 1336-1341.

Gerald, B., 2001. Biologically active compounds from marine organisms. *Phytotherapy Res.*, 15: 89-94.

Iruretagoyena, M., J.A. Tobar, P.A. Gonzalez, 2005. Andrographolide interferes with T-cell activation and reduces experimental autoimmune encephalomyelitis in the mouse. *J Pharmacol Exp Ther.*, 312: 366-372.

Kataky, A., P.J. Handique, 2010. Antimicrobial activity and phytochemical estimation of micropropagated *Andrographis paniculata* (Burm.f) NEES. *Asian J Science and Tech.*, 5: 91-94.

Kokoska, L., Z. Polesny, V. Rada, A. Nepovim, T. Vanek, 2002. Screening of some Siberian medicinal plants for antimicrobial activity. *J Ethnopharmacol.*, 82: 51-53.

Koteswara, R.Y., G. Vimalamma, C.V. Rao, Y.M. Tzeng, 2004. Flavonoids and andrographolides from *Andrographis paniculata. Phytochem.*, 65: 2317-2321.

Kudi, A.C., J.U. Umoh, L.O. Eduvie, J. Gefu, 1999. Screening of some Nigerian medicinal plants for antibacterial activity. *J Ethnopharmacol.*, 67: 225-228.

Leelarasamee, A., S. Trakulsomboon, N. Sittisomwong, 1990. Undetectable anti-bacterial activity of *Andrographis paniculata* (Burma) Wall. ex Ness. *J Med Association* 73: 299-304.

Lene, L., 1996. Microbial metabolites-an infinite source of novel chemistry. *Pure Appl Chem.*, 68: 745-748.

Li, W., X. Xu, H. Zhang, C. Ma, H. Fong, R.V. Breemen, J. Fitzloff, 2007. Secondary metabolites from *Andrographis paniculata. Chem Pharm Bull.*, 55: 455-458.

Matsuda, T., M. Kuroyanagi, S. Sugiyama *et al.*, 1994. Cell differentiation-inducing diterpenes from *Andrographis paniculata* Nees. *Chem Pharm Bull.*, 42: 1216-1225.

Mishra, U.S., A. Mishra, R. Kumari, P.N. Murthy, B.S. Naik, 2009. Antibacterial activity of ethanol extract of *Andrographis paniculata. Ind J Pharm Sci.*, 71: 436-438.

National Committee for Clinical Laboratory Standards (NCCLS), 2003. Methods for dilution antimicrobial susceptibility tests for bacteria that grow aerobically; Approved Standard, 6th edition. M7-A6. NCCLS, Wayne, PA.

Nikaido, H., 2003. Molecular basis of bacterial outer membrane permeability revisited. *Microb Mol Bio Rev.*, 67: 593-656.

Niranjan, A., S.K. Tewari, A. Lehri, 2010. Biological activities of Kalmegh (*Andrographis paniculata* Nees) and its active principles-A review. *Indian J Nat Prod Resour.*, 1: 125-135.

Omar, K., 1974. Surface viable counts with nichrome wire loops. *J Clin Pathol.*, 27: 834-836.

Palombo, E.A., S.J. Semple, 2001. Antibacterial activity of traditional Australian medicinal plants. *J Ethnopharmacol.*, 77: 151-157.

Parvataneni, R., R.L. Koduru, 2010. Antimicrobial activity of the chloroform extracts of the root and the stem of *Andrographis paniculata* Nees. *Int Res J Microb.*, 1: 037-039.

Paul, C.J., V. Arnold, V.B. Dirk, M. Louis, 2006. Anti-infective potential of natural products: How to develop a stronger *in vitro* 'proof-of-concept'. *J Ethnopharmacol.*, 106: 290-302.

Paz, E.A., M.P. Cerdeiras, J. Fernandez, F. Ferreira, P. Moyna, M. Soubes, A. Vazquez, S. Vero, L. Zunino, 1995. Screening of Uruguayan medicinal plants for antimicrobial activity. *J Ethnopharmacol.*, 45: 67-70.

Poonam, K., U.K. Tiwari, A. Shukla, A.K. Gaur, 2010. Chemical constituents isolated from *Andrographis paniculata. Ind J Chem.*, 49: 356-359.

Rahalison, L., M. Hamburger, K. Hostettmann, M. Monod, E. Frenk, 2007. A Bioautographic agar overlay method for the detection of antifungal compounds from higher plants. *Phytochem Anal.*, 2: 199-203.

Roy, S., K. Rao, C. Bhuvaneswari, A. Giri, L.N. Mangamoori, 2010. Phytochemical analysis of *Andrographis paniculata* extract and its antimicrobial activity. *World J Microb Biot.*, 26: 85-91.

Sahalan, A.Z., N. Sulaiman, N. Mohammed, K.M. Ambia, H.H. Lian, 2007. Antibacterial activity of *Andrographis paniculata* and *Euphorbia hirta* methanol extracts. *Jurnal Sains Kesihatan Malaysia* 5: 1-8.

Samy, R.P., M.M. Thwin, P. Gopalakrishnakone, S. Ignacimuthu, 2008. Ethnobotanical survey of folk plants for the treatment of snake bites in southern part of Tamilnadu, India. *J Ethnopharmacol.*, 115: 302-312.

Singha, P.K., S. Roy, S. Dey, 2003. Antimicrobial activity of *Andrographis paniculata. Fitoterapia* 74: 692-694.

Sule, A., Q.U. Ahmed, O.A. Samah, M.N. Omar, 2011a. Bacteriostatic and bactericidal activity of the polar and non-polar extracts of *Andrographis paniculata* against skin disease causing pathogenic bacteria. *J Medicinal Plants Res.*, 5: 7-14.

Sule, A., Q.U. Ahmed, O.A. Samah, M.N. Omar, N.M. Hassan, L.Z.M. Kamal, M.A. Yarmo, 2011b. Bioassay guided isolation of antibacterial compounds from *Andrographis paniculata* (Burm.f.) Wall. ex Nees (Hempedeu bumi). *American J Applied Sci.*, 8: 525-534.

Veronica, G.C., A.R. Scott, 2005. Bioautography and chemical characterization of antimicrobial compound(s) in commercial water-soluble *Annatto* extracts. *J Agri Food Chem.*, 53: 2524-2529.

Voravuthikunchai, S.P., S. Limsuwan, 2006. Medicinal plant extracts as anti-*Escherichia coli* O157:H7 agents and their effects on bacterial cell aggregation. *J Food Prot.*, 69: 2336-2341.

Weiming, C., L. Xiaotian, 1982. Deoxyandrographolide-19beta-D-glucoside from the leaves of *Andrographis paniculata. Planta Med.*, 45: 245-246.

Wen, W.C., K.H. Yueh, L.B. Fong, 2010. Anti-inflammatory activity of new compounds from *Andrographis paniculata* by NF-κB transactivation inhibition. *J Agri Food Chem.*, 58: 2505-2512.

Wiart, C., K. Kumar, M.Y. Yusof, H. Hamimah, Z.M. Fauzi and M. Sulaiman, 2000. Antiviral properties of ent-labdene diterpenes of *Andrographis paniculata* Nees. *Phytother Res.*, 19: 1069-1070.

Xu, Y., R.L. Marshall, T.K.S. Mukkur, 2006. An investigation on the antimicrobial activity of *Andrographis paniculata* extracts and andrographolide *in vitro. Asian J Plant Sci.*, 5: 527-530.

Zaidan, M.R., R.A. Noor, A.R. Badrul *et al.*, 2005. *In vitro* screening of five local medicinal plants for antibacterial activity using disc diffusion method. *Trop Biomed.*, 22: 165-170.

Zakaria, H.M., J.M. Mainen, J.M. Pax., C.K. Modest, S.O.N. Ramadhani, 2007. Antimicrobial activity and brine shrimp toxicity of extracts of *Terminalia brownii* roots and stem. *BMC Comp Alter Med.*, 7: 9.

Zhou, K.L., L.X. Chen, Y.L. Zhuang, N.L. Wang, X.S. Yao, F. Qiu, 2008. Two new ent-labdane diterpenoid glycosides from the aerial parts of *Andrographis paniculata. J Asian Nat Prod Res.*, 10: 939-943.

18

Antibacterial Agents in Textile Industry

Sheila Shahidi[1,*] and Jakub Wiener[2]
[1]Department of Textile, Faculty of Engineering, Islamic Azad University, Arak Branch, Arak,
[2]Department of Textile Chemistry, Faculty of Textile, Technical University of Liberec, Liberec,
[1]Iran
[2]Czech Republic

1. Introduction

With the growing public health awareness of the pathogenic effects, malodors and stain formations caused by microorganisms, there is an increasing need for antibacterial materials in many application areas like medical devices, health care, hygienic application, water purification systems, hospital, dental surgery equipment, textiles, food packaging, and storage.(Shahidi et al, 2007)

The spread of HIV and hepatitis viruses by contact of contaminated materials has created increased pressure for protection of personnel with functional clothing; also, all articles of apparel and home textiles are susceptible to problems of hygiene in normal daily use, for example, socks, sport wear and working clothes as well as mattresses, floor coverings, and shoe linings. Textiles for outdoor use are constantly exposed to the influence of microbes and bacteria. Application of natural antimicrobial agents on textiles dates back to antiquity, when the ancient Egyptians used spices and herbs to preserve mummy warps. Textile goods, especially those made from natural fibers, provide an excellent environment for microorganisms to grow, because of their large surface area and ability to retain moisture. Most textile materials currently used in hospitals and hotels are conductive to cross infection or transmission of diseases caused by microorganisms. Practically every class of chemical compound has been utilized to impart antibacterial activity to textiles. Two different aspects of antimicrobial protection provided by chemical finishes can be distinguished. The first is the protection of the textile user against pathogenic or odour causing microorganisms (hygiene finishes). The second aspect is the protection of the textile itself from damage caused by mould, mildew or rot producing microorganisms. Bacteria are not as damaging to fibres, but can produce some fibre damage, unpleasant odours and a slick, slimy feel. Often, fungi and bacteria are both present on the fabric in a symbiotic relationship. (Heywood, 2003; Bellini, 2001)

Substances added to fibres, such as lubricants, antistatics, natural-based auxiliaries (for example size, thickener and hand modifiers) and dirt provide a food source for

* Corresponding Author

microorganisms. Synthetic fibres are not totally immune to microorganisms, for example polyurethane fibres and coatings can be damaged. Of course, because of evolution, natural fibres are more easily attacked. Wool is more likely to suffer bacterial attack than cotton, and cotton is more likely than wool to be attacked by fungi.

2. Antimicrobial treatments of textile

There are various chemical and physical possibilities that can be considered in the production of antimicrobial fabrics. In practice, the antimicrobial effect is obtained through the application of specific chemical products during the finishing stage, or through the incorporation of these substances into chemical fibres during the spinning process.

These possibilities are:

- The addition of bactericidal substances to the spinning solution, prior to the extrusion stage. substances like Triclosan (2,4,4-hydrophenyl trichloro (II) ether), a member of the antiseptic and disinfectant family.
- A different method for the production of antimicrobial and fungicidal fibres has been adopted by an English company. Its "Stayfresh" fibres exploit the properties of silver and silica, both of which, on coming into contact with water or humidity, arrest the growth of bacterial populations in carpets, fabrics, furniture, mattresses and bed linen, by cutting off a source of their nutrition. As well as having antimicrobial and fungicidal properties, these fibres are safe, non toxic and inorganic because, they guarantee total mildew and fungus control, preventing the propagation of bacteria such as Escherichia coli and Staphylococcus aureus.
- Modification through grafting or other chemical reactions. It is in this sector, that the Institut Textile de France in Ecully has developed the so-called bio textiles. In these products, the chains of molecules containing antiseptic substances are grafted onto the base polymers of the raw fabric. The base polymers are activated by electronic rays and, in the course of the process, they are refracted in given positions, into which is inserted the first graft molecule. The chains of polymers, which grow laterally from the first molecule, confer on the fabric its bactericidal properties. In the event of direct contact, these fabrics act very rapidly against bacteria and their bactericidal property remains intact even after washing.
- Fibre blends.
- Textile finishing treatments with specific active principles. Following heat treatment (drying, condensation), these substances, being incorporated into polymeric and resinogenic finishing products, become fixed to the structure of the textile.
- Plasma coating (sputtering)(Schindler and Houser, 2004; Heywood, 2003)

3. Antimicrobial finishing agents

Man has adopted antimicrobial substances since ancient times, a fact that is demonstrated by their use in Egyptian mummies and in similar applications in other cultures. In this regard, the protection and preservation of fabrics, too, have long fulfilled a role of the utmost importance. The need to protect and preserve is still fundamental in many textile applications today .Antimicrobials are protective agents that, being bacteriostatic, bactericidal, fungistatic and fungicidal, also offer special protection against the various forms of textile rotting. Here it is focused on some of important antibacterial agents that are used in textile finishing.

3.1 Quaternary ammonium

There are numerous antimicrobials suitable for immobilization on polymer surfaces. Quaternary ammonium compounds seem attractive because their target is primarily the microbial membrane and they accumulate in the cell driven by the membrane potential. To maximize efficiency, quaternary ammonium compound is used as monomeric link in the polymeric leash and poly(4- vinylpyridine) (PVP) is usually selected as the carrying polymer. Tiller et al. showed that the surfaces of commercial polymers treated with *N*-alkylated PVP groups were lethal on contact to both Gram-positive and Gram-negative bacteria, and it was also shown that *N*-alkyl chain of six carbon units in length was the most effective. In recent years, trialkyl ammonium chlorides have been reported to possess germicidal effect in dilute aqueous solutions. (Yao et al, ,2008)

Kumar et al showed that mutual radiation grafting of vinylbenzyltrimethylammonium chloride (VBT) onto cotton cellulose is an effective method to incorporate anti-bacterial property onto the cotton cellulose matrix.(Kumar et al, 2005) Shao et al showed that, a novel quaternary ammonium salt, which contains both perfluoroalkyl group and diallyl groups, should be suitable a finishing agent for providing the fabrics with barriers against microorganisms, water, oil, soil and blood. Moreover, the introduction of diallyl groups into the quaternary ammonium salt not only can enhance the antimicrobial activity, but also extend its application fields. It can be applied in two categories of antimicrobial finishes: one category is part of the fiber-forming process and the other category is the one incorporated in the finishing process. It can also be used as a perfluoroalkyl-containing monomer in the polymer field, which is a convenient method incorporating perfluoroalkyl chain in the polymer. (Shao et al, 2003)

3.2 Triclosan

Triclosan (2,4,4-hydrophenyl trichloro (II) ether), a member of the antiseptic and disinfectant family. Triclosan is a halogen containing derivative of phenol, and is used in cosmetics and toothpastes. It has a wide range of action against gram-negative and gram positive bacteria. This compound, thanks to the presence of the acaricide benzyl benzoate, also offers protection against mites and is used in acaricide (spray or powder) formulas, as well as in a solution (25% concentration) for the treatment of scabies. This compound is non toxic. Benzyl benzoate is an acaricide that acts, chemically, directly on the mites.

Due to its antibacterial properties, triclosan has found widespread use in a variety of consumer products including toothpastes, deodorants, soaps, polymers and fibers. (Allmyr et al, 2006)

3.3 Metallic salts

Numerous chemicals have been used to improve the antimicrobial activity of cotton textiles. Many heavy metals are toxic to microbes at very low concentrations either in the free state or in compounds. They kill microbes by binding to intracellular proteins and inactivating them.(Shahidi et al, 2010) Although some other metals, such as copper, zinc and cobalt, have attracted attention as effective antimicrobial agents for textiles, silver is by far the most widely used in general textiles as well as in wound dressings. It has a MIC value of 0.05- 0.1 mg/l against *E. coli.*

Some concerns have been expressed about the development of bacterial resistance to silver.

For synthetic fibers, silver particles can be incorporated into the polymer before extrusion or before nanofiber formation using electro spinning.

The treatment of natural fibers with metals can only be undertaken at the finishing stage and various strategies have been devised to enhance the uptake and durability. Cotton has been pretreated with succinic acid anhydride, which acted as ligand for metal ions to enhance the subsequent adsorption of metallic salts (Ag^+ and Cu^{2+}) and to provide very effective antibacterial activity.

Preparation of nano-sized metals and metal oxides, mainly silver (Ag), titanium dioxide (TiO2), zinc oxide (ZnO) and cooper II oxide (CuO) has enabled the development of a new generation of biocides.

Among these antimicrobial agents, silver has been widely used in many fields because it shows strong biocidal effects on many pathogenic bacteria. In addition, nanosized inorganic particles possess high surface area/volume ratio and display unique physical and chemical properties. Accordingly, the immobilization of silver nanoparticles on various fibers has recently attracted a great deal of attention. Concerning the studies of fiber/silver nanocomposites, most researches have been interest in preparations of ultrafine fiber containing silver nanoparticles. These developments are important and contribute greatly to the textile industry. However, the conventional cotton microfibers are still highly popular in textile markets. Surface modification of cotton microfibers with silver nanoparticles can increase both the price and purpose of the fibers. (Chen & Li Chiang, 2008)

The antimicrobial properties of the silver ion Ag+ have been exploited for a long time in the biomedical field. The significant feature of the silver ion is its broad-spectrum antimicrobial property, which is particularly significant for the polymicrobial colonization associated with biomaterial related infections. The general finding is that bacteria show a low propensity to develop resistance to silver-based products, and therefore both metallic and ionic silver have been incorporated into several biomaterials such as polyurethane, hydroxyapatite (HA) and bioactive glasses.

Silver containing products are also interesting materials for wound repair applications. When metallic silver reacts with moisture on the skin surface or with wound fluids, silver ions are released, damaging bacterial RNA and DNA, thus inhibiting replication. Sustained silver release products have a bactericidal action and manage wound exudates and odour. In particular, Lansdown et al. have shown that silver aids healing in the sterile skin wound in rat models: silver treatment appeared to reduce the inflammatory and granulation tissue phases of healing and induce epidermal repair. (Blaker et al, 2004; Potiyaraj et al, 2007; Bingshe et al, 2007; Chen & Schluesener et al, 2008; Montazer et al, 2012; Ibrahim et al, 2012)

The results of the counting test showed more reduction of survival of bacteria in the case of loading samples with metal salts.

The result of counting test is shown in Figure 1. As it can be seen, no colony of bacteria was found in agar culture for Ag and Cu loaded samples. It means that the bacteria were killed by silver and copper loading of cotton fabric and causes 100 % reduction of bacterial growth. The interaction between silver and copper ions with bacteria can change the metabolic activity of bacteria and eventually causes the death. Also the results related to Nickel and Cobalt loaded samples shown a few amounts of bacteria spread over the agar plate. However, in case of Ti, Sn and Sb loading, it is seen that, more survival bacteria remain and growth in agar culture. The counting test results related to Sb-loaded samples as compared with Sn and Ti, showed better result, and caused fewer bacteria to growth. Although the amount of survival bacteria for Sn-loaded sample as compared with Ti-loaded one are less. In this research work no ultraviolet light were used before bacteria counting test for Ti-loaded sample and all the samples were analyzed in same condition without UV light. So the results related to bacterial counting test for Ti loaded sample shows moderate reduction percentage of bacteria however by using proper UV light, more reduction of bacterial colonies can be maintained.

It can be concluded that, silver and copper salts causes killing of bacteria and percentage reduction of bacteria reach to 100%. It means that, no bacteria can spread over the agar plate. Also the results of antibacterial efficiency for Cu, Ni and Co loaded samples are very good. And the antibacterial activity for Sn and Ti is moderate as compared with the mentioned elements, However better antibacterial efficiency were achieved for Sb treated sample as compared with Ti and Sn. Scanning Electron Microscope (SEM) is the best known and most widely used tool for morphological analyses. SEM micrographs of untreated cotton fabric and metal salt loaded samples are shown in Figure 2. As shown, some new particles were created on the surface of treated cotton fabrics that did not exist on the surface of untreated one. As it is seen, the particles size appears on the surface of Sb and Sn loaded samples are larger than the others but it does not mean that large size of these particles made our samples with more antibacterial efficiency. (Ghoranneviss et al, 2012)

Titanium dioxide (TiO2) photocatalysts, as alternative materials to degrade organic substances for applications, have attracted much attention since the discovery of photo-induced water cleavage on TiO2 electrodes by Fujishima and Honda in the early 1970s. When TiO2 is exposed to ultraviolet light ($\lambda<400$ nm), holes ($h_{vb}+$) and excited electrons ($e_{cb}-$) are generated. The hole is capable of oxidizing water or hydroxide anions into hydroxyl radicals (UOH). UOH is known to be powerful, indiscriminate oxidizing agents to degrade a wide range of organic pollutants, including aromatics and aliphatics, dyes, pesticides and herbicides. In 1985, Matsunaga et al. reported the antibacterial properties of TiO2 for the first time, which attributed to the high redox potential of the surface species, affording non-selective oxidation of bacteria. Since then, TiO2, as the photo-induced antibacterial agent, has attracted increasing interest. With high photo-reactivity, cheapness, non-toxicity and chemical stability, TiO2 is promising for eliminating microorganisms in self-cleaning and self-sterilizing materials. Photo-excited charge carriers, i.e. electrons and holes, may recombine within nanoseconds. The antibacterial efficiency is determined by the competition between the recombination of charge carriers and the transfer of those to the bacteria. A wide range of transition metal ions has been reported to be used as electron acceptor to decrease the e^{-}–h^{+} recombination in the research of photodegradation towards organic substance. Whereas, noble metal, such as Ag, was explored most as antibacterial effect is concerned. (Zhang et al. 2008; Robertson et al. 2005; Matsunaga et al. 1985; Liu et al. 2008 ; Hashemikia et al, 2012)

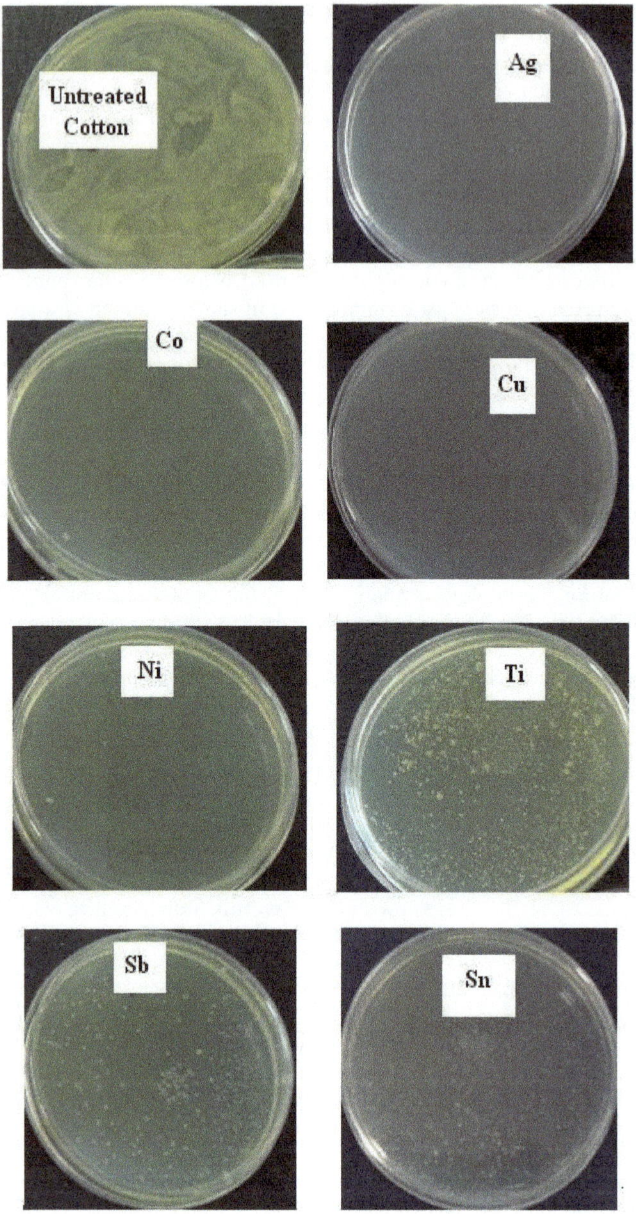

Fig. 1. The bacterial counting test for comparing the antibacterial activity of metallic loaded cotton

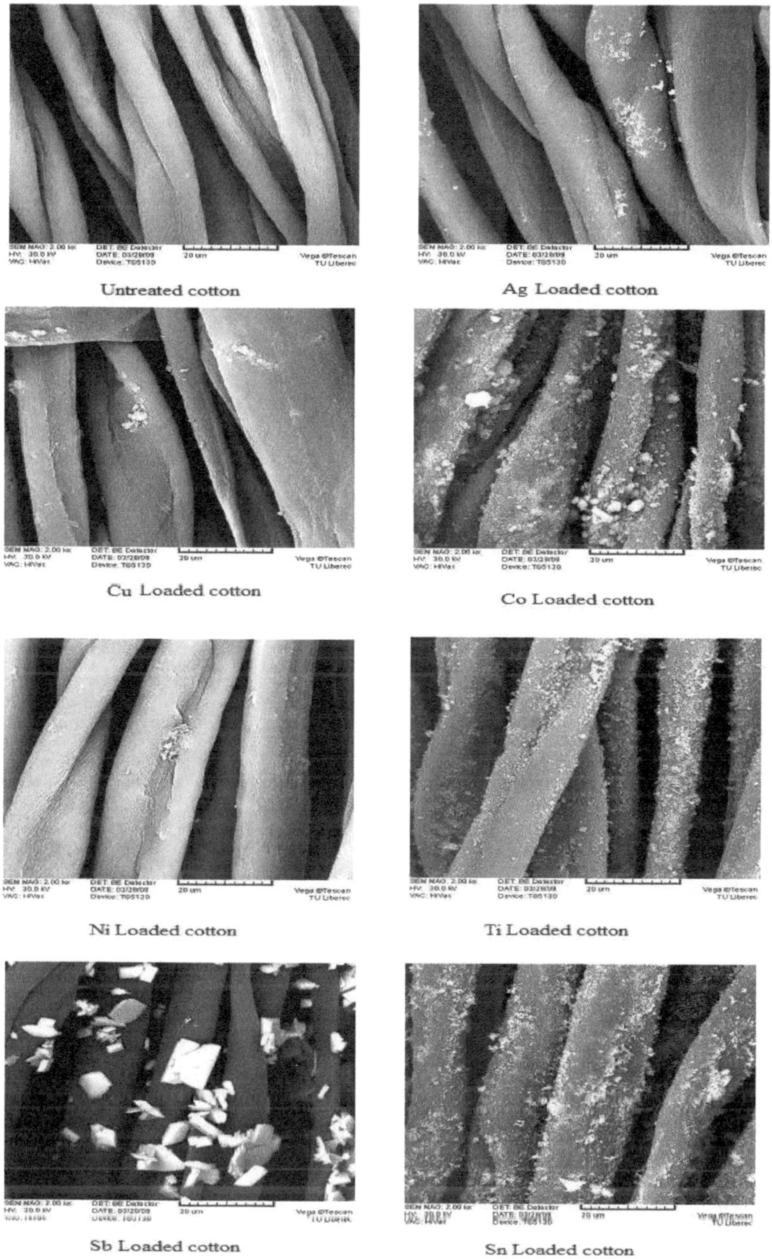

Fig. 2. The SEM images of metallic loaded cotton

The ZnO nanoparticles have been measured to possess probable biological applications as efficient antimicrobial agents, drug carriers, bioimaging probes and possessing cytotoxic behavior for the treatment of cancer. Being a semiconducting material, the band gap between conduction and valance electrons plays a vital role in the generation of reactive oxygen species (ROS), which bring about conformational changes/oxidant injury to the surface of the microorganism membrane. The ZnO nanoparticles, which have positive zeta potential, easily rupture the cell membrane of Escherichia coli (gram negative) on contact and release Zn^{2+} ions, which cause lysosomal and mitochondrial damages. Finally, it is leading to the death of bacterial cells.

The surface defects and morphological changes of ZnO nanoparticles do not play a significant role in the antibacterial activity. That the antibacterial activity depends on the particle size, with an increase in antibacterial activity observed for decreasing size of nanoparticles.

Recently the Krishna Raghupathi et al also reported the properties of antibacterial activity against particles size. This report described the antibacterial activity of ZnO nanoparticles in the range from 212 nm to 12 nm particle size. The antibacterial activity of ZnO nanoparticles is inversely proportional to the size of the nanoparticles. (Krishna Raghupathi et al, 2011; Selvam & Sundrarajan et al, 2012)

3.3.1 Plasma sputtering

However, conventional finishing techniques applied to textiles (dyeing, stain repellence, flame retardance, antibacterial treatments) generally use wet-chemical process steps and produce a lot of wastewater. Plasma treatment, on the other hand, is a dry and eco-friendly technology, which offers an attractive alternative to add new functionalities such as water repellence, long-term hydrophilicity, mechanical, electrical and antibacterial properties as well as biocompatibility due to the nano-scaled modification on textiles and fiber. Moreover, the bulk properties as well as the touch of the textiles remain unaffected.(Shahidi et al, 2010)

In recent years, innovative aspects on the use of coated fabrics have been revealed. Coatings can be applied onto fabrics thus influencing their light reflectivity, electrical conductivity, thermal insulation or for serving decorative purposes. Anti-microbial properties of fabrics are of elevated importance if they are exposed to enhanced biological activity such as in close contact to soil or in a humid environment. In the investigations presented here, the antimicrobial effectiveness of thin films is assessed and the effort of additional finishing for sufficient material protection is determined.

In recent years, physical vapor deposition (PVD) has been applied to modify textile materials due to its inherent merits, such as environmental friendly, various functions and solvent-free process. Sputter coating is one of the most commonly used techniques in PVD, which has been widely used in glass, ceramic and micro-electronic industries.

Sputter coating produces very thin metallic or ceramic coatings on to a wide range of substrates, which can be either metallic or non-metallic in different forms. Sputter coating has also been used to coat textile materials for technical applications. The sputtered atoms have a high energy and when they impinge on any surface, they form a surface coating. The adhesion between the coated layer and the substrate plays a very important role in various applications of the sputter coated materials.(Scholz et al, 2005; Wei et al, 2008; Hegemann et al, 2007; Yuranova et al, 2003 ; Brunon et al, 2011 ; Yuranova et al, 2003)

The advantages of sputtering are the following: simple process, time saving, environmental friendly, and a resulting coating with superior adhesion to substrates.

Deposition of copper on the surface of cotton samples was performed in DC magnetron sputtering, made by Plasma Physics Research Center (Tehran, Iran), by using the setup schematically presented in Figure 3. Copper post cathode was used; also as it can be seen that samples were placed on the anode, and exposed to argon plasma in a cylindrical glass tube. The chamber was evacuated to a pressure of 10^{-5} Torr, using rotary and diffusion pumps, and then argon gas was introduced into the chamber up to a pressure of 0.05 Torr. Voltage was kept at 950 V and the discharge current was about 220 mA.

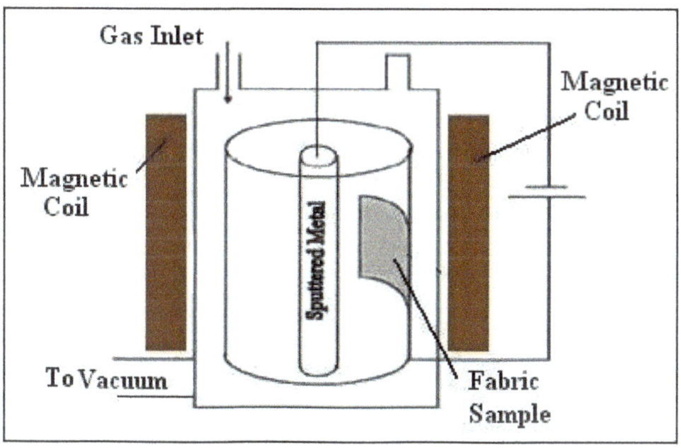

Fig. 3. The schematic view of Plasma sputtering system

Copper particles were deposited on the surface of cotton samples, and the antibacterial has been developed, through incorporation of copper particles on fabric surfaces. The antibacterial properties of the fabrics were connected with the presence of copper on their surface. After plasma treatment, the physical and chemical properties of the fabrics have been examined by surface analysis methods and textile technology tests. Also the antibacterial efficiency was determined by the Halo method.

The agar culture medium is transparent, when the bacterium is inhibited from growth, a transparent area in the form of a halo around the fabric will be observed.

There is no halo observed for untreated cotton fabric. This control test shows that the original cotton fabric does not have any antibacterial properties. Figure 4 illustrate the test results for the untreated and cotton-coated fabric for 30 seconds with S. aureus. (Shahidi et al, 2007; Ghoranneviss et al, 2011)

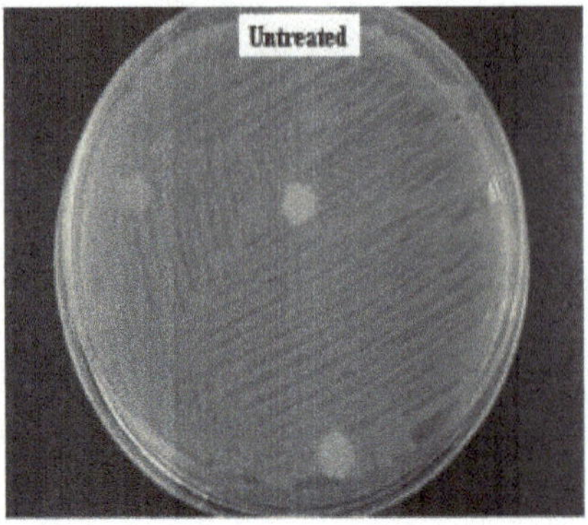

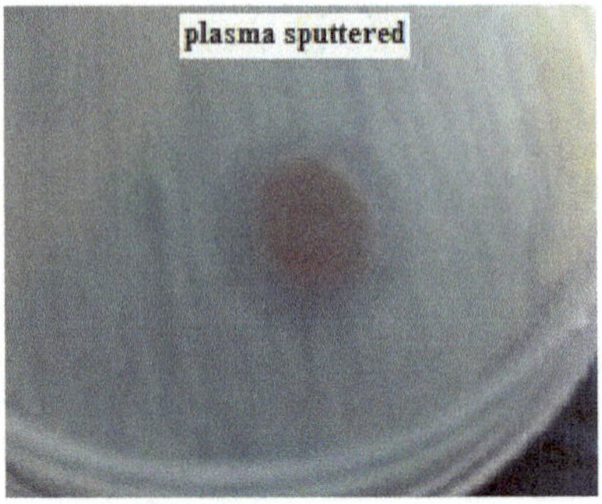

Fig. 4. The inhibition zone of S.aureus around untreated and copper coated cotton.

In the other research work, wool samples have been sputtered by silver particles. The antibacterial counting test was used and the results are shown in Figure 5-8. Both E.coli and S.aureus were used as a bacterial medium. As it is seen, in case of untreated samples, the bacterial colonies cover the completely the agar plate. But after Ag sputtering less amount of bacteria growth in agar plate. However this effect is more significant in case of using s.aureus as bacteria. (Shahidi et al, 2007; Ghoranneviss et al, 2011)

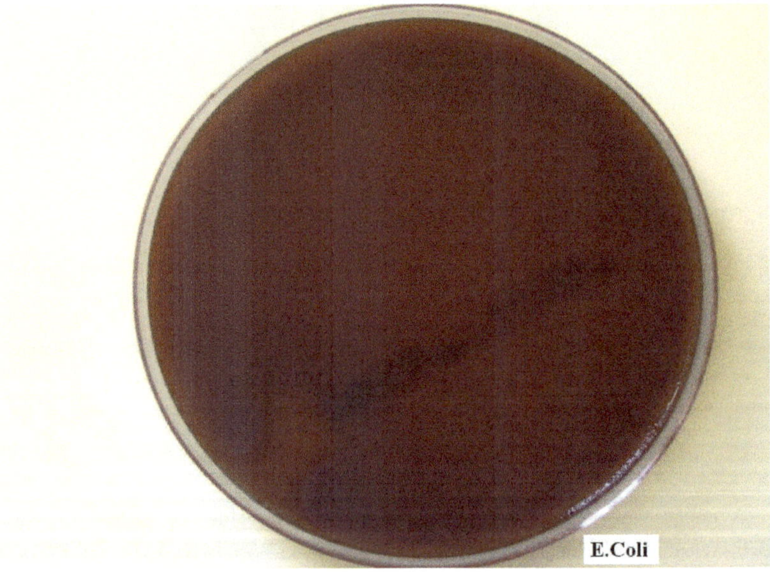

Fig. 5. The bacterial counting test for untreated wool with E. coli

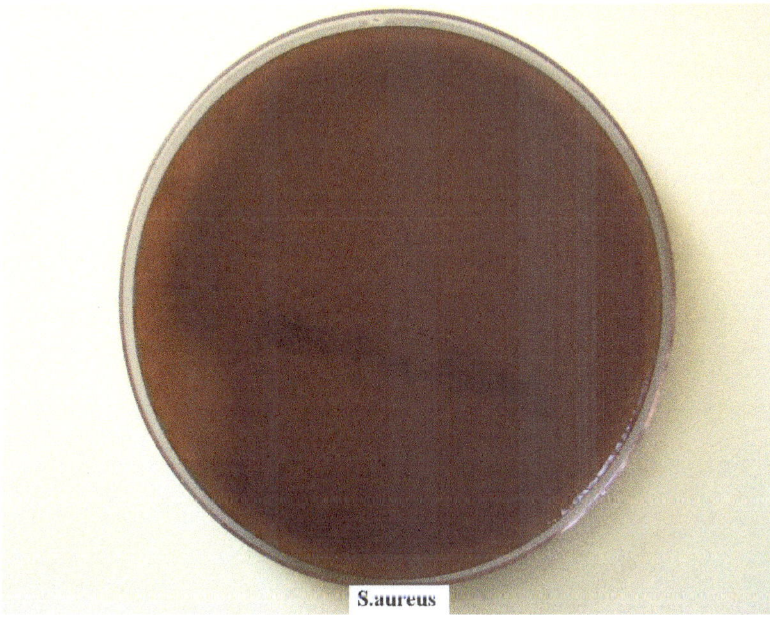

Fig. 6. The bacterial counting test for untreated wool with S.aureus

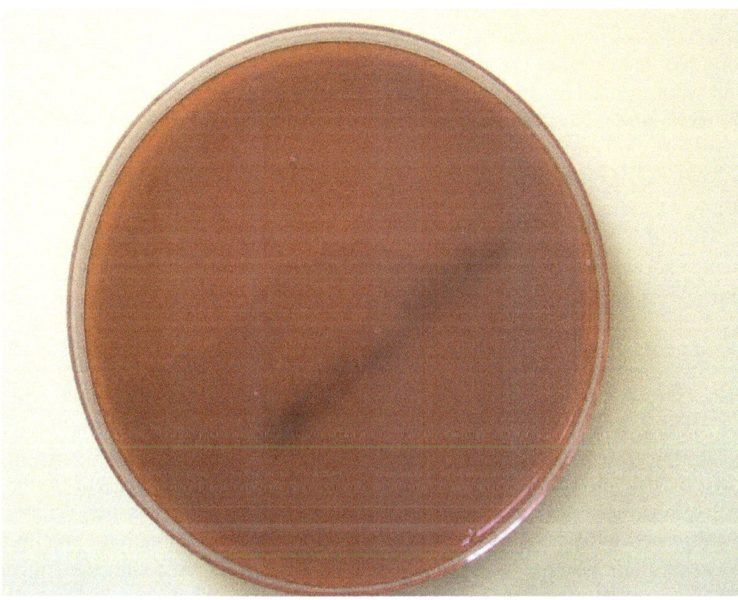

Fig. 7. The bacterial counting test for silver coated wool with E.Coli

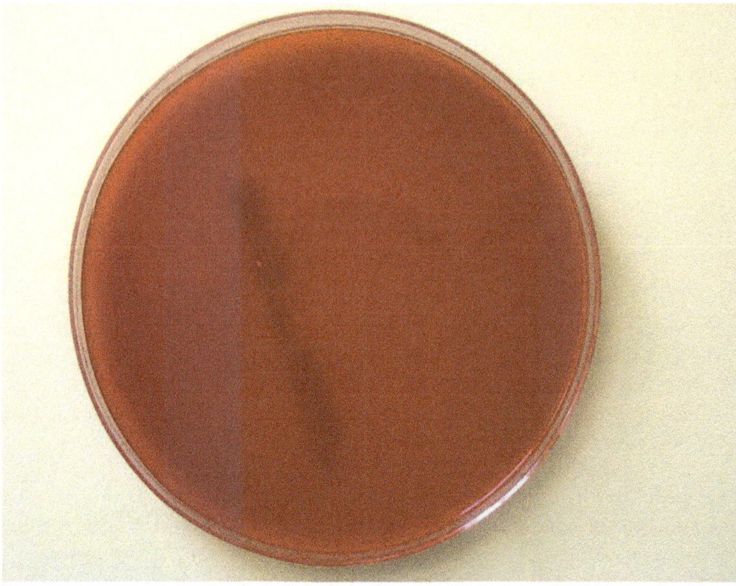

Fig. 8. The bacterila counting test for silver coated wool with S.aureus

3.3.2 Chitosan

Chitosan [poly-_(1-4)-d-glucosamine], a cationic polysaccharide, is obtained by alkaline deacetylation of chitin, the principal exoskeletal component in crustaceans. As the combination of properties of chitosan such as water binding capacity, fat binding capacity, bioactivity, biodegradability, nontoxicity, biocompatibility, acceleration of wound healing and antifungal activity, chitosan and its modified analogs have shown many applications in medicine, cosmetics, agriculture, biochemical separation systems, biomaterials and drug controlled release systems. There are also many studies showing that chitin and chitosan accelerated wound healing in many clinical cases and some types of chitin remedies have already been marketed in Japan. Chitin and chitosan was used in the forms of filament, powder, granule, sponge, and composite with cotton or polyester in most studies. (Yang & Lin, 2004)

Chitosan obtained from the shells of crabs, shrimps and other crustaceans, chitosan is a non-toxic, biodegradable and biocompatible natural polymer, and has long been used as a biopolymer and natural material in the pharmaceutical, medical, papermaking and food processing industries. Because of its polycationic nature, chitosan possesses a good antibacterial property against various bacteria and fungi through ionic interaction at a cell surface, which eventually kills the cell. Previous studies have shown that its antimicrobial activity is influenced by molecular weight (Mw), degree of deacetylation, temperature, pH and cations in solution. Because chitosan is one of the safest and most effective antibacterial agents, it has been widely applied for cotton and other textile antibacterial finishes. (Ye et al, 2005)

It comprises copolymers of glucosamine and N-acetyl glucosamine and has a combination of many unique properties, such as non-toxicity, biocompatibility and biodegradability. Chitosan has got wide application in textile dyeing and finishing as a substitute for the various chemicals used in textile processing . It has been used as a pretreatment agent in dyeing of cotton, in textile printing, wool dyeing and shrink proofing and in durable press finish. (Gupta & Haile, 2007; Knill et al, 2004; Fan et al, 2006)

It is known that chitosan derivatives with quaternary ammonium groups possess high efficacy against bacteria and fungi. It is now widely accepted that the target site of these cationic polymers is the cytoplasmic membrane of bacterial cells. (Ignatova et al, 2007; Ignatova et al, 2006)

Chitosan-based core-shell particle, with chitosan as the shell and a soft polymer as the core, has been designed as a novel antibacterial coating for textiles by Ye et al. The core-shell particles were synthesized via a graft copolymerization of n-butyl acrylate from chitosan in aqueous solution. Properties of the particles, including composition, particle size and distribution, surface charge as well as morphology, were characterized. The treatment of cotton with poly(n-butyl acrylate) (PBA)-chitosan particles confers the fabric with excellent antibacterial property. It is well recognized that chitosan has good antimicrobial activity, especially against the growth of Staphylococcus aureus (S. aureus). Figure 9 shows the result of treated and untreated specimens. As expected, the untreated fabric gave a negligible antibacterial activity of less than 5% while all finished cotton showed over 99% bacterial reduction.

Thus chemical modification of the chitosan through the graft copolymerization does not affect its antimicrobial property. (Ye et al, 2005) Also the TEM images of core-shell particles are shown in Figure 10.

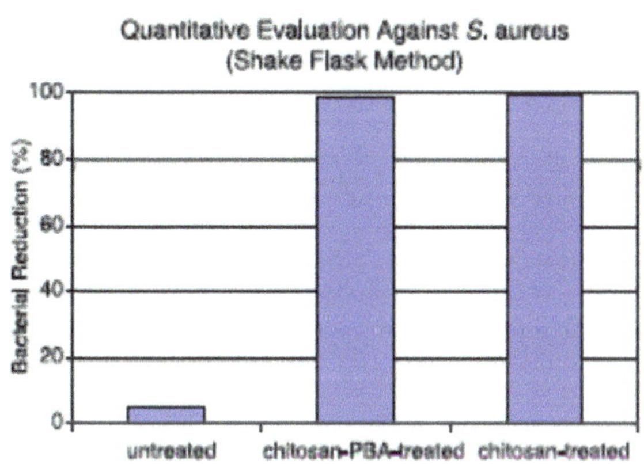

Fig. 9. Comparison of bacterial reduction before and after coating cotton fabrics with chitosan-PBA particles or chitosan solution (after 1 h shaking).

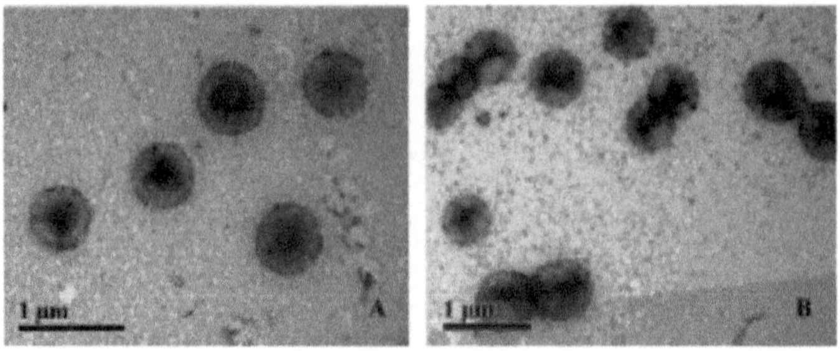

Fig. 10. TEM micrographs of chitosan-PBA particles stained for an appropriate period with 2% PTA solution. (A) Well-defined core-shell particles that consist of PBA cores and chitosan shells; (B) soft PBA-chitosan particles, which deform easily when in contact with each other.

Several mechanisms were proposed for the antimicrobial activity by chitosan:

1. Polycationic structure of chitosan which can be expected to interact with the predominantly anionic components (lipopoly-saccharides and proteins of microorganism surface) resulting in changes in permeability which causes death of the cell by inducing leakage of intracellular components.
2. The chitosan on the surface of the cell can form a polymer membrane which prevents nutrients from entering the cell.
3. The chitosan of lower molecular weight enters the cell, binding to DNA and inhibits RNA and protein synthesis.
4. Since chitosan could adsorb the electronegative substance in the cell and flocculate them, it disturbs the physiological activities of the microorganism leading to death of the cells. (El-tahlawy et al, 2005)

3.3.3 Cyclodextrin

Cyclodextrins are toroidal-shaped cyclic oligosaccharides with a hydrophilic outer surface and an internal hydrophobic hollow interior, which can entrap a vast number of lipophilic compounds into their hydrophobic cavity, depending on their size and molecular structure. The remarkable ability of cyclodextrins to include hydrophobic compounds has been exploited in several fields, spanning from pharmaceuticals to cosmetics, from food manufacturing to commodity

In textile field, a novel functional surface treatment of cotton based on the permanent fixation of cyclodextrin on fabric is receiving increased attention. Some literatures have demonstrated that cyclodextrin fixed to cotton did not affect the hydrophilic properties of cellulose and the immobilized cavities of cyclodextrins did not lose their complexing power to form inclusion complexes with other molecules. (Wang & Cai, 2008)

CDs and their derivatives have been used in the textile domain since the early 1980s. The permanent binding of CDs onto textile fibers offers the advantage that the inclusive properties of CDs towards bioactive molecules become intrinsic to the modified fibers.(El Ghoul et al, 2008)

4. Mechanisms of antimicrobial finishes

Despite the long list of requirements, a variety of chemical finishes have been used to produce textiles with demonstrable antimicrobial properties. These products can be divided into two types based on the mode of attack on microbes. One type consists of chemicals that can be considered to operate by a controlled-release mechanism. The antimicrobial is slowly released from a reservoir either on the fabric surface or in the interior of the fibre. This 'leaching' type of antimicrobial can be very effective against microbes on the fibre surface or in the surrounding environment. However, eventually the reservoir will be depleted and the finish will no longer be effective. In addition, the antimicrobial that is released to the environment may interfere with other desirable microbes, such as those present in waste treatment facilities. The second type of antimicrobial finish consists of molecules that are chemically bound to fibre surfaces. These products can control only those microbes that are present on the fibre surface, not in the surrounding environment. 'Bound' antimicrobials, because of their attachment to the fibre, can potentially be abraded away or become deactivated and lose long term durability. Antimicrobial finishes that control the growth and spread of microbes are more properly called biostats, i.e. bacteriostats, fungistats. Products that actually kill microbes are biocides, i.e. bacteriocides, fungicides. This distinction is important when dealing with governmental regulations, since biocides are strongly controlled.

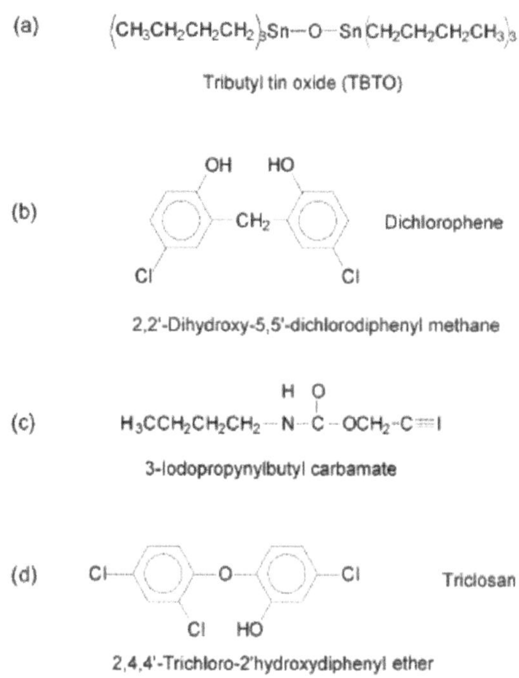

Fig. 11. Controlled release antimicrobials

Textiles with biostatic properties, however, are subject to fewer regulations. The actual mechanisms by which antimicrobial finishes control microbial growth are extremely varied, ranging from preventing cell reproduction, blocking of enzymes, reaction with the cell membrane (for example with silver ions) to the destruction of the cell walls and poisoning the cell from within. In Figure 11 and 12 the chemical structures of some of antimicrobial agents are shown.

(a)

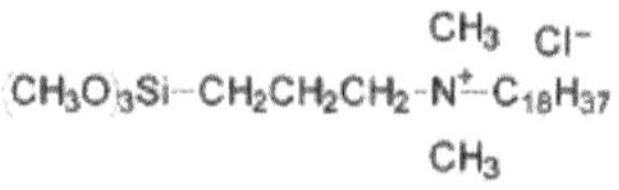

Octadecylaminodimethyltrimethoxysilylpropylammonium chloride

(b)

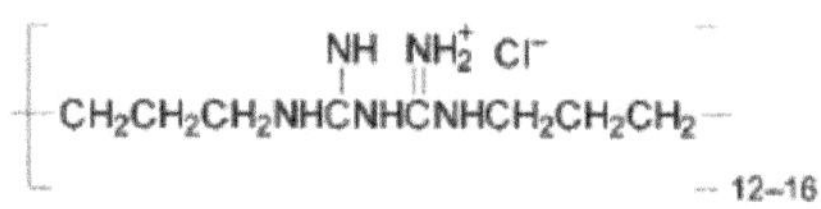

Polyhexamethylene biguanide

Fig. 12. Bound antimicrobials

5. Practical biocides

It is fairly easy to list the desirable properties of an 'ideal' biocide:

1. wide spectrum of effectiveness against both bacteria and fungi;
2. durable for the life of the product;
3. non-toxic to humans at concentrations used - safe to handle and use;
4. colourless and odourless;
5. reasonable cost, and effective at low concentrations;
6. resistant to leaching, weathering and sunlight;
7. no adverse effect on handle or other physical properties of the fabric;
8. compatible with water-repellent and flame-retardant finishes, dyes and other textile chemicals;
9. does not accelerate or catalyse other degenerative processes;
10. applicable using standard textile machinery;
11. withstands processing conditions and temperatures;
12. no environmental problems.

6. Evaluation of antimicrobial finishes

The AATCC Technical Manual12 has a number of test methods that are useful for evaluating antimicrobial finishes on textiles. These tests are summarised in Table 1. Two types of antimicrobial tests are dominant, the agar-based zone of inhibition tests and the bacteria counting tests. The relatively new ISO/DIS 20645 and the corresponding EN ISO

20645 are based on the agar diffusion test and ISO 11721 is a burial test (part 1 for the determination of an antimicrobial finish and part 2 for the determination of the long-term resistance). The main difficulties of these tests are mostly poor reproducibility of the test results and often insufficient correlation between laboratory results and actual conditions in the field. Careful attention to detail and trained laboratory personnel are essential for accurate and repeatable results from these methods.(Schindler & Hauser, 2004)

A more rapid test method, developed by the British Textile Technology Group in the late 1980s, is based on adenosine triphosphate (ATP) luminescence. The growth of microorganisms is assessed by firefly bioluminescent detection and ATP analysis.3

AATCC test method	Comments
Antibacterial activity of textile materials: parallel streak method; test method 147(agar plate test)	Rapid qualitative method for determining antibacterial activity of treated textile materials against both Gram-positive and Gram-negative bacteria. Treated material is placed in nutrient agar that is streaked with test bacteria. Bacterial growth is determined visually after incubation. Antibacterial activity is demonstrated by zones of inhibition on and around the textile.
Antibacterial finishes on textile materials, assessment of: test method 100	Quantitative method for determining the degree of antimicrobial activity of treated textiles. The amount of bacterial growth in inoculated and incubated textiles is determined through serial dilutions and subsequent inoculations of sterile agar. Gram positive and Gram-negative bacteria are used.
Antifungal activity, assessment on textile materials: mildew and rot resistance of textiles; test method 30	Four methods for determining the antifungal assessment on textile properties of treated textiles. One method involves testing fabric properties after burial in soil that contains fungi. In a second method, cellulose fabric is textiles; exposed to *Chaetomium globosum* in an agar plate and the subsequent growth visually determined. The third method exposes textiles to *Aspergillus niger* in an agar plate and visually determines any fungal growth. The fourth method uses a humidity jar to expose textiles to mixture of fungi spores. Any growth on the textile is visually determined
Antimicrobial activity assessment of carpets; test method 174	Methods are given for the qualitative and quantitative determination of antibacterial activity and the qualitative evaluation of antifungal properties of carpet samples using procedures and materials similar to those in the above test methods.

Table 1. Comparison between different AATCC test methods

7. The future

An anti-microbial finish for textiles involving skin contact will need additional safety data concerning this aspect. For manufacturers with biocides with relatively low volumes the cost of generating the necessary data may make ongoing production uneconomical. Acute toxicity data is relatively cheap to generate but sub-acute and other long-term studies are very expensive. It is therefore likely that the number of biocides being produced in the future will diminish and bringing new products to market will be even more expensive. A possible future development would be the micro-encapsulation of biocides. The potential is considerable if the correct performance and economics can be achieved. Benefits could include better durability and greater safety. The search for more cost-effective testing methods will continue.

Overall the need for anti-microbial and hygiene finishes looks set to continue for the foreseeable future. Improving performance and cost-effectiveness, while meeting environmental and toxicity requirements, will continue to challenge those working in this field. (Heywood, 2003)

8. References

Allmyr.M, Margaretha Adolfsson-Erici.M , McLachlan.M.S , Englund.G.S , (2006) Triclosan in plasma and milk from Swedish nursing mothers and their exposure via personal care products, *Science of the Total Environment*, 372, 87-93

Bellini.P, Bonetti.F, Franzetti.E, Rosace.G, Vago.S, (2001) Finishing, ACIMIT

Bingshe.X, Mei.N, Liqiao.W, Wensheng.H, Xuguang.L, (2007) The structural analysis of bio macromolecule wool fiber with Ag-loading SiO2 nano-antibacterial agent by UV radiation, *Journal of Photochemistry and Photobiology A: Chemistry* 188, 98–105

Blaker.J.J, Nazhat.S.N, Boccaccini.A.R, (2004) Development and characterisation of silver-doped bioactive glass coated sutures for tissue engineering and wound healing applications, *Biomaterials*, 25 , 1319–1329

Brunon.C, Chadeau.E, Oulahal.N, Grossiord.C, Dubost.L, Bessueille.F, Simon.F, Degraeve.P, Leonard.D , (2011) Characterization of Plasma Enhanced Chemical Vapor Deposition–Physical Vapor Deposition transparent deposits on textiles to trigger various antimicrobial properties to food industry textiles, *Thin Solid Films*, 519, 5838–5845

Chen.C.Y , Li Chiang.C, (2008) Preparation of cotton fibers with antibacterial silver nanoparticles *Materials Letters*, 62, 3607–3609

Chen.X, Schluesener.H.J , (2008) Nanosilver: A nanoproduct in medical application , *Toxicology Letters* , 176, 1–12

El Ghoul.Y, Blanchemain.N, Laurent.T, Campagne.C, El Achari.A, Roudesli.S, Morcellet.M, Martel.B, Hildebrand.H.F, (2008) Chemical, biological and microbiological evaluation of cyclodextrin finished polyamide inguinal meshes q *Acta Biomaterialia*, 4, 1392-1400

El-tahlawy.K.F, El-bendary.M.A, Elhendawy.A.G, Hudson.S.M, (2005) The antimicrobial activity of cotton fabrics treated with different crosslinking agents and chitosan, *Carbohydrate Polymers* 60, 421–430

Fan.L, Du.Y, Zhang.B, Yang.J, Zhou.J, Kennedy.J.F, (2006) Preparation and properties of alginate/carboxymethyl chitosan blend fibers, *Carbohydrate Polymers*, 65, 447–452

Ghoranneviss.M, Shahidi.S, Anvari.A, Motaghi.Z, Wiener.J,ˇSlamborova.I , (2011) Influence of plasma sputtering treatment on natural dyeing and antibacterial activity of wool fabrics, *Progress in Organic Coatings* , 70, 388-393

Ghoranneviss.M, Shahidi.S, Effect of Various Metallic Salts on Antibacterial Activity and Physical Properties of Cotton Fabrics, *Journal of Industrial Textile*, online published, 2012

Gupta.D, Haile.A, (2007) Multifunctional properties of cotton fabric treated with chitosan and carboxymethyl chitosan, *Carbohydrate Polymers*, 69, 164–171

Hashemikia.S, Montazer.M , (2012) Sodium hypophosphite and nano TiO2 inorganic catalysts along with citric acid on textile producing multi-functional properties, *Applied Catalysis A: General*, 417- 418, 200- 208

Hegemann.D, Mokbul Hossain.M, Balazs.D.J, (2007) Nanostructured plasma coatings to obtain multifunctional textile surfaces, *Progress in Organic Coatings*, 58, 237–240

Heywood.D, Textile Finishing, 2003, Society of Dyers and Colourists

Ibrahim.N.A, Eid.B.M, El-Batal.H, (2012) A novel approach for adding smart functionalities to cellulosic fabrics, *Carbohydrate Polymers*, 87, 744- 751

Ignatova. M, Manolova.N, Rashkov.I , (2007) Novel antibacterial fibers of quaternized chitosan and poly(vinyl pyrrolidone) prepared by electrospinning, *European Polymer Journal* ,43, 1112–1122

Ignatova.M, Starbova.K, Markova.N, Manolova .Nand Rashkov.I, (2006) Electrospun nano-fibre mats with antibacterial properties from quaternised chitosan and poly(vinyl alcohol) , *Carbohydrate Research*, 341, 2098–2107

Knill.C.J, Kennedy.J.F, Mistry.J, Miraftab.M, Smart.G, Groocock.M.R, Williams.H.J, (2004) Alginate fibres modified with unhydrolysed and hydrolysed chitosans for wound dressings , *Carbohydrate Polymers*, 55, 65–76

Krishna Raghupathi, R., Ranjit Koodali, T. & Adhar Manna, C. (2011). Size-dependent bacterial growth inhibition and mechanism of antibacterial activity of zinc oxide nanoparticles. Langmuir, 27, 4020–4028.

Kumar.V, Bhardwaj.Y.K, Rawat.K.P, Sabharwal.S, (2005) Radiation-induced grafting of vinylbenzyltrimethylammonium chloride (VBT) onto cotton fabric and study of its anti-bacterial activities, *Radiation Physics and Chemistry*, 73, 175–182

Liu.X, Zhao.X, Li.B, Cao.C, Dong.Y, Ding.C, Chu.P.K, (2008) UV-irradiation-induced bioactivity on TiO2 coatings with nanostructural surface, *Acta Biomaterialia*, 4, 544–552

Matsunaga.T, Tomoda.R, Nakajima.T, Wake.H, (1985) FEMS *Microbiol. Lett.* 29 , 211.

Montazer.M, Alimohammadi.F , Shamei.A, Rahimi.M.K (2012) In situ synthesis of nano silver on cotton using Tollens' reagent, *Carbohydrate Polymers*, 87, 1706- 1712

Potiyaraj.P, Kumlangdudsana.P, Dubas.S.T, (2007) Synthesis of silver chloride nanocrystal on silk fibers, *Materials Letters* 61 2464–2466

Robertson.J, Robertson.P, Lawton.L, (2005) *Photochem.J. Photobiol., A Chem.* 175 , 51.

Selvam.S, Sundrarajan.M, (2012) Functionalization of cotton fabric with PVP/ZnO nanoparticles for improved reactive dyeability and antibacterial activity, Carbohydrate Polymers 87 , 1419- 1424

Schindler.W.D , Hauser.P.J, Chemical finishing of textiles, woodhead publishing,2004

Scholz.J, Nocke.G, Hollstein.F, Weissbach.A, (2005) Investigations on fabrics coated with precious metals using the magnetron sputter technique with regard to their anti-microbial properties, *Surface & Coatings Technology* , 192 , 252- 256

Shahidi.S, Ghoranneviss.M, Moazzenchi.B, Rashidi.A, Mirjalili.M, (2007) Investigation of Antibacterial Activity on Cotton Fabrics with Cold Plasma in the Presence of a Magnetic Field, *Plasma Process and Polymers*. 4, S1098–S1103

Shahidi.S, Rashidi.A, Ghoranneviss.M, Anvari.A, Rahimi.M.K, Bameni Moghaddam.M, Wiener.J, (2010) Investigation of metal absorption and antibacterial activity on cotton fabric modified by low temperature plasma, *Cellulose* , 17, 627–634

Shao.H, Jiang.L, Meng.W.D, Qing.F.L, (2003) Synthesis and antimicrobial activity of a perfluoroalkyl-containing quaternary ammonium salt, *Journal of Fluorine Chemistry*, 124, 89–91

Wang.J.H, Cai.Z, (2008) Incorporation of the antibacterial agent, miconazole nitrate into a cellulosic fabric grafted with b-cyclodextrin, *Carbohydrate Polymers*, 72, 695–700

Wei.Q, Xu.Q, Cai.Y, Wang.Y, (2008) Evaluation of the interfacial bonding between fibrous substrate and sputter coated copper, *Surface & Coatings Technology*, 202, 4673–4680

Yao.C, Li.X, Neoh.K.G, Shi.Z, Kang.E.T, (2008) Surface modification and antibacterial activity of electrospun polyurethane fibrous membranes with quaternary ammonium moieties, *Journal of Membrane Science*, 320, 259–267

Yang.J.M, Lin.H.T , (2004) Properties of chitosan containing PP-g-AA-g-NIPAAm bigraft nonwoven fabric for wound dressing , *Journal of Membrane Science*, 243, 1–7

Ye.W, Fai Leung.M, Xin.J, Leung Kwong.T, Kam Len Lee.D, Li.P, (2005) Novel core-shell particles with poly(n-butyl acrylate) cores and chitosan shells as an antibacterial coating for textiles *Polymer* 46, 10538–10543

Yuranova.T, Rincon.A.G, Bozzi.A, Parra.S, Pulgarin.C, Albers.P, Kiwi.J, (2003) Antibacterial textiles prepared by RF-plasma and vacuum-UV mediated deposition of silver, *Journal of Photochemistry and Photobiology A: Chemistry*, 161, 27–34

Zhang.W, Chen.Y, Yu.S, Chen.S, Yin.Y (2008) Preparation and antibacterial behavior of Fe3+-doped nano structured TiO2 thin films, *Thin Solid Films* 516, 4690–4694

19

Antibacterial Agents from Lignicolous Macrofungi

Maja Karaman, Milan Matavulj and Ljiljana Janjic
University of Novi Sad, Department of Biology and Ecology, Novi Sad
Serbia

1. Introduction

Since ancient times, the mushrooms have been prized as food as well as source for drugs, giving rise to an increasing interest today ("functional food"). Number of macrofungi is of a medicinal importance and represents an unlimited source of secondary metabolites of high medicinal value while a large number of biologically active molecules are identified in many species of macrofungi throughout the world (Wasser & Weis, 1999; Kitzberger et al., 2007; Barros et al., 2007; Turkoglu et al., 2007; Kim et al., 2008; 2007; Wasser, 2011). In addition, of importance is the amount of produced substances namely, they must be simple for the manufacturing (industrial synthesis) or there must be enough raw material for extraction of active molecules. Such molecules, if chemical groups responsible for biological activity are known, should serve as basic compounds for the synthesis of new molecules.

Lignicolous macrofungi express significant biological effects, including antibacterial activity (Hur et al., 2004; Ishikawa et al., 2005; Kalyoncu et al., 2010) and their secondary metabolites can be easily extracted and identified. It has been found that secondary metabolites are very divergent in structure and play no essential role in their growth and reproduction, but probably have a function in biochemical evolution of a species ensuring its survival (Engler et al., 1998). The presence of these compounds in macrofungi is genetically determined, but also varies as a function of ecological factors and the growth stage of these organisms (Puttaraju et al., 2006). The fungal metabolites of fruiting bodies frequently differ from those of mycelia of submerged cultures or fermentation broth. Moreover, biogenetic pathways are rather dependent on their habitats or geographic origin. The chemical composition of fungal species significantly relies on the strains and sites (substrates) of the fruiting body production. The level of phenolic compounds seems to be very much dependent on the location and stress conditions (Kim et al., 2008). With regard to this, more geographical regions and more habitats should be analyzed in the future.

A great potential of these fungi is found in their use as dietary supplements, regardless active principle. A number of products derived from mushrooms that are sold in the market is untested and of suspicious quality. Since the natural style of life become more and more popular around the world, what means return to the organic, natural food and medicines, many people lack a critical attitude to the so-called ecological products. It would therefore be important to develop food suplements and medicines based on natural resources, but with the necessary scientific confirmation of values of such products.

1.1 Macrofungi

Macrofungi or mushrooms are not taxonomic categories, being most frequently used as terms for fungi with distinctive fruiting bodies, which are usually fleshy and edible, hypogeous or epigeous, large enough to be seen with the naked eye, and picked by hand (Chang and Miles, 2002, Karaman et al., 2012).

Lignicolous (wood-decaying) macrofungi, mostly belonging to the *Polyporaceae* family, are easily noticed, collected and recognized in the field. Taxonomically, these fungi mainly belong to the phyla Basidiomycota and Ascomycota, including about 20,000 known species, widely distributed on Earth. Recent estimations suggest that even more than 1.5 million species of fungi exist on our planet and about 140,000 species belong to macrofungi. However, only 10% of them are explored and 16% are cultured (Chang & Miles, 2004; Mueller, Bills & Foster, 2004).

1.2 Antibiotics and antimicrobial agents

From the beginning until now, the humankind has always been faced with a problem of spreading of infectious diseases. Today, more than 150 compounds make arsenal of antimicrobial substances used in the treatment of infectious diseases. Antibiotics are defined as low molecular weight organic natural products (secondary metabolites or idiolites) made by microorganisms, which are active at low concentrations against other microorganisms. There are estimations that among 12,000 antibiotics known, approximately 55% are produced by Streptomyces, 11% by other Actinomycetes, 12% from other bacteria and 22% from filamentous fungi (Inouye et al., 2004). In its broadest definition an antibacterial is an agent that interferes with the growth and reproduction of bacteria. Unlike antibiotics, antibacterials are not used as medicine for humans or animals, but are now most commonly described as agents used to disinfect surfaces and eliminate potentially harmful bacteria found in products such as soaps, detergents, health and skincare products and household cleaners.

Since Alexander Fleming`s discovery, in 1928, of the first antibiotic, called penicillin, produced by the mold *Penicillium chrysogenum*, a real revolution in medicine with a new era of antibiotics have started. Later, the entire group of β-lactam antibiotics (penicillins and cephalosporins) was discovered, followed by the Waxman`s discovery of streptomycin derived from Streptomyces bacteria, used in a treatment of tuberculosis), and then tetracyclines, quinolones, antifungal metabolites, antiparasitic substances and more recently antiviral drugs such as acyclovir. In 1971, the second significant antibiotic cyclosporin A and C were isolated from fungal organism *Hypocladium inflatum gams* (*Tolypocladium inflatum*) which is the asexual state of the pathogen of beetles *Elaphocordyceps subsessilis* (Petch) G.H. Sung, J.M. Sung & Spatafora). Its immunosupresive activity was revealed in 1976 by J.F. Borel and was approved for use 1983 in order to reduce the risk of organ rejection in transplant surgery (Upton, 2001 as cited in Giovannini, 2006).

1.3 Antibiotic resistance and further perspectives

Today, antibiotic resistance is a serious problem and antibiotics are losing their effectiveness what is especially important and have serious threats for humans whose health is already compromised by stress in modern way of life or by illness (HIV patients, immnocompromised persons that are under chemotherapy). Along with the increasing use of antibiotics and antibiotic agents, the resistance of bacteria to common and more frequently used antibiotics increased, resulting in low respond to the antibiotic treatment. The existance of multidrug-resistant diseases, once felt to be under control, increased as well, tuberculosis, penicillin-resistant pneumonia, resistant malaria (the cause of death of 1.1 million people in 1998), resistant strains of gonorrhea or dysentery caused by Shigella and Salmonella (2.2 million deaths in 1998).

Public concern about infection has been expanded, resulting in a greater public use of a variety of antibacterial agents designed to remove disease-causing organisms from external surfaces before they can enter the body. Today, antibacterials may also be impregnated into sponges, cutting boards, carpeting, and children's toys. However, if used too frequently and indiscriminately, certain antibacterial agents, those that leave trace chemical residues and that target particular processes in the life cycle of bacteria, may select for resistant strains (http://www.tufts.edu/med/apua/about_issue/agents.shtml).

Furthermore, no new class of antibacterial substances has been developed to combat infectious diseases since 1970 (WHO, 2000). It is therefore necessary to find some new compounds to fight against these resistant microorganisms. Then starts the parallel struggle against antibiotic resistance exhibited in the continuous screening of new natural resources of undiscovered antibiotics from the nature. In this manner, the potential of mushrooms have a great advantage, even in comparison to the bacteria. Nowadays it is much more complicated to find new pharmaceutical active substances by chemical synthesis than from the existing and unexplored natural resources. Screenings of biological activities have made great progress in exploring the rich unlimited and undiscovered natural products in order to use it for production of pharmaceutical and agrochemical products (Anke, 1989). Many organisms were studied as potentially new resources of undiscovered bioactive components, among which fungi from the phylum Basidiomycota gave the promising results. In the forties, the pioneers in such research were Anchel, Hervey, Wilkins et al. and Florey et al. 1949, who tested extracts derived from fruiting bodies and mycelia cultures of more then 2000 species, resulting in isolation of a tricyclic diterpene antibiotic (pleuromutilin from *Pleurotus mutilus*). During nineties of the last century many new structures and biological activities were detected (Anke, 1989). Since then, numerous studies have been performed. Today we are witnessing very important struggle not only against microorganisms but also against other human diseases such as cancer, viral and other diseases.

1.4 Antimicrobial substances - Antibiotics from fungi and macrofungi

Microbial metabolites and their derivatives play an important role in the development of medicines. The use of these metabolites has grown extensively over the past century, starting with the Fleming's discovery of penicillin (1924), originally from *Penicillium notatum* filamentous micro-fungus, via Brotzu's discovery of cephalosporins from another fungus, mold *Cephalosporium acremonium* (*Acremonium chrysogenum* now), until today when the Japanese clinics use 30 penicillin derivatives and about 49 derivatives of cephalosporin. Although the metabolites originating from fungi were the main targets of antimicrobial screening, these studies were interrupted for a short time by Waksman's discovery of streptomycin (1945) originating from Actinomycetes. It is believed that the cause of the break helped by the fact that fungi often produce mycotoxins with pronounced cytotoxicity in humans and animals, and one example is the aflatoxin from the mold *Aspergillus flavus*, the most prominent cause of chronic hepatitis that leads to tumor malignancy.

However, in recent years the trend has changed and fungal metabolites have again attracted the attention of pharmacological research. This can be seen from the statistics presenting fungal metabolites increasingly important as bioactive agents and showing that the percentage of medicines versus the metabolites originating from actinomycetes are as it follows (according to the Journal of Antibiotics (I), Tokyo): 13 versus 66% (1983), 16 versus 74% (1990), 38 versus 53% (1994) and 47 versus 44% (2000), while the percentage of metabolites originating from the bacteria remained at about 8%, except 1983 when it was 21%. A similar tendency was observed for metabolites that are registered as patents in Japan, showing that the products from the fungi grew intensively: 11% (1983), over 21% (1990) to 36% (2000), and for the products from actinomycetes decreased sharply from 74% (1983), over 66% (1990) to 48% (2000). According to Tanaka and Omura (1993), 43% of more than 8000 new microbial metabolites were discovered thanks to Japanese scientists. It is possible that the abundance of secondary metabolites of fungi and actinomycetes, compared with bacteria and yeasts, is associated with the characteristics of the environment poor in nutrients. Nutritional limitation further induces secondary metabolism and production of various compounds, in order to exploit scarce nutrients in the best extent possible (Aldered et al., 1999). Taking into account the antibiotic screening, review of Inouye et al., 2004 showed that the number of antifungal metabolites increased significantly, anticancer metabolites - moderately, while the number of antibacterial metabolites decreased in the last ten years. However, the most significant increase was observed in bioactive metabolites of non-antibiotic mode of action, especially regarding the screening of inhibitors of cholesterol synthesis, of which 93% originated from fungi (Yagisawa, 2000).

In this sense it is considered that the eukaryotic fungal metabolites in action in mammalian cells could have far fewer side-effects compared with prokaryotic metabolites. Cultures of micro-organisms usually contain complex mixtures of different compounds, small and large molecular weight, what makes a direct pharmacological screening more difficult, considering the fact that can easily be masked by the activity of other compounds in the mixture. Being sessile organisms, which are in their natural environment constantly exposed to the influence of different competitors (parasitic organisms), it is not surprising that many antibiotics are isolated from fungi (Lindequist et al., 2005). Although today, still only compounds originating from micro-fungi or synthetic medicines have been used, literature data pointing to higher fungi, macro-fungi, primarily Basidiomycetes as natural sources rich in new antimicrobial substances are infrequently found (Suay et al., 2000).

As potential new sources of natural antibiotics, lignicolous mushrooms again become the subject of study (Smania et al., 2001). The fact that humans and animals share common microbial pathogens with fungi (*E. coli, S. aureus* and *P. areuginosa*) has prompted the thought that they produce compounds that may have similar effects in humans (Zjawioni, 2004). In Western Europe, the interest for this group of fungi start with the discovery of antibiotics (penicillin), when a group of scientists with their pioneering research of new antibiotics originating from macrofungi Basidiomycota, led by M. Anchel, A. Hervey, WH Wilkins and Kavanagh, started research of extracts and culture mycelia and fruit body of about 2000 species (Florey et al., 1949). This research has resulted in isolation of antibiotics three-cyclic diterpene pleuromutilin (Kavanagh et al., 1951) from *Pleurotus mutilus* species. Pleuromutilin has demonstrated its antibacterial activity by inhibiting bacterial protein synthesis by interacting with RNA (Lorenzen & Anke, 1998). After that, the first semisynthetic antibiotic tiamulin was produced together with valnemuline, used in veterinary medicine (Egger & Reinshagen, 1976) for the treatment of *Mycoplasma* infections in animals (Lorenzen & Anke, 1998).

Many studies have shown that macrofungi produce many interesting pharmacological substances. By comparing the number of studied fungi with those whose chemical and pharmacological effects are completely unknown, we realized that only a very small, even insignificant fraction of potentially active fungal substances are known. For instance, the illustrative example is the species *Ganoderma lucidum*, witnessing that each species contains many different active components. In addition, production of certain secondary metabolites may depend on the characteristics of the strains (isolates) or culture conditions. Therefore, many scientists coping with this problem are actually trying to find new active compounds to be used in the future. It is clear that only a small number of active compounds studied *in vitro* or *in vivo* on animals as biological models suits the needs of allopathic medicine, defined by chemical composition, precise dosing, toxicology, pharmacodynamics and clinical studies.

Macrofungi need antibacterial and antifungal compounds to survive in their natural environment. Since fungi and humans share common microbial pathogens (e.g. *E. coli*, *S. aureus* and *P. areuginosa)*, antimicrobial compounds that are produced by fungi against microorganisms, can benefit to humans (animals). Compounds of special interest are those that exhibit antibacterial activities against multiresistant bacterial strains (methicillin resistant *S. aureus* - MRSA or vancomycine resistant *Enterococcus* - VRE).

According to a recent biological evaluation, more than 75% of screened polypores showed strong antimicrobial activity inhibiting mostly Gram-positive bacterial strains (*B. subtilis*, *S. aureus* and *M. flavus)*. It was reported that new sesquiterpenoid hydroquinones produced by some species of the European *Ganoderma* genus, named ganomycins, inhibit the growth of methicillin-resistant *S. aureus* and other bacteria (Mothana et al., 2000).

Based on our results of antibacterial screening, 60% methanol and 55% chloroform extracts reached a significant antibacterial activity, giving the diameter of inhibitory zone (>15mmØ) against one or more target bacteria. Gram -negative bacteria were less sensitive to the applied extracts than Gram-positive ones, except *G. lucidum* ethanolic extract (25mg/ml) against *P. aeruginosa* (h) and *E. coli* (ATCC 25922). Three extracts of lignicolous macrofungi *P. betulinus*, *C. versicolor* and *G. lucidum* showed a wide range of activities against all tested Gram-positive and some of Gram-negative bacteria, reaching MIC values mainly at a concentration of 17.5 mg/ml. Unlike methanol, chloroform extracts did not show concentration dependence while the concept of a dose response phenomenon- hormesis (low dose stimulation and high dose inhibition) may be used for explanation of this phenomenon. The precise composition of examined extracts of fungi is unknown and can only be assumed that the effect of crude extracts, which are concentration dependent, is a consequence of complex interactions between cells and mixtures of compounds in the extracts (Karaman et al., 2009a).

In a recent screening of antibacterial activity of water and methanol crude extracts of the species *Meripilus giganteus* against nine species of Gram-positive and four species of Gram- negative bacteria, the most active extract was methanolic extract, inhibiting all the Gram-positive bacteria (mostly *S. aureus*[an], *Rh. equi*, *Bacillus*) and only two Gram-negative ones, *C. perfringens* and *P. aeruginosa*, ATCC strains (Karaman et al., 2009b) The animal strains showed to be the most susceptible analyzed strains, indicating a possible application of this fungus against Gram-positive bacterial infections in animals. Since water extract exhibited only a narrow antibacterial effect, we assumed that the obtained results could not be attributed to the compounds like proteins or polysaccharides. These results are in agreement with the literature data for similar polypore fungi (Lindequist et al., 2005; Zjawioni, 2004), demonstrated sterols and lanostanoid terpenoids as well as phenolic compounds as the main active components responsible for the obtained activity (Turkoglu et al., 2007; Barros et al., 2007; Elmastas et al., 2007).

1.4.1 Antiviral substances

Presented antiviral activity of fungi is related to their whole, complex extracts, but also to the isolated compounds. Agents isolated from fungi can directly cause the inhibition of viral enzymes, the synthesis of viral nucleic acid, or adsorption and absorption of virus in mammalian cells. The most often small molecules are active in the direct antiviral effect, while the indirect effects are mediated by antiviral activity immunostimulative polysaccharides and other complex molecules (Zjawioni, 2004).

1.4.1.1 Low molecular weight compounds with antiviral activity

Several triterpenes from *G. lucidum* (ganoderiol F, ganodermanontriol and ganoderic acid and B) are active antiviral agents against HIV-1 virus. *In vitro* antiviral activity of influenza viruses type A and B was noticed in extracts of mycelium of mushroom *Kuehneromyces mutabilis* (Schaeff.: Fr.) (Singer & AH Sm.), while the extract and two isolated phenolic components from the mushroom *Inonotus hispidus* (Bull.; Fr.) P. Karst, as well as ergosterol peroxide, are present in many different fungal species.

1.4.1.2 High molecular weight compounds with antiviral activity

Water-soluble lignins isolated from *Inonotus obliquus* (Pers.: Fr.) Pilate, inhibit HIV protease with IC 50 value of 2.5 mg/ml. Anti-HIV activity is recorded for the submerged culture media of *L. edodes* and water-soluble lignin isolated from the same fungus. Protein-polysaccharide complex PSK and PSP from *Coriolus versicolor*, also shows antiviral activity on HIV and cytomegalovirus *in vitro*. Inhibition of HIV-1 reverse transcriptase is caused by velutin, protein from *Flammulina velutipes*, which inactivates ribosomes. MD fractions of mushroom *Grifola frondosa* showed general improvement of condition of the patients (85%) who had various symptoms of HIV and other secondary diseases (Zjawioni, 2004).

1.4.2 Antifungal substances

Compounds with antibacterial and antifungal activity of mushrooms assists in their survival in their environment. These substances can be very useful in the treatment of human infections, but the official antibiotic therapeutics in the world market can be only found originating from microfungi so far. Opportunistic fungal infections are always a big problem, especially in immunocompromised patients receiving chemotherapy or in cases of transplantation of organs or bone marrow, as well as in HIV infection. During the last ten years, the interest in compounds that show antifungal activity has been increased. Among them the sordarin (tricyclic diterpene glycoside) was for the first time isolated in 1971 (Hauer and Sigg as cited in Inouye et al., 2004), and slightly more potent zofimarin was isolated for the first time in 1987 (Ogita et al. 1987 as cited in Inouye et al., 2004). In addition, suggestive is xylarin (compound SCH57404) isolated from the lignicolous fungus *Xylaria* sp. (Schneider, 1995). Many derivatisations of sordarin antibiotics have been performed in research groups of the GlaxoSmith Kline company by biotransformation with *Streptomyces avermitilis*, what resulted in the synthesis of GM237354 (Herreros et al., 1998), with the MIC of 90% that was 0.015 mg/ml for isolates of *C. albicans* and 0.12 for *C. tropicalis*. Further development of these compounds has led to the azasordarin group in which the sugar component is replaced by N-substituted morpholine (Herreros et al., 2001 as cited in Inouye et al., 2004).

Several antifungal metabolites with steroid structure have been also isolated from fungi A25822 A and B from *Geotrichum* (Gordee and Butler, 1975 as cited in Inouye et al., 2004) and from *Wallemia sebi*; Mer-NF8054 A and X from the genus *Aspergillus*. The most famous triterpene, favonol isolated from basidiomycetous *Favolashia* sp. (Anke et al., 1995 as cited in Inouye et al., 2004) is a metabolite that exhibited antifungal activity against Ascomycetes, Basidiomycetes, Zygomycetes and Oomycetes, but did not show antibacterial activity. Researchers of Merck Group have discovered four acidic terpenoids from filamentous fungi: ergokonin A (from *Trichoderma koningii*), ascosteroid (from *Ascotricha amphitricha*) arundifungin (steroid from *Arthrinium arundinis*) and enfumafungin (pentacyclic terpenoid from from mould *Trichoderma koningii*), ascosteroid (from ascomycetous *Ascotricha amphitricha*), arundifungin (steroid from mould *Arthrinium arundinis*) and enfumafungin (pentacyclic terpenoid from *Aureobasidium*), which were found to affect the biosynthesis of β-D-glucan but not the biosynthesis of steroids. Among them the best antifungal activity on *Candida* species and species of *Aspergillus* genera showed enfumafungin.

1.5 Chemical nature of antibacterial agents

A large number of pharmacologically active substances like sesquiterpenes (Abraham, 2001), hydroquinones (Mothana et al., 2000), polysaccharides and complexes of polysaccharide-peptide (Liu, 1999), lanostanoide triterpenoids (Shiao, 1992, Leon et al., 2004) steroids (Smania, 2003), nucleosides, alkaloids and vitamins (Paterson, 2006) from fruitbodies of polypore fungi have been detected. Recent studies pronounced phenolic compounds (Turkoglu et al., 2007, Paterson, 2006, Ribeiro et al., 2007) as the main active antioxidative components in fungal extracts (Kityberger et al., 2007; Barros et al., 2007). It is assumed that antibacterial effects exhibited by fungal extracts of different polarites could be related to an overall effect of phenolic compounds (e.g. phenolic acids: caffeic acid, ellagic acid; flavonoids, hydroquinones) detected in similar extracts of the species *G.lucidum, F.velutipes, P.ostreatus* or organic acids (oxalic, malic) previously detected in *L. sulphureus* and *F. hepatica*, as well as terpenoids.

1.5.1 Products of primary metabolism

Polysaccharides. Polysaccharide molecules that form an integral part of the fungal cell wall also exhibit antimicrobial properties (Stamets, 2002). Polysaccharides are the most important components of fungal bioactive substances, proven to provide many medical and therapeutic possibilities (Fan et al., 2006) while their antibiotic effect is often specific to certain microorganisms (Stamets, 2002). Most of these compounds belong to glucans or heteroglycans (Fan et al., 2006). It is believed that the antibacterial and antifungal effects of β-glucan is based on the activation and strengthening of the immune response, and their use is recommended in combination with other antibiotics and immunostimulators in prevention and treatment of infectious diseases, especially immunocompromised individuals (Chen & Seviour, 2007).

Proteins and polypeptides. Proteins that act inhibitory on microorganisms are found frequently in organisms of plant and animal species, whereas their presence is rare in fungi (Wang & Ng, 2006). It is believed that these proteins are often positively charged, and that the mechanism of their action is realized by forming ion channels in cell membranes of microorganisms as well as by competitive binding to host cell polysaccharide receptors (Cowan, 1999). Proteins and peptides are isolated from macrofungi whose antimicrobial effect is limited to a small number of mostly phytopathogenic species (Table 1).

COMPOUNDS	ORIGIN/SOURCE	BIOLOGICAL ACTIVITY/REFERENCE
EXTRACELULAR POLYSACCHARIDES (noncellulose β-glucans)		
LENTINAN	*Lentinus edodes* mycelial extract of *Lentinus edodes*	antifungal: *Candida albicans*, antibacterial: *Mycobacterium tuberculosis, Listeria monocytogenes, S. aureus, M. luteus* i *B. cereus* (Stamets, 2002; Kitzberger et al., 2007; Chen & Seviour, 2007) antiviral: Herpes simplex-a type 1 (Stamets, 2002)
SCHYZOPHYLLAN (SPG)	*Schyzophyllum commune*	antifungal: *Candida albicans*, antibacterial: *S. aureus*. (Stamets, 2002)
KRESTIN (PSK), proteoglycan	*Trametes versicolor*	antifungal effect: *C. albicans* (Stamets, 2002; Kitzberger et al., 2007)
GRIFOLAN (GRN)	*Grifola frondosa* *Lepista nuda*	
INTRACELLULAR POLYSACCHARIDES - containing 1,6-α-D-galactopyranosyl units, substituted on O-2 position with α-L-fucopyranosyl or 3-O-α-D-manopyranosyl-α-L-fucopyranosyl units. Found only in fungi and concerned as a type of reserve materials (Fan et al., 2006)		
FUCOGALACTAN CMP3 (hydrosoluble heteroglucan)	from the mycelium of *Coprinus comatus*	not yet investigated (*C. comatus* showing antibacterial activity) (Fan et al., 2006).
FUCOGALACTAN	*G. applanatum*	
MANOFUCOGALACTANES	*F. velutipes, Polyporus pinicola, P. fomentarius* and *P. igniarius*	not yet investigated, concerned as a reserve material (Fan et al., 2006)
FUCOMANOGALACTANS	*Laetiporus sulphureus*	
GANODERMIN protein, molecular weight ≈15 kDa	*Ganoderma lucidum*	antifungal to phytopathogens *Botrytis cinerea, Fusarium oxysporum* and *Physalospora piricola* (Wang & Ng, 2006)
PLEUROSTRIN Peptide, molecular weight of 7kDa	*Pleurotus ostreatus*	antifungal effect : *Fusarium oxysporum, Mycosphaerella arachidicola* and *Physalospora piricola* (Chu *et* al., 2005)
LYOPHYLLIN	aqueous solution of *Lyophyllum shimeiji*	antifungal effect : *Mycosphaerella arachidicola* and *Physalospora piricola* (Takakura et al., 2001; Wang & Ng, 2006)
TRICHOGIN peptide	*Tricholoma giganteum*	antifungal activity against *Fusarium oxysporum, Mycosphaerella arachidicola* and *Physalospora piricola,* as well as inhibitory effect on HIV-1 reverse transcriptase (Guo et al., 2005)
ERYNGIN peptide, molecular weight of 10kDa	*Pleurotus eryngii*	inhibition of *Fusarium oxysporum* and *Mycosphaerella arachidicola,* its N-terminal end shows certain similarity with antifungal protein liophyllin (Wang & Ng, 2004)
AGROCYBIN peptide, molecular weight of 9 kDa	*Agrocybe dura* *A. cylindracea*	antibacterial effect against Gram + and Gram - bacteria: *B. mycoides, B. subtilis, E. coli, Klebisiella pneumoniae, Mycobacterium pheli, M. smegmatis, Photobacterium fischeri, P. aeruginosa , S. aureus* (Kavanagh et al., 1950) antifungal effect: *Aspergillus niger, Gliomastix convoluta, Memnoinella echinata, Myrothecium verrucaria, Penicillium notatum, Phycomyces blackesleeanus, Stemphylium consortiale* and *Trichomonas mentagrophytes* (Ngai et al., 2005)

Table 1. Polysaccharides, proteins and peptides from macrofungi with antimicrobial effect

Dietary fibers. High molecular weight substances that are excreted without digestion and absorption from the human body are called dietary fibers (Mizuno, 1999). Mushrooms contain these substances, which are composed of β-glucan, chitin and heteropolysaccharide (pectin substances, hemicellulose, polyuronidase, etc..) in the range of 10-50% in dry weight of the substance. Since they absorb harmful substances, hindering their intestinal absorption, dietary fibers are effective in preventing colon and rectal cancers (Mizuno, 1999).

Lectins. Lectins (Latin legere = to take, to choose) are defined as carbohydrate-binding proteins of non-immune origin which agglutinate cells or precipitate polysaccharides or glycoconjugates (Kawagishi, 1995). Many species of plants, animals and microorganisms contain lectins, but the fungal lectin is still not explicitely defined. So far, several lectins were isolated from mushrooms of the genus Polyporales: *Grifola frondosa* (GFL), *Fomes fomentarius* (FFL), *Ganoderma lucidum* (GLLs). Some are isolated from the fruit bodies and some from the mushroom mycelium. GFL is cytotoxic to HeLa cells, and its activity is explained by binding of lectins to carbohydrate parts of the cell by preventing aggregation of cells (Wasser & Weis, 1999).

1.5.2 Products of secondary metabolism

Secondary metabolites produced by a large number of macrofungi have great therapeutic significance. These compounds occur as intermediate products of primary metabolism, but most of them are classified according to the five major metabolic sources (Table 2,3,4). The most productive pathways of synthesis of secondary metabolites are polyketide and mevalonate pathways (Zeidman et al., 2005, from Giovaninni, 2006).

1.5.2.1 Phenolic compounds

Phenols are one of the largest classes of secondary biomolecules, which are characterized by the presence of aromatic rings with hydroxyl group bonded directly to an aromatic hydrocarbon group. Although they are firstly identified in plants (Cowan, 1999), their presence was also observed in fungi (Barros et al., 2008, Mattila et al., 2001, Karaman, 2002, Karaman et al., 2012a). In recent years, there was a causal relationship between the total content of these compounds with biological activities recorded in a large number of macrofungi (Barros et al., 2007), which include anti-inflammatory, antiallergic, anticancer, antihypertensive, antirheumatic and antibacterial activity. Antimicrobial properties of phenolics are explained by the presence of phenol hydroxyl groups, which number is in correlation with their toxicity toward microorganisms (Cowan, 1999). The possible mechanisms of their action include inhibition of extracellular microbial enzymes, deprivation of the substrates required for microbial growth or direct action on microbial metabolism through inhibition of oxidative phosphorylation, by sulfhydryl groups and some non-specific interactions (Cowan, 1999).

It has been shown that the antimicrobial effects of extracts of mushroom *Lactarius deliciosus, Sarcodon imbricatus* and *Tricholoma portentosum* directly correlated with total content of phenols and flavonoids in them (Barros et al., 2007). Extracts of all three fungi showed antibacterial effects on *Bacillus cereus* and antifungal to *Candida neoformans,* while the extract of mushrooms *Lactarius deliciosus* and efficiency demonstrated against *P. aeruginosa* and *Candida albicans*. High content of phenols has been recorded in lignicolous fungi *Meripilus giganteus, G. lucidum* and *Flammulina velutipes* in the form of coumarins and tannins, as well as in *Ganoderma applanatum*, where they were detected in the form of coumarins, flavonoids and tannins (Karaman, 2002, Karaman et al., 2005). Data on the antimicrobial action of these fungi also exist (Karaman et al., 2010). Analyses of extracts of the genus *Ganoderma* species shown the presence of polyphenolic compounds, and antimicrobial properties of these mushrooms explains the activity of compounds of hydrohynon composition - ganomycin A and B (Ofodile et al., 2005 as cited in Mothana et al., 2000).

High concentrations of phenolic acids (> 1.0 mg / g), mainly a high concentration of gallic acid and protocatechuic, could be interpreted as anti-microbial activity of the following species: *L. sulphureus, F. hepatica, P. ostreatus, F. velutipes* and partially *M. giganteus*, which in antimicrobial screening showed moderate activity (Karaman, 2009b). Further studies of mechanisms of antimicrobial components originating from mushrooms could be suggested, including the influence of the protein compounds and organic acids such as oxalic acid, which accumulates in the fruit bodies of brown rot mushrooms, but also malic acid, ellagic acid, or some other compounds.

Flavonoids are hydroxylated phenolic compounds (C6-C3 units associated with the aromatic core) and antimicrobial activity can be explained by their ability to create complexes with extracellular soluble proteins and polypeptides that builds cell wall of microorganisms, as well as disruption of the function of cell membrane (Cowan, 1999). There are only few data dealing with detection of flavonoids (rutin, chrysin, naringin, myrcetin and quercetin) in tericolous (Turkoglu, 2007; Baros et al., 2007) lignicolous fungal species (Kim et al., 2008, Jayakumar et al., 2009). Since flavonoids are phenolics that generally occur in plants acting as antioxidants, antimicrobials, photoreceptors, feeding repellants or UV protectors (Pietta, 2000) we assume that the presence of these metabolites in TP of fungi that generally are in tight connection with wood, could have impact on the expressed bioactivity. Recent studies conducted with mushrooms showed a positive correlation between the TP and antioxidant capacity (Turkoglu, 2007, Ribeiro, 2007), possibly due to their ability to chelate metals, inhibit lipoxygenase and scavenge free radicals. Plotting TP content versus antibacterial activity (Karaman et al., 2010), revealed a good positive correlation between these two parameters , showing higher values for MeOH than CHCl3 extracts against most of the bacteria. By comparing different strains of the same bacteria (*S. aureus*) it was concluded that the effect of TP upon the antibacterial activity may be strain specific.

Worthy of note is the antibacterial activity of fungi against the multidrug-resistant strains of bacteria. New sesquiterpenoid hydroquinone from *Ganoderma pfeiefferi* Bres., called ganomycin (Mothana, et al., 2000) inhibit methicillin-resistant strains of *Staphylococcus aureus* and the growth of other, mainly Gram-positive bacteria. In addition, sterol-type compounds, isolated from the species *G. applanatum* such as 5α-ergost-7-en-3β-ol, 5α-ergost-7, 22-dien-3β-ol, 5.8-epidioxy-5α, 8α-ergost-6,22-dien-3β-ol and another new lanostanoid showed weak activity against many Gram + and Gram - bacteria. Oxalic acid is one of the substances responsible for the antimicrobial effects of mushroom *Lentinula edodes* (Berk.). Chloroform extract of mycelium *L. edodes* has bactericidal properties (Hirasawa et al., 1999).

Tannins are complex polyphenolic compounds that are devided into the two groups: the hydrolizated (esters of phenolic acids and sugars), and condensed (constructed from flavonoid monomers). Antimicrobial activity of tannins is expressed due to their ability to link amino acids in proteins, inactivating adhesions, enzymes and transport proteins of cell membranes of microorganisms (Cowan, 1999), as well as the formation of complexes with metal ions (Biradar et al., 2007). In addition, tannins could form complexes with polysaccharides, affecting microorganisms.

The equivalent of tannic acid was detected in extracts of shiitake mushrooms (*Lentinus edodes*), which show the antibiotic effect against bacteria *M. luteus* and *B. cereus* and the fungus *Candida albicans*, while against the strains of *E. coli* and *S. aureus* did not show the same activity (Kitzberger et al., 2007). While the focus of previous mycochemical (gr. myces=fungi) analysis of *Pleurotus ostreatus* was mainly put on the vitamins and minerals content, indicating a high nutritional value of mushrooms (Mattila et al., 2005), recent research revealed its exceptional antimicrobial and antioxidant effects that are associated with the presence of terpene and phenolic compounds (Iwalokun et al., 2007). The presence of phenols in the form of pyrocatechols, and flavonoids in the form of quercetin, was noted in extracts of fungus *Laetiporus sulphureus*, which explains its strong antioxidant properties (Turkoglu et al., 2006). This study also shows that ethanol extract of *L. sulphureus* exhibits strong antibiotic effect against Gram-positive bacteria (*B. subtilis, B. cereus, M. luteus* and *M. flavus*) and the yeast *Candida albicans*, while its activity against Gram-negative bacteria is much lower.

Coumarins are phenolic compounds of characteristic odor, and, according to the chemical structure, they are lactones built from the benzene and pyrone ring (Cowan, 1999). Despite the antiviral activity of some coumarins and the evidence of their inhibitory effect on the fungus *Candida albicans in vitro* conditions (Cowan, 1999), data on antimicrobial activity of these compounds are scarce. The presence of coumarin in fungi has been established in most genera of Xylariaceae family (Ascomycetes) (Whalley et al., 1999), as well as in certain fungi belonging to lignicolous basidiomycets based on preliminary TLC profiling (Karaman, 2002).

Other agents with weak antibacterial effects found in macrofungi are steroids like 5α-ergosta-7,22-dien-3β-ol or 5,8-epidioxy-5α,8α-ergosta-6,22-dien-3β-ol, isolated from *Ganoderma applanatum* (Pers.) Pat., proved to be weakly active against a number of Gram-positive and Gram-negative bacteria and organic acids like oxalic acid proved to be responsible for the antibacterial effect of *Lentinula edodes* (Berk.) Pegler against *S. aureus* and other bacteria.

Other, non-phenolic, compounds including terpenoids (Leon et al., 2004) and polysaccharides (Tseng et al., 2008) have also been designated as mushroom antioxidants or antimicrobials.

1.5.2.2 Terpenoid compounds

Terpenes are a broad class of lipophilic secondary metabolites whose general chemical structure is $C_{10}H_{16}$. In nature they appear as diterpenes, triterpenes and tetraterpens (carotenoids) - C_{20}, C_{30}, C_{40}, as well as the hemiterpens and sesquiterpens - C_5, C_{15}. If include additional elements (mostly oxygen within the hydroxyl and carbonyl groups), they are called terpenoids (Cowan, 1999). Terpenoids originate from simple acyclic compounds, isoprene and mevalonic acid, and their structure may be acyclic, monocyclic or bicyclic. Basically, their structure is isopentenyl-pyrophosphate (IPP), whose synthesis is realized in two ways, and pathways of synthesis of higher isoprenoids continue on after the isomerization of IPP in DMAPP. For all animal and fungal cells characteristic is the mevalonic pathway of isopentenyl-pyrophosphate synthesis, while most plants, bacteria, actinomycetes and protozoa have non-mevalonic mode of its synthesis (Inouye et al., 2004).

One of the many functions of these compounds is their antimicrobial activity, but the mechanism of action of terpenoids on microorganisms is not fully understood (Cowan, 1999). According to their lipophilic nature, it is assumed to act by disrupting membrane functions of microbial cells (Cowan, 1999), and some authors believe that they may cause increasing of non-specific cell membrane permeability for the antibiotic molecule (Byron et al., 2003). Though plant organisms are thought to be the largest source of triterpenoids, in recent years more and more data indicate the presence of these compounds in some representatives of macrofungi (He et al., 2003, Akihisa et al., 2005; de Silva et al., 2006; Abraham, 2001, Deyrup et al., 2007).

Sesquiterpenes. One of the many strategies that representatives of the higher fungi use to protect themselves against a number of parasites that feed on their fruit bodies is the production of toxins. It is interesting that many of these toxic chemical suits sesquiterpens (Abraham, 2001). For most basidiomycota fungi the presence of sesquiterpens of protoiludane type is characteristic, which originate from humulene, compounds present in a rare fungus, formed by cyclization of farnesyl-pyrophosphate. Of the few ways of humulene transformation, the most important pathway of synthesis of protoiludane, tricyclic compound which, due to the high reactivity caused by the presence of cyclobutane, is further transformed into a series of compounds. Some of these sesquiterpenes show interesting biological activity, and are considered to be a very interesting object of study in terms of medical chemistry. Several groups of sesquiterpenes originating from higher fungi show a greater or lesser antimicrobial effect (Tables 2, 3). It is interesting to note that some representatives of the genera *Russula* and *Lactarius* synthesize sesquiterpene alcohols that are esterifies with fatty acids. These esters do not show strong antibiotic activity, but in the case of mushroom fruit body injury, leads to cleavage of ester bonds and release of alcohols that are highly reactive and therefore very toxic to microorganisms. Therefore, the mentioned esters may be considered as pro-medicines or precursors of compounds that in metabolic processes are transformed into an active form.

Triterpenes. Compounds of triterpene composition are found in many mushroom extracts which showed some antibiotic properties. Genus *Ganoderma* contains about 200 species known for the production of triterpene compounds. Many of these species have found wide application in the prevention and treatment of various diseases due to the numerous biological activities based on the presence of triterpene components (Ofodile et al., 2005). Although thought to be active against bacteria just due to the presence of triterpenes in these fungi, there are data that disagree with such opinions, giving the example of seven different triterpenes isolated from a Vietnamese species *G. collosum*, which showed no antimicrobial effect, but exhibit strong anti-inflammatory activity (Ofodile et al., 2005). Most triterpenes synthesized by species of the genus *Ganoderma* belong to the lanostane type (de Silva et al., 2006). Over 100 compounds from this group have been identified, among them a few newly discovered (Akihisa et al., 2005; de Silva et al., 2006, Jian et al., 2003, Kamo et al., 2003). The review of triterpene compounds isolated from macrofungi is given in Table 3.

Overview of other compounds isolated from macrofungi, which exhibit antimicrobial activity is shown in Tab. 4

COMPOUND	NAME OR CHEMICAL STRUCTURE	ORIGIN	EFFECT (ACTIVITY)
CARYOPHYLLENE	**Naematolin**	*Hypholoma fasciculare*	weak antibacterial
COLLYBIAL	**α,β-unasturated aldehyde**	*Collybia confluens*	low antifungal, high antibacterial (*Bacillus* sp.), high antiviral, cytotoxic, nonselective antibiotic
PROTOILLUDANES (esters of protoilludanol)	**Armillyl orselinate** **Arnamiol** (chlorinated derivatives) **Melleolide B, C, D, E, F, G, H** (everniate-armillarin) **Melleolide I, J** **Radulon A** **Lentinellic acid** methyl-estars of lentinellic acid	*Armillaria mellea* (similar to *A. tabescens*) *Clitocybe elegans* *A. novae-zelandiae* *Radulomyces confluens* *Lentinellus*	prevent trombocite aggregation, cytotoxic, antimicrobial **low antifungal, high antibacterial, cytotoxic** high antifungal , low antibacterial
MARASMANES	**Marasmic acid** hydroxy derivative of marasmic acid **Pilatin** **Velutinal and fatty acid esters**	*Marasmius conigenus* culture – *Flagelloscypha pilatii* contain many Basidiomycota by damage of fruiting-bodies, converting to **Isovelleral**	**antibacterial** less antifungal, cytotoxic and phytotoxic lower antibiotic and cytotoxic high antibacterial, antifungal & cytotoxic
HYDROGRAMMANE (modified marasmic sesquiterpenes)	**10-hydroxy-isovelleral** **Hydrogrammic acid**	*Clitocybe hydrogramma*	antibacterial against *Bacillus* sp., non against *E. coli* and fungi
CUCUMANES		culture –*Macrocystidia cucumis*	antimicrobial and cytotoxic
FOMANNOSANES	**Fomanosin** **Illudosin**	***Fomes annosus*** *Omphalotus olearius* *Omphalotus nidiformis.*	**bactericidal,phytotoxic** antibacterial against Gram + (*Sarcina lutea* and *Bacillus* spp.), non against *E. coli* antifungal
ILLUDANES	**Illudin S (lampterol)** **Illudin M** Hydroxydihydroilludin M **Illudin A, B, C, D i E** **Illudalenol,** **Illudin F, G i H** **Illudin C_2 i C_3** **Illudinic acid**	*Omphalotus olearius* *Lampteromyces japonicus, Omphalotus olivascens* *Clitocybe subilludens* *Pleurotus japonicus* *Omphalotus olearius* *Omphalotus nidiformis* *Coprinus atramentarius* *Agrocybe aegerita*	anticancerogenic properties weak antibiotic activity on *B. subtilis* cytotoxic, antibiotic (*S. aureus*), antifungal
ILLUDALANES (dicoumaric sesquiterpenes)	**Fomajorin D & S** **Illudalic acid** **illudinine** **Candicansol** **Clavicoronic acid**	*Fomes annosus* *Omphalotus olearius* *Clitocybe candicans* *Clavicorona pyxidata* *Mycena leaiana*	antiviral (inhibits reverse transcriptase of viruses causing leukemia in rats -weak antibiotic activity (*Acinetobacter*), high
ISOILLUDANES	**Leaianafulven**		cytotoxic, mutagenic

Table 2. Antimicrobial effects of sesquiterpenoids orginated from macrofungi (according to Abraham, 2001)

Compound	Name or chemical structure	ORIGIN	EFFECT (ACTIVITY)
HIRSUTANES		**Hirsutic acid C**	*Stereum hirsutum*
		Complicatic acid	*Stereum complicatum - culture*
			Pleurotus hypnophilus
PLEUROTELANES pleurotelic skeleton, created by modification of hypnophillin		**Hypnophillin** Pleurotelic acid Pleurotellol	
			Coriolus consors
		Coriolin A, B, C	
		Hypnophillin 1-desoxyhipnophyilin	*Lentinus crinitus-*
			Gloeostereum incarnatum - culture
		Gloeosteretriol **Incarnal** (dehydro-hirsutanol A)	
			Macrocystidia cucumis
CUCUMANES		**Cucumins A-H**	
			Merulius tremellosus - culture
		Merulidial	
MERULANES ISOLACTARANES **TRITERPENOIDES**			
		Meruliolactone Stereopolide Dihydrostereopolide	*Stereum purpureum* – culture, *Merulius tremellosus*
TRITERPENES	Lanostane-type	*G. applanatum* *G lucidum*	(de Silva et al., 2006)
		Lanostane-type, fatty acids lanostane and ergostane derivatives	*Fomes*
Triterpenoid lactons		**Fomlactons A, B, C**	*Fomes cajanderi*
Triterpenic glycosides		**Kolocosides A, B, C, D**	common in plants and lichens, so far only three representatives found:
		Fuscoatroside **Enfumafungin** - WF11605	*Xylaria* from Hawaiian Islands
Triterpenoid saponins		glycosides with *betulin* as a aglyconic component	*P. ostreatus*
		Favolon (with variable cyclic structure and method of substitution)	*Favolaschia*

Table 3. Antimicrobial effects of sesquiterpenoids and triterpenoids from macrofungi (according to Abraham, 2001)

1.6 Extraction methods

Extraction procedures are important in assessing good antibacterial activities of extracts. Macrofungi are commonly collected either randomly or by locals in geographical areas or forest habitats where the fruiting bodies are found. Initial screenings of fungi for possible antibacterial activities usually begin by using crude aqueous or alcohol extractions. Since the majority of the identified components of mushrooms are active against microorganisms, they are mostly obtained through initial ethanol or methanol extraction.

Water-soluble compounds, such as polysaccharides and polypeptides, including lectins, are commonly more effective as inhibitors of virus adsorption and cannot be identified in the screening techniques commonly used. Tannins and terpenoids are occasionally obtained by treatment with less polar solvents.

For alcoholic extraction, the intact mature fruiting bodies or their segments are brush cleaned, air-dried to constant mass and pulverized, and then soaked in methanol or ethanol for extended periods (24-72h). The resultant filtrated extracts are then filtered and washed, concentrated under reduced pressure at low temperature to avoid destroying of any thermo-labile antimicrobial agents present in the extract and redissolved in the alcohol (or 5% DMSO) to a determined concentration. Water extractions, generally used distilled water, blending of slurry, filtration and centrifugation (approximately 15,000 for 30 min) multiple times for clarification.

Compounds	Origin/Source	Biological activity	Reference
β-methoxyacrylates **strobilurins** and **oudemansins**	cultures of *Oudemansiella mucida, Xerula malanotricha* and *Xerula longipes*	- antifungal activity against a large number of saprotrophic and phytopatogenic fungi, inhibiting the process of respiration	Anke et al., 1979; Anke et al., 1983
Polyenes **xerulin, dihydroxerulin** and **xerulinic acid**	*Xerula malanotricha*	- antimicrobial, anticancer, antiviral and anti-inflammatory activity - inhibition of cholesterol biosynthesis and cytotoxic effect	Negishi et al., 2000; Kuhnt et al., 1990
Agrocybolacton	cultures of representatives of the genus *Agrocybe*	- moderate antibacterial activity against Gram-positive bacteria *B. subtilis* and *M. smegmatus*	Rosa et al., 2003
Lentionine (1,2,3,5,6-enthatiocyclocheptane) and its disulfide derivate	*Lentinus edodes*	antibacterial antifungal effect	Hirasawa et al., 1999)
Cinnabarine	*Pycnoporus cinnabarinus*	antibacterial (*B. subtilis S. aureus*) antifungal effect	Shitu et al., 2006
Laschiatrion new antibiotic with steroid skeleton	submerged cultures of the genus *Favolaschia*	- *in vitro* antifungal activity against some human pathogens - antibacterial and citotoxic effects not detected	Anke et al., 2004

Table 4. Other compounds from macrofungi with antimicrobial activity

1.7 Evaluation of antibacterial activity

1.7.1 Techniques used in research of new substances

Basidiomycota and fungi in general, represent an inexhaustible source of new substances, even though each species contains hundreds of active metabolites. Therefore, test systems for research of new substances must be fully simplified, fast, efficient and as cheap as possible (Hostettmann et al., 1997, as cited in Giovaninni, 2006). In addition, biotests (bioassays) must be sufficiently sensitive to detect the activity of substances in low concentrations, in the so-called solid (crude) extracts.

Crude products can be used in antimicrobial testing disc-diffusion and broth-dilution assays to test for antibacterial properties including bioautography according to standard procedures (NCCLS or CLSI procedures). The use of standard cultures of familiar characteristics is recommended though several precautions have to be taken into account. In a recent study the differences between two screening methods applied were not statistically significant (t-test at level $p < 0.05$). Both *Meripilus* extracts analyzed (water and methanol) showed wider inhibition zones in disc-diffusion method, indicating that it is more appropriate for the testing of polar extracts (Karaman et al., 2009b). Similar results were confirmed for extracts of the genus *Fomes* although showed broader inhibitory zones using the method of "wells", compared with inhibitory zones obtained by disc-diffusion method. For other extracts, however, the disk-diffusion method could be recommended, indicating that polarity of active substances in extract influence on results obtained in particular method applied.

MIC and MBC determination is used to quantify antimicrobial activity using the two-fold dilution method according to CLSI guidelines. The MIC is defined as the lowest concentration preventing visible growth while complete absence of growth is considered as the MBC. The lower MIC or MBC values with respect to the extract concentration indicate a higher activity, implying better quality of the extract. To confirm MBCs, aliquots of the experimental suspensions (100µl) could be sub-cultured on Müeller Hinton agar plates incubated overnight.

Potent source of antibacterial agents is the species *M. giganteus* (50mg/ml), showing high activity against both groups of bacteria reaching MIC values in a wide range of concentrations (<17.5 -1125µg/ml). Various activities have been detected among different strains of *S. aureus*, indicating that fungal extracts are target specific on intraspecific level (strain specific).

Antibacterial assay may be performed in 96-well micro-plates instead of tubes. If 5% DMSO is applied for dissolving a negative control with 0.5% DMSO must be used to ensure that DMSO did not affect bacterial growth. Results are recorded after incubation at 35-37°C for 18-24h and all the samples should be tested in triplicate.

Bioautography is one of the most effective tests for detection of antimicrobial metabolites, considering the fact that it localizes the place of the active component, therefore enabling the isolation of the active component precisely. Bioautography may be the direct, when microorganisms grow directly on the TLC plate, then contact, when the active compound is transferred from the TLC plates to inoculated agar and agar-spill-over (so-called immersion bioautography), when the inoculated agar medium is spilled over the TLC plate (Rahalison et al., 1991). In the bioautography agar overlay method, the drug to be evaluated is adsorbed onto the TLC plate and the inoculum is laid onto the plate as a very thin layer (1 mm). The advantage of this method is that the amount of sample being used is very small and that the fractionalisation of the crude extracts on its different components simplifies the identification of active compound.[26]

In our recent work, the TLC chemical profile of the analyzed species of lignicolous macrofungi showed that they are rich in phenols, although the differences in the number and quality of the extracted compounds have been noticed. Comparing the TLC profiles, fungi can be classified into three groups according to the obtained retention factor e.g. Rf values representing the distance traveled by the compound divided by the distance traveled by the solvent: 1) three species: *C. versicolor, G. lucidum* and *G. applanatum* contain compounds with similar (Rf = 0.68, Rf = 0.69, Rf = 0.70, respectively), 2) five species *M. giganteus, L. sulphureus, F. velutipes, F. hepatica* and *P. ostreatus* showed a small amount of eluated compounds and intense fluorescence at the start line after the spraying, 3) the species *P. betulinus* expressed with three spots in the MeOH extracts (Rf = 0.62, Rf = 0.65, Rf = 0.68), which extinguished fluorescence in the UV 254th (Karaman, 2009c).

Furthermore we made slight modifications of the standard procedure of bioautography in the same study using the following: soft (top) agar (0.7% Nutrient agar) which was mixed with freshly prepared inoculum of bacteria (0.5Mac Farland optical density) and with the aqueous solution of tetrazolium red dye 0.1% w/v (1mg/ml)- 2,3,5-triphenyltetrazolium chloride (TTC, Sigma) (3:1:0.1). The strain *S. aureus*^{an} was used as the indicator organism. Amoxicillin (64μg/ml) was used as positive control. Approximately 10μl of the solution of each extract was applied on a TLC plates (silica gel 60, F 254, DC-Plastikfolien, 0.2 mm thick, Merck, Germany) for about 2h, equally prepared as a reference plate for chemical analysis. Bioautography test plate was developed in the same tank using the pre-determined mobile phase which was removed from the plate by drying with a stream of cool air from a heating gun. Separated spots were visualised under UV light and marked by pencil (Figure 2A). Developed plates were placed upside-down in the petri dishes containing bottom agar (nutrient agar, Torlak, Belgrade). Soft agar (07% Nutrient agar) was melted and poured into sterile tubes (100 ml) in which the dye and bacteria were added quickly. That mixture was flowed over the chromatograms in the petri dishes. After the agar has solidified, the plates were inverted and incubated at 35°C for 24h. The clear zones on the chromatogram indicate areas of inhibition zones on the red background where bacteria are present. Comparing clearing zones with reference TLC plate according to Rf values the most active components of crude fungal extracts could be approximately detected (Fig. 1B).

Bioautography results showed many antibacterial compounds against animal strain of *S. aureus* that were mostly present in the polar region of the bioautogram. According to detected clearing zones, chloroform extracts were more active corresponding to more detected UV absorptive substances along the chromatogram. However, these substances were not active in methanolic extracts on bioautogram for *C. versicolor* and *P. betulinus*.

Developing system: toluene-ethyl acetate – 90% formic acid (5:4:1 v/v/v). **Detection:** 366 nm UV light without spraying. **Extracts:** lane 1- *M. giganteus* (MeOH), lane 2- *L. sulphureus* (MeOH), lane 3- *C. versicolor* (MeOH), lane 4- *F. velutipes* (MeOH), lane 5- *G. lucidum* (EtOH), lane 6- *G. applanatum* (MeOH), lane 7- *P. tigrinus* (MeOH), lane 8- *P. betulinus* (MeOH), lane 9- *P. ostreatus* (MeOH), lane 10- *F. hepatica* (MeOH), lane 2´- *L. sulphureus* ($CHCl_3$), lane 3´- *C. versicolor* ($CHCl_3$), lane 4´- *F. velutipes* ($CHCl_3$), lane 6´- *G. applanatum* ($CHCl_3$), lane 7´- *P. tigrinus* ($CHCl_3$), lane 8´- *P. betulinus* ($CHCl_3$) **B: Bioautogram of extracts for *S. aureus*[a]. Extracts:** lane 1- *M. giganteus* (MeOH), lane 2- *L. sulphureus* (MeOH), lane 4- *F. velutipes* (MeOH), lane 3- *C. versicolor* (MeOH), lane 6- *G. applanatum* (MeOH), lane 5- *G. lucidum* (EtOH), lane 7- *P. tigrinus* (MeOH), lane 8- *P. betulinus* (MeOH), lane 9- *P. ostreatus* (MeOH), lane 10- *F. hepatica* (MeOH), lane 2´- *L. sulphureus* ($CHCl_3$), lane 3´- *C. versicolor* ($CHCl_3$), lane 4´- *F. velutipes* ($CHCl_3$), lane 6´- *G. applanatum* ($CHCl_3$), lane 7´- *P. tigrinus* ($CHCl_3$), lane 8´- *P. betulinus* ($CHCl_3$).

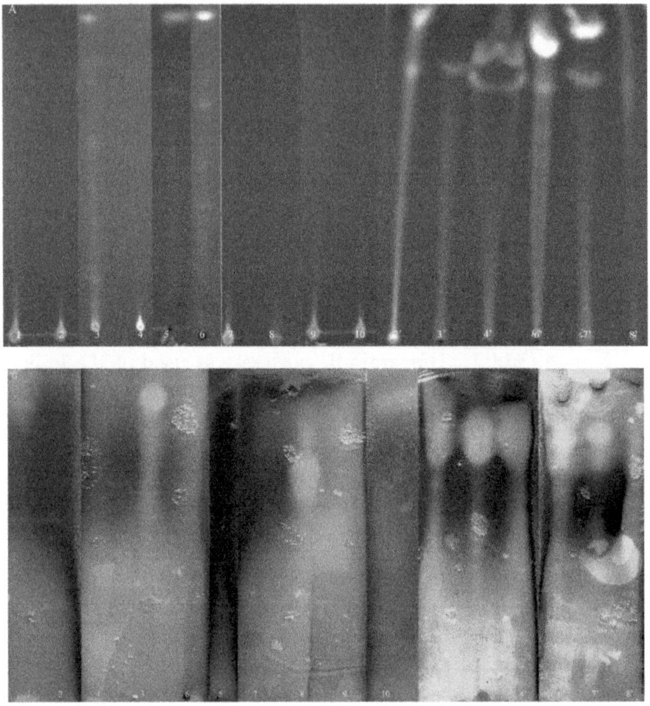

Fig. 1. **A:** TLC separation of crude extracts (methanol - MeOH and chloroform - $CHCl_3$) of selected lignicolous species prepared for bioautography assay and **B:** bioautogram of extracts for Gram- positive bacteria *S. aureus,* animal strain

1.8 Target organisms

Bacillus subtilis is a Gram + bacteria, non-pathogenic to humans and can be used as a model organism in similar tests, since the representative of the same genus, bacteria *B. anthracis* is responsible for the disease anthrax, which is characterized by the appearance of edema, hemorrhage and tissue necrosis. It is common in some animals, often used as a biological weapon in bioterrorism. If an extract shows activity against *B.subtilis*, it is possible to be active against *B. anthracis* and possibly against other pathogenic Gram + bacteria such as specieses of the genera *Staphylococcus* and *Streptococcus.*

Escherichia coli. *E. coli*, Gram - bacteria, inhabits the gastro-intestinal tract of humans and warm-blooded animals, making their normal indigenous microflora. In immuno-suppressed patients, however, it can cause infections, sometimes fatal (Giovannini, 2006). Gram - bacteria cause more problems than Gram +, as a result of their different cell wall structure. Since penicillin and cephalosporin antibiotics belong to the group that act at the level of cell wall synthesis, the exploration of new types of antibiotics is very important for group of Gr- organisms.

C. albicans belongs to Deuteromycota, representing yeasts forming pseudo-mycelia. It lives as a part of the normal human microflora, especially in the mucosa of the mouth and vagina. In immuno-suppressed individuals (AIDS, chemotherapy, inadequate nutrition and poor hygiene), or after prolonged use of antibiotics, it can cause disease called candidiasis, which is the most common caused by *C. albicans* as the most widespread species. It may affect almost any tissue, starting with simple children's thrush, and ending as the systemic infections. Most commonly it is manifested in the form of slimy mucus. *C. albicans*, is very convenient target organism in the detection of new antifungal drugs.

2. Determination of active substances

In the last decades of the 20th century, the study of macrofungi was intensified, including the research of structurally different metabolites (polysaccharides, glycoproteins, proteo-glucans, terpenoids, fatty acids, proteins, lectins, etc..) originating from the primary or secondary metabolism of fungi, as well as different biological activities that they express. Metabolites from fungal fruit bodies or spores themselves are substantially different from those that come from extracellular liquid of the medium in which submerged mycelium was grown or from cells of the culture. Since the phenomenon of multidrug-resistance of microorganisms is on the rise, the studies of macrofungi increased in range, in spite of the fact that they are very slow growing organisms. The value of macrofungi and the dietary supplements, originating from these organisms, grows each year on the world market. They are very safe and considered as the factors useful in the daily diet, especially for people suffering from various diseases.

Natural-products chemists further purify active chemicals from crude extracts by a variety of methods. The chemical structures of the purified material can then be analyzed. Techniques for further chemical analysis include chromatography, bioautography, radioimmunoassay, various methods of structure identification, or modern techniques such as atom bombardment mass spectrometry, Gas chromatography-mass spectrometry, high-performance liquid chromatography, capillary zone electrophoresis, nuclear magnetic resonance spectroscopy, and X-ray crystallography.

3. Conclusion

The presented results indicate that extracts from lignicolous macrofungi could be used in the prevention and treatment of Gram-positive bacterial infections resistant to antibiotics in animals (humans), although further toxicity assays (*in vivo*) must be performed before its application. The fact that fungi can have bactericidal properties with low cytotoxicity to the animal host underscores their usefulness as natural sources of human or veterinary medicines.

Also, the results obtained should stimulate further studies of other, so far unexplored, species such as *M. giganteus* and *P. tigrinus*, since current knowledge of the antibacterial activities or chemical composition of their active agents is not capable of fulfilling the expectations.

4. Acknowledgment

This work is fully supported by the project No 172058 of Ministry of Education and Science of Republic of Serbia

5. References

Abraham, W.R. (2001). Bioactive sesquiterpenes produced by fungi: are they useful for humans as well. *Current Medical Chemistry*, 8: 583-606.

Ajith, T.A. & Janardhanan K.K. (2007). Indian Medicinal Mushrooms as a source of antioxidants and antitumor agents. *Journal of Clinical Biochemistry and Nutrition*, 40, pp. 157-162.

Akisha T, Tagata M, Ukiya M, Tokuda H, Suzuki T, Kimura Y. (2005): Oxygenated Lanostane-Type Triterpenoids from Fungus *Ganoderma lucidum*. *Journal of Natural Products*. 68:559-563.

Aldred, D., Magan, N., Lane B. S. (1999). Influence of water activity and nutrients on growth and production of squalestatin S1 by a *Phoma* sp. *Journal of Applied Microbiology*, Vol.87, No. 6, pp. 842-848.

Anke, T., Besl, H., Mocek, U., Steglich, W. (1979): Antibiotics from basidiomycetes. IX. Oudemansin, an antifungal antibiotic from Oudemansiella mucida (Schrader ex Fr.) Hoehnel (Agaricales). *The Journal of Antibiotics*, 32 (11): 1112-1117.

Anke, T., Besl, H., Mocek, U., Steglich, W. (1983): Antibiotics from basidiomycetes. XVIII. Strobilurin C and oudemansin B, two new antifungal metabolites from Xerula species (Agaricales). *The Journal of Antibiotics*, 36 (6): 661-666.

Anke, T., Werle, A., Kapre, R., Sterner, O. (2004): Laschiatrion, a New Antifungal Agent from a Favolaschia Species (Basidiomycetes) Active against Human Pathogens. The Journal of Antibiotics, 57 (8): 496-501.

Asatiani, M., Elisashvili, V., Wasser, S.P., Reznick, A.Z., Nevo, E. (2007). Antioxidant activity of submerged cultured mycelium extracts of higher Basidiomycetes Mushrooms. *International Journal of Medicinal Mushrooms*, Vol.9, pp. 151-158.

Asatiani, M.D.; Kachlishvili, E.T.; Khardziani, T.S.; Metreveli, E.M.; Mikiashvili, N.A.; Songulashvili, G.G. et al. (2008). Basidiomycetes as a source of antioxidants, lectins, polysaccharides and enzymes. *Journal of Biotechnology*, Vol.136S, pp. S717-S742.

Barros, L.; Calhelha, R.C.; Vaz, J.A.; Ferreira, I.C.F.R.; Baptista, P.; Esteviinho, L.M. (2007). Antimicrobial activity and bioactive compounds of Portugese wild edible mushrooms methanolic extracts. *European Food Research and Technology*, Vol.225, pp. 151-156,

Barros, L.; Cruz, T.; Baptista, P.; Estevinho, L.M.; Ferreira, I.C.F.R. (2008). Wild and commercial mushrooms as source of nutrients and nutraceuticals. *Food and Chemical Toxycology*, Vol.46, No.8, (August), pp. 2742-2747.

Bendini, A.; Bonoli, M.; Cerretani, L.; Biguzzi, B.; Lercker, G.; Toshi, T.G. (2003). Liquid-liquid and solid-phase extractions of phenols from virgin olive oil and their separation by chromatographic and electrophoretic methods. *Journal of Chromatography A*, Vol.985, No.1-2, pp. 425-433.

Berger-Bachi, B. (2002). Resistence mechanism of Gram-positive bacteria. Mini review. *International Journal of Medicinal Microbiology*, Vol.292, pp. 27-35.

Berghe, D.A.; Vlietinck, A.J. (1991). Screening Methods for Antimicrobial and Antiviral Agents from Higher Plants. *Methods in Plant Biochemistry*, Vol.6, pp. 47-69.

Biradar, Y.S., S. Jagatap, K.R. Khandelwal and S.S. Singhania (2008). Exploring of antimicrobial activity of triphala mashi-an ayurvedic formulation. *Evidence-based Complementary and Alternative Medicine*, 5: 107-113.

Calabrese, E.J.; Baldwin, L.A. (2001). The scientific foundation of hormesis. *Critical Reviews in Toxicology*. Vol.31, pp. 349-691

Ćetković, G.S.; Djilas, S.M.; Čanadanović, J.M.; Tumbas, V.T. (2004). Antioxidant properties of marigold extracts. *Food Research International*, Vol.37, pp. 643-650,

Cetto, B. (1979). Der grosse Pilzführer. BLV Verlagsgesellschaft, NSIB , Wien, Austria.

Cheesman, K.H.; Bearis, A.; Esterbauer, H. (1988). Hydroxyl-radical-induced iron catalyzed degradation of 2-deoxyribose. *Biochemical Journal*, Vol.252, No.3, pp. 649-653.

Chen, J., Seviour, R. (2007): Medicinal importance of fungal - (1→ 3), (1→ 4) - glucans. *Mycological research*, 3: 635-652.

Chu, K. T., Xia, L., Ng, T. B. (2005) : Pleurostrin, an antifungal peptide from the oyster mushroom. *Peptides*, 26 (11): 2098-2103.

Clinical and Laboratory Standards Institute. Methods for dilution susceptibility test for bacteria that grow aerobically. 6th edition. Approved standard. (2003). Clinical and Laboratory Standards Institute, NSIB , Wayne, USA

Courtecuisse, R. & Duhem, B. (1995). Mushrooms & toadstools of Britain and Europe. Harper Collins Publishers, NSBI , London, England.

Cowan, M.M. (1999). Plant products as antimicrobial agents. Clinical Microbiologicy Reviews. Vol.12, No.4, (October), pp. 564-582,

Cui, Y.; Kim, D.S.; Park, K.C. (2005). Antioxidant effect of Innonotus obliquus. *Journal of Ethnopharmacology*, Vol.96, No.1-2, pp. 79-85.

de Silva, E. D., van der Sar, S. A., Santha, R. G. L., Wijesundera, R. L. C., Cole, A. L. J., Blunt, J. W., Munro, M. H. G. (2006): Lanostane Triterpenoids from the Sri Lankan Basidiomycete Ganoderma applanatum. *Journal of Natural Products*, 69: 1245-1248.

Deyrup, S.T.; Gloer, J.B.; O'Donnell, K.; Wicklow, D.T. (2007). Kolokosides A-D: Triterpenoid Glycosides from a Hawaiian Isolate of Xylaria sp. *Journal of Natural Products*, Vol.70, No.3, pp. 378-382.

Dubost, N.J.; Ou, B.; Beelman, R.B. (2007). Quantification of polyphenols and ergothioneine in cultivated mushrooms and correlation to total antioxidant capacity. *Food Chemistry*, Vol.105, pp. 727-735.

Egger, H. & Reinshagen, H. (1976). New pleuromutili derivatives with enhanced antimicrobial activity. II. Structure-activity correlations. *Journal of Antibiotics*, Vol.29, pp. 923-927.

Elmastas, M.; Isildak, O.; Turkekul, I.; Temur, N. (2007). Determination of antioxidant activity and antioxidant compounds in wild edible mushrooms. *Journal of Food Composition and Analysis*, Vol.20, pp. 337-345.

Engler, M.; Anke, T.; Sterner, O. (1998). Production of Antibiotics by Collybia nivalis, Omphalotus olearius, a Favolashia and a Pterula species on natural substrates. *Zeitschrift für Naturforschung C*, Vol.53, No.5-6, pp. 318-324

Fan, J. M., Zhang, J. S., Tang, Q. J., Liu, Y. F., Zhang, A. Q., Pan, Y. J. (2006): Structural elucidation of a neutral fucogalactan from the mycelium of Coprinus comatus. *Carbohydrate Research*, 341: 1130–1134.

Ferreira, I.C.F.R.; Barros, L.; Abreu, R.M.V. (2009). Antioxidants in Wild Mushrooms. *Current Medicinal Chemistry*, Vol.16, No.12, pp. 1543-1560.

Florey, H.W.; Chain, W.; Heatley, A.; Jennings, M.A.; Sanders, A.G.; Abraham, E.P.; Florey, M.E. (1949). Antibiotics. Oxford University Press, London, England.

Fukumoto, L. & Mazza, G. (2000). Assessing antioxidant and prooxidant activities of phenolic compounds. *Journal of Agricultural and Food Chemistry*, Vo.44, No.8, pp. 3597-3604.

Gentry, D.R.; Wilding, I.; Johnson, J. M.; Chen, D.; Remlinger, K.; Richards, C. et al. (2010). A rapid microtiter plate assay for measuring the effect of compounds on Staphylococcus aureus membrane potential. Journal of Microbiological Methods, Vol.83, No.2, (November), pp. 254-256.

Giovaninni, I. S. (2006). Cultivated Basidiomycetes as a source of new products: - in vitro cultivation development, - selection of strains resistant to Trichoderma viride, - search for new active compounds, - factors influencing plasticity in Grifola frondosa. Universite de Neuchatel, Faculte des Sciences, Neuchatel, Switzerland.

Grace, G.L.; Yue, K.P.F.; Gary, M.K.; Tse, P.C.L.; Clara, B.S.L. (2006). Comparative Studies of Various Ganoderma Species and Their Different Parts with Regard to Their Antitumor and Immunomodulating Activities In Vitro. *Journal of Alternative and Complementary Medicine*, Vol.12, No.8, pp. 777-789.

Griffin, S.P. & Bhagooli, R. (2004). Measuring antioxidant potential in corals using the FRAP assay. *Journal of Experimental Marine Biology and Ecology*, Vol.302, pp. 201-211.

Gunde-Cimerman, N. & Cimerman, A. (1995). Pleurotus fruiting bodies contain the inhibitor of HMG CoA reductase- lovastatin. *Experimental Mycology*. Vol.19, No.1, pp. 1-6.

GuoY., Wang H., Ng T.B. (2005): Isolation of trichogin, an antifungal protein from fresh fruiting bodies of the edible mushroom Tricholoma giganteum. *Peptides*, 26: 575–580.

Halliwell, B. & Gutteridge, J.M.C. (2007). Free radicals in biology and medicine. Biosciences, Oxford University Press, Oxford, England.

He, J., Feng, X., Lu, Y., Zhao, B. (2003): Fomlactones A-C, Novel Triterpene Lactones from Fomes cajanderi. *Journal of Natural Products*, 66: 1249-1251.

Hirasawa, M., Shouji, N., Neta, T., Fukushima, K., Takada, K. (1999). Three kinds of antibacterial substances from *Lentinus edodes* (Berk.) Sing. (Shiitake, an edible mushroom). *International Journal of Antimicrobial Agents*, 11: 151–157.

Hirasawa, M.; Shouji, N.; Neta, T.; Fukushima, K.; Takada, K. (1999). Three kinds of bacterial substances from Lentinus edodes (Berk) Sing. (Shiitake an edible mushroom). *International Journal of Antimicrobial Agents*, Vol.11, No.2, pp. 151-157.

Hur, J.M.; Yang, C.H.; Han, S.H.; Lee, S.H.; You, Y.O.; Park, J.C.; Kim, K.J. (2004). Antibacterial effect of Phellinus linteus against methicillin-resistant Staphylococcus aureus. *Fitoterapia*, Vol.75, pp. 602-605.

Inouye, S., Abe, S.h., Yamagushi, H. (2004). Fungal terpenoid Antibiotics and Enzyme Inhibitors. In: Handbook of fungal Biotechnology. Arora D, editor, 2nd ed. New York: Marcel Dekker;, pp. 379-400.

Ishikawa, N.K.; Yamaji, K.; Ishimoto, H.; Miura, K.; Fukushi, Y.; Takahashi, K.; Tahara, S. (2005). Production of enokipodins A,B,C and D: a new group of antimicrobial metabolites from mycelial culture of Flammulina velutipes. *Mycoscience,* Vol.46, pp. 39-45.

Jayakumar, T.; Thomas, P.A.; Geraldine, P. (2009). In vitro antioxidant activities od an ethanolic extract of the oyster mushroom, Pleurotus ostreatus. *Innovaative Food Science and Emerging Technologies,* Vol.10, No.2, pp. 228-234.

Jian, H.; Xiao-Zhang, F.; Yang, L.; Bin, Z. (2003). FomLactones A-C, Novel Triterpene Lactones from Fomes cajanderi. *Journal of Natural Products,* Vol.66, pp. 1249-1251.

Kalyoncu, F.; Oskay, M.; Sağlam, H.; Erdoğan, T.F.; Tamer, A.U. (2010). Antimicrobial and antioxidant activities of mycelia of 10 wild mushroom species. *Journal of Medicinal Food.* Vol.13, No.2, pp. 415-419.

Kamo, T.; Asanoma, M.; Shibata, H. & Hirota, M. (2003). Anti-inflamantory lanostane-type acids from *Piptoporus betulinus. Journal of Natural Products,* 66, pp. 1104-1106.

Karaman A.M. (2009c). Autochtonous fungal species of Basidiomycotina - potential resources of naturally active substances. PhDThesis. University of Novi Sad.

Karaman M, Novakovic M, Matavulj M. (2012b). Fundamental fungal strategies in restoration of natural environment. In: Vazquez, Silva editors. Fungi: Types, environmental impact and role in disease. New York: Nova Science Publishers Inc; In press.

Karaman M., Vesic, M, Stahl, M, Novakovic M., Janjic Lj., Matavuly M. (2012a): "Bioactive Properties of Wild-Growing Mushroom Species *Ganorderma applanatum* (Pers.) Pat. from Fruska Gora Forest (Serbia)". RPMP Vol. 32: "Ethnomedicine and Therapeutic Validation", pp. 361-377.

Karaman, A.M.; Matavulj, N.M. (2005): Macroelements and heavy metals in some lignicolous and tericolous fungi. *Proceedings of Natural Scieneces,* Matica Srpska Novi Sad, 108, 255-267.

Karaman, M. (2002). "Content of Macroelements and Heavy Metals in sporocarps of dominately present Basidiomycotina fungi from the Fruska gora Mountain and their antioxidative activity". Master Degree. University of Novi Sad. Faculty of Natural Sciences and Mathematics. Department of Biology and Ecology.

Karaman, M., Jovin, E., Malbaša, R., Matavuly, M., Popović, M. (2010). Medicinal and Edible Lignicolous Fungi as Natural Sources of Antioxidative and Antibacterial agents. *Phytotherapy Research;* Vol.24, No.10, pp. 1473-1481.

Karaman, M., Mimica-Dukić, N., Knežević, P., Svirčev, Z., Matavulj, M. (2009a): Antibacterial properties of selected lignicolous mushrooms and fungi from northern Serbia. *International Journal of Medicinal Mushrooms,* Vol.11, No.3, pp. 269-279.

Karaman, M.; Kaišarević, S.; Somborski, J.; Kebert, M.; Matavuly, M. (2009b): Biological activities of the lignicolous fungus Meripilus giganteus (Pers.:Pers.) Karst. *Archives of Biological Sciences,* Vol.61, No.4, pp. 353-361.

Kavanagh F., Hervey, A. & Robbins (1950): Antibiotic substances from Basidiomycetes. VI.Agrocybe dura. *Proceedings of Natural Academy Sciences* U S A. 36: 102-106.

Kavanagh, F.; Hervey, A.; Robbins, W.J. (1951). Antibiotic substances from basidiomycetes. VIII. Pleurotus mutilus (Fr) Sacc. and Pleurotus passeckierianus Pilat. *Proceedings of Natural Academic Science;* 37, pp. 570-574.

Kim, H.W. & Kim, B.K. (1999). Biomedicinal triterpenoids of Ganoderma lucidum (Curt.:Fr.)P. Karst. (aphyllophoromicetidae). *International Journal of Medicinal Mushrooms,* 1, pp. 121-138.

Kim, M.Y.; Seguin, P.; Ahn, J.K.; Kim, J.J.; Chun, S.C.; Kim, E.H.; Seo, S.H.; Kang, E.Y.; Kim, S.L. ; Park, Y.J. ; Ro, H.M. & Chung, I.M. (2008). Phenolic compound concentration and antoxidant activities of edible and medicinal mushrooms from Korea. *Journal of Agricultural and Food Chemistry*; Vol.56, No.16, pp. 7265-7270.

Kitzberger, C.S.G.; Smania, JrA.; Pedrosa, R.C. & Ferreira S.R.S. (2007). Antioxidant and antimicrobial activities of shiitake (Lentinula edodes) extracts obtained by organic solvents and superficial fluids. *Journal of Food Engineering*; 80, pp. 631- 638.

Kryger, K.; Sosulski, F. & Hogge, L. (1982). Free, esterified, and insoluble-bound phenolic acids, *Journal of Agricultural and Food Chemistry*, 30, pp. 330-334.

Kuhnt, D., Anke, T., Besl, H., Bross, M., Herrmann, R., Mocek, U., Steffan, B., Steglich, W. (1990): Antibiotics from basidiomycetes. XXXVII. New inhibitors of cholesterol biosynthesis from cultures of Xerula melanotricha Dörfelt. *The Journal of Antibiotics*, 43 (11): 1414-1420.

Lee, J.S. (2005). Effects of *Fomes fomentarius* supplementation on antioxidant enzyme activities, blood glucose, and lipid profile in streptozotocin-induced diabetic rats. *Nutritional Research*; 25: 187–195.

Lee, S.Y. & Rhee, H.M. (1990). Cardiovascular effects of mycelium extract of Ganoderma lucidum: inhibition of sympathetic outflow as a mechanism of its hypotensive action. *Chemical & Pharmacological Bulletin (Tokyo)*; Vol.38, No.5, pp. 1359-1364.

Leon, F.; Quintana, J.; Rivera, A.; Estevez, F. & Bermejo, J. (2004). Lanostanoide triterpenes from Laetiporus sulphureus and apoptosis induction on HL-60 Human myeloid leukaemia cells. *Journal of Natural Products*, 67, pp. 2008-2011.

Lindequist, U.; Niedermeyer, T.H.J. & Julich, W.D. (2005). The pharmacological potential of mushrooms. *Evidence-based Complementary and Alternative Medicine*; Vol.2, No.3, pp. 285-299.

Liu, F., Ooi, V.E.C. & Chang, S.T. (1997). Free radical scavenging activities of mushroom polysaccharide extracts. *Life Sciences*, Vol.60, No.10, pp. 763-771.

Liu, G.T. (1999). Recent advances in research of pharmacology and clinical application of Ganoderma P. Karst. species (Aphyllophoromycetdeae) in China. *International Journal of Medicinal Mushrooms*, 1, pp. 63-67.

Liu, X.T., Winkler, A.L., Schwan, W.R., Volk, T.J., Rott M., Monte A. (2010). Antibacterial Compounds from Mushrooms II: Lanostane Triterpenoids and an Ergostane Steroid with Activity Against Bacillus cereus Isolated from Fomitopsis pinicola. *Planta Medica*, 76(5), pp. 464-466.

Lo, K.M. & Cheung, C.K. (2005). Antioxidant activity of extracts from the fruiting bodies of Agrocybe aegerit var. alba. *Food Chemistry*, 89, pp. 533-539.

Lorenzen, K. & Anke, T. (1998). Basidiomycetes as a sources for new bioactive natural products. *Current Organic Chemistry*, 2, pp. 329-364.

Magae, Y. & Ohara, S. (2006): Structure-activity relationship of triterpenoid saponins on fruiting body induction in Pleurotus ostreatus. *Bioscience, Biotechnology and Biochemistry* 70: 1979–1982.

Magan, N. ; Hope, R. ; Cairns, V. & Aldred, D. (2003): Post-harvest fungal ecology: Impact of fungal growth and mycotoxin accumulation in stored grain. *European Journal of Plant Pathology*, 109, pp. 723–730.

Mau, J.L., Lin, H.C., & Chen, C.C. (2002). Antioxidant properties of several medicinal mushrooms. *Journal of Agricultural and Food Chemistry*, 50, 6072-6077.

Moser, M. Agarisc and Boleti. Stuttgart: Gustav Fisher Verlag, 1978.

Mothana, R.A.A.; Jansen, R.; Julich, W.D. & Lindequist, U. (2000). Ganomycin A and B, new antimicrobial farnesyl hydroquinones from the Basidiomycete Ganoderma pfeifferi. *Journal of Natural Products,* 63, pp. 416-418.

Negishi, E., Alimardanov, A., Xu, C. (2000): An efficient and stereoselective synthesis of xerulin via Pd-catalyzed cross coupling and lactonization featuring (E)-Iodobromoethylene as a novel two-carbon synthon. *Organic Letters,* 2 (1): 65-67.

Ngai, P.H.; Zhao, Z. & Ng, T.B. (2005). Agrocybin, an antifungal peptide from edible mushroom Agrocybe cilindracea. *Peptides,* Vol .26, No.2, pp. 191-196.

Ofodile, L.N.; Uma, N.U.; Kokubun, T.; Grayer, R.J.; Ogundipe, O.T., Simmonds, M.S.J. (2005). Antimicrobial activity of some Ganoderma species from Nigeria. *Phytotherapy Research,* Vol.19, No.4, pp. 310-313.

Orrù, B., A., R., - Fruciano, E. (2002) Giuseppe Brotzu and the Discovery of Cephalosporins. In: 8th European Conference of Medical and Health Libraries, 16-21 Settembre 2002, Colonia (Germania).

Park, Y.K., Kim, I.T., Park, H.J., & Choi, J.W. (2004). Anti-inflammatory and Anti-nociceptive effects of the Methanol extract of Fomes fomentarius. *Biological & Pharmacological Bulletin;* 27(10): 1599-1593.

Park, Y.K., Koo, M.H., Ikegaki, M., & Contado JL. (1997). Comparison of the flavonoid aglycone contents of Apis mellifera propolis from various regions of Brazil. *Brazilian Archives of Biology and Technology;* 40(1): 97-106.

Paterson, R.R.M. (2006). Ganoderma –a therapeutic fungal biofactory. *Phytochemistry,* 67, pp. 1985-2001.

Performance Standards for Antimicrobial Susceptibility Testing. (2005). Clinical Laboratory Standards Institute CLSI, NSBI , Wayne, USA

Pietta, P.G. (2000). Flavonoids as Antioxidants. Reviews. *Journal of Natural Products;* 63, pp. 1035-1042.

Puttaraju, N.G., Venkateshaiah, S.U., Dharmesh, S.M., Urs, S.M.N., Somasundaram, R. (2006). Antioxidant activity of indigenous Edible Mushrooms. *Journal of Agricultural and Food Chemistry* 54, pp. 9764-9772.

Ren, G., Liu, X.Y., Zhu, H.K., Yang, S.Z., Fu, C.X. (2006): Evaluation of cytotoxic activities of some medicinal polypore fungi from China. *Fitoterapia;* 77, pp. 408-410.

Ribeiro, B., Valentao, P., Baptista, P., Seabra, R., Andrade, P.B. (2007). Phenolic compounds organic acids profiles and antioxidative properties of beefsteak fungus (Fistulina hepatica). *Food Chemical Toxicology,* 45, pp. 1805-1813.

Rosa, L.H., Machado, K.M.G., Jacob, C.C., Capelari, M., Rosa, C.A., Zani, C.L. (2003). Screening of Brazilian Basidiomycetes for Antimicrobial Activity. *Memórias do Instituto Oswaldo Cruz.;* 98(7):967-974.

Rosecke, J., Pietsch, M., Konig, W.A. (2000). Volatile constituents of wood-rotting Basidiomycetes. *Phytochemistry,* 54, pp. 747-750.

Shiao, M.S. (1992). Triterpenoid Natural Products in the Fungus Ganoderma lucidum. Journal of Chinese Chemical Society, 39, pp. 669-674.

Shimada M, Akamatsu Y, Tokimatsu T, Mii K, Hattori, T. (1997). Possible biochemical roles of oxalic acids as a low molecular weight compound involved in brown-rot and white-rot wood decay . *Journal of Biotechnology* 53: 103-113.

Shittu, O. B., Alofe, F. V., Onawunmi, G. O., Ogundaini, A. O., Tiwalade, T. A. (2006): Bioautographic Evaluation of Antibacterial Metabolite Production by Wild Mushrooms. *African Journal of Biomedical Research,* 9: 57 62.

Smania, JrA, Monache, F.D., Loguericio-Leite, C., Smania, E.F.A., Gerber, A.L. (2001). Antimicrobial activity of Basidiomycetes. *International Journal of Medicinal Mushrooms*, 3, pp. 87-93.

Soler-Rivas, C., Espin, J.C., Wichers, H.J. (2000). An easy and fast test to compare total free radical scavenger capacity of foodstuffs. *Phytochemical Analysis*, 11, pp. 330-338.

Stadtler, M. & Sterner, O. (1998). Production of bioactive secondary metabolites in the fruit bodies of macrofungi as a response to injury. *Phytochemistry*, Vol.49, No.4, pp. 1013-1019.

Stamets, P. (2002): Novel antimicrobials from mushrooms. *Herbal Gram*, 54: 2-6.

Suay, I., Arenal, F., Asensio, F.J., Basilio, A., Cabello, M.A., Diez, M.T., Garcia, J.B., Gonzales del Val, A., Gorrochategui, J., Hernandez, P., Pelaez, F., Vicente, M.F. (2000). Screening of basidiomycetes for antimicrobial activities. *Antonie van Leewenhook*, 78, pp. 129-139.

Taga, M.S., Miller, E.E., Pratt, D.E. (1984). Chia seeds as a source of natural lipid antioxidants. *Journal of the American Oil Chemist's Society*, 61, pp. 928-993.

Takakura, Y., Kuwata, S., Inouye, Y. (2001): Antimicrobial protein from Lyophyllum shimeji. Available via: http://www.patentstorm.us.

Tanaka, Y. & Omura, S. (1993): Agroactive Compounds of Microbial Origin. *Annual Review of Microbiology*, Vol. 47: 57-87

Tseng, Y.H., Yang, J.H., Mau, J.L. (2008). Antioxidant properties of polysaccharides from Ganoderma tsugae. *Food Chemistry*, 107, pp. 732-738.

Turkoglu, A., Duru, M.E., Mercan, N., Kivrak, I., Gezer, K. (2007). Antioxidant and antimicrobial activities of Laetiporus sulphureus (Bull) Murrill. *Food Chemistry*, 101, pp. 267-273.

USDA Database for the Flavonoid Content of Selected Foods 2003, accessed May 2009. http://www.nal.usda.gov/fnic/foodcomp/Data/Flav/flav.html

Wang, H., Ng, T.B. (2004): Eryngin, a novel antifungal peptide from fruiting bodies of the edible mushroom Pleurotus eryngii. *Peptides*, 25 (1): 1-5.

Wang, H., Ng, T.B. (2006): Ganodermin, an antifungal protein from fruiting bodies of the medicinal mushroom Ganoderma lucidum. *Peptides*, 27: 27-30.

Wasser, S.P. & Weis, A.L. (1999). Medicinal properties of substances occurring in higher Basidiomycetes mushrooms: current perspectives (review). *International Journal of Medicinal Mushrooms*.;1,31-62.

Wasser, S.P. (2011). Current findings, future trends and unsolved problems in studies of medicinal mushrooms. *Applied Microbiology and Biotechnology*, 89, pp. 1323-1332.

Whalley, A.J.S. & Edwards, R.L. (1999). The Xylariaceae: A Case Study in Biological and Chemical Diversity. Published online in IUPAC. Available via Dialog. http://www.iupac.org/symposia/proceedings/phuket97/whalley.htmL. Accessed 9th Jun 2009

Wu, Y. & Wang, D. (2009). A new class of natural glycopeptides with sugar moiety-dependent antioxidant activities derived from Ganoderma lucidum fruiting bodies. *Journal of Proteome Research*., Vol.8, No.2, pp. 436–442.

Yang, J.H., Lin, H.C., Mau, J.L. (2002). Antioxidant properties of several commercial mushrooms. *Food Chemistry*, 77, pp. 229-235.

Zhang, C.R., Yang, S.P., Yue, J.M. (2008). Sterols and trterpenoids from the spores of Ganoderma lucidum. *Natural Product Research*, 22, pp. 1137-1142.

Zjawiony, J.K. (2004). Biologically active compounds from Aphyllophorales (polypore) Fungi. *Journal of Natural Products*; 67, pp. 300-310.

20

Silver Nanoparticles: Real Antibacterial Bullets

G. Thirumurugan and M. D. Dhanaraju
Research Lab, GIET School of Pharmacy, Chaitanya Nagar, Rajahmundry, AP India

1. Introduction

One of the first and most natural questions to ask when starting to deal with nanoparticles is: "why are nanoparticles so interesting"? Why even bother to work with these extremely small structures when handling and synthesis is much more complicated than that of their macroscopic counterparts. The answer lies in the nature of and unique properties possessed by nanostructures. Nanoparticles possess a very high surface to volume ratio. This can be utilized in areas where high surface areas are critical for success. Over the past few decades, Metal nanoparticles, whose structures exhibit significantly novel and distinct physical, chemical, and biological properties, and functionality due to their nanoscale size, have elicited much interest. Especially in biological and pharmaceutical sector nanostructure materials are attracting a great deal of attention because of their potential for achieving specific processes and selectivity. Decreasing the dimension of nanoparticles has pronounced effect on the physical properties that significantly differ from the bulk material. Moreover, there are several reasons for the use of silver nanoparticles in nanotechnology as well as in medical and pharmaceutical field. (i) First of all, silver compounds have been used in medicine throughout the history of civilization. (Patra, 2008; Klasen, 2000; Lansdown, 2002) (ii) It is easy to synthesize silver nanoparticles by several simple, economically cheap, safe and reliable methods such as wet chemical, physical and biological; (iii) it can be synthesized from sizes of 2-500 nm by changing the reaction parameters; (iv) it can be easily synthesized with different shapes (spheres, rods, tubes, wires, ribbons, plate, cubic, hexagonal, triangular) using templates and changing reaction conditions; (v) due to the presence of a negative charge on the surface, they are highly reactive, which helps to modify the surface of silver nanoparticles using several biomolecules. Due to the strong interaction between the metal surface and thiol/amine containing molecules (organic molecules, DNA, protein, enzyme etc.) the surface of SNPs can be easily modified; (Bhattacharya, 2007) (vi) SNPs can be easily characterized due to the presence of the characteristic surface plasmon resonance (SPR) bands; (Daniel and Astruc, 2004) due to the presence of a unique optical as well as electronic behavior, these metal particles can be used in biosensors and molecular imaging; (Oghabian, 2010) due to its strong antimicrobial activity, it has found variety of application in different fields (Fig. 1).

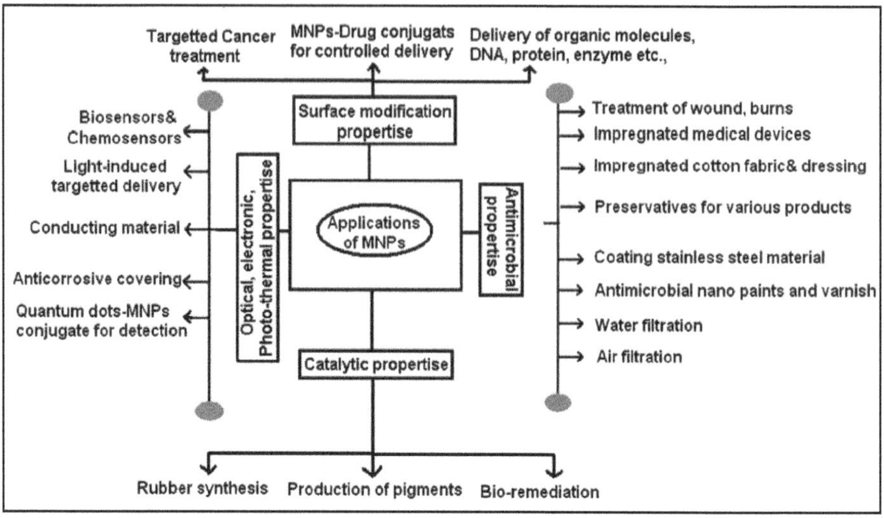

Fig. 1. Applications of metal nanoparticles in various fields (G.Thirumurugan, 2011).

The synthesis of monodispersed metal nanoparticles with different size and shape has been challenge in nanotechnology. Although various physical and chemical methods are extensively used to produce monodispersed nanoparticles, the stability and the use of toxic chemicals is the subject of paramount concern. Moreover, the use of toxic chemicals on the surface of nanoparticles and non-polar solvents in the synthesis procedure limits their applications in clinical and pharmaceutical field (Oghabian, 2010) Therefore, development of clean, biocompatible, non-toxic and eco-friendly methods for silver nanoparticles synthesis deserves merit.

In this chapter, we will discuss an overview of silver nanoparticle preparation involving physical, chemical method and biological method, mechanism and advantages and disadvantages of the above methods. We provide various antibacterial mechanisms of silver nanoparticles to reduce antibiotic resistance and incorporation of SNPs on cotton fabrics and conjugation of SNPs on pharmaceutical compounds. Finally, we will discuss site-specific, antibacterial drug delivery of SNPs due to its unique surface modification, photo-thermal properties.

2. Synthesis of silver nanoparticles

2.1 Physical and chemical method

There are various physical and chemical approach widely used for the synthesis of silver nanoparticles, such as reduction in solution, (Goia, 1998) chemical and photochemical reactions in reverse micelles, (Taleb, 1997) thermal decomposition of metal compounds, (Esumi, 1990) radiation assisted, (Henglein, 2001) electrochemical, (Rodriguez-Sanchez, 2000) sonochemical, (Zhu, 2000) microwave assisted process (Isabel Pastoriza-Santos, 2002).

Most frequently preparation of silver nanoparticles is carried out by chemical reduction method. Borohydrate, citrate, ascorbate, and elemental hydrogen are commonly used reductants for the synthesis of silver nanoparticles. The reduction of metal ions (Me^+) like silver (Ag^+ or gold (Au^+) in aqueous solution generally yields colloidal metal with particle diameters of several nanometers (Wiley, 2005). Initially, the reduction of various complexes with metal (Ag^+) ions leads to the formation of metal atoms (Ag^0), which is followed by agglomeration into oligomeric clusters (Kapoor, 2002). These clusters eventually lead to the formation of colloidal Metal particles (Kapoor, 2002). For example, while formation of colloidal silver particles, when the colloidal particles are much smaller than the wavelength of visible light, the solutions have a yellow color with an intense band in the 380–400 nm range and other less intense or smaller bands at longer wavelength in the absorption spectrum (Cao, 2002). This band is attributed to collective excitation of the electron gas in the particles, with a periodic change in electron density at the surface (surface Plasmon absorption), (Gutiérrez, 1993).

The synthesis of silver nanoparticles in this project will be based on a wet chemical method. The starting point of the synthesis is the production of a silver nitrate (AgNO3) solution. When silver nitrate is dissolved it splits into a positive silver ion (Ag^+) and a negative nitrate ion (NO_3^-). In order to turn the silver ions into solid silver, the ions have to be reduced by receiving an electron from a donator. A flowchart illustrating the reduction of the silver ions by addition of an electron can be seen in Equation 1. The flowchart of Equation 2 illustrates the reduction of (Ag^+) in a solution of ethanol. After the silver germ has been formed it starts to grow and continue the growth until the equilibrium between the final nanoparticles and the (Ag^+) of the solution is reached (Chou, 2005).

$$Ag^+_{(aq)} + e^- \rightarrow Ag_{(s)} \tag{1}$$

$$2Ag^+_{(aq)} + C_2H_5OH{+}H_2O \rightarrow 2Ag_{(s)} + C_2H_5O_2^- + 3H^+ \tag{2}$$

The chemical reaction is the sodium borohydride reduction of silver nitrate:

$$AgNO_3 + NaBH_4 \rightarrow Ag + \tfrac{1}{2}H_2 + \tfrac{1}{2}B_2H_6 + NaNO_3 \tag{3}$$

The preparation of silver nanoparticles in briefly, A 10-mL volume of 1.0 mM silver nitrate was added dropwise (about 1 dropsecond) to 30 mL of 2.0 mM sodium borohydride solution that had been chilled in an ice bath. The reaction mixture was stirred vigorously on a magnetic stir plate. The solution turned light yellow after the addition of 2 mL of silver nitrate and a brighter yellow, when all of the silver nitrate had been added. The entire addition took about three minutes, after which the stirring was stopped and the stir bar removed. The clear yellow colloidal silver is stable at room temperature stored in a transparent vial for as long as several weeks or months. Reaction conditions including stirring time and relative quantities of reagents (both the absolute number of moles of each reactant as well as their relative molarities) must be carefully controlled to obtain stable yellow colloidal silver. A large excess of sodium borohydride is needed both to reduce the ionic silver and to stabilize the silver nanoparticles. The possibility of aggregation during the synthesis, colloidal silver solution turns darker yellow, violet, and then grayish. Adsorption of borohydride plays a key role in stabilizing growing silver nanoparticles by providing a particle surface charge as shown in the schematic diagram in Figure 2. There must be enough borohydride to stabilize the particles as the reaction proceeds. However, later in the reaction too much sodium borohydride increases the overall ionic strength and aggregation will occur (Van Hyning, 2001). The aggregation can also be brought about by addition of electrolytes such as NaCl. Nanoparticles are kept in suspension by repulsive electrostatic forces between the particles owing to adsorbed borohydride (Fig. 2). Salt shields the charges allowing the particles to clump together to form aggregates.

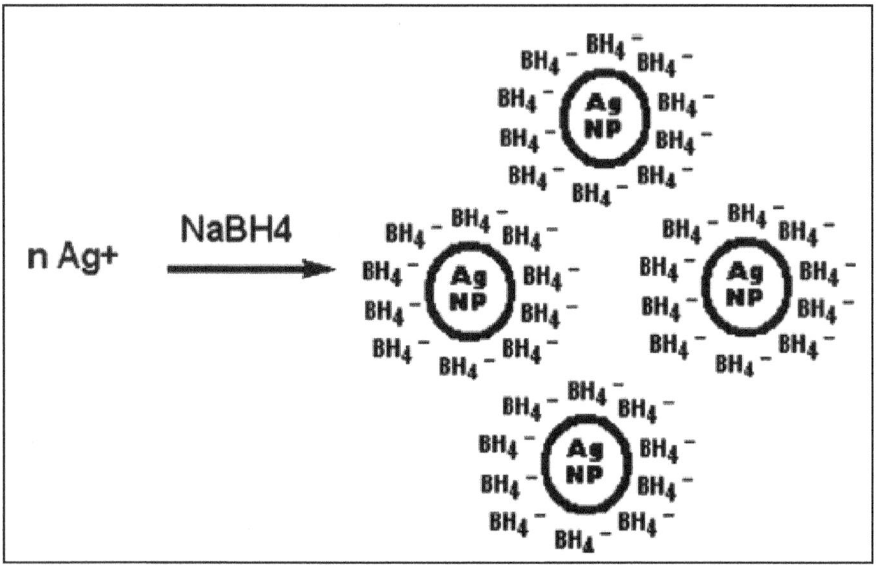

Fig. 2. Repulsive forces separate Ag nanoparticles (NP) with adsorbed borohydride (G.Thirumurugan, 2011).

2.2 Biological method of silver nanoparticle synthesis

Though various chemical and biochemical methods are being explored for silver nanoparticle production (Wiley, 2005), microbes, plants are also very effective in this process. Various microbes (Sharma, 2006; Mann, 1984; Beveridge, 1997), plants (Shankar, 2004; Gardea-Torresdey, 2002) are known to reduce the metals [Table 1], most of them are found to be spherical particles as reported earlier (Chen, 2003; Ahmad, 2005). Extracts from microbes act both as reducing and capping agents in metal nanoparticles synthesis. The reduction of metal ions by combinations of biomolecules found in these extracts such as enzymes or proteins, amino acids, polysaccharides, and vitamins (Jagadeesh, 1981) is environmentally benign, yet chemically complex.

Bio-recovery of silver metals from solution, a process referred to as "biosorption", occurs by either active or passive mechanisms. Active metal transformation processes require viable microbes, enzymatically catalyzing the alteration of the metal, leading to sequestration or concentration. One possible (passive) role of the microorganisms is in providing a multitude of nucleation centers; establishing conditions for obtaining highly disperse nanoparticle systems. In addition, they slow down aggregation, or entirely prevent it by immobilizing the particles, and providing viscous medium (*Sun,* 2002). Thus produced nanoparticles have highly intricate architectures and are ordered during assembly. In some cases, the particles have a well-defined shape formed within an arrow size range and have orientational and geometrical symmetry (Sarikaya, 1999). In case of silver nanoparticle production, the resistance conferred by bacteria to silver is determined by the *'sil'* gene in plasmids (Silver, 2003) while a nitrate-dependent reductase and a shuttle quinine extracellular process were reported for the reduction of silver ions by several Fusarium oxysporum strains (Duran, 2005). The extract of unicellular green algae Chlorella vulgaris was used to synthesize single-crystalline Ag nanoplates at room temperature (Jianping Xie, 2007). Proteins in the extract provide dual function of $Ag+$ reduction and shape-control in the nano silver synthesis. The carboxyl groups in aspartic and or glutamine residues and the hydroxyl groups in tyrosine residues of the proteins were suggested to be responsible for the $Ag+$ ion reduction (Jianping Xie, 2007). Carrying out the reduction process by a simple bifunctional tripeptide Asp-Asp-Tyr-OMe further identified the involvement of these residues. This synthesis process gave small Ag nanoplates with low polydispersity in good yield (>55%) (Gole, 2001). Balaji, 2009 reported FTIR spectroscopic studies on silver nanoparticles obtained from the fungus, Cladosporium cladosporioides. Their study confirmed that the carbonyl groups from the amino acid residues and peptides of proteins have strong ability to bind silver. The proteins could possibly forma coat covering the metal nanoparticles to prevent their agglomeration and aid in its stabilization in the medium. Hence, the biological molecules could possibly function in the formation and stabilization of the silver nanoparticles in aqueous medium. Gole, 2001 reported that proteins can bind to silver nanoparticles either through free amine groups in the proteins and possibly play a role in stabilization of the silver nanoparticles by surface-bound proteins. Moreover, Vigneshwaran, 2006 explained the synthesis of metal nanoparticles by using fungal mycelium, in the a rotary shaker, metal ions in solution were adsorbed on the surface of the mycelia through interactions with chemical functional groups such as carboxylate anion, carboxyl and peptide bond of proteins, and hydroxyl of saccharides (Lin, 2005) found on the mycelia. The mycelia, matted together, was more immobile, and more capable of binding Me^+ than that of the external cellular substances that distributed in the inter-mycelial space, then most of the Me^+ was *in situ* reduced to Me^0 by reducing sugars from the saccharides (Gole, 2001) on the mycelia. In the mean time, stronger adsorptive groups such as the carbonyl group on the extracellular substances could further adsorb the particles located on the surface of the mycelia, resulting in capping these nanoparticles, while rocking. When other Me^+ in the solution was rocked on to this overlay and was bound and reduced to Me^0 on the surface of the layer and these Me^0 might be possibly further coated with the other extra cellular substances; this process was repeated continuously until these substances distributing in the inter-mycelial space was used up.

Plant extracts from live alfalfa, the broths of lemon grass, geranium leaves and others have served as green reactants in silver nanoparticle synthesis (Shankar, 2004; Gardea-Torresdey,

2002). Using plants for nanoparticle synthesis can be advantageous over other biological processes because it eliminates the elaborate process of maintaining cell cultures and can also be suitably scaled up for large-scale nanoparticle synthesis (Shenton, 1999)

3. Anti bacterial effect of silver nanoparticles

Due to the outbreak of the infectious diseases caused by different pathogenic bacteria and the development of antibiotic resistance the pharmaceutical companies and the researchers are searching for new antibacterial agents free of resistance and cost. In the present scenario silver nanoparticles have emerged up as novel antimicrobial agents owing to their high surface area to volume ratio and its unique chemical and physical properties. The use of silver nanoparticles can be exploited in various fields, particularly medical and pharmaceutical due to their low toxicity to human cells, high thermal stability and low volatility (Silver, 2003). This has resulted in a broad array of studies in which silver nanoparticles have played a role as drug and as well as superior anti bacterial agent. The highest synergistic antibacterial activity was observed with silver nanoparticles combined antibiotics (Raymond Wai-Yin Sun, 2005). silver nanoparticle incorporated cotton fabrics showed antibacterial activity (Shahverdi, 2007), and silver nanoparticle containing poly vinyl nano- fibres shows efficient antibacterial property (Duran, 2007), it can be used in silver dressings, creams, gel effectively reduce the bacterial infections in chronic wound (Jun, 2007; Richard, 2002; Leaper, 2006). Siver nanoparticles are reported to show better wound healing capacity, better cosmetic appearance and scarless healing when tested using an animal model (Ip, 2006). Kumar et al., 2008 investigated an eco-friendly method for synthesis of metal nanoparticles embedded paint from using vegetable oil. The paint depicts excellent antibacterial activity and in future this paint can be used for efficient antimicrobial coating agent to coat various surfaces such as wood, glass, walls. Silver has been used in water and air filtration to eliminate microorganisms, additionally the $Fe_3 O_4$ attached Ag nanoparticles can be used for the treatment of water and easily removed using magnetic field to avoid contamination in the environment (Kumar et al., 2008).

4. Silver nanoparticles and antibiotic resistance

Antibiotic resistance is a type of drug resistance where a microorganism has developed the ability to survive exposure to an antibiotic. The volume of antibiotic prescribed is the major factor in increasing rates of bacterial resistance rather than compliance with antibiotics. The four main mechanisms by which microorganisms exhibit resistance to antimicrobials are: Drug inactivation or modification (e.g. enzymatic deactivation of Penicillin G in some penicillin-resistant bacteria through the production of β-lactamases) and .alteration of target site(e.g. alteration of Penicillin-binding proteins (PBPs) —the binding target site of penicillins—in Methicillin-resistant *Staphylococcus aureus* (MRSA) and other penicillin-resistant bacteria). Alteration of metabolic pathway(e.g. some sulfonamide-resistant bacteria do not require para-aminobenzoic acid (PABA), an important precursor for the synthesis of folic acid and nucleic acids in bacteria inhibited by sulfonamides. Instead, like mammalian cells, they turn to utilizing preformed folic acid) and reduced drug accumulation: by decreasing drug permeability and/or increasing active efflux (pumping out) of the drugs across the cell surface [Figure 3].

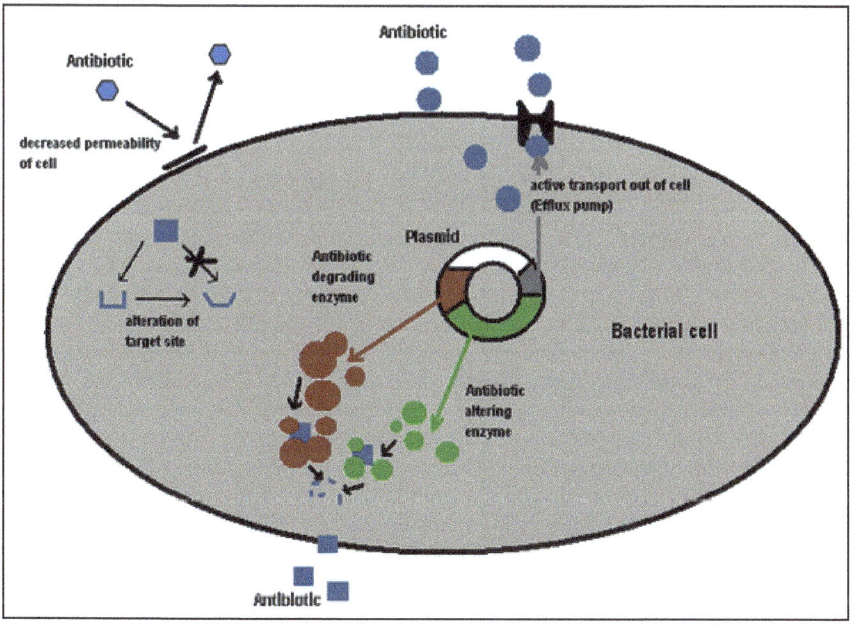

Fig. 3. Various mechanisms of bacterial resistance against antibacterials (G. Thirumurugan, 2011).

Therefore, an alternative way to overcome the antibiotic and drug resistance of various micro organisms is needed desperately, especially in medical devices, pharmaceutical etc. The nano size allowed expansion of the contact surface of silver with the microorganisms, and this nano scale has applicability for medical devices and pharmaceutical by surface coating agents. Kim et al., 2007 studied antibacterial mechanism of silver nanoparticles for certain microbial species. The peptidoglycan layer is a specific membrane feature of bacterial species and not mammalian cells. Therefore, if the antibacterial effect of silver nanoparticles is associated with the peptidoglycan layer, it will be easier and more specific to use silver nanoparticles as an antibacterial agent. Sondi and Salopek-Sondi, 2007 reported that the antibacterial activity of silver nanoparticles on Gram-negative bacteria was dependent on the concentration of Ag nanoparticle, and was closely associated with the formation of 'pits' in the cell wall of bacteria. Then, Ag nanoparticles accumulated in the bacterial membrane caused the permeability, resulting in cell death and they reported degradation of the membrane structure of micro organism with silver nanoparticles. Kim et al., 2007 suggested that the antimicrobial mechanism of Ag nanoparticles is related to the formation of free radicals and subsequent free radical-induced membrane damage. The free radicals may be derived from the surface of silver nanoparticles and be responsible for the antibacterial activity. In proteomic and biochemical studies, nano molar concentrations of AgNPs have killed E.coli cells within minutes possibly due to immediate dissipation of the proton motive force (Lok, 2006). This action is similar to that found for antibacterial activities of Ag^+ ions (Dibrov, 2002). For example, low concentrations of Ag^+ ion result in massive proton leakage through the Vibrio cholerae membrane (Dibrov, 2002). This proton leak might be happening from either any Ag^+ -modified membrane protein or any Ag^+-modified phospholipids bilayer. The phenomenon causes deenergization of the membrane and consequently cell death (Dibrov, 2002). Shahverdi et al., 2007 studied the combined effect of silver nanoparticles with different antibiotics against S.aureus and E.coli using the disk diffusion method. The antibacterial activities of penicillin G, amoxicillin, erythromycin, clindamycin, and vancomycin increased in the presence of Ag-NPs against both test strains.

5. Silver nanoparticles incorporated cotton fabrics

The current interest is to development of efficient, non-toxic, durable and cost effective antibacterial finishing textiles with increased application in medical, healthcare, hygienic products as well as protective textiles materials. However the ability of cotton fibres to absorb large amount of moisture makes them more prone to microbial attack under certain conditions of humidity and temperature. Cotton may act as a nutrient, becoming suitable medium for bacterial and fungal growth (Rosemary, 2006). Therefore, cotton fibres are treated with numerous chemicals to get better antibacterial cotton textiles. Among the various antibacterial agents, silver nanoparticles have shown strong inhibitory and antibacterial activity, has no negative effect on the human body (Gao, 2008). These particles can be incorporated in several kinds of materials such as clothes. These clothes with silver nanoparticles are sterile and can be used to prevent or to minimize infection with pathogenic bacteria. Nowadays, metal based topical dressings have been widely used as a treatment for infections in burns, open wounds, and chronic ulcers (Panyala, 2008). Incorporation of silver naoparticles was carried out by physical means, before being used; cotton fabrics were washed, sterilized and dried. These were submerged in an Erlenmeyer flask containing silver nanoparticles and agitated at 600 rpm for 24 hrs and dried at 70° C followed by curing at 150 ° C. The schematic representation of the formation of silver nanoparticles on cotton fabrics is presented in Scheme 1.

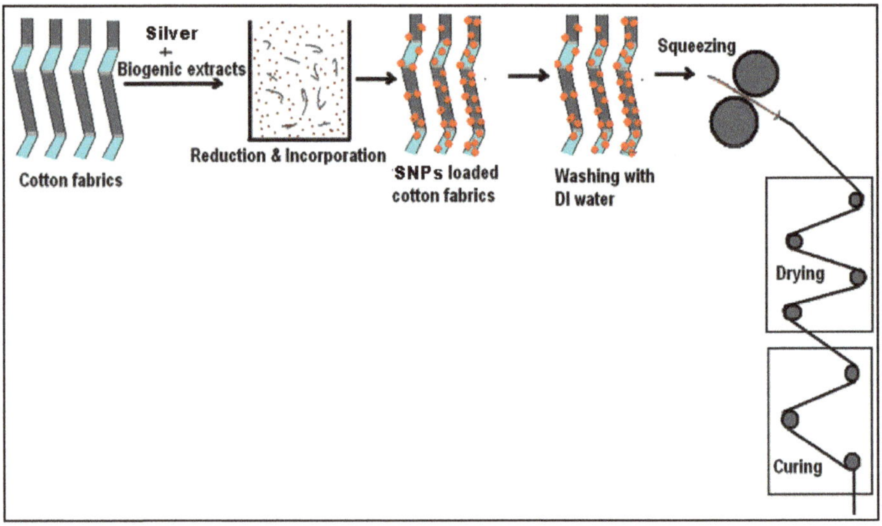

Scheme 1. Incorporation of silver nanoparticles on cotton fabrics (G.Thirumurugan, 2011).

The antibacterial properties and the toxicity of metals to micro-organisms is well known, thus, now a days, silver is used in different kinds of formulations like surface coating agents, wound dressing, etc., (Shahverdi, 2007). The silver dressings make use of delivery systems that release silver in different concentrations. But different factors like the distribution of silver in the dressing, its chemical and physical form, affinity of dressing to moisture also influence the killing of micro organisms (Lansdown, 2002). In this direction, metal nanocomposite fibres were prepared containing silver nanoparticles incorporated inside the fabric but from the scanning electron microscopic study it was concluded that the silver nanoparticles incorporated in the sheath part of fabrics possessed significant antibacterial property compared to the fabrics incorporated with silver nanoparticles in the core part (Chopra, 2007). Similar results were obtained by using silver nanoparticles on polyester nonwovens. It is also reported that silver nanoparticles coated textile fabrics possess antibacterialactivity against S.aureus (Shahverdi, 2007).

6. Silver nanoparticles in antibacterial drug delivery

Drug delivery system provide useful adjuncts for therapeutics including drugs, nucleic acids and proteins, with variety or roles like improving poor solubility, enhancing invivo stability, optimizing the biodistribution and pharmacokinetics of drugs. In recent years, interest has been stimulated by capability of the metal nanoparticles like AgNPs to bind a wide range of organic molecules, their low toxicity, and their strong and tunable optical absorption. This has resulted in a broad array of studies in which silver nanoparticles have played a role as drug and vaccine carriers into target cells or specific tissues. Furthermore, the unique chemical, physical, and photo-physical properties of silver nanoparticles can be exploited in innovative ways to control the transport and controlled release of pharmaceutical compounds (Skirtach, 2006). Generally, this has been achieved by modifying the surface of the silver nanoparticles so that they can bind to the specific targeting drugs or other biomolecules. But direct conjucation of metal nanoparticle with drugs also possible, it has been shown that conjugates of metal nanoparticles with antibiotics provide promising results in the treatment of intracellular infections (Skirtach, 2006). The conjugation of silver nanoparticles in antibiotic can increase the effectiveness of drug delivery to target some cases. Generally, exact dose is required to kill the pathogens but the amount of antibiotic used in therapy is much higher than the actual dose required. The excess amount of antibiotic can cause adverse effects. Therefore, this conjugation of antibiotic with silver nanopaticles would be helpful to improve antibiotic efficacy. Silver nanoparticles can be directly conjugated with antibiotics or other drug molecules via ionic or covalent bonding, or by physical absorption. For example, Drug has been conjugated to silver nanoparticles [Figure 4]. The cytotoxic effect of free drug is about seven times lower than that of drug conjugated silver nanoparticles. Saha et al., 2007, conjugated directly different type of antibiotic to non-functionalized spherical metal nanoparticles, conjugated form showed greater degree of antibacterial activity with stability than free antibiotics. However, the conjugated form showed some aggregation after conjugation, a situation that other workers consider very deleterious. Therefore, it is likely that modification of the surface of the metal nanoparticles to prevent aggregation would improve the efficacy of such drug delivery systems further.

Surface chemistry of nanomaterial plays an important role, to improve the stability of metal nanoparticles and prevent their aggregation during the conjugation process between biomolecules and nanoparticles. Compared with other drug release materials, the unique surface plasmonic properties of the silver particles make it possible to observe the drug release process in living cells by surface enhanced Raman scattering (SERS) method. Jing Yang et al., 2009, found that silver nanoparticles can be used to control the release of drug in living cells. The reason may be that silver nanoparticles can hold the surrounding drug molecules to its surface until a monolayer is formed. The way drug absorbing on the silver surfaces plays an important role in their drug delivery effect in living cells. Figure 5, depicts the SERS spectra of drug in (a) solution and (b) living cells and viability of cells treated with different concentrations of drug and silver nanoparticles. (a) Pure drug; (b) Drug and silver nanoparticle complex; (c) pure silver nanoparticles.

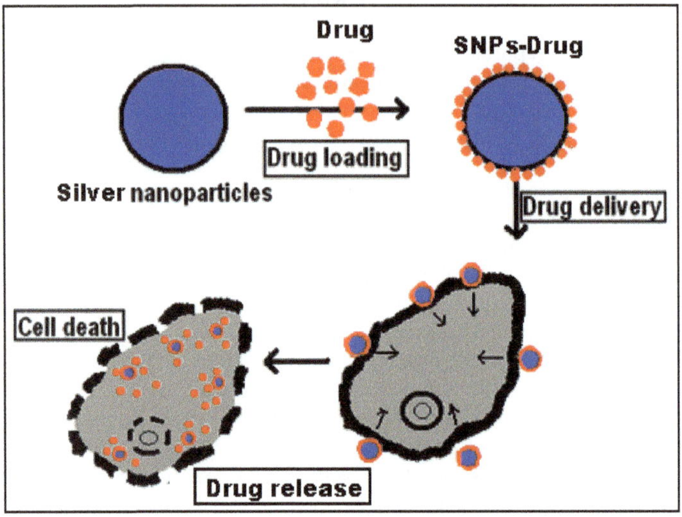

Fig. 4. Cytotoxic effect of drug conjugated silver nanoparticles (G.Thirumurugan, 2011).

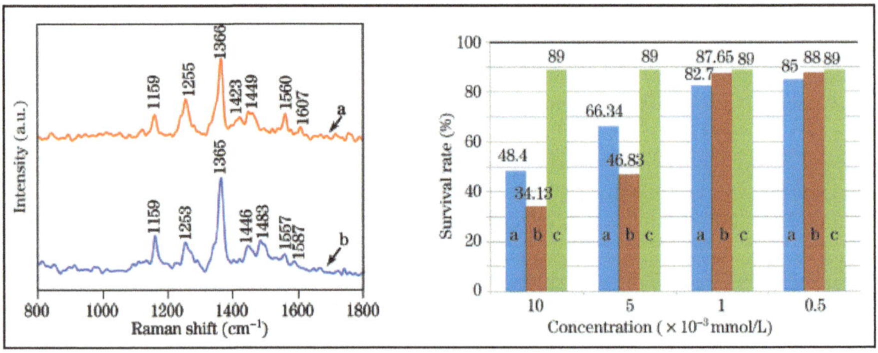

Fig. 5. Left side shows SERS spectra of drug in (a) solution and (b) living cells and right side shows viability of cells treated with different concentrations of drug and silver nanoparticles. (a) Pure drug; (b) Drug and silver nanoparticle complex; (c) pure silver nanoparticles.

In addition to the surface chemistry of SNPs, their physical properties could be exploited for delivery applications (Asadishad, 2010). The release of a drug from silver nanoparticles could proceed via internal stimuli (pH or glutathione mediated) or also via external stimuli with the application of light. Silver nanoparticles of various shapes can undergo a strong plasmon resonance with light; therefore light induced plasmonic heating may be exploited to release a chemical payload which had been attached to the silver nanoparticles. This may be provided an interesting approach to deliver pharmaceutical compound directly into the cytoplasm or nucleus of target cells. Due to optical properties silver nanoparticles, light sensitive molecule can be attached onto silver nanoparticles in which SNPs serves as a substrate. In this case, light sensitive and fully reversible conformation-changing molecule had been attached onto the silver naoparticles (Jain, 2007). The conformation has been changed from a closed form to an open form when it is irradiated by UV light and the process can be reversed by the application of visible light or heat. This light mediated metal nanoparticle conjugate system could be very effective in the controlled release to treat selected conditions (Jain, 2007). Cheng, 2008, prepared the microcapsules via layer-by-layer technique to encapsulate fluorescein-labeled dextran. The capsule-shells were doped with metal nanoparticles, which response against near infra red (NIR) light. FITC-dextran released upon laser (1064) treatment due to rupture of the shell [Figure 6].

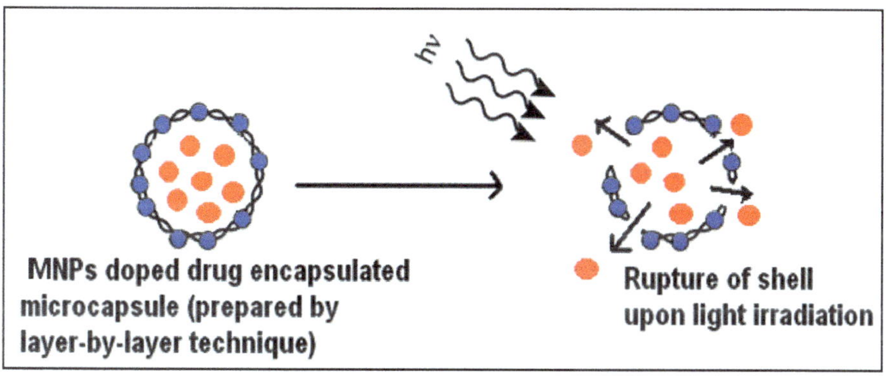

Fig. 6. Light- mediated drug release (G.Thirumurugan, 2011).

7. Conclusion

Increasing awareness towards green chemistry and biological processes has led to a desire to develop an environment-friendly approach for the synthesis of non toxic nanoparticles. Unlike other processes in physical and chemical methods, which involve hazardous chemicals, microbial biosynthesis of nanoparticles is cost-effective and eco friendly approach. Therefore, microbes regarded as potential bio factories for nanoparticles synthesis and serves as a new generation anti bacterial agent with their unique chemical and physical properties. The silver nanoparticle have also found diverse applications in the form of wound dressings, coating medical devices, silver nanoparticles impregnated textile fabrics, silver nanoparticls incorporated pharmaceutical compounds, etc. The presence of a negative charge on the surface, they are highly reactive, which helps to modify the surface of silver nanoparticles using several biomolecules that leads to loading of SNPs with drug or genes, offers the targeted and controlled release. In particular, the combination of silver nanopartcilcles and laser irradiation to control the release of drugs and genes has provided useful therapeutic benefits.

8. References

Ahmad, A,; Senapati, S,; Khan, M. I,; Kumar, R,; Sastry, M. (2005). Extra/Intracellular Biosynthesis of Gold Nanoparticles by a Novel Alkalotolerant Fungus, Trichothecium sp, J Biomed Nanotechnol. 1, 47-53.

Asadishad, B,; Vossoughi, M,; Alemzadeh, I. (2010). Folate-Receptor-Targeted Delivery of Doxorubicin Using Polyethylene Glycol-Functionalized Gold Nanoparticles, Industrial & Engineering Chemistry Research. 49(4), 1958–1963.

Balaji, D.S,; Basavaraja, S,; Deshpande, R,; Mahesh, B.D,; Prabhakar, B.K,; Venkataraman, A. (2009). Extracellular biosynthesis of functionalized silver nanoparticles by strains of Cladosporium cladosporioides fungus, Coll Surf B: Bio interf. 68, 88-92.

Beveridge, T.J,; Hughes, M.N,; Lee, H,; Leung, K.T,; Poole, R.K,; Savvaidis, I,; Silver, S and Trevors, J.T. (1997). Metal-microbe interactions: Contemporary approaches, Advances in Microbial Physiology. 38, 177- 243.

Bhattacharya, R,; Patra C. R,; Verma R,; Kumar S,; Greipp P. R and Mukherjee P. (2007). Gold Nanoparticles Inhibit the Proliferation of Multiple Myeloma Cells. Adv. Mater, 19, 711.

Cao,; YunWei Charles,; Jin,; Rongchao,; Mirkin,; Chad A. (2002). Nanoparticles with Raman Spectroscopic Fingerprints for DNA and RNA Detection, Science, 297, 1536-1540.

Chen, J. C,; Lin Z. H and Ma, X. X. (2003). Evidence of the production of silver nanoparticles via pretreatment of Phoma sp.3.2883 with silver nitrate, Letters in Applied Microbiology. 37, 105–108.

Cheng, Y,; Anna, C.S,; Meyers, J.D,; Panagopoulos, I,; Fei, B,; Burda, C. (2008). Deep Penetration of a PDT Drug into Tumors by Noncovalent Drug-Gold Nanoparticle Conjugates, J.Am.Chem.Soc. 130 (32), 10643–10647.

Chopra. (2007). The increasing use of silver-based products as antimicrobial agents: a useful development or a cause for concern, Antimicrob Chemother. 59, 587–90.

Chou, K-S,; Lu, Y-C,; and Lee, H-H. (2005). Effect of alkaline ion on the mechanism and kinetics of chemical reduction of silver, Materials Chemistry and Physics. 94, 429-433.

Daniel, M.-C. and D. Astruc. (2004). Gold nanoparticles: assembly, supramolecular chemistry, quantum-size-related properties, and applications toward biology, catalysis, and nanotechnology. Chemical reviews, 104(1): p. 293-346.

Dibrov, P,; Dzioba, J,; Gosinl, K.K,; Hase, C.C. (2002). Chemiosmotic mechanism of antimicrobial activity of Ag+ in Vibrio cholerae, Antimicrob Agents Chemother. 46, 2668.

Duran, N,; Marcarto, P.D,; DeSouza, G.I.H,; Alves, O.L,; Esposito, E. (2007). Antibacterial Effect of Silver Nanoparticles Produced by Fungal Process on Textile Fabrics and Their Effluent Treatment, J Biomed Nanotechnol. 3, 203–8.

Duran, N,; Marcato, P.D,; Alves, O.L,; DeSouza, G.I.H,; Esposity, E. (2005). Mechanistic aspects of biosynthesis of silver nanoparticles by several *Fusarium oxysporum* strains, J. Nanobiotech. 3, 8.

Esumi, K,; Tano, T,; Torigoe, K,; Meguro, K. (1990). Preparation and characterization of bimetallic palladium-copper colloids by thermal decomposition of their acetate compounds in organic solvents. Chem. Mater, 2(5), 564- 567.

Gao, Y,; Cranston, R. (2008). Recent Advances in Antimicrobial Treatments of Textile,Text. Res. J. 78, 60–72.

Gardea-Torresdey, Parsons, J.G,; Gomez, E,; Peralta-Videa, J,; Troiani, H.E,; Santiago, P,; JoseYacaman, M. (*2002*). Formation and Growth of Au Nanoparticles Inside Live Alfalfa Plants, Nano let. 2(4), 397-401.

Goia D. V and Matijevic E. (1998). Preparation of Monodispersed Metal Particles, New J. Chem. 22, 1203-1215.

Gole, A,; Dash, C,; Ramachandran, V,; Sainkar, S.R,; Mandale, A.B,; Rao, M. (2001). Pepsin−Gold Colloid Conjugates: Preparation, Characterization, and Enzymatic Activity, Langmuir. 17, 1674- 9.

Gutiérrez, M. and Henglein A. (1993). Formation of colloidal silver by "push-pull" reduction of Ag+. J. Phys. Chem. 97, 11368.

Henglein, A. (2001). Reduction of Ag (CN)2" on silver and platinum colloidal nanoparticles. Langmuir, 17, 2329-2333.

Ip, M,; Lui, S.L,; Poon, V.K.M,; Lung, I,; Burd, A. (2006). Antimicrobial activities of silver dressings: an in vitro comparison, J Med Microbiob. 55, 59–63.

Isabel Pastoriza-Santos and Luis M. Liz-MarzJn. (2002). Synthesis of Silver Nanoprisms in DMF. Langmuir, 18, 2888.

Jagadeesh M. S and Seehra, M. S. (1981). Principal magnetic susceptibilities of MnO and their temperature dependence, Phys. Rev. B. 23, 1185.

Jain, P.K,; El-Sayed, I.H,; El-Sayed, M.A. (2007). Au nanoparticles target cancer, NanoToday. 2, 18–29.

Jianping Xie,; Jim Yang Lee and Daniel I.C. Wang. (2007). Synthesis of Single-Crystalline Gold Nanoplates in Aqueous Solutions through Biomineralization by Serum Albumin Protein, J. Phys. Chem. C. 111 (28), 10226- 10232.

Jing yang,; Hong Wang,; Zhuyuan Wang,; Xuebin tan,; Chunyuan Song,; Ruohu Zhang,; Jin Li,; Yiping Cui. (2009). Interaction between antitumor drug and silver nanoparticles: combined fluorescence and surface enhanced Raman scattering study, Chinese Optics Letters. 7(10).

Jun, J,; Yuan-Yuan, D,; Shao-hai, W,; Shao-feng, Z,; Zhong-yi, W. (2007). Preparation and characterization of antibacterial silver containing nano fibers for wound dressing applications, JUS-China Med Sci. 4(2), 52- 4.

Kapoor, M.P.; Yang, Q.; Inagaki, S. (2002). Self-Assembly of Biphenylene-Bridged Hybrid Mesoporous Solid with Molecular-Scale Periodicity in the Pore Walls. J. Am. Chem. Soc, 124, 15176-15177.

Kim, J.S,; Kuk, E,; Yu, K.N,; Kim, J.H,; Park, S.J,; Lee, H.J. (2007). Antimicrobial effects of silver nanoparticles, Nanomed Nanotechnol Biol Med. 3, 95-101.

Klasen, H. J. (2000). Historical review of the use of silver in the treatment of burns. Early uses. Burns, 26, 11730.

Kumar, A,; Vemula, P.K,; Ajayan, P.M,; John, G. (2008). Silver-nanoparticle-embedded antimicrobial paints based on vegetable oil, Nature Materials. 7(3), 236–41.

Lansdown, A.B. (2002). Silver. 2: Toxicity in mammals and how its products aid wound repair, Journal of Wound Care. 11(5), 173–177.

Lansdown, A.B. (2002). Silver: its antibacterial properties and mechanism of action. J. Wound Care. 11, 125.

Leaper, D.L. (2006). Silver dressings: their role in wound management, Int Wound J. 3(4), 282–94.

Lin, Z,; Wu, J,; Xue, R,; Yong, Y. (2005). Spectroscopic characterization of Au3+ biosorption by waste biomass of Saccharomyces cerevisiae, Spectrochim. Acta Part A. 61, 761–765.

Lok, C-N,; Ho, C-M,; Chen, R,; He, Q-Y,; Yu, W-Y,; Sun, H. (2006). Proteomic analysis of the mode of antibacterial action of silver nanoparticles, J Proteome Res. 5, 916.

Mann, S,; Frankel, R.B,; Blakemore, R.P. (1984). Structure, Morphology, and Crystal Growth of Bacterial Magnetite, Nature. 310, 405- 407.

Oghabian, M. A and Farahbakhsh, N. M. (2010). Potential use of nanoparticle based contrast agents in MRI: a molecular imaging perspective, J. Biomed. Nanotechnol, 6, 203.

Panyala, N.R,; Pena-Mendez, E.M,; Havel, J. (2008). Silver or silver nanoparticles: A hazardous threat to the environment and human health? J Applied Biomedicine. 6(3), 117–129.

Patra C. R,; Bhattacharya R,; E. Wang, and Katarya A. (2008).Targeted Delivery of Gemcitabine to Pancreatic Adenocarcinoma Using Cetuximab as a Targeting Agent. Cancer Re, 68, 1970.

Raymond Wai-Yin Sun,; Rong Chen,; Nancy P.-Y.Chung,; Chi-Ming Ho,; Chen-Lung Steve Lin and Chi-Ming Che. (2005). Silver nanoparticles fabricated in Hepes buffer exhibit cytoprotective activities toward HIV-1 infected cells, Chem.Commun. 5059–5061.

Richard, J.W,; Spencer, B.A,; McCoy, L.F,; Carina, E,; Washington, J,; Edgar, P. (2002). J Burns Surg Wound Care. 1, 11–20.

Rodriguez-Sanchez, L,; Blanco, M. C. and Lopez-Quintela, M. A. (2000).Electrochemical Synthesis of Silver Nanoparticles. J. Phys.Chem. B, 104, 9683-9688.

Rosemary, M.J,; Mac Laren, I,; Pradeep, T. (2006). Investigations of the antibacterial properties of ciprofloxacin and SiO2, Langmuir. 22, 10125.

Saha, B,; Bhattacharya, J,; Mukherjee, A,; Ghosh, A.K,; Santra, C.R,; Dasgupta, A.K,; Karmakar, P. (2007). In vitro structural and functional evaluation of gold nanoparticles conjugated antibiotics, Nanoscale Res. Lett. 2, 614–622.

Sarikaya, M,; Fong, H,; French, D.W,; Humbert, R. (1999). Biomimetic assembly of nanostructured materials, Mat. Sci. Forum. 293, 83–98.

Shahverdi, A.R,; Fakhimi, A,; Shahverdi, H.R,; Minaian, S. (2007). Synthesis and effect of silver nanoparticles on the antibacterial activity of different antibiotics against Staphylococcus aureus and Escherichia coli, Nanomed: Nanotechnol. Biol Med. 3 (2), 168–71.

Shankar, S.S,; Rai, A,; Ahmad, A,; Sastry, M. J. (2004). Rapid synthesis of Au, Ag, and bimetallic Au core-Ag shell nanoparticles using Neem (Azadirachta indica) leaf broth, J Colloid Interf Sci. 275, 496-502.

Sharma, V. K,; Nevecna, T,; Zboril, R. (2006). Silver colloid nanoparticles: synthesis, characterization, and their antibacterial activity, J. Phys. Chem. B. 110, 16248-16253.

Shenton, W,; Douglas, T,; Young, M,; Stubbs, G,; Mann, S. (1999). Inorganic–Organic Nanotube Composites from Template Mineralization of Tobacco Mosaic Virus, Adv Mater. 11,253.

Silver, S. (2003). Bacterial silver resistance: molecular biology and uses and misuses of silvercompounds, FEMS Microbiol. Rev. 27 (2–3), 341–353.

Skirtach, A.G,; Javier, A.M,; Kreft, O,; Köhler, K,; Alberola, A.P,; Möhwald, H,; Parak, W.J,; Sukhorukov, G.B. (2006). Laser-induced release of encapsulated materials inside living Cells, Angew. Chem. 118(28), 4728–4733.

Sondi, B,; alopek-Sondi. (2007). Silver nanoparticles as antimicrobial agent: a case study on E. coli as a model for Gram-negative bacteria, J Colloid Interface. 275, 177–182.

Sun Y and Y. Xia. (2002). Shape-Controlled Synthesis of Gold and Silver Nanoparticles, Science. 298, 2176–2179.

Taleb, A,; Petit, C,; Pileni, M. P. (1997). Synthesis of Highly Monodisperse Silver Nanoparticles from AOT Reverse Micelles: A Way to 2D and 3D Self-Organization. Chem. Mater, 9, 950-959.

Thirumurugan, G and Dhanaraju.M.D. (2011). Novel Biogenic *Metal Nanoparticles* for *Pharmaceutical Applications*, Adv. Sci. Lett, 4, 339-348.

Thirumurugan, G,; Satya Veni, V,; Ramachandran, S,; Seshagiri Rao, J. V. L. N. and Dhanaraju, M. D. (2011). Superior wound healing effect of topically delivered silver nanoparticle formulation using eco-friendly potato plant pathogenic fungus: synthesis and characterization, J. Biomed. Nanotechnol. 7, 659- 666.

Van Hyning, D. L,; Klemperer, W. G and Zukoski, C. F. (2001). Silver nanoparticle formation: Predictions and verification of the aggregative growth model, Langmuir 17, 3128-3135.

Vigneshwaran, N,; Kathe, A. A,; Varadarajan, P.V,; Nachane, R.P,; Balasubramanya, R.H. (2006). Biomimetics of silver nanoparticles by white rot fungus, Phaenerochaete chrysosporium, Coll Surf B: Interf. 53, 55- 59.

Wiley, B.J,; Sun, Y,; Mayers, B and Xia, Y. (2005). Shape-Controlled Synthesis of Metal Nanostructures: The Case of Silver, Chem. Eur. J. 11, 454.

Zhu, J. J,; Koltypin, Y and Gedanken, A. (2000). A General Sonochemical Method for the preparation of Nanophased Selenides: the synthesis of ZnSe. Chem. Mater, 12, 73.

Permissions

The contributors of this book come from diverse backgrounds, making this book a truly international effort. This book will bring forth new frontiers with its revolutionizing research information and detailed analysis of the nascent developments around the world.

We would like to thank Varaprasad Bobbarala, for lending his expertise to make the book truly unique. He has played a crucial role in the development of this book. Without his invaluable contribution this book wouldn't have been possible. He has made vital efforts to compile up to date information on the varied aspects of this subject to make this book a valuable addition to the collection of many professionals and students.

This book was conceptualized with the vision of imparting up-to-date information and advanced data in this field. To ensure the same, a matchless editorial board was set up. Every individual on the board went through rigorous rounds of assessment to prove their worth. After which they invested a large part of their time researching and compiling the most relevant data for our readers. Conferences and sessions were held from time to time between the editorial board and the contributing authors to present the data in the most comprehensible form. The editorial team has worked tirelessly to provide valuable and valid information to help people across the globe.

Every chapter published in this book has been scrutinized by our experts. Their significance has been extensively debated. The topics covered herein carry significant findings which will fuel the growth of the discipline. They may even be implemented as practical applications or may be referred to as a beginning point for another development. Chapters in this book were first published by InTech; hereby published with permission under the Creative Commons Attribution License or equivalent.

The editorial board has been involved in producing this book since its inception. They have spent rigorous hours researching and exploring the diverse topics which have resulted in the successful publishing of this book. They have passed on their knowledge of decades through this book. To expedite this challenging task, the publisher supported the team at every step. A small team of assistant editors was also appointed to further simplify the editing procedure and attain best results for the readers.

Our editorial team has been hand-picked from every corner of the world. Their multi ethnicity adds dynamic inputs to the discussions which result in innovative outcomes. These outcomes are then further discussed with the researchers and contributors who give their valuable feedback and opinion regarding the same. The feedback is then collaborated with the researches and they are edited in a comprehensive manner to aid the understanding of the subject.

Apart from the editorial board, the designing team has also invested a significant amount of their time in understanding the subject and creating the most relevant covers. They scrutinized every image to scout for the most suitable representation of the subject and create an appropriate cover for the book.

The publishing team has been involved in this book since its early stages. They were actively engaged in every process, be it collecting the data, connecting with the contributors or procuring relevant information. The team has been an ardent support to the editorial, designing and production team. Their endless efforts to recruit the best for this project, has resulted in the accomplishment of this book. They are a veteran in the field of academics and their pool of knowledge is as vast as their experience in printing. Their expertise and guidance has proved useful at every step. Their uncompromising quality standards have made this book an exceptional effort. Their encouragement from time to time has been an inspiration for everyone.

The publisher and the editorial board hope that this book will prove to be a valuable piece of knowledge for researchers, students, practitioners and scholars across the globe.

List of Contributors

Renaud Condé, Martha Argüello, Javier Izquierdo, Raúl Noguez, Miguel Moreno and Humberto Lanz
Centro de Investigación Sobre Enfermedades Infecciosas, Instituto Nacional de Salud Pública, Mexico

Olgica Stefanović, Ivana Radojević, Sava Vasić and Ljiljana Čomić
Labaratory of Microbiology, Department of Biology and Ecology, Faculty of Science, University of Kragujevac, Kragujevac, Serbia

Tomaž Bratkovič
Department of Pharmaceutical Biology, Faculty of Pharmacy, University of Ljubljana, Ljubljana, Slovenia

Nataša Radić
Department of Pharmaceutical Biology, Faculty of Pharmacy, University of Ljubljana, Ljubljana, Slovenia AB Inovacije d.o.o., Mirna, Slovenia

Mirjana Bukvić Krajačić
GlaxoSmithKline Research Centre Zagreb, Zagreb, Croatia Galapagos Research Center Ltd., Zagreb, Croatia

Miljenko Dumić
Department of Biotechnology, University of Rijeka, Rijeka, Croatia

André Silvério and Maria Lopes
Department of Microbiology, Faculty of Pharmacy, University of Lisbon, Portugal

Johannes Bodenstein and Karen Du Toit
Discipline of Pharmaceutical Sciences, University of KwaZulu-Natal (Westville Campus), Durban, South Africa

Varaprasad Bobbarala
Translational Research Institute of Molecular Sciences (TRIMS), Visakhapatnam, AP, India

Chandrasekhar K. Naidu
Department of Botany, College of Science and Technology, Andhra University, Visakhapatnam, India

Aphichart Karnchanatat
The Institute of Biotechnology and Genetic Engineering, Chulalongkorn University, Bangkok, Thailand

Kamila Myszka and Katarzyna Czaczyk
Poznań University of Life Sciences, Poland

Chirlei Glienke
Department of Genetics, Federal University of Parana (UFPR), Setor de Ciências Biológicas, Centro Politécnico, Curitiba, Paraná, Brazil

Daiani Savi, Vania Aparecida Vicente and Fabiana Tonial
Department of Basic Pathology, Federal University of Parana (UFPR), Setor de Ciências Biológicas, Centro Politécnico, Curitiba, Paraná, Brazil

Beatriz H. L. N. Sales Maia
Department of Chemistry, Federal University of Parana (UFPR), Setor de Ciências Exatas, Centro Politécnico, Curitiba, Paraná, Brazil

Yvelise Maria Possiede
Department of Biology, Federal University of Mato Grosso do Sul, Campo Grande, Mato Grosso do Sul, Brazil

Josiane Gomes-Figueiredo
Department of Genetics, Federal University of Parana (UFPR), Setor de Ciências Biológicas, Centro Politécnico, Curitiba, Paraná, Brazil Department of Basic Pathology, Federal University of Parana (UFPR), Setor de Ciências Biológicas, Centro Politécnico, Curitiba, Paraná, Brazil

Ménonvè Atindehou, Rizwan Aslam, Jean-François Chich, Youssef Haïkel, Francis Schneider and Marie-Hélène Metz-Boutigue
Biomatériaux et Ingénierie Tissulaire, University of Strasbourg, Strasbourg, France

Pintilie Lucia
National Institute for Chemical-Pharmaceutical, Research and Development, Bucharest, Romania

Amy L. Stockert and Tarek M. Mahfouz
The Raabe College of Pharmacy, Ohio Northern University, USA

Saeed Rahim, Amin Salem Milani and Shahriar Shahi
Dental and Periodontal Research Center, Faculty of Dentistry, Tabriz University of Medical Sciences,Tabriz, Iran

Negin Ghasemi
Department of Endodontics, Faculty of Dentistry, Tabriz University of Medical Sciences,Tabriz, Iran

Ivana D. Radojević, Olgica D. Stefanović and Ljiljana R. Čomić
Department of Biology and Ecology, Faculty of Science, University of Kragujevac, Kragujevac, Republic of Serbia

Verica V. Glođović, Gordana P. Radić and Srećko R. Trifunović
Department of Chemistry, Faculty of Science, University of Kragujevac, Kragujevac, Republic of Serbia

Jelena M. Vujić
Faculty of Agronomy, University of Kragujevac, Čačak, Republic of Serbia

V. G. Papatsiros and C. Billinis
School of Veterinary Medicine, University of Thessaly, Greece

Qamar Uddin Ahmed
Department of Pharmaceutical Chemistry, Faculty of Pharmacy, Malaysia

Othman Abd. Samah and Abubakar Sule
Department of Biomedical Science, Faculty of Allied Health Sciences, International Islamic University Malaysia, Kuantan, Pahang, Malaysia

Sheila Shahidi
Department of Textile, Faculty of Engineering, Islamic Azad University, Arak Branch, Arak, Iran

Jakub Wiener
Department of Textile Chemistry, Faculty of Textile, Technical University of Liberec, Liberec, Czech Republic

Maja Karaman, Milan Matavulj and Ljiljana Janjic
University of Novi Sad, Department of Biology and Ecology, Novi Sad, Serbia

G. Thirumurugan and M. D. Dhanaraju
Research Lab, GIET School of Pharmacy, Chaitanya Nagar, Rajahmundry, AP, India